CLINICAL PRACTICE GUIDELINES

Examination and Intervention for Rehabilitation

REVISIONS BY
DAVID DEPPELER, PT, OCS, FAAOMPT

ORIGINAL WORK BY
CAROL SCHUNK, PT, PsyD
KELLY REED, PT, OCS, COMT

Clinical Practice Guidelines
Examination and Intervention for Rehabilitation

Copyright © 2008 Therapeutic Associates, Inc. All rights reserved.

Therapeutic Associates, Inc. grants permission for photocopying for limited personal or internal use. This consent does not extend to other kinds of copying, such as copying for general distribution, for advertising or promotional purposes, for creating new collective works, or for resale.

For Information
Therapeutic Associates, Inc., Guideline Permissions Dept.
11481 SW Hall Blvd., Suite 201, Portland, Oregon, 97223.

Orders & Customer Service: (800) 219-8835

CareConnections and Therapeutic Associates are registered trademarks of Therapeutic Associates, Inc.

The author has made every effort to ensure the accuracy of the information herein. However, appropriate information sources should be consulted, especially for new or unfamiliar procedures. It is the responsibility of every practitioner to evaluate the appropriateness of a particular opinion in the context of actual clinical situations and with due considerations to new developments. The authors, editors, and the publisher cannot be held responsible for any typographical or other errors found in this book.

Therapeutic Associates, Inc. is a physical therapy company that dates back to the 1950s, but our mind set is always now and in the future.

Our physical and occupational therapists are professionals dedicated to educating, training, and treating people according to the principles of tested medicine. Decades of experience and knowledge of the healing process allows us to serve each patient's unique condition and goals for recovery. We have a rich history of successfully managing injury and impairment as well as a progressive view toward wellness through physical activity and maintaining a healthy lifestyle. From diagnosis to discharge, and with each procedure, treatment technique, and word of encouragement in between, we strive to help people reach their best.

www.therapeuticassociates.com

ISBN: 1-888629-09-6

Printed in the United States of America

CARE CONNECTIONS — OTHER PRODUCTS

CareConnections is a **Web-based suite of rehabilitation medical management services**. CareConnections uses combinations of tools to assist providers and payers with the medical management of patients and clinical services. These tools are the:

CareConnections Outcomes System
- A functionally based patient data collection system that compares clinical outcomes to similar groups of clinics and provider submitted episodes of care. Outcome reports provide valuable clinical information and management data that can be used to promote best practices, improve quality of care, and add value for those responsible for the costs of care.

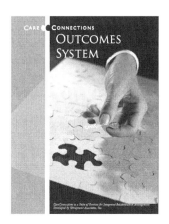

CareConnections Patient Satisfaction Monitoring
- A standardized survey for patients, allowing them to provide valuable feedback about their provider experience. All results can be submitted for benchmarking against therapy sites from around the country.

CareConnections Prior Authorization/Advice System (PAS)
- PAS ties it all together as a tool that permits 24/7 Web-based dissemination and acquisition of utilization management information. PAS delivers prospective utilization of care in the form of an appropriate number of visits per specific patient condition along with an appropriate CareConnections Treatment Guideline. PAS provides concurrent utilization management based upon initial measures and continued monitoring using the CareConnections Outcomes System and provider requests for additional treatment. It also provides retrospective utilization management in the form of CareConnections Outcome reports and benchmarked utilization statistics.

The entire suite of CareConnections management tools present powerful, yet cost effective systems for today's healthcare world. Providers and payers alike can benefit from CareConnections' component parts or their integrated ability to serve the needs of both value-based and outcome-oriented care to all rehabilitation patients.

Visit **www.careconnections.com/Products/** for more information and to order.

ORDER OTHER BOOKS AND DVDS

CareConnections Therapy Referral Handbook $35.00
NEW Third Edition, Available 2008!
- The Therapy Referral Handbook lists "Considerations for Referral" by anatomical region, plus single-page treatment summaries for over 100 diagnoses. The Handbook is a great tool for educating physicians, nurse practitioners, physician assistants, case managers, and payers. If you are involved in claims review or as a case manager, you need a reference on therapy.

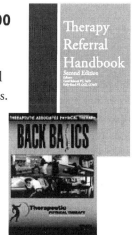

Back Basics DVD $795.00
Back Basics, an educational video produced by Therapeutic Associates, is designed to improve manual material handling safety and reduce back injuries in the workplace.

ORDER FORM

Qty	Product	Price	Total
	Clinical Practice Guidelines: Examination And Intervention For Rehabilitation (Third Edition)	$179.00	
	Therapy Referral Handbook: (Third Edition) *See below for quantity discount rates*	$35.00	
	Customize the Handbook cover with our clinic logo—minimum order of 40 books required [One-time set-up fee]	$100.00	
	Back Basics DVD	$795.00	

Subtotal _____
(See chart below) Shipping & handling _____
Total _____

Shipping and Handling

All orders will ship via UPS Ground to the continental US.
Alaska and Hawaii customers, please call for shipping and handling rates.

No of Items	S&H fee	No of Items	S&H fee
1	$10.95	4	$16.95
2	$12.95	5	$18.95
3	$14.95	6 +	Please call

Therapy Handbook Quantity Discounts

Quantity	Discount	Price/Book
1–9	0%	$35.00
10–39	15%	$29.75
40–74	25%	$26.25
75 +	30%	$24.50

INFORMATION

Customer Name _____
Company _____
Address 1 _____
Address 2 _____
City _____ State _____ Zip _____
Contact Phone _____
E-mail Address _____

Therapeutic Associates, Inc. respects your privacy. We will not distribute your personal information to anyone.

PAYMENT

Please bill my credit card: ❑ MasterCard ❑ Visa ❑ Discover
Card No _____
Expiration Date (month/year) _____
Signature _____

❑ Check enclosed, made payable to: Therapeutic Associates, Inc.

PLACE AN ORDER

By Internet
www.careconnections.com/Order

By Phone
Phone in your order at
(800) 219-8835

By Mail
Mail this form to:
CareConnections
ATTN: Order Processing
11481 SW Hall Blvd., Suite 201
Portland, OR 97223

By Fax
Copy this form and fax it to
(503) 639-9699

INFORMATION AND SUPPORT

E-mail
info@taiweb.com

Mail & Phone
CareConnections
11481 SW Hall Blvd., Suite 201
Portland, OR 97223
(800) 219-8835
(503) 443-6156
(503) 639-9699 (fax)

Customer Service Hours
8 am–5 pm Pacific Time

©2008 Therapeutic Associates, Inc.
All prices subject to change without notice

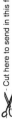
Cut here to send in this form

TABLE OF CONTENTS

INTRODUCTION
Contributors vii
What's New About This Book ix
How To Use This Book x
  Summary Overview x
  Examination x
  Goals/Outcomes xi
  Intervention xi
Discharge Planning and Patient Responsibility xii
A Note on ICD-9 Code Reporting: Level of Detail xiii

FOOT AND ANKLE   1
Achilles Tendinitis 3
Achilles Tendon Repair 9
Ankle Enthesopathy 15
Ankle Fracture 21
Ankle Sprain/Instability 27
Biomechanical Lower Extremity Dysfunction 33
Bunion 39
Diabetic Foot 43
Foot Care Guidelines for The Diabetic Patient 49
Foot Contusion 51
Foot Reconstruction 57
Orthotics: Answers to Commonly Asked Questions 63
Orthotics: Choosing the Right Shoe 65
Orthotics: Your New Orthotics 67
Plantar Fasciitis 69
Posterior Tibialis Tendinitis (Shin Splints) 75

KNEE   81
Accelerated Anterior Cruciate Ligament Reconstruction 83
Iliotibial Band Syndrome 89
Knee Arthroscopy 95
Knee Contusion 101
Knee Degenerative Joint Disease 105
Knee Enthesopathy 111
Knee Hypomobility/Infrapatellar Contracture Syndrome (IPCS) 117

Knee Sprain/Strain...123
Meniscal Repair..129
Meniscus Tear (Without Surgery)...135
Patellar Tendinitis..141
Patellofemoral Syndrome..147
Posterior Cruciate Ligament Reconstruction...153
Total Knee Replacement—Inpatient...159
Total Knee Replacement—Outpatient...163

HIP — 169

Hip Degenerative Joint Disease..171
Hip Fracture/Total Hip Replacement—Outpatient....................................177
Hip Fracture/Total Hip Replacement—Inpatient.......................................183
Hip Soft Tissue Pain...187
Hip Sprain/Strain...193

LUMBAR SPINE — 199

Ankylosing Spondylitis..201
Low Back General Pain...209
Lumbar Disc Pathology...219
Lumbar Fracture..227
Lumbar Spondylolysis with Myelopathy..235
Lumbar Surgery—Inpatient...243
Pelvic Floor Dysfunction...249
Postoperative Rehabilitation of The Lumbar Spine...................................255
Postural Dysfunction..263
Sacroiliac Dysfunction..271
Spinal Stenosis..279
Spondylolisthesis...285

CERVICAL/THORACIC SPINE — 293

Cervical/Thoracic General Pain..295
Cervical Disc Pathology..301
Cervical Spondylolysis with Myelopathy..308
Cervical Stenosis...313
Compression Fracture...319
Craniovertebral Stability Tests...325
Objective Measurement of Forward Head Posture....................................327
Osteoporosis...329
Postoperative/Postfracture Rehabilitation of the Cervical/Thoracic Spine...335
Rib Dysfunction...341
Scoliosis...347
Thoracic Outlet Syndrome..353
Whiplash Syndrome...359

TMJ/HEADACHE/STRESS — 365

Headache 367

Postoperative Rehabilitation of the Temporomandibular Joint
  (Orthognathic, Arthroplasty, or Arthroscopic) 373

Relaxation and Stress Management 381

Stress Management 384

Temporomandibular Dysfunction 389

SHOULDER — 397

Adhesive Capsulitis 399

Biceps Tendon Rupture 405

Humerus Fracture 411

Labrum Tear 417

Postoperative Rehabilitation for Shoulder Instability 423

Postoperative Rehabilitation of the Rotator Cuff 429

Postoperative Total Shoulder Arthroplasty 435

Shoulder Anterior Dislocation 441

Shoulder Bursitis 447

Shoulder Degenerative Joint Disease 455

Shoulder Fracture 461

Shoulder Joint Pathology 467

Shoulder Sprain/Strain 475

Shoulder Tendinitis 483

ELBOW — 491

Elbow Fracture (Closed) 493

Elbow/Hand Enthesopathy (Other Disorders of the Synovium, Tendon,
  and Bursa) 498

Elbow Joint Pathology 506

Elbow Sprain/Strain 511

Lateral Epicondylitis 517

Medial Epicondylitis 523

Ulnar Nerve Lesion 530

WRIST/HAND — 535

Carpal Tunnel Syndrome 537

DeQuervain's Tendinitis 543

Flexor Tendon Repair 549

Hand Arthropathy 557

Hand Fracture 561

Postoperative Carpal Tunnel Release 565

Postoperative DeQuervain's Syndrome 571

Postoperative Dupuytren's Fasciectomy 577

Proximal Interphalangeal Joint Injuries Collateral Ligament Sprain 583

Proximal Interphalangeal Joint Injuries Dorsal Dislocation 589

Reflex Sympathetic Dystrophy of the Upper Extremity 593

Wrist Fracture 599

Wrist Sprain/Strain 605

TABLE OF CONTENTS   V

RETURN TO SPORT   609

Ankle Sprain/Instability—Return To Sport 611
Anterior Cruciate Ligament Reconstruction—Return To Sport 613
Elbow/Shoulder Injury—Return To Tennis 615
Exercise Sequence: Elbow/Shoulder Injury—Return To Tennis 617
Hamstring Injury—Return To Sport 621
Hip Pain In Runners—Return To Sport 623
Exercise Sequence: Hip Pain In Runners—Return To Sport 625
Upper Extremity Injury—Return To Throwing 627
Exercise Sequence: Upper Extremity Injury—Return To Throwing 629
Walking Program—Walking For The Health Of It 635
Patient Information Sheet: Walking For The Health Of It 637
Activity Questionnaire for Runners/Walkers 639

GENERAL MEDICINE   641

Amputations 643
Time of Fitting the Prosthesis 649
Arthritis 653
Geriatric Rehabilitation 659
Muscle Weakness—General 663
Vestibular Rehabilitation 667
Wound Management 673

NEUROLOGICAL CONDITIONS   681

Cerebral Vascular Accident 683
Guillain-Barré Syndrome 693
Multiple Sclerosis 699
Parkinson's Disease 705

Appendix 711

Index 729

CONTRIBUTORS

Steve Allen, PT, OCS, FAAOMPT
THERAPEUTIC ASSOCIATES LIBERTY LAKE
Spokane, WA

Gale Anderson, PT, MS, OCS, FAAOMPT
THERAPEUTIC ASSOCIATES MT SPOKANE
Mead, WA

Steve Barsotti, PT
THERAPEUTIC ASSOCIATES TUALATIN
Tualatin, OR

Jeffrey Blanchard, PT, MS
VALLEY PHYSICAL THERAPY AND SPORTS REHABILITATION
Salem, OR

Robert Bowker, PT, GCS
PROVIDENCE SAINT JOSEPH MEDICAL CENTER
Burbank, CA

Timothy O. Brinker, PT, OCS, FAAOMPT
THERAPEUTIC ASSOCIATES HILLSBORO
Portland, OR

Todd Cadby, PT, MS, ATC

Ken Call, MS, PT, DPT
THERAPEUTIC ASSOCIATES WEST KENNEWICK
Kennewick, WA

Lee Ann Carlson, PT
THERAPEUTIC ASSOCIATES RICHLAND
Richland, WA

H. Patrick Corrigan, PT
THERAPEUTIC ASSOCIATES SAINT HELENS
St. Helens, OR

Rick Costain, PT
THERAPEUTIC ASSOCIATES MID VALLEY
Albany, OR

Julianne Courtenay, PT
PROVIDENCE OCCUPATIONAL HEALTH CENTER
Burbank, CA

Alison Davis, MPT
PROVIDENCE SAINT JOSEPH MEDICAL CENTER
Burbank, CA

Michael Deegan, DPT
THERAPEUTIC ASSOCIATES HILLSBORO
Hillsboro, OR

David Deppeler, PT, OCS, FAAOMPT
THERAPEUTIC ASSOCIATES CLINICAL EDUCATION
Portland, OR

David Directo, PT
THERAPEUTIC ASSOCIATES OUTPATIENT CLINIC
Santa Clarita, CA

Julie Dresch, PT, MS
THERAPEUTIC ASSOCIATES FAIRWOOD
Renton, WA

Amy Eckenroch, PT

Karen Walz, PT, MA, OCS, FAAOMPT
THERAPEUTIC ASSOCIATES REDMOND
Redmond, OR

Alice Engelmann, OTR

Paul Groschel, PT, MS
THERAPEUTIC ASSOCIATES YELM
Yelm, WA

Julie Gross, PT, MS, ARTIC
THERAPEUTIC ASSOCIATES CLACKAMAS
Clackamas, OR

Janet Hamilton, MA, PTA, CSCS

Chuck Hanson, PT, OCS
THERAPEUTIC ASSOCIATES NORTH LAKE
Seattle, WA

Chris Hoekstra, PT, DPT, OCS, FAAOMPT
THERAPEUTIC ASSOCIATES SHERWOOD
Sherwood, OR

Valerie Hunter, PT, CHT
PROVIDENCE SAINT JOSEPH OCCUPATIONAL HEALTH
CENTER
Burbank, CA

Evan Jones, PT, OCS
VALLEY PHYSICAL THERAPY AND SPORTS REHABILITATION
Salem, OR

Jeff Jones, PT, OCS
THERAPEUTIC ASSOCIATES CENTRAL PHYSICAL THERAPY
Roseburg, OR

Mike Jones, PT
THERAPEUTIC ASSOCIATES EAST PORTLAND
Portland, OR

Rick Jusko, PT
THERAPEUTIC ASSOCIATES CANYON PARK
Bothell, WA

Teri Kato, PT
THERAPEUTIC ASSOCIATES WEST SEATTLE
Seattle, WA

Wendy Katsiotis, PT
PROVIDENCE SAINT JOSEPH MEDICAL CENTER
Burbank, CA

Marci Keefer-Hutchison, PT, MS, ATC
THERAPEUTIC ASSOCIATES VALLEY KEIZER
Keizer, OR

Steve Kennoy, DPT
PROVIDENCE SAINT JOSEPH MEDICAL CENTER
Burbank, CA

Barbara Kleine, PT
PROVIDENCE SAINT JOSEPH MEDICAL CENTER
Burbank, CA

Lynn Leech, PT

Jennifer Lesko, PT, MS
THERAPEUTIC ASSOCIATES QUEEN ANNE
Seattle, WA

Jennifer Lorengo, PT, DPT
THERAPEUTIC ASSOCIATES WEST KENNEWICK
Kennewick, WA

Roman Lu, PT, OCS, CMPT
THERAPEUTIC ASSOCIATES HILLSBORO
Hillsboro, OR

Mark McCurdy, PT, COMT
THERAPEUTIC ASSOCIATES CLACKAMAS
Clackamas, OR

David McHenry, DPT
THERAPEUTIC ASSOCIATES NORTH PORTLAND
Portland, OR

Eric E. Medley, PT, MS, CSCS
THERAPEUTIC ASSOCIATES GRANTS PASS
Grants Pass, OR

Jennifer O. Medley, PT, MS
THERAPEUTIC ASSOCIATES GRANTS PASS
Grants Pass, OR

Jim Moore, PT, OCS, ATC, FAAOMPT
THERAPEUTIC ASSOCIATES, WANDERMERE
Spokane, WA

Jodie Padgett, PT, DPT
THERAPEUTIC ASSOCIATES SHERWOOD
Sherwood, OR

Martha Patterson, OTR, CHT

Christine Porter, PT
PROVIDENCE SAINT JOSEPH MEDICAL CENTER
Burbank, CA

Kelly Reed, PT, OCS, COMT
THERAPEUTIC ASSOCIATES CEDAR HILLS
Portland, OR

Jennie Ritchie, PT, MBA
PROVIDENCE SAINT JOSEPH MEDICAL CENTER
Burbank, CA

Mary Ann Seeger, PT, MS
THERAPEUTIC ASSOCIATES Vestibular and Balance Specialist
Portland, OR

Carol Schunk, PT, PsyD

Bradley Schwin, PT, MS
THERAPEUTIC ASSOCIATES WEST EUGENE
Eugene, OR

David Standifer, PT
THERAPEUTIC ASSOCIATES CENTRAL POINT
Medford, OR

Nancy Tam, OTR, CHT

William Temes, PT, MS, OCS, FAAOMPT
Eugene, OR

Mikki Townsend

Mike Waller, PT

Roger Wegley, PT, GDMT
THERAPEUTIC ASSOCIATES BALLARD
Seattle, WA

WHAT'S NEW ABOUT THIS BOOK

Welcome to the latest edition of Therapeutic Associates, Inc. Clinical Practice Guidelines. We've added 21 new treatment guidelines and updated visit ranges for all diagnostic codes. These changes are based on new billing data from hundreds of Physical Therapists over the past few years. Many of the guidelines have revised content and updated reference lists.

Visit Range Determination

Five years of billing and treatment outcomes data were used to establish appropriate visit ranges for each guideline. Data was grouped by guideline according to primary diagnosis. Descriptive statistics were calculated for number of visits per treatment episode, and quartiles were used to eliminate extreme values to arrive at a more representative visit range.

For example, 7571 episodes were analyzed for the *Cervical Disc Pathology* guideline. Measures of dispersion suggested a fairly uniform data population. A lower quartile of 6 and an upper quartile of 12 were calculated for both the billing and treatment outcomes data sets. After being reviewed for appropriateness by clinical experts, the guideline visit range was adjusted from 7–14 visits to 6–12.

New Treatment Guidelines

This same wealth of data was used to determine the need for new treatment guidelines. The following guidelines have been added:

Ankle Enthesopathy
Biceps Tendon Rupture
Bunion
Cervical Spondylolysis with Myelopathy
Elbow and Hand Enthesopathy
Elbow Fracture
Elbow Joint Pathology
Foot Contusion
Hand Arthropathy
Hand Fracture
Hip Sprain/Strain
Humerus Fracture

Knee Contusion
Knee Enthesopathy
Labrum Tear
Lumbar Spondylolysis with Myelopathy
Meniscus Tear
Muscle Weakness—General
Shoulder Joint Pathology
Ulnar Nerve Lesion
Wrist Sprain/Strain

Electronic Version

An electronic version of this publication will be available in 2008.

The incredible initial work of Carol Schunk and Kelly Reed has been preserved. This work is still largely credited to their initial efforts.

Special thanks to the Aurelius Capellan and Steve Pearson for their relentless dedication to the creation and production of this book.

–David Deppeler

HOW TO USE THIS BOOK

Although the face of *CareConnections Clinical Practice Guidelines* (formerly *Therapeutic Associates, Inc. Clinical Practice Guidelines*) has changed, the "how to" has stayed the same. APTA's *Guide to Physical Therapists Practice* ("The Guide") aims to describe all reasonable current Physical Therapy practice. These Clinical Practice Guidelines attempt to narrow the focus to the current examination and treatment principles that seem to result in the best outcomes. The focus is broad enough to allow for individual clinical judgment. As the profession of Physical Therapy evolves, so will these Clinical Practice Guidelines. We welcome your feedback. All Clinical Practice Guidelines reference Preferred Practice Patterns from The Guide.

To maximize the application and utilization of the guidelines the following information should be reviewed:

SUMMARY OVERVIEW

The Summary pages provide a synopsis of the guideline. All information is from the corresponding guideline and is intended to be a quick reference. Many clinicians have utilized the Summaries as an educational tool for third-party payers or referral sources, as justification for intervention during utilization review, or as instructional marketing material. The format is concise to facilitate easy access to the information.

- The number of visits is presented in a range that includes acute and subacute phases of treatment. The therapist's judgement is always a consideration in the determination of the appropriate frequency and duration of treatment.
- Circumstances requiring additional visits provide instances when a patient may need treatment in excess of the range of visits listed. If additional circumstances are present, documentation must support medical necessity.

EXAMINATION

The initial section, "Examination," contains the KEY areas for the History and Systems Review and the Tests and Measures applicable for the diagnostic group. The following items should be noted:

- Items are not intended to be all-inclusive but are intended to provide a selection of tests that can contribute to the information base when a therapist establishes a treatment plan or sets appropriate goals/outcomes. Therapists will need to use clinical judgement with consideration of severity, irritability, acuity, and patient's medical history when selecting tests. Often the outcome of one test will be a crucial factor in the selection of additional assessment tools.
- Tests and measures are not presented in the order of occurrence in a physical examination but are alphabetized as in The Guide. It is assumed that therapists have a personal system of assessment and the tests and measures will be conducted in an order that is in accordance with the flow of the examination.
- Clinics may want to develop an initial patient questionnaire to obtain the information addressed in the History and Systems Review. The data collected will be similar for many diagnostic groups and can provide a framework for discussion between therapist and patient.
- Information regarding patient's functional activity tolerance is essential in determining the value of therapeutic intervention. All guidelines recommend assessing activity levels prior to and following intervention to assist clinical decision-making and goal setting.
- Current functional level is best assessed through the utilization of a standardized functional outcome measurement tool. Results will provide quantifiable baseline information and

will identify specific limitations. If the same tool is administered at discharge, functional outcomes can be assessed to determine the efficacy of intervention.

- A visual analog scale is suggested to measure pain. It is a validated scale and can be administered at intake and discharge to provide outcome data. There are other valid pain assessment tools that could be substituted.

GOALS/OUTCOMES

Goals/outcomes presented are specific, quantifiable, and functional. This is the only way the therapist can assess the efficacy of intervention. The therapist may modify goals to accommodate specific patient characteristics.

- Functional goal statement in the guidelines is not intended to be used verbatim but is to be adapted to match specific functional limitation and previous activity level identified by the patient during assessment.
- Patient's goals provide information and are incorporated when establishing rehabilitation goals.
- Terminologies such as *increase*, *decrease*, or *improve* are used infrequently, as they do not reflect measurable outcome necessary to justify intervention.
- Range-of-motion goal values have been rounded to the nearest 5 degrees, except in cases where rounded values do not distinguish from baseline values.

INTERVENTION

Intervention is divided into four sections: Coordination, Communication, and Documentation; Patient Instruction; Direct Intervention; and Functional Carryover.

- Coordination, Communication, and Documentation is standard for all guidelines based on The Guide. When applicable, provisions specific to the diagnosis are included in the guideline.
- Patient Instruction is emphasized to highlight patient's responsibility in the rehabilitation process.
- References for basic anatomy and biomechanical influences are suggested, in addition to handout material and daily activity carryover. Actual handouts are not included, as most clinics have material specific to their practice, and there are numerous commercially available products.
- Functional Considerations remind the clinician of the focus on function. Educating patients on the relationship of their condition to daily activities enhances the partnership in rehabilitation. This concept is emphasized again in the Functional Carryover section.
- In most guidelines, treatment is divided into Acute and Subacute Phases. The patient's acuity level is dependent upon the achievement of goals/outcomes for each phase. In some cases a patient may enter therapy in the subacute phase and follow the guideline from that point forward.
- Direct Interventions are categorized based on The Guide. The guidelines provide ideas and direction, yet allow for individual clinical preference.
- *Manual therapy* is defined broadly to represent a variety of treatment procedures. This will allow therapists with differing orientations to utilize the guidelines without being restricted by definition.
- In some cases commercial equipment is suggested, however, inclusion of a brand name in the guideline is not intended to be an endorsement. Selection of equipment is dependent upon therapist preference and availability.

- The exercise program can also serve as a template for a home exercise program. Given the importance of patient responsibility in recovery, a home program is introduced early in the therapy program.
- A range of the number of therapy sessions is suggested for each phase of treatment. These numbers can be adjusted to reflect geographic and referral patterns. Duration is indicated in some cases. Clinical judgement on the achievement of goals/outcomes will be the ultimate factor for frequency and duration decisions. Circumstances requiring additional visits are listed under discharge planning. When treatment duration significantly exceeds the facility standard, exceptional factors should be well documented.
- Complications may arise during treatment that influence the applicability of the guideline. Therapist clinical judgement will always override the guideline when patients do not follow an expected pattern of recovery.

DISCHARGE PLANNING AND PATIENT RESPONSIBILITY

Discharge from therapy is the therapist's decision, based upon the progress of the patient. The guidelines provide criteria and factors associated with discharge planning.
- Criteria for discharge do not always mean the patient has reached rehabilitation goals. Given the restraints of some coverage systems, discharge may occur prior to full return to functional status.
- As stated above, in some cases there are circumstances that influence a patient's recovery. The most common reasons are listed.
- Home programs are initiated with the first therapy session and must include ongoing assessments of compliance. At discharge, the program is finalized and, when possible, a transition to functional activities is recommended.
- Monitoring is a shared task between the patient and therapist. By educating the patient in expectations and possible complications, the therapist is available as an ongoing resource for the patient.

A NOTE ON ICD-9 CODE REPORTING: LEVEL OF DETAIL

Diagnosis codes are either three-digit codes (category codes), four-digit codes (subcategory codes), or five-digit codes (subclassification codes). ICD-9-CM conventions require diagnosis codes to be assigned at their highest number of digits available (i.e., a code is invalid if it has not been coded to the full number of digits required for that code).

Not all codes require a 4th or 5th digit. For your convenience, each Clinical Practice Guideline includes a listing of one or more appropriate ICD-9 codes. These diagnosis codes are listed at their lowest level of specificity.

    NOTE: The individual provider is ultimately responsible for determining which diagnostic codes require 4th or 5th digits.

For example, ICD-9 code 724—"Other and unspecified disorders of back"—is a category code and requires a 4th digit. The four-digit subcategory codes available under this category code are:

724.0	Spinal stenosis, other than cervical
724.1	Pain in thoracic spine
724.2	Lumbago
724.3	Sciatica
724.4	Thoracic or lumbosacral neuritis or radiculitis, unspecified
724.5	Backache, unspecified
724.6	Disorders of sacrum
724.7	Disorders of coccyx
724.8	Other symptoms referable to back
724.9	Other unspecified back disorders

Eight of these four-digit subcategory codes are at their highest level of specificity. 724.0 and 724.7, however, also require a 5th digit. If 724.0 is selected, a 5th digit code is required:

724.00	Spinal stenosis, unspecified region
724.01	Thoracic region
724.02	Lumbar region
724.09	Other

Example A.
The ICD-9 code list for Clinical Practice Guideline Shoulder Fracture includes 812—"Fracture of humerus." This means that all valid subcategory (four-digit) and subclassification (five-digit) codes beginning with "812" are appropriate diagnoses under this guideline.

Example B.
The ICD-9 code list for Clinical Practice Guideline Flexor Tendon Repair includes 883.2—"Open wound of finger(s) with tendon involvement." This means that not all four-digit subcategory codes under category 883—"Open wound of finger(s)"—are applicable to this guideline, and since 883.2 does not require a 5th digit, it is at the highest level of specificity.

Example C.
The ICD-9 code list for Clinical Practice Guideline Medial Epicondylitis includes 726.31—"Medial epicondylitis." This diagnosis code has five digits and indicates that 1) not all four-digit subcategory codes under category 726—"Peripheral enthesopathies and allied syndromes"—are applicable to this guideline, and 2) not all five-digit subclassification codes under subcategory 726.3—"Enthesopathy of elbow region"—are applicable to this guideline.

XIV ICD-9 CODE REPORTING

Foot and Ankle

CARE CONNECTIONS *Clinical Practice Guidelines*

FOOT AND ANKLE

Achilles Tendinitis	3
Achilles Tendon Repair	9
Ankle Enthesopathy	15
Ankle Fracture	21
Ankle Sprain/Instability	27
Biomechanical Lower Extremity Dysfunction	33
Bunion	39
Diabetic Foot	43
Foot Care Guidelines for The Diabetic Patient	49
Foot Contusion	51
Foot Reconstruction	57
Orthotics: Answers to Commonly Asked Questions	63
Orthotics: Choosing the Right Shoe	65
Orthotics: Your New Orthotics	67
Plantar Fasciitis	69
Posterior Tibialis Tendinitis (Shin Splints)	75

FOOT AND ANKLE   1

2   FOOT AND ANKLE

ACHILLES TENDINITIS
SUMMARY OVERVIEW

ICD-9

726.71   727.00   727.01   727.06

APTA Preferred Practice Pattern: 4D, 4E, 4F, 4J

EXAMINATION

- History and Systems Review
- Tests and Measures
  Systems review per APTA's *Guide to Physical Therapy Practice*
  - Gait, locomotion, and balance
  - Muscle performance
  - Orthotic, protective and support devices
  - Pain
  - Posture
  - ROM
- Establish Plan of Care

GOALS/OUTCOMES

- Pain: 2/10 or less
- Normal gait pattern without assistive device on all surfaces
- Foot and ankle ROM
- Strength: 5/5 on manual muscle test or equivalent to uninvolved leg for gastrocnemius and soleus
- Return to previous functional status for ADLs and vocational, recreational, and sports activities as identified by patient
- Independence in a progressive home exercise program emphasizing function

INTERVENTION
NUMBER OF VISITS: 6–11

- Patient Instruction
  - Basic Anatomy and Biomechanics
  - Handouts
  - Functional Considerations

- Direct Interventions
  - Acute Phase: 2–4 Visits
  - Subacute/Chronic Phase: 4–7 Visits
- Functional Carryover

DISCHARGE PLANNING AND PATIENT RESPONSIBILITY

- Criteria for Discharge
  - All goals/outcomes achieved with the exception of return to previous functional status for recreational and sports activities
  - Patient demonstrates understanding of proper footwear, orthotics, and training schedule to prevent exacerbation of symptoms
- Circumstances Requiring Additional Visits
  - History of additional lower-extremity pathology
  - Presence of other medical conditions
  - Severe obesity
  - Chronicity or severity of condition
  - Ongoing aggravating risk factors (e.g., repetitive motion)
- Home Program
  - Flexibility exercises
  - Gastrocnemius stretch in subtalar neutral
  - Strengthening exercises
  - Toe flexors
  - Posterior tibialis
  - Gastrocnemius
  - Soleus
  - Fitness walking/running/other sport progression as appropriate
  - Plyometrics as appropriate
  - Contrast bath or use of cryotherapy after exercise or increased activity as needed
- Monitoring

SUMMARY OVERVIEW | FOOT AND ANKLE | ACHILLES TENDINITIS   3

ACHILLES TENDINITIS

ICD-9

726.71	Achilles bursitis or tendinitis
727.00	Synovitis and tenosynovitis, unspecified
727.01	Synovitis and tenosynovitis in diseases classified elsewhere
727.06	Tenosynovitis of foot and ankle

APTA Preferred Practice Pattern: 4D, 4E, 4F, 4J

EXAMINATION

History and Systems Review

- History of current condition
  - Location of symptoms
  - Aggravating factors
  - Accompanying lower-extremity symptoms
- Past history of current condition
  - Lower-extremity problems
- Other tests and measures to date
- Functional status and activity level (current/prior)
- Patient's functional goals

Tests and Measures

Systems review per APTA's *Guide to Physical Therapy Practice*

- Gait, locomotion, and balance
  - Antalgic gait
  - Premature heel off
  - Excessive pronation/supination
- Muscle performance
  - Palpation
    - Periosteum vs. tenoperiosteal junction vs. tendon vs. tenovaginitis (sheath) vs. musculotendinous junction
    - Rule out plantar fascia aggravation
  - Primarily plantarflexion with resistance as appropriate (manual vs. weight-bearing vs. repetitions of hops for provocation)
- Orthotic, protective and support devices
  - Footwear analysis
    - Look for source of friction from dress or sport footwear
    - Look for wear patterns indicating heel whip or excessive pronation
- Pain
  - Measured on visual analog scale

- Posture
  - Biomechanical screening
    If screen is positive, a full biomechanical assessment may be indicated. See *Biomechanical Lower Extremity Dysfunction* Guideline.
  - Static stance
    - Relaxed calcaneal posture
  - General lower-extremity alignment
  - Specific foot alignment
    - Subtalar neutral calcaneal position
    - Forefoot to rearfoot alignment
- ROM
  - Dorsiflexion with knee extended and flexed, (passive)
  - Plantarflexion (passive)

Establish Plan of Care

- Based on history, tests, and measures

GOALS/OUTCOMES

- Pain: 2/10 or less
- Normal gait pattern without assistive device on all surfaces
- Foot and ankle ROM:
  - Plantarflexion: 40°
  - Dorsiflexion: 10° in subtalar neutral with knee extended, 15° with knee flexed
  - Ratio of inversion to eversion: 2:1
- Strength: 5/5 on manual muscle test or equivalent to uninvolved leg for gastrocnemius and soleus
- Return to previous functional status for ADLs and vocational, recreational, and sports activities as identified by patient
- Independence in a progressive home exercise program emphasizing function

INTERVENTION
NUMBER OF VISITS: 6–11

Coordination, Communication, and Documentation

- Provision of services between admission and discharge that facilitate cost-effective and efficient integration or reintegration to home, community, or work
- Documentation of therapeutic intervention is required for each episode of care and serves as the basic foundation for communication
- Coordination and additional communication will depend on the patient's impairment and home/work/community/leisure situation and requirements. Such services may include:
  - Case management
  - Coordination of care and collaboration with those integral to the patient's rehabilitation program
  - Coordination and monitoring of the delivery of available resources
  - Referrals to other health-care professionals
  - Identification of resources, support groups, or advocacy services
  - Provision of educational or training information
  - Technical assistance
- Specific coordination and communication provisions:
  - Referral for biomechanical orthotics

Patient Instruction

Basic Anatomy and Biomechanics
- Location and attachments of the Achilles tendon and calf muscles, as well as their function
- Review the history of current condition
- Consequences of triceps suræ tightness and foot/ankle weakness
- The need to stretch and strengthen the ankle and Achilles tendon through rehabilitation
- Pertinent Gray's Anatomy (Gray. 1995. 884–886)

Handouts
- Cryotherapy and contrast baths
- Ankle joint ROM exercises
- Gastrocnemius and soleus stretching and strengthening exercises

Functional Considerations
- Walking/running as appropriate for the patient's symptoms, motor performance, and foot support
- Proper footwear, heel cups, heel lifts, or orthotics
- Use of cryotherapy and stretching after activity

Direct Interventions

Acute Phase: 2–4 Visits
- Therapeutic exercise and home program
  - ROM of ankle, including ankle pumps and ankle circles
  - Graded gastrocnemius and soleus stretching in subtalar neutral
  - Instruction regarding gait pattern with proper load (assistive device as needed)
  - Cardiovascular exercise via bike, swimming, or upper body ergometer as appropriate to maintain conditioning level
- Functional training
  - Activity level
    - Rest and cessation of running, jumping, and athletic activities
    - Protection
      a. Heel lifts or pads
      b. Very limited barefoot walking
  - Cryotherapy: Every 2–3 hours for up to 20 minutes per session
- Manual therapy techniques
  - Soft-tissue techniques
    - Soft-tissue mobilization to gastrocnemius and soleus
    - Friction massage to Achilles tendon, dependent on severity of inflammation
- Electrotherapeutic modalities
  - Electrical stimulation
  - Iontophoresis
- Physical agents and mechanical modalities
  - Whirlpool baths: Cold or contrast
  - Pulsed ultrasound
  - Phonophoresis
- Goals/outcomes
  - Pain: 4/10 or less
  - Full weight-bearing gait pattern with orthotics or assistive devices as needed
  - Foot and ankle ROM:
    - Plantarflexion: 30°

FOOT AND ANKLE | ACHILLES TENDINITIS

- Dorsiflexion: 5° in subtalar joint neutral with knee extended, 15° with knee flexed

Subacute/Chronic Phase: 4–7 Visits

- Therapeutic exercise and home program
  - Flexibility exercises
    - Gastrocnemius, soleus, and Achilles tendon
    - Toe flexors
    - Plantar fascia
  - Strengthening exercises with resistive band, manual resistance, and closed chain exercises
    - Toe and heel raises
    - BAPS
    - Stationary bicycle
    - Treadmill
    - Stair machine
  - Progressive gait training for stance stability and control of excessive pronation as appropriate
  - Step progression to hopping and jumping as tolerated (plyometrics goal)
    - SportCord™ for forward, backward, and sideways lunges
- Functional training
  - Activity level
    - Graded walking/running activities
    - Protection as needed with activity
      a. Heel cups
      b. Heel pads
      c. Orthotics
      d. Taping
  - Cryotherapy after activity as needed for edema or pain (self management)
- Manual therapy techniques
  - Soft-tissue techniques
    - Deep friction to specific lesion site in Achilles tendon or calf muscle
    - Myofascial release to the gastrocnemius and soleus muscles as indicated for increased tissue length and elasticity
  - Joint mobilization
    - As indicated to restore normal foot and ankle ROM
- Therapeutic devices and equipment
  - Functional biomechanics

- Integration of specific structural or biomechanical components that may relieve symptoms, including the choice of shoes or custom biomechanical orthotics to control excessive compensatory pronation
- Electrotherapeutic modalities
  - Electrical stimulation
- Physical agents and mechanical modalities
  - Cryotherapy as needed
  - Ultrasound
  - Phonophoresis
- Goals/outcomes
  - Pain-free, normal gait pattern without assistive device on all surfaces
  - Strength: 5/5 on manual muscle test or equivalent to uninvolved leg for gastrocnemius and soleus
  - Foot and ankle ROM:
    - Plantarflexion: 40°
    - Dorsiflexion: 10° in subtalar neutral with knee extended, 15° with knee flexed
    - Ratio of inversion to eversion: 2:1
  - Pain: 2/10 or less

Functional Carryover

- Instruction is given regarding specific training errors that may exacerbate symptoms
- Counsel patient regarding cross-training options

DISCHARGE PLANNING AND PATIENT RESPONSIBILITY

Criteria for Discharge

- All goals/outcomes achieved with the exception of return to previous functional status for recreational and sports activities
- Patient demonstrates understanding of proper footwear, orthotics, and training schedule to prevent exacerbation of symptoms

Circumstances Requiring Additional Visits

- History of additional lower-extremity pathology
- Presence of other medical conditions
- Severe obesity
- Chronicity or severity of condition
- Ongoing aggravating risk factors (e.g., repetitive motion)

Home Program

- Flexibility exercises
- Gastrocnemius stretch in subtalar neutral
- Strengthening exercises
- Toe flexors
- Posterior tibialis
- Gastrocnemius
- Soleus
- Fitness walking/running/other sports progression as appropriate
- Plyometrics as appropriate
- Contrast bath or use of cryotherapy after exercise or increased activity as needed

Monitoring

- Patient is to recheck/call at 2 weeks post-discharge to report progression toward previous functional status for recreational and sports activities
- If necessary, schedule a 4 week follow-up at clinic to monitor objective parameters and progress the home exercise program

REFERENCES

1. American Physical Therapy Association. *Guide To Physical Therapist Practice.* Alexandria, VA: APTA; 1997.
2. Cailliet R. *Foot And Ankle Pain.* 2nd ed. Philadelphia, PA: FA Davis; 1983.
3. Curwin S, Stanish WO. *Tendinitis: Its Etiology and Treatment.* Lexington, MA: DC Heath; 1984.
4. Gray H; Williams PL, ed. *Gray's Anatomy.* 38th ed. New York, NY: Churchill Livingstone; 1995.
5. Hart A, Hopkins C, Ford B. *ICD-9-CM Expert For Physicians, Volumes 1&2.* 7th ed. USA: Ingenix; 2005.
6. Kessler R, Hertling D. *Management of Common Musculoskeletal Disorders: Physical Therapy Principles and Methods.* 2nd ed. Philadelphia, PA: Harper & Row; 1990.
7. Magee DJ. *Orthopedic Physical Assessment.* 2nd ed. Philadelphia, PA: WB Saunders; 1987.
8. Rodgers MM. Dynamic foot biomechanics. *J Orthop Sports Phys Ther.* 1995;21(6):306-316.
9. Sammarco GJ. *Rehabilitation of The Foot And Ankle.* St. Louis, MO: Mosby-Yearbook; 1995.
10. Scioli MW. Achilles tendinitis. *Orthop Clin North Am.* 1994;25:177-182.

ACHILLES TENDON REPAIR
SUMMARY OVERVIEW

ICD-9

727.67   959.7

APTA Preferred Practice Pattern: 4D, 4E, 4F, 4J

EXAMINATION

- History and Systems Review
- Tests and Measures
  Systems review per APTA's *Guide to Physical Therapy Practice*
  - Anthropometric characteristics
  - Gait, locomotion, and balance
  - Muscle performance
  - Pain
  - ROM
  - Sensory integrity
- Establish Plan of Care

GOALS/OUTCOMES

- Strength: 4/5 in all major groups
- Talocrural ROM
- Unassisted normal gait pattern with maximized propulsive phase on all surfaces and stairs
- Neuromuscular/balance/proprioceptive reactions equal to uninvolved side
- Pain: 2/10 or less
- Return to previous functional status for ADLs and vocational, recreational, and sports activities as identified by patient
- Independence in a progressive home exercise program emphasizing function

INTERVENTION
NUMBER OF VISITS: 5–14

- Patient Instruction
  - Basic Anatomy and Biomechanics
  - Handouts
  - Functional Considerations
  - Description of Surgical Procedure
- Direct Interventions
  - Protection Phase: 2–7 Visits
  - Progressive Phase: 3–7 Visits
- Functional Carryover

DISCHARGE PLANNING AND PATIENT RESPONSIBILITY

- Criteria for Discharge
  - Patient has achieved all rehabilitation goals except full return to recreation
- Circumstances Requiring Additional Visits
  - History of additional lower-extremity pathology
  - Other medical or postoperative complications
  - Chronicity or severity of condition
  - Delayed healing
- Home Program
  - Flexibility exercises
  - Achilles tendon
  - Gastrocnemius and soleus
  - Other lower-extremity muscles as appropriate
  - Strengthening exercises
  - Heel raises and other functional closed-chain exercises
  - Water exercise, including swimming
  - Cycling
  - Running/fitness walking progression
  - Plyometrics
  - Home instruction regarding the use of cryotherapy after activity
- Monitoring

SUMMARY OVERVIEW | FOOT AND ANKLE | ACHILLES TENDON REPAIR

ACHILLES TENDON REPAIR

ICD-9

727.67	Nontraumatic rupture of achilles tendon
959.7	Other and unspecified injury to knee, leg, ankle, and foot

APTA Preferred Practice Pattern: 4D, 4E, 4F, 4J

EXAMINATION

History and Systems Review

- History of current condition
  - Date of surgical procedure and postoperative course
  - Weight-bearing status
- Past history of current condition
  - History of previous lower-extremity problems
- Past medical/surgical history
  - History of systemic disease
- Functional status and activity level (current/prior)
- Patient's functional goals

Tests and Measures

Systems review per APTA's *Guide to Physical Therapy Practice*

- Anthropometric characteristics
  - Comparative girth measurement
    - Figure 8: Circumferential measurement using bony landmarks just inferior to the medial and lateral malleoli, tubercle of the navicular, and peroneal sulcus and cuboid bone (just proximal to the tuberosity of the fifth metatarsal)
    - Malleolar level: Circumferential measurement just inferior to the medial and lateral malleoli
    - Metatarsophalangeal joint level: Circumferential measurement around forefoot at the metatarsophalangeal joints
    - Mid-calf: Circumferential measurement of calf girth at a measured distance superior to lateral malleolus
- Gait, locomotion, and balance
  - Premature heel off
  - Excessive pronation/supination
  - Focus on propulsion

- Muscle performance
  - Plantarflexors
  - Dorsiflexors
  - Invertors
  - Evertors
- Pain
  - Measured on visual analog scale
- ROM
  - Talocrural ROM
  - Rear foot and mid-tarsal inversion and eversion
- Sensory integrity
  - Proprioceptive testing
  - Weight shift
  - BAPS
  - Balance/reach test
    - Unilateral stance balancing, reaching with opposite leg
    - Unilateral stance balancing, reaching with arms

Establish Plan of Care

- Based on history, tests, and measures

GOALS/OUTCOMES

- Strength: 4/5 in all major groups
- Talocrural ROM:
  - Dorsiflexion: 10° in subtalar neutral with knee extended, 15° with knee flexed
  - Plantarflexion: 40°
- Unassisted normal gait pattern with maximized propulsive phase on all surfaces and stairs
- Neuromuscular/balance/proprioceptive reactions equal to uninvolved side
- Pain: 2/10 or less
- Return to previous functional status for ADLs and vocational, recreational, and sports activities as identified by patient
- Independence in a progressive home exercise program emphasizing function

INTERVENTION
NUMBER OF VISITS: 5–14

Coordination, Communication, and Documentation
- Provision of services between admission and discharge that facilitate cost-effective and efficient integration or reintegration to home, community, or work
- Documentation of therapeutic intervention is required for each episode of care and serves as the basic foundation for communication
- Coordination and additional communication will depend on the patient's impairment and home/work/community/leisure situation and requirements. Such services may include:
  - Case management
  - Coordination of care and collaboration with those integral to the patient's rehabilitation program
  - Coordination and monitoring of the delivery of available resources
  - Referrals to other health-care professionals
  - Identification of resources, support groups, or advocacy services
  - Provision of educational or training information
  - Technical assistance
- Specific coordination and communication provisions:
  - May request operative report and surgeon's specific postoperative rehabilitation protocol

Patient Instruction

Basic Anatomy and Biomechanics
- Hinge motion at the mortise vs. supination/pronation contributed by subtalar and midtarsal joints
- The role of the plantarflexors to break forward momentum and also perform propulsion
- Review the mechanism of injury, the consequences of Achilles tendon and triceps suræ tightness, and foot and ankle weakness
- Pertinent Gray's Anatomy (Gray. 1995. 713–729, 733–734)

Handouts
- Home exercise program
  - Flexibility
    - Gastrocnemius
    - Soleus

- Other lower quadrant muscles as indicated
  - Motor performance
    - Tubing
    - Closed-kinetic chain exercise
    - Gait drills
- Home contrast bath

Functional Considerations
- Instructions regarding protection and progression of gait on stairs, uneven ground, hopping, jumping, and sudden stops and starts
- Critical elements of tissue healing post-repair with description of normal timing for progressive resistive exercise program and ankle strengthening through resistance tubing and closed-chain exercise

Description of Surgical Procedure
- Review of operative procedure in relation to joint biomechanics, rehabilitation, and function

Direct Interventions

Protection Phase: 2–7 Visits
- Therapeutic exercise and home program
  - Manual resistive exercises to foot and ankle
  - General lower-extremity stretches as indicated
  - Gastrocnemius and soleus stretching to a maximum of 10–15° of dorsiflexion (gradual progression)
  - Foot and ankle resistance exercise using bands/tubing
  - Neuromuscular/balance/proprioceptive reeducation
  - Gait training (partial weight bearing or full weight bearing)
    - Heel lift or cam walker to maximize comfortable propulsion in terminal stance if appropriate
    - Progress to full weight bearing out of protective device
  - Cardiovascular exercise with upper or lower body ergometer
- Manual therapy techniques
  - Soft-tissue techniques
    - Friction to surgical scar and tendon repair
    - Myofascial techniques to the gastrocnemius and soleus muscles
  - Joint mobilization
    - Talocrural dorsiflexion, plantarflexion
    - Rearfoot and midfoot inversion/eversion

FOOT AND ANKLE | ACHILLES TENDON REPAIR

- Electrotherapeutic modalities
  - Electrical stimulation for pain control and edema reduction
- Physical agents and mechanical modalities
  - Cryotherapy for edema
  - Pulsed ultrasound progressing to continuous ultrasound
- Goals/outcomes
  - Full-weight-bearing, normal gait pattern with assistive device as needed
  - Ankle ROM:
    - Dorsiflexion: 5° in subtalar joint neutral with knee extended, 10° with knee flexed
    - Plantarflexion: 30°
  - Pain: 5/10 or less
  - Strength: Minimum of 3/5 in all major muscle groups

Progressive Phase: 3–7 Visits
- Therapeutic exercise and home program
  - Manual resisted exercises
  - Continuation of ankle flexibility exercises
  - Progressive closed chain, calf strengthening and ankle stabilizer strengthening
  - Ergometry (pedal under midfoot prior to 10–12 weeks postoperative), progressing into treadmill, ski machine, or stair machine for endurance as tolerated
  - Neuromuscular/balance/proprioceptive reeducation
  - Progressive walking/running activities on all surfaces
- Manual therapy techniques
  - Mobilization as indicated
    - Ankle
    - Rearfoot
    - Midfoot
- Electrotherapeutic modalities
  - Electrical stimulation for inflammation reduction
- Physical agents and mechanical modalities
  - Cryotherapy after exercise
- Goals/outcomes
  - Unassisted, normal gait pattern with maximized propulsive phase on all surfaces and stairs
  - Strength: 4/5 in all major muscle groups
  - Return to full ADLs and vocational function
  - Pain: 2/10 or less
  - Neuromuscular/balance/proprioceptive reactions equal to uninvolved side

Functional Carryover
- Gait pattern progression
- Protected (backward trunk lean) gait progressed to propulsive gait
- Brisk walking
- Running
- Running progression into sprints, start/stop, Figure 8, carioca, and function-specific footwork; functional combination of such exercises as squatting and heel raises added to rehabilitation regime
- Counseling regarding cross-training options during progression toward recreational and sport goals

DISCHARGE PLANNING AND PATIENT RESPONSIBILITY

Criteria for Discharge
- Patient has achieved all rehabilitation goals except full return to recreation. May be discharged with:
  - ROM: 8° dorsiflexion in subtalar neutral with knee extended
  - Strength: 4+/5 in all major muscle groups
  - Functional status: Previous functional level for ADLs and vocational activities, progression toward recreational and sport goals

Circumstances Requiring Additional Visits
- History of additional lower-extremity pathology
- Other medical or postoperative complications
- Chronicity or severity of condition
- Delayed healing

Home Program
- Flexibility exercises
- Achilles tendon
- Gastrocnemius and soleus
- Other lower-extremity muscles as appropriate
- Strengthening exercises
- Heel raises and other functional closed chain exercises
- Water exercise, including swimming
- Cycling
- Running/fitness walking progression
- Plyometrics
- Home instruction regarding the use of cryotherapy after activity

Monitoring
- Patient is to recheck/call at 1 month post-discharge to ensure expected progression toward all rehabilitation goals
- Schedule clinic follow-up as deemed necessary to monitor objective parameters and progress home program

REFERENCES

1. American Physical Therapy Association. *Guide To Physical Therapist Practice.* Alexandria, VA: APTA; 1997.

2. Blake RL, Ferguson HJ. Achilles tendon rupture: a protocol for conservative management. *J Am Podiatr Med Assoc.* 1991;81:486-489.

3. Buchgraber A, Passler HH. Percutaneous repair of Achilles tendon rupture: immobilization versus functional postoperative treatment. *Clin Orthop Rel Res.* August 1997:113-122.

4. Carter TR, Fowler PJ, Blokker C. Functional postoperative treatment of Achilles tendon repair. *Am J Sports Med.* 1992;20:459-462.

5. Gray H; Williams PL, ed. *Gray's Anatomy.* 38th ed. New York, NY: Churchill Livingstone; 1995.

6. Hart A, Hopkins C, Ford B. *ICD-9-CM Expert For Physicians, Volume 1&2.* 7th ed. USA: Ingenix; 2005.

7. Kissel CG, Blacklidge DK, Crowley DL. Repair of neglected Achilles tendon ruptures: procedure and functional results. *J Foot Ankle Surg.* 1994;33(1):46-52.

8. Kuwada GT. Diagnosis and treatment of Achilles tendon rupture. *Clin Podiatr Med Surg.* 1995;12:633-652.

9. Landvater SJ, Renstrom P. Complete Achilles tendon ruptures. *Clin Sports Med.* 1992;11:741-758.

10. Mascaro TB, Swanson LE. Rehabilitation of the foot and ankle. *Orthop Clin North Am.* 1994;25:147-160.

ANKLE ENTHESOPATHY
SUMMARY OVERVIEW

ICD-9

726.70

APTA *Preferred Practice Pattern:* **4E, 4D, 4I**

EXAMINATION

- History and Systems Review
- Tests and Measures
  Systems review per APTA's *Guide to Physical Therapy Practice*
  - Gait, locomotion, and balance
  - Joint integrity and mobility
  - Muscle performance
  - Orthotics, protective and supportive devices
  - Pain
  - Posture
- Establish Plan of Care

GOALS/OUTCOMES

- Pain: 2/10 or less
- Normal gait pattern without assistive device on all surfaces
- Foot and ankle ROM
- Strength: 5/5 on manual muscle test or equivalent to uninvolved leg for gastroc and soleus
- Return to previous functional status for ADLs and vocational, recreational, and sports activities as identified by patient
- Independence in a progressive home exercise program emphasizing function

INTERVENTION
NUMBER OF VISITS: 5–9

- Patient Instruction
  - Basic Anatomy and Biomechanics
  - Handouts
  - Functional Considerations
- Direct Interventions
  - Acute Phase: 1–3 Visits
  - Subacute Phase: 4–6 Visits
- Functional Carryover

DISCHARGE PLANNING AND PATIENT RESPONSIBILITY

- Criteria for Discharge
  - All goals/outcomes achieved with the exception of return to recreation and sports activities
  - Patient demonstrates understanding of proper footwear and orthotics
  - Patient demonstrates understanding of training guidelines to prevent exacerbation of symptoms, including recognizing signs of fatigue and allowing recovery time
- Circumstances Requiring Additional Visits
  - Severe degenerative changes
  - History of other pathology of lower extremity
  - Presence of other medical conditions
  - Chronicity or severity of condition
  - Postoperative complications
  - Ongoing repetitive aggravating factor
- Home Program
  - Muscle flexibility and lengthening exercises
  - Strengthening exercises
  - Cardiovascular endurance
  - Balance and coordination training
  - Plyometrics for return to sport as appropriate
  - Cryotherapy after activity as needed
- Monitoring

SUMMARY OVERVIEW | FOOT AND ANKLE | ANKLE ENTHESOPATHY

ANKLE ENTHESOPATHY

ICD-9
    726.70   Enthesopathy of ankle and tarsus, unspecified
APTA Preferred Practice Pattern: 4E, 4D, 4I

EXAMINATION

History and Systems Review
- History of current condition
  - Location of symptoms
  - Aggravating factors
  - Accompanying lower-extremity symptoms
- Past history of current condition
  - Other lower-extremity problems
- Other tests and measures
- Medications
- Past medical/surgical history
- Functional status and activity level (current/prior)
- Patient's functional goals

Tests and Measures
Systems review per APTA's *Guide to Physical Therapy Practice*
- Gait, locomotion, and balance
  - Antalgic gait, premature heel off, excessive pronation or supination
- Joint integrity and mobility
  - Long axis extension
  - Anteroposterior glide
  - Talar rock
  - Side tilt
  - Rotation
  - Side glide
  - First ray and tarsal bone mobility
- Muscle performance (including strength, power, and endurance)
  - Plantarflexors, secondary plantarflexors, dorsiflexors, intrinsics
  - Eccentric/concentric muscle contractions
- Orthotics, protective and supportive devices
  - Footwear analysis
    - Wear patterns, current bracing (donning/doffing, proper fit)
- Pain
  - Measured on visual analog scale

- Posture
  - Biomechanical/lumbar screen
  - Static stance
    - Relaxed calcaneal posture
    - Position in space (frontal, sagittal plane)
  - Lower-extremity observation and alignment
  - Specific foot alignment
    - Subtalar neutral alignment
    - Forefoot to rearfoot alignment
  - ROM (including muscle length)
    - Active dorsiflexion (knee flexed, knee extended, passive range, and overpressures)
    - Active plantarflexion (passive and overpressures)
    - Active inversion and eversion (passive and overpressures)
    - Toe flexion, extension, abduction, adduction

Establish Plan of Care
- Based on history, tests, and measures

GOALS/OUTCOMES
- Pain: 2/10 or less
- Normal gait pattern without assistive device on all surfaces
- Foot and ankle ROM:
  - Plantarflexion: 20–40° (20–30° needed for normal gait)
  - Dorsiflexion: 6–15° (6–10° needed for normal gait)
  - Ratio of inversion to eversion: 2:1, subtalar neutral 6° inversion/eversion
- Strength: 5/5 on manual muscle test or equivalent to uninvolved leg for gastroc and soleus
- Return to previous functional status for ADLs and vocational, recreational, and sports activities as identified by patient
- Independence in a progressive home exercise program emphasizing function

INTERVENTION
NUMBER OF VISITS: 5–9

Coordination, Communication, and Documentation
- Provision of services between admission and discharge that facilitate cost-effective and efficient integration or reintegration to home, community, or work
- Documentation of therapeutic intervention is required for each episode of care and serves as the basic foundation for communication
- Coordination and additional communication will depend on the patient's impairment and home/work/community/leisure situation and requirements. Such services may include:
  - Case management
  - Coordination of care and collaboration with those integral to the patient's rehabilitation program
  - Coordination and monitoring of the delivery of available resources
  - Referrals to other health-care professionals
  - Identification of resources, support groups, or advocacy services
  - Provision of educational or training information
  - Technical assistance
- Specific coordination and communication provisions

Patient Instruction

Basic Anatomy and Biomechanics
- Foot anatomy
  - Rearfoot, midfoot, forefoot
    - Allows for both flexibility and rigidity
  - Planes of motion
    - Sagittal, frontal, and transverse
    - Triplanar motion: pronation/supinate
  - 26 bones: 7 tarsals, 5 metatarsals, 14 phalanges
  - Arches: Plantar arch, metatarsal arch, lateral arch
- Subtalar neutral
  - Head of talus is aligned with the navicular
- Windlass mechanism
  - Dorsiflexion through the foot increases medial longitudinal foot through hindfoot supination

Handouts
- Commercially available products, such as:
  - Ankle anatomy handouts, foot/ankle models

- Exercises as per handouts
- Cryotherapy and contrast baths
- Self-mobilization or massage techniques
- Home program
- Specific home program for ankle/foot mobility, flexibility, and strengthening
  - Flexibility
    - Gastrocnemius/soleus stretching in subtalar neutral
  - Strengthening
    - Foot intrinsics
    - Gastrocnemius, soleus, posterior tibialis
  - Plyometrics, return to sport as appropriate
  - Contrast bath or cryotherapy after exercise as needed

Functional Considerations
- Posture (sitting, standing, sleeping, driving)
  - Utilize rest positions, avoid prolonged weight bearing/standing
  - Decrease activity, alter ADLs to decrease inflammation
  - Weight management
- Assistive devices
  - Crutches, canes to decrease effects of pain during weight bearing
  - Taping
  - Bracing, temporary or permanent orthotics
- Proper supportive footwear

Direct Interventions

Acute Phase: 1–3 Visits
- Therapeutic exercise and home program
  - Increase ROM of ankle: Ankle pumps and circles
  - Muscle flexibility of the gastrocnemius and soleus in subtalar neutral
  - Instruction on gait mechanics (assistive device as appropriate)
  - Cardiovascular exercise (bike, swim, upper body ergometer) as appropriate
- Functional training
  - Activity level
    - Rest and cessation of aggravating factors (prolonged standing, walking, running, jumping, sports)
    - Protection
      a. Arch supports or orthotics
      b. Supportive footwear

FOOT AND ANKLE | ANKLE ENTHESOPATHY   17

- Cryotherapy: Every 2–3 hours up to 20 minutes per session
- Manual therapy
  - Soft-tissue mobilizations as indicated to decrease inflammation and improve blood flow
  - Joint mobilizations: Gentle Grade I/II ankle mobilizations to increase range as appropriate
- Modalities as indicated to decrease pain and inflammation
  - Electrical stimulation
  - Iontophoresis
  - Pulsed ultrasound
- Goals/outcomes
  - Pain: 4/10 or less
  - Full weight-bearing gait pattern with orthotics or assistive devices as appropriate
  - Foot and ankle ROM:
    - Plantarflexion: 40°
    - Dorsiflexion: 10°
    - Ratio of inversion to eversion: 2:1, subtalar neutral 6° inversion/eversion

Subacute Phase: 4–6 Visits

- Therapeutic exercise and home program
  - Continue muscle flexibility and lengthening exercises
  - Strengthening exercises
    - Concentric and eccentric contraction
      a. Manual resistance, resistive band, closed chained
  - Cardiovascular endurance
    - Continue bike, swim, may add treadmill, elliptical as tolerated
  - Balance and coordination training
    - Controlled twisting, turning, lateral weight shifting
    - Even and uneven surfaces in subtalar neutral
    - Rocker, wobble, BAPS board
- Functional training
  - Activity level
    - Walking/running activities
      a. Educate patient on recognizing signs of muscle fatigue and joint stress or aggravation and how to modify appropriately
    - Protection as needed with increase in activity
    - Cryotherapy as needed after activity
- Manual therapy techniques
  - Soft-tissue techniques as indicated to increase tissue length

- Deep tissue massage, deep friction, myofascial release
- Joint mobilization techniques as indicated to improve joint play
  - Sustained or oscillation Grade III/IV techniques
  - Mobilizations with movement to increase ROM and decrease pain that occurs with motion
- Inhibition techniques
  - Hold-Relax, Contract-Relax, Agonist Contraction, Hold-Relax with agonist contraction
- Modalities as appropriate to promote tissue healing and reeducation
  - Electrical stimulation
  - Neuromuscular stimulation
  - Continuous ultrasound
- Goals/outcomes
  - Pain: 1/10 or less
  - Full weight-bearing gait pattern without pain or assistive device on all surfaces
  - Strength: 5/5 manual muscle test all planes
  - Foot and ankle ROM: WNL

Functional Carryover

- Integration of home exercise program into vocational environment
- Completion of ergonomic adjustments to home, automobile, and vocational areas
- Incorporation of proper posture and body mechanics to avoid exacerbation of symptoms
- Recognition/avoidance of activities that increase or exacerbate radiating symptoms

DISCHARGE PLANNING AND PATIENT RESPONSIBILITY

Criteria for Discharge

- All goals/outcomes achieved with the exception of return to recreation and sports activities
- Patient demonstrates understanding of proper footwear and orthotics
- Patient demonstrates understanding of training guidelines to prevent exacerbation of symptoms, including recognizing signs of fatigue and allowing recovery time

Circumstances Requiring Additional Visits

- Severe degenerative changes
- History of other pathology of lower extremity
- Presence of other medical conditions
- Chronicity or severity of condition
- Postoperative complications
- Ongoing repetitive aggravating factor

Home Program

- Muscle flexibility and lengthening exercises
  - Gastrocnemius in subtalar neutral
- Strengthening exercises
  - Posterior tibialis, gastrocnemius, intrinsics
- Cardiovascular endurance
  - Walking, running, sport progression as tolerated
  - Bike, swim, treadmill, elliptical
- Balance and coordination training
- Plyometrics for return to sport as appropriate
- Cryotherapy after activity as needed

Monitoring

- Patient is to recheck at 2 weeks post-discharge to report progression towards previous functional status and/or return to sport
- Schedule a follow-up at clinic to monitor objective parameters and progress home exercise program as deemed necessary

REFERENCES

1. American Physical Therapy Association. *Guide to Physical Therapist Practice.* Alexandria, VA: APTA; revised 2003

2. Hart A, Hopkins C, Ford B. *ICD-9-CM Expert For Physicians, Volumes 1&2.* 7th ed. USA: Ingenix; 2005.

3. Kisner C, Colby LA. *Therapeutic Exercise: Foundation Aand Techniques.* 4th ed. Philadelphia, PA: F.A. Davis; 2002:180-91, 563-87.

4. Magee, DJ. Orthopedic physical assessment, 4th ed. Philadelphia, PA: Saunders; 2002, 765-839

5. McPoil T, Mueller M, Reischl S, Tomaro J. *Taking Care of Your Foot and Ankle.* Available at: http://www.apta.org/AM/Template.cfm?Section=Logout&TEMPLATE=/CM/HTMLDisplay.cfm&CONTENTID=24759. Accessed August 28, 2007.

6. Placzek, JD, Boyce KA. *Orthopaedic Physical Therapy Secrets.* Philadelphia, PA: Hanley & Belfus, Inc; 2001:439-55.

7. Saunders Website. *Ankle Model and Bracing.* http://www.thesaundersgroup.com/index.asp?PageAction=PRODSEARCH&txtSearch=ankle&btnSearch=GO&Page=1. Accessed August 28, 2007.

ANKLE FRACTURE
SUMMARY OVERVIEW

ICD-9

824 825 827

APTA Preferred Practice Pattern: 4D, 4H, 4J

EXAMINATION

- History and Systems Review
- Tests and Measures
  Systems review per APTA's *Guide to Physical Therapy Practice*
  - Anthropometric characteristics
  - Gait, locomotion, and balance
  - Muscle performance
  - Pain
  - Posture
  - ROM
  - Sensory integrity
- Establish Plan of Care

GOALS/OUTCOMES

- Pain: 2/10 or less
- Foot and ankle ROM
- Edema: Less than 1 cm Figure 8 girth difference between limbs
- Transition to normal footwear
- Functional joint ROM of midtarsal joints, first ray, and fifth ray
- Return to functional status and activity level (current/prior) for ADLs and vocational, sport, and recreational activities as identified by patient
- Normal gait pattern without assistive devices on all surfaces
- Strength: 5/5 on manual muscle test or equivalent to uninvolved leg
- Improved neuromuscular/balance/proprioceptive awareness for stability and reduction of risk for future injury
- Independence in a progressive home exercise program emphasizing function

INTERVENTION
NUMBER OF VISITS: 6–15

- Patient Instruction
  - Basic Anatomy and Biomechanics
  - Handouts
  - Functional Considerations
- Direct Interventions
  - Postoperative/Immobilization Phase: 3–6 Visits, 6–8 Weeks Post-Fracture
  - Functional Strengthening Phase: 3–9 Visits, 9–12 Weeks Post-Fracture
- Functional Carryover

DISCHARGE PLANNING AND PATIENT RESPONSIBILITY

- Criteria for Discharge
  - Patient has achieved all goals/outcomes with possible exceptions listed in guidelines
  - Functional status: Prior to attainment of previous level for ADLs and vocational activities, progression toward recreational and sports activities if progress is present
- Circumstances Requiring Additional Visits
  - History of additional lower-extremity pathology
  - Multiple fracture sites
  - Presence of other medical conditions
  - Postoperative complications
  - Delayed fracture healing/union
  - Severe obesity
- Home Program
  - Flexibility exercises
  - Contrast bath and/or use of cryotherapy, especially after exercise or increased activity, to reduce edema and control pain
  - Strengthening exercises
  - Running progression
  - Plyometrics
- Monitoring

ANKLE FRACTURE

ICD-9

824	Fracture of ankle
825	Fracture of one or more tarsal and metatarsal bones
827	Other, multiple, and ill-defined fractures of lower limb

APTA Preferred Practice Pattern: 4D, 4H, 4J

EXAMINATION

History and Systems Review

- History of current condition
  - Date and type of fracture/surgical procedure
  - Post injury/postoperative course (progression of weight-bearing/functional activity level)
  - Current home exercise program
- Past history of current condition
  - History of ankle sprain, fracture, instability
  - History of other lower-extremity problems
- Functional status and activity level (current/prior)
- Patient's functional goals/outcomes

Tests and Measures

Systems review per APTA's *Guide to Physical Therapy Practice*

- Anthropometric characteristics
  - Comparative girth measurements
    - Figure 8: Circumferential measurement using bony landmarks just inferior to the medial and lateral malleolus, tubercle of the navicular, and peroneal sulcus and cuboid bone (just proximal to the tuberosity of the fifth metatarsal)
    - Malleolar level: Circumferential measurement just inferior to the medial and lateral malleolus
    - Metatarsophalangeal joint level: Circumferential measurement around forefoot at the metatarsophalangeal joints
- Gait, locomotion, and balance
  - Weight-bearing tolerance
  - Quality of gait
  - Assistive devices

- Muscle performance
  - Plantarflexors
  - Dorsiflexors
  - Invertors
  - Evertors
- Pain
  - Measured on visual analog scale
- Posture
  - Static stance position
  - General lower-extremity alignment
  - Specific foot alignment
- ROM
  - Talocrural: Dorsiflexion, plantarflexion (passive/active)
  - Subtalar/midtarsal: Inversion, eversion (passive/active)
  - Hallux: Dorsiflexion (passive/active)
- Sensory integrity
  - Proprioceptive tests
  - Weight shift
  - Stork stand
  - BAPS
  - Balance/reach test
    - Unilateral stance balancing, reaching with opposite leg
    - Unilateral stance balancing, reaching with arms

Establish Plan of Care

- Based on history, tests, and measures

GOALS/OUTCOMES

- Pain: 2/10 or less
- Foot and ankle ROM:
  - Plantarflexion: 40°
  - Dorsiflexion: 10° in subtalar neutral with knee extended, 15° with knee flexed
  - Ratio of inversion to eversion: 2:1
  - Hallux dorsiflexion: 60°

- Edema: less than 1 cm Figure 8 girth difference between limbs
- Transition to normal footwear
- Functional joint ROM of midtarsal joints, first ray, and fifth ray
- Return to functional status and activity level (current/prior) for ADLs and vocational, sport, and recreational activities as identified by patient
- Normal gait pattern without assistive devices on all surfaces
- Strength: 5/5 on manual muscle test or equivalent to uninvolved leg
- Improved neuromuscular/balance/proprioceptive awareness for stability and reduction of risk for future injury
- Independence in a progressive home exercise program emphasizing function

INTERVENTION
NUMBER OF VISITS: 6–15

Coordination, Communication, and Documentation
- Provision of services between admission and discharge that facilitate cost-effective and efficient integration or reintegration to home, community, or work
- Documentation of therapeutic intervention is required for each episode of care and serves as the basic foundation for communication
- Coordination and additional communication will depend on the patient's impairment and home/work/community/leisure situation and requirements. Such services may include:
  - Case management
  - Coordination of care and collaboration with those integral to the patient's rehabilitation program
  - Coordination and monitoring of the delivery of available resources
  - Referrals to other health-care professionals
  - Identification of resources, support groups, or advocacy services
  - Provision of educational or training information
  - Technical assistance
- Specific coordination and communication provisions:
  - Referral to social worker as needed if functional status and living arrangements warrant assistance

Patient Instruction

Basic Anatomy and Biomechanics
- Hinge motion at the mortise vs. supination/pronation motion contributed by subtalar and midtarsal joints
- Time frame for weight-bearing progression
- Pertinent Gray's Anatomy (Gray. 1995. 721)

Handouts
- Home contrast bath
- Home exercise program
  - Straight and bent knee/calf flexibility exercises
  - Ankle rubber band/resistive tubing exercises
  - Closed-kinetic chain functional exercise progression
  - Gait training to reduce limp and improve stance stability (stepping exercise)

Functional Considerations
- Amount of walking as appropriate to the patient's weight-bearing allowance and other signs and symptoms
- Ankle support or appropriate protective devices are provided for protection/compression
- Functional progression regarding stairs, varied terrain, vigor of loading (walking vs. running vs. jumping) is covered with patient appropriate to SIN (severity, irritability, nature)

Description of Surgical Procedure
- Location and function of surgical hardware
- Postoperative edema management
- Review of operative procedure and relation to joint biomechanics, rehabilitation, and function

Direct Interventions

Postoperative/Immobilization Phase: 3–6 Visits, 6–8 Weeks Post-Fracture
- Therapeutic exercise and home program
  - Gastrocnemius and soleus lengthening in subtalar neutral
  - Gait training to maximize stance stability and tibial translation in gait
  - Stationary bike riding for improved metabolism and increased endurance

- BAPS for controlled ROM, ankle stabilizer strengthening, and neuromuscular/balance/proprioceptive reeducation
- Progressive resistive exercises
- Closed-kinetic chain functional progression as appropriate for patient's tolerance and functional roles
- Aquatic therapy
- Manual therapy techniques
  - Joint mobilization: Progress grade of mobilization for return to function
    - Talocrural dorsiflexion
    - Subtalar and midtarsal motion
    - Hallux dorsiflexion
  - Soft-tissue techniques
    - Proximal and distal tibiofibular ligaments are assessed for stability and addressed as appropriate
    - Venous drainage massage as needed
- Electrotherapeutic modalities
  - Electrical stimulation
- Physical agents and mechanical modalities
  - Ultrasound
  - Cold whirlpool as needed for edema reduction and pain control
- Goals/outcomes
  - Ankle ROM:
    - Plantarflexion: 20°
    - Dorsiflexion: 5° with knee extended, 10° with knee flexed
  - Strength: 4/5 on manual muscle test
  - Pain: 5/10 or less
  - Normal gait pattern with assistive devices as needed

Functional Strengthening Phase: 3–9 Visits, 9–12 Weeks Post-Fracture

- Therapeutic exercise and home program
  - Manual resistive exercise
    - Dorsiflexor and evertor strengthening for stance stability
    - Plantarflexor and invertor strengthening for enhanced propulsion
  - Progression of resistive tubing exercises at home
  - BAPS progressed to larger range and may include weighted resistance
  - Stair machine, elliptical, bicycle ergometry, or treadmill for improved endurance and function

- Functional progression tailored to individual's household and vocational demands, for example:
    - Step up/step down
    - Heel raises
    - Lunges
    - Squats
  - Plyometrics as appropriate
- Manual therapy techniques
  - Joint mobilization: Increase vigor of joint mobilizations for:
    - Talocrural plantarflexion/dorsiflexion
    - Rearfoot and midfoot supination/pronation
    - Hallux dorsiflexion
    - Mobilization at syndesmosis and proximal tibiofibular joint may be indicated
- Electrotherapeutic modalities
  - Electrical stimulation for controlling or reducing edema
- Physical agents and mechanical modalities
  - Cryotherapy
  - Whirlpool
  - Ultrasound
- Goals/outcomes
  - Foot and ankle ROM:
    - Plantarflexion: 40°
    - Dorsiflexion: 10° in subtalar neutral with knee extended, 15° with knee flexed
    - Ratio of inversion to eversion: 2:1
    - Hallux dorsiflexion: 60°
  - Pain: 2/10 or less
  - Strength: 5/5 on manual muscle test or equivalent to uninvolved leg
  - Functional ROM of midtarsal joints, first ray, and fifth ray
  - Improved neuromuscular, balance, proprioceptive awareness for stability and reduction of risk for future injury

Functional Carryover

- Instruction is given regarding appropriate use of and tapering off of external support as appropriate
- Elevation, compression, and application of cold are reviewed for edema control in home activities
- Dorsiflexion range performed in sitting is encouraged
- Gait pattern progression is reviewed from protected to normal walking pace, to brisk walking, to running
- Running progression (sprints, start/stop, Figure 8, carioca, and function-specific footwork and functional combination of squatting, heel raises, etc.) is added to rehabilitation regime as appropriate

DISCHARGE PLANNING AND PATIENT RESPONSIBILITY

Criteria for Discharge

- Patient has achieved all goals/outcomes except may be discharged at:
  - ROM: 8° dorsiflexion in subtalar neutral with knee extended
  - Strength: 4+/5
- Functional status: Prior to attainment of previous level for ADLs and vocational activities, progression toward recreational and sports activities if progress is present

Circumstances Requiring Additional Visits

- History of additional lower-extremity pathology
- Multiple fracture sites
- Presence of other medical conditions
- Postoperative complications
- Delayed fracture healing/union
- Severe obesity

Home Program

- Flexibility exercises
  - Gastrocnemius/soleus stretching
  - Hands and knees "heel sit" for plantarflexion
  - Controlled ankle roll for supination stretching
- Contrast bath and/or use of cryotherapy, especially after exercise or increased activity, to reduce edema and control pain
- Strengthening exercises
  - Resistive tubing
  - Heel raises
  - Continued step-training exercises

- Running progression
  - Forward running
  - Forward sprinting
  - Start/stop
  - Figure 8
  - Cutting
  - Carioca
  - Multidirectional starts/stops
- Plyometrics

Monitoring

- Patient is to recheck/call at 2 weeks post-discharge to ensure expected return to function and continued healing.
- As necessary, schedule 4 week clinic follow-up to monitor objective parameters (edema, ROM, motor performance, functional capabilities) and adapt the program for targeted patients

REFERENCES

1. American Physical Therapy Association. *Guide To Physical Therapist Practice*. Alexandria, VA: APTA; 1997.

2. Becker HP, Rosenbaum D, Kriese T, Gengross H, Claes L. Gait asymmetry following successful surgical treatment of ankle fractures in young adults. *Clin Orthop Rel Res*. February 1995:262-269.

3. Donatelli RA. Normal biomechanics of the foot and ankle. *J Orthop Sports Phys Ther*. 1985;7(3):91-95.

4. Gray H; Williams PL, ed. *Gray's Anatomy*. 38th ed. New York, NY: Churchill Livingstone; 1995.

5. Gross MT. Lower extremity screening for skeletal malalignment: suggestions for orthotics and shoewear. *J Orthop Sports Phys Ther*. 1995;21(6):389-405.

6. Hart A, Hopkins C, Ford B. *ICD-9-CM Expert For Physicians, Volume 1&2*. 7th ed. USA: Ingenix; 2005.

7. Howell DW. Therapeutic exercise and mobilization. In: Hunt GC, ed. *Physical Therapy of the Foot and Ankle*. New York, NY: Churchill Livingston; 1988:257.

8. Kaltenborn F. *Mobilization of The Extremity Joints*. 3rd ed. Oslo, Norway: Olaf Norlis Bokhandel; 1985:114-137.

9. Kegerreis S. The construction and implementation of functional progressions as a component of athletic rehabilitation. *J Orthop Sports Phys Ther*. 1983;5(1):14-19.

10. Kessler RM. The ankle and hindfoot. In: Kessler RM, Hertling D, eds. *Management of Common Musculoskeletal Disorders: Physical Therapy Principles and Methods*. Philadelphia, PA: Harper & Row; 1983:448.

11. Lentell G, Bass B, Lopez D, et al. The contribution of proprioceptive deficits, muscle function and anatomic laxity to functional instability of the ankle. *J Orthop Sports Phys Ther*. 1995;21(4):206-215.

12. Maitland GD. *Subjective Examination In Vertebral Manipulation*. 5th ed. Oxford, England: Butterworth-Heinemann; 1986:43-92.

13. Maitland GD. *Peripheral Manipulation*. 3rd ed. Oxford, England: Butterworth-Heinemann; 1992:265.

14. Mascaro TB, Swanson LE. Rehabilitation of the foot and ankle. *Orthop Clin North Am*. 1994;25:147-160.

15. Rockar PA. The subtalar joint: anatomy and joint motion. *J Orthop Sports Phys Ther*. 1995;21(6):361-372.

16. Rodgers MM. Dynamic foot biomechanics. *J Orthop Sports Phys Ther*. 1995;21(6):306-316.

17. Seto JL, Brewster CE. Treatment approaches following foot and ankle injuries. *Clin Sports Med*. 1994;13:695-718.

18. Tatro-Adams D, McGann SF, Carbone W. Reliability of the figure-of-eight method of ankle measurement. *J Orthop Sports Phys Ther*. 1995;22(4):161-163.

ANKLE SPRAIN/INSTABILITY
SUMMARY OVERVIEW

ICD-9
> 837   845

APTA Preferred Practice Pattern: **4D, 4E, 4F, 4I, 4J**

EXAMINATION

- History and Systems Review
- Tests and Measures
  Systems review per APTA's *Guide to Physical Therapy Practice*
  - Anthropometric characteristics
  - Gait, locomotion, and balance
  - Joint integrity and mobility
  - Muscle performance
  - Pain
  - Posture
- Establish Plan of Care

GOALS/OUTCOMES

- Pain: 2/10 or less
- Foot and ankle ROM
- Weight bearing to allow return to previous functional status for ADLs and vocational, sport, and recreational activities as identified by patient
- Normal gait pattern without assistive devices on all surfaces
- Strength: 5/5 on manual muscle test or equivalent to uninvolved leg on functional tests
- Edema reduction to allow patient to wear normal footwear
- Neuromuscular/balance/proprioceptive reeducation for improved stability and reduction of risk for future injury
- Independence in a progressive home exercise program emphasizing function

INTERVENTION
NUMBER OF VISITS: 5–10

- Patient Instruction
  - Basic Anatomy and Biomechanics
  - Handouts
  - Functional Considerations

- Direct Interventions
  - Acute Phase: 1–3 Visits
  - Subacute Phase: 4–7 Visits
- Functional Carryover

DISCHARGE PLANNING AND PATIENT RESPONSIBILITY

- Criteria for Discharge
  - Patient has achieved all rehabilitation goals with possible exceptions listed in guidelines
- Circumstances Requiring Additional Visits
  - Positive ankle drawer
  - Positive talar tilt
  - Positive Telos stress test
  - Positive peroneal subluxation
  - History of additional lower-extremity pathology
  - Previous history of chondral defect
  - Tests positive for peroneal tendon injury or positive dural tension signs
  - Atypical load sensitivity, signifying possible chondral lesion of talus or tibia
  - Presence of other medical conditions
  - Chronicity or severity of condition
  - Severe obesity
- Home Program
  - Flexibility exercises
  - Gastrocnemius/soleus stretching
  - Hands and knees "heel sit" for plantarflexion
  - Controlled ankle roll for supination stretching
  - Contrast bath and/or use of cryotherapy, especially after exercise or increased activity, to reduce edema and control pain
  - Strengthening exercises
  - Resistive tubing
  - Heel raises
  - Running progression
  - Plyometrics
- Monitoring

SUMMARY OVERVIEW | FOOT AND ANKLE | ANKLE SPRAIN/INSTABILITY   27

ANKLE SPRAIN/INSTABILITY

ICD-9

837	Dislocation of ankle
845	Sprains and strains of ankle and foot

APTA Preferred Practice Pattern: 4D, 4E, 4F, 4I, 4J

EXAMINATION

History and Systems Review

- History of current condition
  - Edema, discomfort, and discoloration after injury
  - Sense of instability
- Past history of current condition
  - History of sprains/instability
  - History of other lower-extremity problems
- Other tests and measures
  - X-rays
  - Telos stress tests
  - Imaging
- Functional status and activity level (current/prior)
- Patient's functional goals

Tests and Measures

Systems review per APTA's *Guide to Physical Therapy Practice*

- Anthropometric characteristics
  - Comparative girth measurements
    - Figure 8: Circumferential measurement using bony landmarks just inferior to the medial and lateral malleolus, tubercle of the navicular, and peroneal sulcus and cuboid bone (just proximal to the tuberosity of the fifth metatarsal)
    - Malleolar level: Circumferential measurement just inferior to the medial and lateral malleolus
- Gait, locomotion, and balance
  - Including functional tests as appropriate
  - Weight-bearing tolerance
  - Quality of gait pattern
  - Assistive devices
  - Neuromuscular/balance/proprioceptive tests
    - Mirror posturing
    - Stork stand

- BAPS
- Balance/reach test
  a. Unilateral stance balancing, reaching with opposite leg
  b. Unilateral stance balancing, reaching with arms
- Joint integrity and mobility
  - Palpation of ligamentous structures
    - Anterior talofibular
    - Calcaneofibular
    - Posterior talofibular
    - Anterior tibiofibular
    - Deltoid
  - Stress tests
  Comparison with uninvolved leg is necessary for accurate assessment. These tests are appropriate only when acuteness of injury allows. Specific tissue tension tests for the posterior talofibular, calcaneofibular and posterior tibiofibular ligaments may also be performed as appropriate.
    - Ankle drawer
    While stabilizing the distal tibia and fibula just proximal to the talocrural joint with one hand, grasp the calcaneus posteriorly with the other hand. The testing hand pulls the calcaneus directly anteriorly. The thumb of the stabilizing hand at the distal tib-fib joint can palpate the talar dome's translation anterior. This tests the integrity of the anterior talofibular and anterior tibiofibular ligaments.
    - Talar tilt
    The stabilizing hand is on the medial and posterior aspect of the tibia with the thenar eminence over the medial malleolus. The testing hand moves the calcaneus and cuboid into a supinated position (plantarflexion, inversion and adduction). This tests the integrity of the lateral ligamentous structures in the ankle, primarily the anterior talofibular and calcaneofibular ligaments.

- Muscle performance
  - Inversion/eversion (being sensitive to possible presence of peroneal tendon subluxation with eversion movement)
  - Plantarflexion/dorsiflexion
- Pain
  - Measured on visual analog scale
- Posture
  - Standing alignment noting:
    - Typical posturing of support and center of gravity over base
    - Presence of malalignment in sagittal, frontal or transverse planes
    - Particularly note tibial and foot posture (ie, genu recurvatum, cavus or supinated foot type at risk for mechanical instability)

Establish Plan of Care
- Based on history, tests, and measures

GOALS/OUTCOMES
- Pain: 2/10 or less
- Foot and ankle ROM:
  - Plantarflexion: 40°
  - Dorsiflexion: 10° in subtalar neutral with knee extended, 15° with knee flexed
  - Ratio of inversion to eversion: 2:1
- Weight bearing to allow return to previous functional status for ADLs and vocational, sport, and recreational activities as identified by patient
- Normal gait pattern without assistive devices on all surfaces
- Strength: 5/5 on manual muscle test or equivalent to uninvolved leg on functional tests
- Edema reduction to allow patient to wear normal footwear
- Neuromuscular/balance/proprioceptive reeducation for improved stability and reduction of risk for future injury
- Independence in a progressive home exercise program emphasizing function

INTERVENTION
NUMBER OF VISITS: 5–10

Coordination, Communication, and Documentation
- Provision of services between admission and discharge that facilitate cost-effective and efficient integration or reintegration to home, community, or work
- Documentation of therapeutic intervention is required for each episode of care and serves as the basic foundation for communication
- Coordination and additional communication will depend on the patient's impairment and home/work/community/leisure situation and requirements. Such services may include:
  - Case management
  - Coordination of care and collaboration with those integral to the patient's rehabilitation program
  - Coordination and monitoring of the delivery of available resources
  - Referrals to other health-care professionals
  - Identification of resources, support groups or advocacy services
  - Provision of educational or training information
  - Technical assistance
- Specific coordination and communication provisions:
  - Possible referral re: further diagnostics if patient demonstrates poor load tolerance and marked amount of pain

Patient Instruction

Basic Anatomy and Biomechanics
- Hinge motion at the mortise vs. supination/pronation motion contributed by subtalar and midtarsal joints
- History of current condition and importance of protection and rehabilitation of the stabilizing structures
- Distinction between passive supporting structures (ligamentous and bony) vs. dynamic structures (muscle)
- Pertinent Gray's Anatomy (Gray. 1995. 720–722)

Handouts
- Home contrast baths
- Cryotherapy, compression, elevation
- Home exercise program
  - Straight and bent-knee calf flexibility exercises

FOOT AND ANKLE | ANKLE SPRAIN/INSTABILITY

- o Ankle resistive band/resistive tubing exercises
- o Gait retraining to reduce limp and improve stance stability (stepping exercise)
- o Functional progression exercise sheet

Functional Considerations

- Amount of walking and use of assistive devices as appropriate to the patient's weight-bearing tolerance and acuteness of injury
- Ankle support, or appropriate protective device, is provided for protection/compression
- Functional progression regarding stairs, varied terrain, and vigor of loading (walking vs. running vs. jumping) is covered with patient appropriate to SIN (severity, irritability, nature)

Direct Interventions

Acute Phase: 1–3 Visits

- Use the PRICE program:
  - o **P**rotection: Aircast®, Stromgren
  - o **R**est : As needed, especially in diagnosed Grade III sprain per physician
  - o **I**ce: Acute, every 2 hours for 20–30 minutes per session; Subacute, 1–2 times a day
  - o **C**ompression: Aircast®, Stromgren elastic bandage
  - o **E**levation: During treatment in clinic and at home when at rest
- Therapeutic exercise and home program
  - o Ambulation as appropriate with weight bearing as tolerated unless pain or gait quality necessitates toe touch weight bearing or non-weight bearing
  - o AROM during hydrotherapy
  - o Encourage maximum pain-free foot and ankle ROM every two hours
- Manual therapy techniques
  - o Soft-tissue techniques
    - Venous drainage massage
    - Friction massage to affected ligament
  - o Grade I–II joint mobilization
- Electrotherapeutic modalities
  - o Electrical stimulation (for edema reduction and pain control)
- Physical agents and mechanical modalities
  - o Cryotherapy
  - o Pulsed ultrasound

- Goals/outcomes
  - o Pain: 5/10 or less
  - o Decrease edema to allow patient to wear normal footwear
  - o Prevent decrease in ROM
  - o Achieve normal gait pattern with ambulatory aids as needed
  - o Strength: 4/5 on manual muscle test

Subacute Phase: 4–7 Visits

- Therapeutic exercise and home program
  - o Manual resistive exercise
    - Dorsiflexors and evertors for stance stability
    - Plantarflexors for propulsion
  - o Progression to resistive tubing exercises at home
  - o Ankle and foot flexibility
    - Focus on gastrocnemius and soleus muscle lengthening
  - o Gait training to maximize stance stability and tibial translation in gait
  - o Stationary cycling for improved metabolism and increased endurance
  - o Neuromuscular/balance/proprioceptive reeducation
    - BAPS
    - Single-leg stance
    - Balance/reach activities
  - o Stair machine/treadmill with functional progression of speed and variety of approaches (forward, backward, and sideways) as appropriate for return to household or athletic function
  - o Step training, initially for improved stair-climbing capabilities and progressing into loaded forward, backward, and diagonal step ups. This can progress into plyometrics and hopping/jumping training (refer to *Ankle Sprain/Instability Return to Sport* guideline)
  - o Other exercise equipment for functional-specific training may include: slide board, Profitter, ski machine, Total Gym®
- Manual therapy techniques
  - o Joint mobilization
    - Maximize talocrural dorsiflexion
    - Improve subtalar and midtarsal joint supination for return to function
    - Improve pronation to enhance mechanical advantage of peroneal muscle groups for ankle stability
  - o Soft-tissue techniques

30   ANKLE SPRAIN/INSTABILITY | FOOT AND ANKLE

- Friction massage to affected ligaments
- Venous drainage massage
- Electrotherapeutic modalities
  - Electrical stimulation
- Physical agents and mechanical modalities
  - Ultrasound over affected ligament structures
  - Cryotherapy
- Goals/outcomes
  - Ankle ROM:
    - Plantarflexion: 40°
    - Dorsiflexion: 10° in subtalar neutral with knee extended, 15° with knee flexed
  - Strength: 5/5 on manual muscle test or equivalent to uninvolved leg on functional tests
  - Pain: 2/10 or less

Functional Carryover

- Instruction regarding appropriate use of and tapering off of external support as appropriate
- Ambulation progression
- Protected to normal walking pace
- Brisk walking
- Running
- Running progression into sprints, start/stop, Figure 8, carioca, and function-specific footwork, functional combination of squatting, heel raises, etc., added to rehabilitation regime
- Progression into simulated function (such as squat lift, rebounding drills/jumping, golf swing, etc.)

DISCHARGE PLANNING AND PATIENT RESPONSIBILITY

Criteria for Discharge

- Patient has achieved all rehabilitation goals except may be discharged at:
  - Strength: 4+/5 on manual muscle test
  - ROM: 8° dorsiflexion in subtalar neutral with knee extended
  - Functional status: Previous level for ADLs and vocational activities, progression toward recreational and sports activities

Circumstances Requiring Additional Visits

- Positive ankle drawer
- Positive talar tilt
- Positive Telos stress test
- Positive peroneal subluxation
- History of additional lower-extremity pathology
- Previous history of chondral defect
- Tests positive for peroneal tendon injury or positive dural tension signs
- Atypical load sensitivity, signifying possible chondral lesion of talus or tibia
- Presence of other medical conditions
- Chronicity or severity of condition
- Severe obesity

Home Program

- Flexibility exercises
- Gastrocnemius/soleus stretching
- Hands and knees "heel sit" for plantarflexion
- Controlled ankle roll for supination stretching
- Contrast bath and/or use of cryotherapy, especially after exercise or increased activity, to reduce edema and control pain
- Strengthening exercises
- Resistive tubing
- Heel raises
  - Continued step training exercises
- Running progression
  - Forward running
  - Forward sprinting
  - Start/stop
  - Figure 8
  - Cutting
  - Carioca
  - Multidirectional start/stops
- Plyometrics

Monitoring

- Patient is to recheck/call at 2 weeks post-discharge to ensure expected return to function, continued healing, and progression toward attaining all rehabilitation goals

REFERENCES

1. American Physical Therapy Association. *Guide To Physical Therapist Practice*. Alexandria, VA: APTA; 1997.

2. Boruta PM, Bishop JO, Braly WG, Tullos HS. Acute lateral ankle ligament injuries: a literature review. *Foot Ankle*. 1990;11:107-113.

3. Burroughs P, Dahners LE. The effect of enforced exercise on the healing of ligament injuries. *Am J Sports Med*. 1990;18:376-378.

4. Cyriax J. *Textbook of Orthopaedic Medicine*. 8th ed. Tindall, England: Bailliere; 1982.

5. Diamond JE. Rehabilitation of ankle sprains. *Clin Sports Med*. 1989;8:877-890.

6. Freeman MAR. Treatment of ruptures of the lateral ligament of the ankle. *J Bone Joint Surg*. 1965;47B:661-668.

7. Frost HM, Hanson CA. Technique for testing the drawer sign in the ankle. *Clin Orthop Rel Res*. 1977;123:49-51.

8. Gray H; Williams PL, ed. *Gray's Anatomy*. 38th ed. New York, NY: Churchill Livingstone; 1995.

9. Hart A, Hopkins C, Ford B. *ICD-9-CM Expert For Physicians, Volume 1&2*. 7th ed. USA: Ingenix; 2005.

10. Karlsson J, Ericksson BI, Renstrom P. Subtalar instability of the foot: a review and results after surgical treatment. *Scand J Med Sci Sports*. 1998;8(4):191-197.

11. Kegerris S. The construction and implementation of functional progression as a component of athletic rehabilitation. *J Orthop Sports Phys Ther*. 1983;5(1):14-19.

12. Kessler RM, Hertling D. *Management of Common Musculoskeletal Disorders: Physical Therapy Principles and Methods*. Philadelphia, PA: Harper & Row; 1983.

13. Lynch SA, Renstrom PA. Treatment of acute lateral ankle ligament rupture in the athlete: conservative versus surgical treatment. *Sports Med*. 1999;27(1):61-71.

14. Malone TR, Hardaker MT. Rehabilitation of foot and ankle injuries in ballet dancers. *J Orthop Sports Phys Ther*. 1990;11(8):355-361.

15. Nitz AJ, Dobner JJ, Kersey D. Nerve injury and grades II and III ankle sprains. *Am J Sports Med*. 1985;13:177-182.

16. Roy S, Irvin R. *Sports Medicine*. Englewood Cliffs, NJ: Prentice-Hall; 1983:391.

17. Smith RW, Reischl SF. Treatment of ankle sprains in young athletes. *Am J Sports Med*. 1986;14:465-471.

18. Wilkerson GB, Horn-Kingery HM. Treatment of the inversion ankle sprain: comparison of different modes of compression and cryotherapy. *J Orthop Sports Phys Ther*. 1993;17(5):240-246.

BIOMECHANICAL LOWER EXTREMITY DYSFUNCTION
SUMMARY OVERVIEW

ICD-9

355.5	355.6	715.95	715.96	715.97	719.47	719.57	719.66	719.7	720.2
726.5	726.64	726.7	728.71	733.10	733.14	733.15	733.16	733.19	735.0
735.2	754.69	754.71							

APTA Preferred Practice Pattern: 4A, 4B, 4C, 4D, 4E, 4F, 4G, 4H, 4I, 4J, 4K, 5D, 6B

EXAMINATION

- History and Systems Review
- Tests and Measures
  Systems review per APTA's *Guide to Physical Therapy Practice*
  - Gait, locomotion, and balance
  - Motor function
  - Orthotics, protective and supportive devices
  - Pain
  - Posture
  - ROM
  - Special tests
- Establish Plan of Care

GOALS/OUTCOMES

- Pain: 0/10
- Normal gait pattern with orthotics as indicated
- Proper lower quarter biomechanical alignment
- Flexibility and joint ROM for daily activity
- Strength: Manual muscle test grade of 5/5 or equivalent to uninvolved leg on functional closed-kinetic chain test
- Return to previous functional status for ADLs and vocational, recreational, and sports activities as identified by patient
- Independence in a progressive home exercise program emphasizing function

INTERVENTION
NUMBER OF VISITS: 5–11

- Patient Instruction
  - Basic Anatomy and Biomechanics
  - Handouts
  - Functional Considerations
  - Description of Surgical Procedure
- Direct Interventions
  - Acute Phase: 1–4 Visits
  - Subacute Phase: 4–7 Visits
- Functional Carryover

DISCHARGE PLANNING AND PATIENT RESPONSIBILITIES

- Criteria for Discharge
  - Patient is able to wear biomechanical orthotics for all activities without discomfort
  - Patient has achieved rehabilitation goals with the exception of return to previous functional status for recreational and sports activities
- Circumstances Requiring Additional Visits
  - Severe inflammatory process
  - Severely restricted lower-extremity ROM
  - Presence of other medical conditions, especially diabetes
  - Delayed healing
  - Chronicity or severity of condition
  - Ongoing aggravating risk factors (such as repetitive motion)
- Home Program
  - Continue flexibility and strengthening home exercise program as instructed
  - Modify activity level as needed and modify shoe wear as recommended
  - Continue orthotics utilization according to therapist recommendations
- Monitoring

SUMMARY OVERVIEW | FOOT AND ANKLE | BIOMECHANICAL LE DYSFUNCTION   33

BIOMECHANICAL LOWER EXTREMITY DYSFUNCTION

ICD-9

355.5	Tarsal tunnel syndrome
355.6	Lesion of plantar nerve
715.95	Osteoarthrosis, unspecified whether generalized or localized, pelvic region and thigh
715.96	Osteoarthrosis, unspecified whether generalized or localized, lower leg
715.97	Osteoarthrosis, unspecified whether generalized or localized, ankle and foot
719.47	Pain in joint, ankle and foot
719.57	Stiffness of joint, not elsewhere classified, ankle and foot
719.66	Other symptoms referable to joint, lower leg
719.7	Difficulty in walking
720.2	Sacroiliitis, not elsewhere classified
726.5	Enthesopathy of hip region
726.64	Patellar tendinitis
726.7	Enthesopathy of ankle and tarsus
728.71	Plantar fascial fibromatosis
733.10	Pathologic fracture, unspecified site
733.14	Pathologic fracture of neck of femur
733.15	Pathologic fracture of other specified part of femur
733.16	Pathologic fracture of tibia or fibula
733.19	Pathologic fracture of other specified site
735.0	Hallux valgus (acquired)
735.2	Hallux rigidus
754.69	Other valgus deformities of feet
754.71	Talipes cavus

APTA Preferred Practice Pattern: 4A, 4B, 4C, 4D, 4E, 4F, 4G, 4H, 4I, 4J, 4K, 5D, 6B

EXAMINATION

History and Systems Review

- History of current condition
  - Footwear/orthotics
  - Aggravating factors
- Past history of current condition
  - History of previous injury that may be biomechanically related to the current diagnosis
  - Previous orthotics
- Functional status and activity level (current/prior)
- Patient's functional goals

Tests and Measures

Systems review per APTA's *Guide to Physical Therapy Practice*

- Gait, locomotion, and balance
  - Biomechanical assessment
    - Assess quality, quantity, and symmetry of motion in sagittal, transverse, and frontal planes at the hips, knees, subtalar joint, and midtarsal joint as well as the lumbar and thoracic spine
    - Assess for patterns of limping or compensation
    - Use appropriate assistive devices as needed
- Motor function
  - Lunge distance
  - Single-leg squat excursion
  - Hopping
- Orthotics, protective and supportive devices
  - Footwear analysis
    - Wear patterns indicating heel whip or excessive pronation
    - Shoe style and structure in relation to biomechanical needs
- Pain
  - Measured on visual analog scale

34   BIOMECHANICAL LE DYSFUNCTION | FOOT AND ANKLE

- Posture
  - Static stance position
    - Calcaneal varus/valgus
    - Genu varus/valgus/recurvatum
    - ASIS and PSIS height and alignment
  - General lower-extremity alignment
    - Femoral anteversion/retroversion
    - Genu varus/valgus
    - Patellar alignment
    - Tibial torsion
    - Leg length in supine, long sitting, and standing positions
  - Specific foot alignment (nonweight-bearing)
    - Subtalar neutral position
    - Forefoot to rearfoot alignment
    - First-ray alignment
- ROM
  - General lower-extremity muscle flexibility
    - Hamstrings: Isolation of medial component
    - Gluteals
    - Hip flexors
    - Quadriceps
    - Hip abductors
    - Gastrocnemius/soleus
  - Specific foot/ankle ROM
    - Talocrural dorsiflexion/plantarflexion
    - Subtalar joint inversion/eversion
    - Midtarsal joint inversion/eversion
    - First ray dorsiflexion/plantarflexion
    - Hallux dorsiflexion
- Special tests
  - Rule out other joints as primary cause of symptoms
    - Lumbar spine
    - Sacroiliac joint
    - Hip
    - Knee

Establish Plan of Care
- Based on history, tests, and measures

GOALS/OUTCOMES
- Pain: 0/10
- Normal gait pattern with orthotics as indicated
- Proper lower quarter biomechanical alignment
- Flexibility and joint ROM for daily activity
  - Thomas test showing full hip extension and knee flexion to at least 70°

- Straight-leg raise to at least 80°
- Ober test showing adduction to the level of the plinth
- Ankle dorsiflexion to 10° in subtalar neutral with knee extended, 15° with knee flexed
- Hallux dorsiflexion of at least 60°
- Ratio of inversion to eversion: 2:1
- Strength: Manual muscle test grade of 5/5 or equivalent to uninvolved leg on functional closed-kinetic chain test
- Return to previous functional status for ADLs and vocational, recreational, and sports activities as identified by patient
- Independence in a progressive home exercise program emphasizing function

INTERVENTION
NUMBER OF VISITS: 5–11

Coordination, Communication, and Documentation
- Provision of services between admission and discharge that facilitate cost-effective and efficient integration or reintegration to home, community, or work
- Documentation of therapeutic intervention is required for each episode of care and serves as the basic foundation for communication
- Coordination and additional communication will depend on the patient's impairment and home/work/community/leisure situation and requirements. Such services may include:
  - Case management
  - Coordination of care and collaboration with those integral to the patient's rehabilitation program
  - Coordination and monitoring of the delivery of available resources
  - Referrals to other health-care professionals
  - Identification of resources, support groups, or advocacy services
  - Provision of educational or training information
  - Technical assistance
- Specific coordination and communication provisions:
  - Referral for biomechanical orthotics
  - Referral for biomechanically sound footwear

FOOT AND ANKLE | BIOMECHANICAL LE DYSFUNCTION

Patient Instruction

Basic Anatomy and Biomechanics
- Clinician references for anatomy and biomechanics (Hunt GC. 1988; Root, et al. 1977)
- Pertinent Gray's Anatomy (Gray. 1995. 700–702, 728, 884)
- Role of abnormal biomechanics in the cause/exacerbation of injuries, including excessive or prolonged pronation, shoe choices, and training protocols

Handouts
- *Answers to Commonly Asked Questions About Orthotics*
  A good reference for discussing foot orthotics with a patient (see page 63)
- *Your New Orthotics*
  The basics of care, cleaning, and break-in (see page 67)
- *Choosing The Right Shoe*
  The basics of shoe construction and shape and their relation to assisting the orthotics in controlling excessive foot motion (see page 65)
- Home exercise program
  - Specific lower-extremity flexibility exercises as determined by initial evaluation
  - Gait retraining to reduce limp if present

Functional Considerations
Many painful foot conditions can be successfully managed by a comprehensive, conservative approach that includes:
- Proper biomechanical orthotics support
- Instruction in proper activity protocols
- Exercise to strengthen weak structures and increase flexibility in tight structures

Description of Surgical Procedure
- Review of operative procedures and relation to joint biomechanics, rehabilitation, and function

Direct Interventions

Acute Phase: 1–4 Visits
- Therapeutic exercise and home program
  - Stretching exercises:
    Areas to be addressed will be determined by the initial evaluation
  - Strengthening exercises performed in a closed-kinetic chain position, focused on muscles that are primary decelerators of pronation
    - Soleus
    - Gastrocnemius
    - Quadriceps
    - Posterior tibialis
    - Gluteals
  - Gait training to decrease antalgic patterns and improve neuromuscular/balance/proprioceptive reeducation
    - Balance beam walking: Forward and backward
    - Crouch walk
    - Carioca
    - Backward walking: Incline and flat surfaces
- Manual therapy techniques
  - Soft-tissue techniques
    - Friction massage
    - Soft-tissue mobilization and stretching as indicated by positive findings in biomechanical examination
  - Specific joint mobilization techniques as indicated in biomechanical examination
- Therapeutic devices and equipment
  - Temporary orthotics
    - May be constructed to provide short-term alleviation of symptoms and to further assess the efficacy of orthotics intervention
  - Permanent orthotics
    - Non-weight-bearing, neutral position plaster casts should be made if it is determined that biomechanical orthotics are appropriate. See *Physical therapy of the foot and ankle* (Hunt. 1988:15) Chapter 11, for further information on casting techniques.
    - Determine appropriate posting for adequate biomechanical support on the basis of these casts and the biomechanical evaluation
    - Casts will be sent to an appropriate orthotics lab where they will be fabricated according to therapist directions
- Electrotherapeutic modalities
  - Electrical stimulation
  - Iontophoresis
- Physical agents and mechanical modalities
  - Cryotherapy
  - Ultrasound

- Goals/outcomes
  - Flexibility and joint ROM
    - Thomas test showing 10° hip flexion and knee flexion to at least 50°
    - Straight-leg raise to at least 60°
    - Ober test showing adduction to within 3" of the level of the plinth
    - Ankle dorsiflexion to 5° in subtalar neutral with knee extended, 10° with knee flexed
    - Hallux dorsiflexion of at least 50°
  - Strength: Manual muscle test grade of 4/5
  - Pain: 2/10 or less
  - Restore proper lower quarter biomechanical alignment

Subacute Phase: 4–7 Visits

- Therapeutic exercise and home program
  - Self-massage and mobilization techniques for use at home
  - Progression of closed-kinetic chain and flexibility exercises
    - Squats
    - Lunges
      a. Anterior
      b. Lateral
      c. Posterior
      d. Rotational
    - Step up/step down
    - Single-leg balance and reach drills
      a. Anterior reach, both arms at waist height
      b. Anterior reach, opposite leg
      c. Posterior reach, opposite leg
      d. Lateral reach, opposite leg
      e. Rotational reach, opposite leg
  - Progression to full activity with use of orthotics
  - Instructions to avoid training errors
- Manual therapy techniques
  - Soft-tissue techniques
    - Soft-tissue mobilization
    - Friction massage
  - Progression of joint mobilization as indicated
- Therapeutic devices and equipment
  - Adjust temporary orthotics to minimize symptoms
  - Permanent orthotics
    - Orthotics are visually evaluated when they arrive from the lab, and the posting is compared to the prescription in the patient's record

- Orthotics are modified to fit the shoe, and recommendations on changes in footwear are made as needed
- Patient is instructed on "breaking-in" the orthotics to avoid discomfort or blistering
- Patient is instructed on proper care and cleaning of the orthotics and is notified of any manufacturer's warranties
- Physical agents and mechanical modalities
  - Thermal modalities prior to and cryotherapy following exercise as appropriate
- Goals/outcomes
  - Pain: 0/10
  - Normal gait pattern with orthotics as indicated
  - Restore proper lower quarter biomechanical alignment
  - Flexibility and joint ROM for daily activity:
    - Thomas test showing full hip extension and knee flexion to at least 70°
    - Straight-leg raise to at least 80°
    - Ober test showing adduction to the level of the plinth
    - Ankle dorsiflexion to 10° in subtalar neutral with knee extended, 15° with knee flexed
    - Hallux dorsiflexion of at least 60°
    - Ratio of inversion to eversion: 2:1
  - Strength: Manual muscle test grade of 5/5 or equivalent to uninvolved leg on functional closed-kinetic chain test
  - Pain-free functional status for ADLs and vocational activities

Functional Carryover

- Long-term impact of continued biomechanical stress, for example: The influence of frequent wearing of high-heeled dress shoes or unsupportive footwear in contributing to poor bony alignment of the foot and leg in spite of the presence of well-made orthotics
- Counseling regarding cross-training options for physical activities that do not place undue stress on the tissues of the lower quarter

DISCHARGE PLANNING AND PATIENT RESPONSIBILITIES

Criteria for Discharge

- Patient is able to wear biomechanical orthotics for all activities without discomfort
- Patient has achieved rehabilitation goals with the exception of return to previous functional status for recreational and sports activities

Circumstances Requiring Additional Visits

- Severe inflammatory process
- Severely restricted lower-extremity ROM
- Presence of other medical conditions, especially diabetes
- Delayed healing
- Chronicity or severity of condition
- Ongoing aggravating risk factors (such as repetitive motion)

Home Program

- Continue flexibility and strengthening home exercise program as instructed
- Modify activity level as needed and modify shoe wear as recommended
- Continue orthotics utilization according to therapist recommendations

Monitoring

- Modify orthotics as needed
- Patient is to call at 2 weeks post-discharge to ensure expected return to previous level of activity and to report status of orthotics wear

REFERENCES

1. American Physical Therapy Association. *Guide To Physical Therapist Practice.* Alexandria, VA: APTA; 1997.
2. Coughlin M, Mann R. *Surgery of The Foot and Ankle.* St. Louis, MO: CV Mosby; 1993.
3. Gould JA III. *Orthopedic and Sports Physical Therapy.* 2nd ed. St Louis, MO: CV Mosby; 1990.
4. Gray G. *Lower Extremity Functional Profile.* Adrian, MI: Wynn Marketing; 1995.
5. Gray H; Williams PL, ed. *Gray's Anatomy.* 38th ed. New York, NY: Churchill Livingstone; 1995.
6. Gross MT. Lower quarter screening for skeletal malalignment: suggestions for orthotics and shoewear. *J Orthop Sports Phys Ther.* 1995;21(6):389-405.
7. Hart A, Hopkins C, Ford B. *ICD-9-CM Expert For Physicians, Volume 1&2.* 7th ed. USA: Ingenix; 2005.
8. Hunt GC, McPoll, TG, eds. *Physical Therapy of The Foot And Ankle.* New York, NY: Churchill Livingstone; 1988:15.
9. McPoil TG, Schuitt D. Management of matatarsalgia secondary to biomechanical disorders: a case report. *Phys Ther.* 1986;66:970.
10. McPoil TG, Hunt GC. Evaluation and management of foot and ankle disorders: present problems and future directions. *J Orthop Sports Phys Ther.* 1995;21(6):381-388.
11. Rockar PA. The subtalar joint: anatomy and joint motion. *J Orthop Sports Phys Ther.* 1995;29(6):361-372.
12. Root ML, Orien WP, Weed JH, Hughes RJ. *Biomechanical Examination of The Foot.* Los Angeles, CA: Clinical Biomechanics Corporation; 1971.
13. Root ML, Orien WP, Weed JH. *Normal and Abnormal Function of The Foot.* Los Angeles, CA: Clinical Biomechanics Corp; 1977.
14. Tomaro JE, Butterfield SL. Biomechanical treatment of traumatic foot and ankle injuries with the use of foot orthotics. *J Orthop Sports Phys Ther.* 1995;21(6):373-380.

BUNION
SUMMARY OVERVIEW

ICD-9

727.1

APTA Preferred Practice Pattern: 4I

EXAMINATION
- History and Systems Review
- Tests and Measures
  Systems review per APTA's *Guide to Physical Therapy Practice*
  - Gait, locomotion, and balance
  - Integument integrity
  - Joint integrity and mobility
  - Muscle performance
  - Orthotics, protective and supportive devices
  - Pain
  - Posture
  - ROM
- Establish Plan of Care

GOALS/OUTCOMES
- ROM
- Muscle performance/strength
- Gait assessment and proprioceptive testing
- Pain: 2/10 or less
- Return to previous functional status for ADLs and recreational, vocational, and sports activities as identified by the patient
- Proper footwear and/or orthotics
- Independence in a home exercise program emphasizing function and strength of surrounding joints and muscles

INTERVENTION
NUMBER OF VISITS: 6–11

- Patient Instruction
  - Basic Anatomy and Biomechanics
  - Handouts
  - Functional Considerations
- Direct Interventions
  - Acute Phase: 3–5 Visits
  - Subacute Phase: 3–6 Visits
- Functional Carryover

DISCHARGE PLANNING AND PATIENT RESPONSIBILITY
- Criteria for Discharge
  - Normal ankle ROM, first metatarsal phalangeal joints 30° extension for gait
  - Gait assessment: Unassisted, pain-free normal gait pattern on all surface
  - Pain: 2/10 or less
  - Return to previous functional status for ADLs
  - Demonstrates knowledge of proper footwear, padding, and/or orthotics
  - Home exercise program independence
- Circumstances Requiring Additional Visits
  - Severe degenerative changes
- Home Program
  - Protection of joint and soft tissues with proper footwear and/or orthotics, application of padding
  - Flexibility exercises
  - Strengthening and proprioceptive training of surrounding musculature
- Monitoring

SUMMARY OVERVIEW | FOOT AND ANKLE | BUNION   39

BUNION

ICD-9
   727.1   Bunion
APTA Preferred Practice Pattern: 4I

EXAMINATION

History and Systems Review
- History of current condition
- Past history of current condition
- Other tests and measures
- Medications
- Past medical/surgical history
- Functional status and activity level (current/prior)
- Patient's functional goals

Tests and Measures
Systems review per APTA's *Guide to Physical Therapy Practice*
- Gait, locomotion, and balance
  - Observation of gait mechanics with or without use of assistive device
  - Willingness to weight bear
  - Proprioceptive testing and weight shifting
- Integument integrity
  - Bony malformation, degree of
  - Skin characteristics including temperature and color
  - Tolerance to palpation
- Joint integrity and mobility
  - First ray and metatarsal phalangeal joints posture and mobility, including stress tests
  - Ankle/foot mobility including talocrural and mid tarsals
- Muscle performance
  - Ankle plantarflexors, dorsiflexors, invertors, evertors
  - Toe flexors and extensors
- Orthotics, protective and supportive devices
- Pain
  - Measured on visual analog scale
- Posture
  - Observation in stance, alignment, position, symmetry between joints static and dynamic
- ROM (including muscle length)
  - Active and passive joint movement
  - Functional ROM including squats and heel raises

Establish Plan of Care
- Based on history, tests, and measures

GOALS/OUTCOMES
- ROM
  - Great toe metatarsal phalangeal joints extension: 30–60°
- Muscle performance/strength
  - 5/5 all major muscle groups
- Gait assessment and proprioceptive testing
  - Unassisted, pain-free gait pattern on all surfaces
- Pain: 2/10 or less
- Return to previous functional status for ADLs and recreational, vocational, and sports activities as identified by the patient
- Proper footwear and/or orthotics
- Independence in a home exercise program emphasizing function and strength of surrounding joints and muscles

INTERVENTION
NUMBER OF VISITS: 6–11

Coordination, Communication, and Documentation
- Provision of services between admission and discharge that facilitate cost-effective and efficient integration or reintegration to home, community, or work
- Documentation of therapeutic intervention is required for each episode of care and serves as the basic foundation for communication
- Coordination and additional communication will depend on the patient's impairment and home/work/community/leisure situation and requirements. Such services may include:
  - Case management
  - Coordination of care and collaboration with those integral to the patient's rehabilitation program
  - Coordination and monitoring of the delivery of available resources
  - Referrals to other health-care professionals

40   BUNION | FOOT AND ANKLE

- Identification of resources, support groups, or advocacy services
- Provision of educational or training information
- Technical assistance

Patient Instruction

Basic Anatomy and Biomechanics
- Anatomy of foot/ankle
- Biomechanics of ankle/foot and relationship of symptoms to:
  - Joint dysfunction due to bursa irritation
  - Muscle weakness or imbalance
  - Effects of hallux valgus on lower extremity biomechanics and gait

Handouts
- Home program: Specific for joint protection and pain and inflammation control with a gradual return to activity
- Protection through proper footwear: Wide, low-heeled, soft-material shoes
- Protection with orthotics and bunion pads
- Ankle/foot AROM exercises, ankle and intrinsic foot strengthening

Functional Considerations
- Alteration of ADLs requiring standing and walking
- Avoidance of prolonged postures
- Pre-operative consideration such as occupation and current health status
- Body mechanic instruction for activities such as lifting, pushing, pulling

Direct Interventions

Acute Phase: 3–5 Visits
- Ankle/foot AROM and flexibility
- Aerobic/endurance conditioning including bike or swimming
- Instruction regarding use of protective splints or padding and avoidance of skin breakdown
- Shoe modifications and instruction to avoid barefoot walking
  - Modifications including wide, low-heeled shoes and/or orthotics

- Provide and instruct in use of assistive device as needed for joint protection
- Manual therapies such as soft-tissue mobilization and gentle Grade I/Grade II mobilizations for pain relief
- Primary use of cryotherapy in the first 3–4 days

Subacute Phase: 3–6 Visits
- Joint and tissue protection, reassess footwear, protective padding, or orthotics and alter as necessary
- Progress ROM exercises and initiate proprioceptive training and strengthening of surrounding musculature
- Cryotherapy as needed

Functional Carryover
- Integration of home exercise program into vocational environment
- Completion of ergonomic adjustments to home, automobile, and vocational areas
- Incorporation of proper posture and body mechanics to avoid exacerbation of symptoms
- Recognition/avoidance of activities that increase or exacerbate radiating symptoms

DISCHARGE PLANNING AND PATIENT RESPONSIBILITY

Criteria for Discharge
- ROM: Normal ankle ROM, first metatarsal phalangeal joints 30° extension for gait
- Gait assessment: Unassisted, pain-free, normal gait pattern on all surface
- Pain: 2/10 or less
- Return to previous functional status for ADLs
- Demonstrates knowledge of proper footwear, padding, and/or orthotics
- Home exercise program independence

Circumstances Requiring Additional Visits
- Severe degenerative changes
  - History of other pathology
  - Presence of other medical conditions
  - Postoperative complications

Home Program

- Protection of joint and soft tissues with proper footwear, orthotics, and/or application of padding
- Flexibility exercises
  - Gastrocnemius, soleus, and Achilles
  - Other lower-extremity muscles as appropriate
- Strengthening and proprioceptive training of surrounding musculature

Monitoring

- Patient is to recheck/call at 1 month post-discharge to ensure proper fit and support of footwear and protective padding
- Assess progression towards all rehabilitation goals and function during ADLs
- Follow up with physician if it becomes difficult to wear shoes or participate in ADLs for alternative treatment, i.e. injections or surgery

REFERENCES

1. American Physical Therapy Association. *Guide to Physical Therapist Practice*. Alexandria, VA: APTA; revised 2003.
2. Hart A, Hopkins C, Ford B. *ICD-9-CM Expert For Physicians, Volume 1&2*. 7th ed. USA: Ingenix; 2005.
3. Magee D. *Orthopedic Physical Assessment*, 4th ed. Philadelphia, PA: Saunders; 2002.
4. Placzek JD, Boyce DA. *Orthopedic Physical Therapy Secrets*. Philadelphia, PA: Hanley & Belfus, Inc; 2001.

DIABETIC FOOT
SUMMARY OVERVIEW

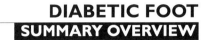

ICD-9
    250.8   707.10   707.13   707.14   707.15   707.19
APTA Preferred Practice Pattern: **5E, 6B, 7A, 7B, 7C, 7D, 7E**

EXAMINATION
- History and Systems Review
- Tests and Measures
  Systems review per APTA's *Guide to Physical Therapy Practice*
  - Anthropometric characteristics
  - Gait, locomotion, and balance
  - Integumentary integrity
  - Joint integrity and mobility
  - Muscle performance
  - Orthotics, protective and supportive devices
  - Pain
  - Posture
  - Sensory integrity for neurological examination
  - Ventilation, respiration, and circulation
- Establish Plan of Care

GOALS/OUTCOMES
- Adequate skin integrity to tolerate functional weight-bearing loads
- Patient demonstration of the essentials of self-inspection, foot care, and proper choice of footwear
- Independence in a progressive home exercise program emphasizing function
- Ankle ROM
- Weight-bearing tolerance to allow return to ADLs and vocational, recreational, and sports activities
- Stance stability and normal gait pattern to minimize pathomechanics and achieve independence
- Strength: A minimum of 4/5 on foot and ankle manual muscle tests
- Pain: 2/10 or less

INTERVENTION
NUMBER OF VISITS: 2–10

- Patient Instruction
  - Basic Anatomy and Biomechanics
  - Handouts
  - Functional Considerations
- Direct Interventions
  - Acute Phase: 1–6 Visits
  - Progressive Phase: 1–4 Visits
- Functional Carryover

DISCHARGE PLANNING AND PATIENT RESPONSIBILITY
- Criteria for Discharge
  - All rehabilitation goals achieved with the exception of return to previous functional level for recreational and sports activities
- Circumstances Requiring Additional Visits
  - Cognitive limitations
  - Severe obesity
  - History of additional lower-extremity pathology
  - Presence of other medical conditions
- Home Program
  - General flexibility exercises for the calf, digits, and lower quadrant
  - Independent self-care program
  - Gait training drills
- Monitoring

DIABETIC FOOT

ICD-9

250.8	Diabetes with other specified manifestations
707.10	Ulcer of lower limb, unspecified
707.13	Ulcer of ankle
707.14	Ulcer of heel and midfoot
707.15	Ulcer of other part of foot
707.19	Ulcer of other part of lower limb

APTA Preferred Practice Pattern: 5E, 6B, 7A, 7B, 7C, 7D, 7E

EXAMINATION

History and Systems Review

- History of current condition
  - Onset, type, and history of diabetic involvement
  - Current footwear and any history of supports, orthotics, etc.
- Past history of current condition
  - Sensory loss
  - Previous plantar ulcers
  - Neuropathic fractures
  - Vision loss
  - Vascular disease
  - Prior treatment for lower-extremity problems
- Other tests and measures
  - Nutrition
- Medications
- Functional status and activity level (current/prior)
- Social habits
  - Health risks
  - Level of physical fitness
- Social history
- Family history
- Living environment
- Occupation/employment
- Patient's functional goals

Tests and Measures

Systems review per APTA's *Guide to Physical Therapy Practice*

- Anthropometric characteristics
  - Girth
    - Figure 8: Circumferential measurement using bony landmarks just inferior to the medial and lateral malleolus, tubercle of the navicular, and peroneal sulcus and cuboid bone (just proximal to the tuberosity of the fifth metatarsal)
    - Malleolar level: Circumferential measurement just inferior to the medial and lateral malleolus
    - Metatarsophalangeal joint level: Circumferential measurement around forefoot at the metatarsophalangeal joints
- Gait, locomotion, and balance
  - Gait characteristics
    - Noting mechanics and load at heel strike or high ground reactive force occurrence
    - Use of orthotics, protective and supportive devices
- Integumentary integrity
  - Calluses
  - Ulcerations
    - Measurement of open area
    - Tunneling or margination
    - Exudate, odor, percentage of necrotic tissue
    - Stage of ulcer
  - Pigment
    - Ecchymosis
- Joint integrity and mobility
  - Foot abnormalities
    - Pes planus
    - Pes cavus
    - Hammertoes
    - Claw toes
    - Hallux valgus
  - Mobility of foot to accommodate weight-bearing forces
    - Talocrural dorsiflexion
    - Subtalar joint motion
    - Hallux extension
- Muscle performance
  - Posterior tibialis
  - Anterior tibialis

- Peroneus tertius
- Gastrocnemius
- Soleus
- Foot intrinsics
- Orthotics, protective and supportive devices
  - Footwear analysis
    - Shoe fit: Adequate length, width (especially in toe box)
    - Stability/support: Appropriate degree of motion control and cushioning provided
- Pain
  - Measured on visual analog scale
- Posture
  - Static stance
  - Dynamic
  - General lower-extremity alignment/foot type
  - Specific foot alignment
    - Rigid forefoot
    - Plantarflexed first ray
- Sensory integrity for neurological examination
  - Light touch (Semmes-Weinstein > 5.07 SW monofilament at risk for ulceration)
  - Temperature
  - Pain
- Ventilation, respiration, and circulation
  - Palpation of peripheral pulses (popliteal, posterior tibialis, and dorsalis pedis)
  - Blood pressure (ankle/arm index < 0.70 indicative of moderate to severe vascular disease [LoGerfo, Coffman. 1992;3:289–309.])
  - Capillary filling

Establish Plan of Care
- Based on history, tests, and measures

GOALS/OUTCOMES
- Adequate skin integrity to tolerate functional weight-bearing loads
- Patient demonstration of the essentials of self-inspection, foot care, and proper choice of footwear
- Independence in a progressive home exercise program emphasizing function
- Ankle ROM:
  - Plantarflexion: 40°
  - Dorsiflexion: 10° in subtalar neutral with knee extended, 15° with knee flexed

- Weight-bearing tolerance to allow return to ADLs and vocational, recreational, and sports activities
- Stance stability and normal gait pattern to minimize pathomechanics and achieve independence
- Strength: A minimum of 4/5 on foot and ankle manual muscle tests
- Pain: 2/10 or less

INTERVENTION
NUMBER OF VISITS: 2–10

Coordination, Communication, and Documentation
- Provision of services between admission and discharge that facilitate cost-effective and efficient integration or reintegration to home, community, or work
- Documentation of therapeutic intervention is required for each episode of care and serves as the basic foundation for communication
- Coordination and additional communication will depend on the patient's impairment and home/work/community/leisure situation and requirements. Such services may include:
  - Case management
  - Coordination of care and collaboration with those integral to the patient's rehabilitation program
  - Coordination and monitoring of the delivery of available resources
  - Referrals to other health-care professionals
  - Identification of resources, support groups, or advocacy services
  - Provision of educational or training information
  - Technical assistance
- Specific coordination and communication provisions:
  - Referral for biomechanical orthotics
  - Referral for biomechanically sound footwear
  - Referral to social worker or home health agency
  - Referral to internal medicine or other specialty physician for systemic disease management as needed

Patient Instruction

Basic Anatomy and Biomechanics
- Normal foot mechanics
- Common areas of ulceration due to high pressure
- Benefit of exercise for improved glucose tolerance and cardiovascular fitness. This may reduce risk for cardiovascular disease and other complications of diabetes.
- Pertinent Gray's Anatomy (Gray. 1995. 713)

Handouts
- General conditioning exercises
- Foot and calf flexibility
- Gait retraining
- Foot care measures
- Footwear

Functional Considerations
It is imperative that the patient understand the preventive role the following activities play in achieving his or her functional status:
- Self-inspection using mirrors
- Skin care
- Footwear

Direct Interventions

Acute Phase: 1–6 Visits
Superficial ulcers involving only the skin will be the limit of treatment discussed in this guideline.
- Therapeutic exercise and home program
  - Active ankle and foot ROM that does not disturb the lesion's healing
  - Gait training with assistive devices as indicated to minimize high pressure
  - Flexibility exercises for tight muscles of the lower quadrant
  - Skin self-inspection program
- Manual therapy techniques
  Limited to maintaining functional range in uninvolved areas of the foot and ankle
  - Soft-tissue mobilization
  - Joint mobilization
- Wound management
  - Sterile whirlpool
  - Peroxide cleansing

  - Topical antibacterial agent with a thin gauze dressing for acute skin lesions as appropriate
- Electrotherapeutic modalities
  - Electrical nerve stimulation for healing of ulcers as appropriate
- Goals/outcomes
  - Pain: 5/10 or less
  - Intact skin
  - Independent, normal gait pattern with assistive device as necessary
  - Independent, home self-care for cleansing and dressing changes
  - Improved weight-bearing tolerance to allow return to ADLs and vocational activities

Progressive Phase: 1–4 Visits
- Therapeutic exercise and home management
  - Instruction in home soft-tissue and joint-mobilization techniques
  - Ergometry for cardiovascular effect
- Functional training
  - Functional progression, including gait training and ADLs, to minimize undue load or shear forces on the foot
  - Integration of structural biomechanical components that may relieve symptoms, including the choice of shoes/custom biomechanical orthotics to control:
    - Excessive compensatory pronation
    - Shear forces
    And to provide:
    - Maximum shock absorption
    - Accommodation
- Manual therapy techniques
  - Soft-tissue techniques
  - Joint mobilization
  - General passive stretching for calf and forefoot/digit flexibility
- Wound management
  - As appropriate for pain or edema
  - Sterile whirlpool
  - Peroxide cleansing
  - Topical antibacterial agent with a thin gauze dressing for acute skin lesions as appropriate
- Electrotherapeutic modalities
  - Electrical nerve stimulation for healing of ulcers as appropriate

- Goals/outcomes
  - Intact skin
  - Independence in a progressive home exercise program emphasizing function
  - Independence in self-inspection and skin care
  - Functional ankle ROM: 40° plantarflexion, 10° dorsiflexion
  - Strength: Foot/ankle to a minimum of 4/5
  - Independent normal gait pattern
  - Demonstrated knowledge regarding appropriate footwear selection

Functional Carryover

- Patient is counseled regarding long-term benefits of exercise, self-inspection, and appropriate footwear
- Guidelines are given regarding need for medical follow-up
- Appropriate referral is made to home health or social work as necessary for transition into the home

DISCHARGE PLANNING AND PATIENT RESPONSIBILITY

Criteria for Discharge

- All rehabilitation goals achieved with the exception of return to previous functional level for recreational and sports activities

Circumstances Requiring Additional Visits

- Cognitive limitations
- Severe obesity
- History of additional lower-extremity pathology
- Presence of other medical conditions

Home Program

- General flexibility exercises for the calf, digits, and lower quadrant
- Independent self-care program
- Gait training drills

Monitoring

- Patient is to recheck/call at 2 weeks post-discharge to ensure expected return to function, continued healing, and progression toward attaining all rehabilitation goals
- A clinic follow-up at 6–12 weeks is advised for patients deemed at risk due to insensitivity, newly healed lesions, or unstable home environment

REFERENCES

1. American Physical Therapy Association. *Guide To Physical Therapist Practice.* Alexandria, VA: APTA; 1997.
2. Gray H; Williams PL, ed. *Gray's Anatomy.* 38th ed. New York, NY: Churchill Livingstone; 1995.
3. Gross MT. Lower quarter screening for skeletal malalignment: suggestions for orthotics and shoewear. *J Orthop Sports Phys Ther.* 1995;21(6):389-405.
4. Hart A, Hopkins C, Ford B. *ICD-9-CM Expert For Physicians, Volume 1&2.* 7th ed. USA: Ingenix; 2005.
5. Jette DU. Physiological effects of exercise in diabetes. *Phys Ther.* 1984;63:339-342.
6. LoGerfo, Coffman. Cited in Mueller M. Etiology, evaluation and treatment of the neuropathic foot. *Crit Rev Phys Rehab Med.* 1992;3:289-309.
7. Lundeberg TC, Erikssan SV, Malm M. Electrical nerve stimulation improves healing of diabetic ulcers. *Ann Plastic Surg.* 1992;29:328-331.
8. Mueller M, Minor S, Diamond J, Blair V. Relationship of foot deformity to ulcer location in patients with diabetes mellitus. *Phys Ther.* 1990;70:356-362.
9. Nawoczenski DA, Birke JA, Graham SL, Koziateck E. The neuropathic foot: a management scheme. A case report. *Phys Ther.* 1989;69:287-291.
10. Sims DS, Cavanagh PR, Ulbriecht JS. Risk factors in the diabetic foot: recognition in management. *Phys Ther.* 1988;68:1887-1902.
11. Tatro-Adams D, McGann SF, Carbone W. Reliability of the figure-of-eight method of ankle measurement. *J Orthop Sports Phys Ther.* 1995;22(4):161-163.

FOOT CARE GUIDELINES FOR THE DIABETIC PATIENT

SELF-INSPECTION

- Inspect all surfaces of feet daily for signs of skin irritation
- Feel for areas of increased temperature
- Palpate plantar surface for tenderness
- Inspect socks and shoes before donning for worn areas or foreign objects
- Replace worn socks and avoid use of obsolete footwear
- Report problems early to a medical professional

SKIN CARE

- Remove excess callus by lightly sanding before bathing rather than by cutting with blade
- Hydrate skin daily by brief soaking or bathing followed by application of an emollient
- Trim nails straight across monthly; thickened nails may require professional assistance
- Keep superficial wounds clean and rested by removing weight from foot
- Report large or slowly healing (no signs of healing within 2–3 days) wounds to a medical professional

FOOTWEAR SELECTION

- A low-wedge, crepe-soled shoe with a high, rounded toe box, moldable upper (leather or nylon mesh), and adjustable closure (straps or laces) is the preferred style
- Fit shoes to the shape and size of your feet
- Choose shoes with extra depth if insoles are to be added
- Never walk barefoot, including inside the house
- Break in new shoes slowly (less than 2 hours a day for first week)
- Repair or replace worn insoles or shoes

FOOT CONTUSION
SUMMARY OVERVIEW

ICD-9

719.47   719.57   729.5   924.20   924.3

APTA Preferred Practice Pattern: **7B**

EXAMINATION

- History and Systems Review
- Tests and Measures
  Systems review per APTA's *Guide to Physical Therapy Practice*
  - Anthropometric characteristics
  - Circulation
  - Functional screen
  - Gait, locomotion, and balance
  - Integumentary integrity
  - Joint integrity and mobility
  - Muscle performance
  - Pain
  - Posture
  - ROM
  - Sensory integrity
- Establish Plan of Care

GOALS/OUTCOMES

- Edema: Less than 1 cm Figure-8 girth difference between limbs
- Transition to normal footwear
- ROM: Foot/ankle
- Ratio of inversion to eversion 2:1
- First metatarsophalangeal extension: 60°
- Normal gait pattern without assistive device on all surfaces, including stairs
- Foot and ankle strength: 5/5 in manual muscle test or equivalent to uninvolved leg on closed-kinetic chain functional tests
- Return to previous functional status for ADLs and vocational, recreational, and sports activities as identified by patient
- Independence in a progressive home exercise program emphasizing function

INTERVENTION
NUMBER OF VISITS: 5–13

- Patient Instruction
  - Basic Anatomy and Biomechanics
  - Handouts
  - Home Program
  - Functional Considerations
- Direct Interventions
  - Acute Phase: 2–7 Visits
  - Subacute Phase: 3–6 Visits
- Functional Carryover

DISCHARGE PLANNING AND PATIENT RESPONSIBILITY

- Criteria for Discharge
  - Patient able to wear normal footwear
  - Patient has achieved functional goals with the exception of return to previous functional status for recreational activity and sports
- Circumstances Requiring Additional Visits
  - Severe degenerative changes
  - History of other pathology
  - Presence of other medical conditions
  - Cognitive limitations
  - Excessive environmental barriers to discharge
  - Obesity
- Home Program
  - Ankle/calf muscle flexibility for adequate dorsiflexion, plantarflexion, inversion, eversion ROM for gait and necessary functional activities
  - Strength intrinsic and extrinsic to the foot including closed chain adequate for functional skill mix of patient
  - Gait progression (with assistive device if necessary) and include stairs, varied terrain. Also may include running if progress and patient's work/recreational roles require
  - May include contrast bath, ice or heat appropriate to level of swelling/inflammation and/or stiffness
  - Balance and proprioceptive training appropriate to skill mix and tolerance
- Monitoring

SUMMARY OVERVIEW | FOOT AND ANKLE | FOOT CONTUSION   51

FOOT CONTUSION

ICD-9

719.47	Pain in joint, ankle and foot
719.57	Stiffness of joint, not elsewhere classified, ankle and foot
729.5	Pain in limb
924.20	Contusion of foot
924.3	Contusion of toe

APTA Preferred Practice Pattern: **7B**

EXAMINATION

History and Systems Review

- History of current condition
  - Mechanism of injury
  - Location/presence of swelling, discoloration
  - Any sense of instability
- Past history of current condition
- Pervious diagnostic procedures
- Medications
- Past medical/surgical history
- Functional status and activity level (current/prior)
- Patient's functional goals

Tests and Measures

Systems review per APTA's *Guide to Physical Therapy Practice*

- Anthropometric characteristics
  - Girth at malleolei or metatarsal heads
- Circulation
  - Pedal pulses, capillary filling test
  - Note any ecchymosis or findings suggestive of venous congestion or ischemia
- Functional screen
  - Squats, balance reach, hops as appropriate for degree of injury and irritability
- Gait, locomotion, and balance
  - Need for assistive device
  - Walking analysis
  - Balance activities
  - Load tolerance (run or hop as tolerated)
- Integumentary integrity
  - Skin integrity, ecchymosis
- Joint integrity and mobility
  - Ligament integrity tests as needed (ankle, subtalar joint, mid-tarsal)

- Muscle performance (including strength, power, and endurance)
  - Manual muscle test ankle and foot
  - Functional test of calf raises, hopping, etc.
- Pain
  - Measured on visual analog scale
- Posture
  - Center of gravity to base of support
  - Foot type
- ROM (including muscle length)
  - Ankle
  - Subtalar joint
  - Midtarsal joints
  - Metatarsal phalangeal joints and digits
- Sensory integrity
  - Note areas of hypo- or hyperaesthesia

Establish Plan of Care

- Based on history, tests, and measures

GOALS/OUTCOMES

- Edema: Less than 1 cm Figure 8 girth difference between limbs
- Transition to normal footwear
- ROM: Foot/ankle
  - Plantarflexion: 40°
  - Dorsiflexion: 10° in subtalar neutral with knee extended, 15° with knee flexed
- Ratio of inversion to eversion: 2:1
- First metatarsophalangeal extension: 60°
- Normal gait pattern without assistive device on all surfaces, including stairs
- Foot and ankle strength: 5/5 in manual muscle test or equivalent to uninvolved leg on closed-kinetic chain functional tests

- Return to previous functional status for ADLs and vocational, recreational, and sports activities as identified by patient
- Independence in a progressive home exercise program emphasizing function

INTERVENTION
NUMBER OF VISITS: 5–13

Coordination, Communication, and Documentation
- Provision of services between admission and discharge that facilitate cost-effective and efficient integration or reintegration to home, community, or work
- Documentation of therapeutic intervention is required for each episode of care and serves as the basic foundation for communication
- Coordination and additional communication will depend on the patient's impairment and home/work/community/leisure situation and requirements. Such services may include:
  - Case management
  - Coordination of care and collaboration with those integral to the patient's rehabilitation program
  - Coordination and monitoring of the delivery of available resources
  - Referrals to other health-care professionals
  - Identification of resources, support groups, or advocacy services
  - Provision of educational or training information
  - Technical assistance
- Specific coordination and communication provisions
  - Referral for support stocking, ankle support as needed
  - Radiology or orthopedic referral if fracture or Grade II–III ligament injury suspected. Likely requires boot immobilization and weight-bearing precautions for proper healing.

Patient Instruction

Basic Anatomy and Biomechanics
- Foot and ankle anatomy diagram (Anatomical Chart Company)
- Foot/ankle model

Handouts
- Commercially available products, such as:
  - Krames Communications (1100 Grundy Lane, San Bruno, CA 94066):
    - *Ankle Owners Manual*
    - *Understanding Ankle Sprains*

Home Program
- Home program to address impairments in mobility, strength, stability, balance, or load tolerance. Also address function limitations with progressive nature and dosage of exercise.

Functional Considerations
- Posture
  - Discuss RICE in acute phase, need for support hose as needed for pressure normalization
- Assistive devices
  - Straight cane, crutch(s), walking staff as needed for load reduction. Consider compressive stocking and/or ankle support as needed to control swelling and provide necessary stability for function.
- Precautions
  - Recommend avoiding excessive stairs, uneven terrain, or prolonged periods on feet in more acute phase
- Alteration of ADLs
  - Monitor and adjust for time on feet, terrain, ROM requirements for functional activities to stay in therapeutic range while necessary
- Avoidance of prolonged postures
  - Differentiate between postures that, when sustained, promote gradual range gains vs. those that are too vigorous or cause abnormal biomechanical stress to injured soft tissues
- Positioning for relief of symptoms
  - May recommend using a rocking chair or rolling foot on a kickball or soccer ball for mobilization in pain-free range (pain inhibition via mechanoreceptor stimulation)
- Body mechanics
  - Instruction in proper stride length, squatting depth, height of heel raises to encourage healing and functional progress
- Training recommendations
  - For high level athletes, recommend cross training that reduces load and motion demands of the injured

foot/ankle. Consider bike vs. running, swimming, upper body ergometry for cardio.

Direct Interventions

Acute Phase: 2–7 Visits
- Electrotherapeutic modalities
  - Electrical stimulation
    - Reduced inflammation/swelling
    - Reduced pain
- Physical agents and mechanical modalities
  - Ultrasound
  - Cryotherapy
    - Reduced inflammation/swelling
    - Reduced pain
- Manual therapy techniques
  - Venous drainage massage
  - Friction massage to promote ligament/tendon healing
- Therapeutic exercise
  - Maintain/improve foot and ankle ROM
  - Improve weight bearing tolerance
- Gait training with proper assistive as needed
- Home exercise instruction
  - To reduce inflammation, maintain ROM, and normalize gait appropriate for ADLs, work, and appropriate recreational activities

Subacute Phase: 3–6 Visits
- Electrotherapeutic modalities
  - Electrical stimulation
    - Reduced inflammation/swelling
    - Reduced pain
- Physical agents and mechanical modalities
  - Ultrasound
  - Cryotherapy
    - Reduced inflammation/swelling
    - Reduced pain
- Manual therapy techniques
  - Venous drainage massage
  - Friction massage for ligament/tendon healing
  - ASTYM to promote collagen healing as appropriate
- Therapeutic exercise
  - Open chain foot ankle strengthening
  - Stretching/self-mobilization for foot and ankle
- Therapeutic activities
  - Closed chain range progressions
  - Closed chain load progression

- Sports-specific skill progressions
- Balance and proprioceptive training
- Gait training
  - Stairs, uneven ground, varied terrain
  - Running as appropriate
- Therapeutic devices and equipment
  - Compression stocking, ankle support as appropriate
- Home exercise program
  - Specific to proper vigor, range, frequency for patient's impairments and functional limitations

Functional Carryover
- Integration of home exercise program into vocational environment
- Completion of ergonomic adjustments to home, automobile, and vocational areas
- Incorporation of proper posture and body mechanics to avoid exacerbation of symptoms
- Recognition/avoidance of activities that increase or exacerbate radiating symptoms

DISCHARGE PLANNING AND PATIENT RESPONSIBILITY

Criteria for Discharge
- Patient able to wear normal footwear
- Patient has achieved functional goals with the exception of return to previous functional status for recreational activity and sports

Circumstances Requiring Additional Visits
- Severe degenerative changes
- History of other pathology
- Presence of other medical conditions
- Cognitive limitations
- Excessive environmental barriers to discharge
- Obesity

Home Program
- Ankle/calf muscle flexibility for adequate dorsiflexion, plantarflexion, inversion, eversion ROM for gait and necessary functional activities
- Strength intrinsic and extrinsic to the foot including closed chain adequate for functional skill mix of patient
- Gait progression (with assistive device if necessary) and include stairs and varied terrain. Also may include

running if progress and patients work/recreational roles require.

- May include contrast bath, ice, or heat appropriate to level of swelling/inflammation and/or stiffness
- Balance and proprioceptive training appropriate to skill mix and tolerance

Monitoring

- Phone call to physical therapist as needed for follow-up questions. Appointment with physician if residual impairments limiting essential functional activity persist

REFERENCES

1. American Physical Therapy Association. *Guide To Physical Therapist Practice.* Alexandria, VA: APTA; 2003
2. *Foot Contusion,* Available at: http://www.mdadvice.com/library/sport/sport138.html. Accessed August 28, 2007.
3. Giza E, Fuller C, Junge A, Dvorak J. Mechanisms of foot and ankle injuries in soccer. *Am J Sports Med.* July-August 2003;31(4):550-4.
4. Hamilton WC. Injuries of the ankle and foot. *Emerg Med Clin North Am.* May 1984;2(2):361-89.
5. Hart A, Hopkins C, Ford B. *ICD-9-CM Expert For Physicians, Volume 1&2.* 7th ed. USA: Ingenix; 2005.
6. Hubbard TJ, Denegar CR. Does cryotherapy improve outcomes with soft tissue injury?. *J Athl Train.* September 2004;39(3):278-79.
7. Thorsson O, Lilja B, Nilsson P, Westlin N. Immediate external compression in the management of an acute muscle injury. *Scand J Med Sci Sports.* June 1997;7(3):182-90.
8. Wilkin LD, Merrick MA, Kirby TE, Devor ST. Influence of therapeutic ultrasound on skeletal muscle regeneration following blunt contusion. *Int J Sports Med.* January 2004;25(1):73-7.

FOOT RECONSTRUCTION
SUMMARY OVERVIEW

ICD-9

| 726.7 | 728.5 | 735.0 | 735.2 | 735.4 | 735.5 | 735.8 | 736.73 | 754.62 |
| 824.8 | 838.0 |

APTA Preferred Practice Pattern: **4B, 4C, 4D, 4E, 4F, 4H, 4I, 4J, 6B**

EXAMINATION

- History and Systems Review
- Tests and Measures
  Systems review per APTA's *Guide to Physical Therapy Practice*
  - Anthropometric characteristics
  - Gait, locomotion, and balance
  - Muscle performance
  - Pain
  - Posture
  - ROM
  - Sensory integrity
  - Ventilation, respiration, and circulation
- Establish Plan of Care

GOALS/OUTCOMES

- Edema: Less than 1 cm Figure-8 girth difference between limbs
- Transition to normal footwear
- Pain-free foot and ankle ROM
- Normal gait pattern without assistive device on all surfaces, including stairs
- Foot and ankle strength: 5/5
- Pain: 2/10 or less
- Improved neuromuscular/balance/proprioceptive awareness for stability and reduction of risk for future injury
- Return to previous functional status for ADLs and vocational, recreational, and sports activities as identified by patient
- Independence in a progressive home exercise program emphasizing function

INTERVENTION
NUMBER OF VISITS: 6–14

- Patient Instruction
  - Basic Anatomy and Biomechanics
  - Functional Considerations
  - Description of Surgical Procedure
- Direct Interventions
  - Acute Phase: 1–2 Visits
  - Subacute Phase: 2–6 Visits
  - Progressive Phase: 3–6 Visits
- Functional Carryover

DISCHARGE PLANNING AND PATIENT RESPONSIBILITY

- Criteria for Discharge
  - Patient has achieved all goals/outcomes with possible exceptions listed in guideline
- Circumstances Requiring Additional Visits
  - History of additional lower-extremity pathology
  - Multiple fracture sites
  - Presence of other medical conditions
  - Postoperative complications
  - Severe obesity
  - Delayed healing
- Home Program
  - Calf flexibility
  - Ankle strengthening exercises using resistive band
  - Midfoot and forefoot self-mobilization
  - Gait progression
  - Closed-kinetic chain sequence
  - Running/walking/other sport progression as appropriate
  - Plyometrics as appropriate
- Monitoring

FOOT RECONSTRUCTION

ICD-9

726.7	Enthesopathy of ankle and tarsus
728.5	Hypermobility syndrome
735.0	Hallux valgus (acquired)
735.2	Hallux rigidus
735.4	Other hammer toe (acquired)
735.5	Claw toe (acquired)
735.8	Other acquired deformities of toe
736.73	Cavus deformity of foot, acquired
754.62	Talipes calcaneovalgus
824.8	Closed fracture of ankle, unspecified
838.0	Closed dislocation of foot

APTA Preferred Practice Pattern: 4B, 4C, 4D, 4E, 4F, 4H, 4I, 4J, 6B

EXAMINATION

History and Systems Review

- History of current condition
  - Date and type of procedure
  - Sensory changes
  - Postoperative progression and treatment
    - Transitions in weight-bearing status to date
    - Complications
- Past history of current condition
  - Lower-extremity problems
- Functional status and activity level (current/prior)
- Patient's functional goals

Tests and Measures

Systems review per APTA's *Guide to Physical Therapy Practice*

- Anthropometric characteristics
  - Comparative girth measurements
    - Figure 8: Circumferential measure using bony landmarks just inferior to the medial and lateral malleolus, tubercle of the navicular, and peroneal sulcus and cuboid bone (just proximal to the tuberosity of the fifth metatarsal)
    - Malleolar level: Circumferential measurement just inferior to the medial and lateral malleolus
    - Metatarsophalangeal joint (MPJ) level: Circumferential measurement taken at the joint lines from the first to fifth

- Gait, locomotion, and balance
  - Weight-bearing tolerance
  - Propulsive ability
  - Assistive devices
  - Excessive/inadequate pronation
- Muscle performance
  Resistance as allowed by postoperative recovery
  - Ankle dorsiflexion, plantarflexion
  - Foot and ankle inversion, eversion
  - Toe flexion, extension
- Pain
  - Measured on visual analog scale
- Posture
  - Static stance position
    - Calcaneal varus/valgus
    - Arch height/Feiss line
    - Forefoot abductus/adductus
  - General lower-extremity alignment
  - Specific foot alignment (non-weight bearing)
    - Subtalar neutral position
    - Forefoot to rearfoot alignment
- ROM
  - Talocrural: Dorsiflexion, plantarflexion
  - Rearfoot: Inversion, eversion
  - Midtarsal joint: Inversion, eversion (2:1 ratio)
  - MPJ and phalangeal: Flexion, extension, especially hallux extension
- Sensory integrity
  - Sensation as indicated
- Ventilation, respiration, and circulation
  - Pulses as indicated

Establish Plan of Care
- Based on history, tests, and measures

GOALS/OUTCOMES
- Edema: Less than 1 cm Figure-8 girth difference between limbs
- Transition to normal footwear
- Pain-free foot and ankle ROM:
  - Plantarflexion: 40°
  - Dorsiflexion: 10° in subtalar neutral with knee extended, 15° with knee flexed
  - Ratio of inversion to eversion: 2:1
  - First MPJ extension: 60°
- Normal gait pattern without assistive device on all surfaces, including stairs
- Foot and ankle strength: 5/5
- Pain: 2/10 or less
- Improved neuromuscular/balance/proprioceptive awareness for stability and reduction of risk for future injury
- Return to previous functional status for ADLs and vocational, recreational, and sports activities as identified by patient
- Independence in a progressive home exercise program emphasizing function

INTERVENTION
NUMBER OF VISITS: 6–14

Coordination, Communication, and Documentation
- Provision of services between admission and discharge that facilitate cost-effective and efficient integration or reintegration to home, community, or work
- Documentation of therapeutic intervention is required for each episode of care and serves as the basic foundation for communication
- Coordination and additional communication will depend on the patient's impairment and home/work/community/leisure situation and requirements. Such services may include:
  - Case management
  - Coordination of care and collaboration with those integral to the patient's rehabilitation program
  - Coordination and monitoring of the delivery of available resources
  - Referrals to other health-care professionals

- Identification of resources, support groups, or advocacy services
  - Provision of educational or training information
  - Technical assistance
- Specific coordination and communication provisions:
  - Referral for biomechanical orthotics
  - Referral to home health agency or social worker as needed

Patient Instruction

Basic Anatomy and Biomechanics
- Hinge motion at mortise vs. supination/pronation motion contributed by subtalar and midtarsal joints
- Time frame for weight-bearing and resistance progression

Handouts
- Home contrast bath
- Home exercise program
  - Self-mobilization of the forefoot and digits
  - Foot and ankle active ROM exercises
  - Ankle rubber band resistance exercises
  - Closed-kinetic chain functional exercise progression
  - Gait training

Functional Considerations
- Education regarding the amount of walking and weight-bearing appropriate for healing
- Recommendations relative to compressive garments and foot and ankle elevation for edema
- Functional progression regarding stairs, varied terrain, and vigor of loading

Description of Surgical Procedure
- Review of surgical technique of osteotomies, fusions, and tendon procedures in relation to rehabilitation and daily activities

Direct Interventions

Acute Phase: 1–2 Visits
Therapeutic intervention at acute phase is limited due to immobility and protection.
- Therapeutic exercise
  - Gait training with assistive device
  - ROM exercises for non-involved joints as appropriate

FOOT AND ANKLE | FOOT RECONSTRUCTION   59

- Physical agents and mechanical modalities
  - Edema control
- Goals/outcomes
  - Partial weight-bearing normal gait pattern with assistive devices
  - Prevent decrease in ROM
  - Pain: 5/10 or less

Subacute Phase: 2–6 Visits

Weight-bearing restrictions, pain, or edema limit the patient's functional level.

- Therapeutic exercise and home program
  - Active and resistive ROM to uninvolved areas as appropriate
  - Assisted and active ROM to involved areas as appropriate
  - Upper body ergometry for fitness as appropriate
  - Sitting BAPS
    - Encourage maximum pain-free dorsiflexion in subtalar neutral in sitting position
  - Gait training
    - Load limited as appropriate for improved standing stability and weight transfer
- Manual therapy techniques
  - Soft-tissue techniques
    - Venous drainage massage
    - Scar massage to surgical incisions
  - Joint mobilization
    - Grade I–II mobilization (primary focus on dorsiflexion)
- Electrotherapeutic modalities
  - Electrical stimulation
- Physical agents and mechanical modalities and mechanical modalities
  - Cryotherapy
  - Pulsed ultrasound
- Goals/outcomes
  - Control and reduce edema to transition to normal footwear
  - Pain: 3/10 or less
  - Improve weight-bearing tolerance
  - Full ROM in non-operative areas
  - ROM of involved joints:
    - Plantarflexion: 30°
    - Dorsiflexion: 5° with knee extended
    - First MPJ extension: 50°

Progressive Phase: 3–6 Visits

- Therapeutic exercise and home program
  - Functional progression as appropriate
    - Step up/step down
    - Mini squats
    - Lunges
    - Heel raises
    - Toe raises
  - Ergometry
  - Treadmill
  - Ankle resistive band
  - Neuromuscular/balance/proprioceptive reeducation exercises
    - Balance board or BAPS
    - Slide bench: Impulse loading limited
    - Profitter
    - Gait drills
      a. Balance beam walk, forward and backward
      b. Carioca
      c. Toe walk, heel walk
    - Balance/reach
      a. Involved leg stance, reaching forward, backward, and laterally with uninvolved leg to maximum distance
      b. Involved leg stance, reaching forward and to sides with one or both arms to shoulder, waist, or floor height, as appropriate, to maximum distance
- Manual therapy techniques
  - Joint mobilization
    Progressive mobilization as appropriate for procedure performed
    - Talocrural: Emphasize ankle dorsiflexion
    - Subtalar
    - Midtarsal joints: Emphasize first ray plantarflexion
    - Digits: Emphasize hallux extension and lesser (2nd–5th) MPJ flexion
  - Soft-tissue techniques
    - Soft-tissue mobilization
    - Scar mobilization
- Therapeutic devices and equipment
  - Functional biomechanics
    - Integration of specific structural or biomechanical components that may relieve symptoms including the choice of shoes and/or custom biomechanical orthotics to control excessive compensatory pronation

- Electrotherapeutic modalities
  - Electrical stimulation
- Physical agents and mechanical modalities
  - Ultrasound
  - Cryotherapy
- Goals/outcomes
  - Pain-free foot and ankle ROM:
    - Plantarflexion: 40°
    - Dorsiflexion: 10° in subtalar neutral with knee extended, 15° with knee flexed
    - Ratio of inversion to eversion: 2:1
    - First MPJ extension: 60°
  - Ankle stabilizer and forefoot stabilizer strength to 5/5 for stance stability and propulsion
  - Transition to normal footwear
  - Normal gait pattern without assistive device on all surfaces, including stairs
  - Pain: 2/10 or less
  - Improved neuromuscular, balance, proprioceptive awareness for stability and reduction of risk for future injury

Functional Carryover

- Instructions for proper transitioning from supports and assistive devices
- Recommendations to create opportunities in the workplace and home to couple exercise with functional activity (such as stretching postures)
- Appropriate progressions in functional activity

DISCHARGE PLANNING AND PATIENT RESPONSIBILITY

Criteria for Discharge

- Patient has achieved all goals/outcomes, except may be discharged with:
  - ROM: 8° dorsiflexion in subtalar neutral with knee extended
  - Strength: 4+/5
  - Functional status: Prior to attainment of previous functional status for recreational and sports activities if progress is present

Circumstances Requiring Additional Visits

- History of additional lower-extremity pathology
- Multiple fracture sites
- Presence of other medical conditions
- Postoperative complications
- Severe obesity
- Delayed healing

Home Program

- Calf flexibility
- Ankle strengthening exercises using resistive band
- Midfoot and forefoot self-mobilization
- Gait progression
  - Stepping exercise
- Closed-kinetic chain sequence
  - Step ups
  - Lunges
  - Squats
  - Heel raises
  - Step downs
- Running/walking/other sports progression as appropriate
- Plyometrics as appropriate

Monitoring

- Patient is to recheck/call at 2 weeks post-discharge to ensure continued healing and expected return to previous functional status

FOOT AND ANKLE | FOOT RECONSTRUCTION   61

REFERENCES

1. American Physical Therapy Association. *Guide To Physical Therapist Practice.* Alexandria, VA: APTA; 1997.

2. Clark N, Sherman R. Soft-tissue reconstruction of the foot and ankle. *Orthop Clin North Am.* 1993;24:489-503.

3. Donatelli RA. Normal biomechanics of the foot and ankle. *J Orthop Sports Phys Ther.* 1985;7(3):91-95.

4. Gooch JL, Gieringer SR, Akau CK. Sports medicine 3: lower extremity injuries. *Arch Phys Med Rehab.* 1993;74(suppl):S438-442.

5. Gray G. *Lower Extremity Functional Profile.* Adrian, MI: Wynn Marketing; 1995.

6. Gray H; Williams PL, ed. *Gray's Anatomy.* 38th ed. New York, NY: Churchill Livingstone; 1995.

7. Hart A, Hopkins C, Ford B. *ICD-9-CM Expert For Physicians, Volume 1&2.* 7th ed. USA: Ingenix; 2005.

8. Howell DW. Therapeutic exercise and mobilization. In: Hunt GC, ed. *Physical Therapy of the Foot and Ankle.* New York, NY: Churchill Livingston; 1988:257.

9. Kaltenborn F. *Mobilization of The Extremity Joints.* 3rd ed. Oslo, Norway: Olaf Norlis Bokhandel; 1985:114-137.

10. Kegerreis S. The construction and implementation of functional progressions as a component of athletic rehabilitation. *J Orthop Sports Phys Ther.* 1983;5(1):14-19.

11. Kessler RM. The ankle and hindfoot. In: Kessler RM, Hertling D, eds. *Management of Common Musculoskeletal Disorders: Physical Therapy Principles and Methods.* Philadelphia, PA: Harper & Row; 1983:448.

12. Lentell G, Baas B, Lopez D, et al. The contributions of proprioceptive deficits, muscle function, and anatomic laxity to functional instability of the ankle. *J Orthop Sports Phys Ther.* 1995;21(4):206-215.

13. Maitland GD. *Subjective Examination In Vertebral Manipulation.* 5th ed. Oxford, England: Butterworth-Heinemann; 1986:43-92.

14. Maitland GD. *Peripheral Manipulation.* 3rd ed. Oxford, England: Butterworth-Heinemann; 1992:265.

15. Mascaro TB, Swanson LE. Rehabilitation of the foot and ankle. *Orthop Clin North Am.* 1994;25:147-160.

16. Rodgers MM. Dynamic foot biomechanics. *J Orthop Sports Phys Ther.* 1995;21(6):306-316.

17. Sangeorzan BJ, Hansen ST Jr. Early and late posttraumatic foot reconstruction. *Clin Orthop Rel Res.* June 1998:86-91.

18. Saxema A, O'Brien T. Postoperative physical therapy for podiatric surgery. *J Am Podiatr Med Assoc.* 1992;82:417-423.

19. Seto JL, Brewster CE. Treatment approaches following foot and ankle injuries. *Clin Sports Med.* 1994;13:695-718.

20. Tatro-Adams D, McGann SF, Carbone W. Reliability of the figure-of-eight method of ankle measurement. *J Orthop Sports Phys Ther.* 1995;22(4):161-163.

ORTHOTICS

ANSWERS TO COMMONLY ASKED QUESTIONS ABOUT ORTHOTICS

What are orthotics?

Biomechanical foot orthotics (more correctly termed *orthoses*) are devices that are worn inside the shoes and are designed to change the weight-bearing pattern of the foot in an effort to alleviate symptoms in the feet, legs, hips, or low back. The devices are custom-made from a neutral-position, plaster-cast mold of your feet and are adjusted specifically to accommodate your particular biomechanical alignment.

How do I know WHETHER I need orthotics?

Typically this will be determined by your physician, your physical therapist, or a biomechanical specialist. Generally speaking, if you have pain in your legs or feet that doesn't seem to respond to rest and gets worse with increased activity, you may want to consider a biomechanical evaluation.

What is a biomechanical evaluation?

A biomechanical evaluation is an assessment of your lower-extremity flexibility, muscle performance, and alignment along with a visual analysis of the way you walk and/or run. Sometimes a video camera is used in this analysis. This assessment must be performed by someone who is skilled in biomechanics and is essential for determining whether orthotics are needed and, if so, what style. This evaluation will take about 45 minutes to one hour.

What will be the overall cost of the orthotics, including the evaluation?

The total charge for the evaluation, the orthotics devices, fitting, and minor adjustments is determined by the individual facility. You may be required to pay a portion of the cost the day you are casted for the orthotics. The balance of the charge may be due in 2–3 weeks when you are fitted with the orthotics and receive instructions on their use and break-in. The evaluation and casting together take about an hour; count on spending fifteen minutes to half an hour on the second visit when your orthotics are fitted to your shoes.

How long will the orthotics last?

Generally speaking, the plastic shell of the orthotics will last anywhere from 2–5 years or more, depending on your body weight and activity level. The topcover, padding, and any softer parts of the orthotics will probably need to be refurbished every 12–18 months. This refurbishing does not require you to be recasted or reevaluated; the orthotics are sent to the lab where it was made and is refurbished there at a minimal cost.

Will I have to wear a "special shoe"?

In most cases, no. The orthotics take up about ⅛–¼" of vertical space in your shoe, so in most cases lace-up shoes are recommended. However, if you need orthotics to fit in your dress shoes, make sure to let us know so we can try to accommodate your needs. It is always best to bring a few pairs of shoes with you when you are being evaluated for orthotics. By looking at your shoes, we can determine wear patterns, decide what style of orthotics will best suit your needs, and make recommendations on choices of footwear that may alleviate your symptoms.

How long will I have to wear the orthotics?

Orthotics are not a "cure" for poor biomechanical alignment any more than glasses are a "cure" for bad eyesight. If you remove your glasses, your vision is still impaired. Likewise, if you remove your orthotics, your feet and legs will return to their previous state of alignment. For the orthotics to help you they should be worn as much as possible, especially for more active pursuits like walking or running.

Will my feet change as I age?

Most people will experience an increase of one-half to one full shoe size after they reach adulthood. This is especially true of women of childbearing years. Generally, though, your biomechanical alignment will undergo only minor changes over the years. It is a good idea to be reevaluated if your symptoms return. Your orthotics may have fatigued, or your biomechanical alignment may have changed.

Will my insurance cover the cost of the biomechanical evaluation and orthotics?

It is very difficult for us to know exactly what your particular insurance policy will cover; therefore, **we strongly recommend that you contact your insurance company to discuss this matter prior to having the biomechanical evaluation**. We will be happy to assist you in any way we can; however, it is your responsibility to determine your particular insurance coverage.

ORTHOTICS

CHOOSING THE RIGHT SHOE

When treating patients with foot or ankle pain, the therapist often wishes to make suggestions and offer guidance to the patient on the selection of shoes. This becomes even more important when the therapist is fitting the patient with orthotics to correct faulty biomechanics.

A few general rules to assist the patient in properly sizing a shoe are helpful in most cases. Most people buy their shoes too short and too narrow, and many people fail to realize that the foot continues to spread in both length and width with age, childbearing, and weight gain. A good test for proper length is to allow a thumb's width between the longest toe and the end of the toe box when you're standing fully weighted. To assess proper width is a little more difficult, since many styles have pointed toe boxes. When you're standing fully weighted, the widest part of the foot (the metatarsal heads) should not splay significantly over the footbed of the shoe. Generally, you should shop for shoes at the end of the day, wearing the same style of socks you intend to wear with that shoe. For patients with metatarsal pain, hammertoes, corns, or bunions, a deeper toe box will allow the forefoot more room and may alleviate the onset of symptoms late in the day as the feet naturally swell. Patients with forefoot pathology should be encouraged to buy lace-up style shoes with extra depth and width, avoiding the slip-on, pointed-toe styles as much as possible. Many patients will balk at this advice, but with proper guidance from the therapist they should understand the reasoning for the adjustment. Stylish, pointed shoes may still be worn for short periods of time, when activity will be kept to a minimum.

Athletic shoe choices are much more challenging, as the manufacturers may change a model drastically from one season to the next or discontinue it entirely. There are several things to consider when a therapist assists a patient in the choice of appropriate athletic footwear. A good source of up-to-date information is *Runner's World* magazine, which publishes a spring and fall shoe review issue. Although this magazine reviews primarily running shoes, the information is valuable for other shoe types as well.

Understanding the basics will help the therapist guide the patient in the appropriate direction. First, a few definitions:

Last Shape and Construction

Shoes are built on a structure called a last, which is shaped like a foot. The last shape can be one of three basic styles: curved, semicurved, or straight.

  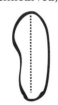 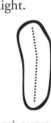

curved lasted *straight lasted* *semi-curved lasted*

A straight-lasted shoe will appear very straight when viewed from the sole. Turn the shoe over and notice that a line bisecting the heel of the shoe will intersect a line bisecting the forefoot of the shoe in a straight alignment. A curved-lasted shoe will have the same bisections intersecting at an angle. A semicurved-lasted shoe will be aligned somewhere in between. The shape of the shoe is significant for the therapist trying to provide motion control with the shoe. The straighter the last, the stronger the motion control. This is advantageous for a patient who is a severe overpronator and who requires maximum motion control. A curved-lasted shoe has the opposite effect, offering maximum cushioning but little motion control. A patient with high arch contours and who does not overpronate would benefit from this structure of shoe.

Last construction also plays a role in the motion-controlling ability of the shoe. When the innersole of the shoe is removed, the structure of the last can be observed. There are three basic structures of lasts: Board lasted, slip lasted, and combination lasted. A slip-lasted structure is suspected when a line of slip stitching can be observed in the shoe from heel to toe. Combination-lasted shoes are somewhat more common for running shoes, offering a combination of rearfoot motion control and forefoot flexibility. They are suspected when a board is visible from the heel to the metatarsal head area and slip stitching is visible from the metatarsal heads to the end of the toe box. Unfortunately, some shoe manufacturers are covering the last construction with a layer of cloth, slip-stitched from heel to toe, thus making the determination of the last construction more difficult.

Outsole

Common outsole materials include carbon rubber (durable but heavy) and blown rubber (light but not durable). Generally, the heavier patients, or those who require more motion control, will benefit from the increased durability of the carbon rubber material.

Midsole

This is the material between the outsole and insole; in essence, the shock absorber. A myriad of materials are in use here, and new ones come on the market regularly. Ethylene vinyl acetate (EVA) is perhaps the most common; it is frequently used in multiple densities to achieve the desired effects of motion control and shock absorption. Many shoe manufacturers are now including other shock-absorbing devices in the midsole, including

air chambers and gel chambers. The best way to stay abreast of new materials is to check the semiannual shoe review issue in *Runner's World* magazine.

In addition to receiving advice on proper fit, patients should be counseled regarding proper frequency of replacing shoes. A general rule of thumb is to replace the shoes worn most frequently about every 6–9 months, depending on body weight and activity level. Athletic shoes should be replaced about every 6 months or approximately every 500 miles (running or walking). Though the outersole may not appear worn at this point, the midsole material is starting to lose its ability to absorb shock. Worn athletic shoes may be used for a short time in less active pursuits, to make them more cost-effective.

The choice of proper footwear for the patient's specific biomechanical needs is an important part of reducing the risk of reinjury or further overuse injury caused by inappropriate biomechanical support. It would be beneficial for the patient to receive this guidance from the therapist at the time of evaluation to further facilitate a speedy recovery.

	Severe Overpronator or Heavier, High-Mileage, Moderate Overpronator	Moderate Overpronator	Mild Overpronator	Underpronator
Curved lasted				x
Semicurved		x	x	x
Straight	x			
Slip lasted			x	x
Combination lasted		x	x	x
Board lasted	x			
Extra depth	Any patient with hammertoes, bunions, or corns			
Wide toe box	Any patient with forefoot pain			

ORTHOTICS

YOUR NEW ORTHOTICS

The following instructions are designed to help you understand the role of your new orthotics and to help you safely make the transition to wearing them. **Remember, orthotics are only one piece of the puzzle. To achieve the best results, continue any stretching exercises you were given by the therapist, wear supportive shoes with plenty of toe room, and exercise sensibly.**

Breaking in Your New Orthotics

Orthotics are designed to control the motions of your foot and to support your foot in a better position for bearing your body weight. Since they were constructed from a mold of your foot, they should fit the contours of your foot fairly closely, but due to the motion-controlling nature of the device, you may feel pressure in some areas of your foot. It is important to allow your feet and legs some time to get used to these new contours, so a slow break-in schedule is recommended.

- *The first day*, you should wear your orthotics for only 1 hour, preferably NOT an active hour.
- *Day 2*, you can increase your wearing time to 2 hours, still during sedentary activities only.
- *Day 3*, increase your time to 3 hours, and gradually begin to increase your activity level.

With each day, increase the wearing time 1 hour until you are able to wear them for a full 8 hours. At this time, if the orthotics are comfortable for a typical 8-hour period, you may begin more vigorous activity. Walking, running, or other exercise programs should be resumed slowly at first to allow the feet and legs to accommodate to the new position. A good rule of thumb is to decrease the activity time to ¼ of what you were previously doing and slowly build back to full intensity over a period of a couple of weeks. **Failure to follow the recommended break-in schedule may result in increased discomfort or blisters.**

Care of Your New Orthotics

Your new orthotics are made of a durable plastic material, covered with a moisture-resistant topcover of naugahyde. They can be easily cleaned with a moistened soft cloth and a mild soap. They should not be exposed to excessive heat from a heat vent, blow-dryer, clothes dryer, or being left in a hot car. **The plastic is heat moldable, so heat will change the shape of the device and therefore its ability to control your foot motions.** The devices are

durable and should last for several years, depending on your body weight and activity level. Over time, the plastic will fatigue and will eventually need to be replaced. Your therapist can help you determine when this is necessary. The topcover, posting, and any padding material will probably need replacement every 12–18 months. Simply bring your orthotics back to your therapist, who will send it back to the lab for refurbishing for a nominal charge. You may find you need additional pairs of orthotics for different styles of shoes. Additional orthotics can be fabricated from the original casts in most cases, at a reduced charge. Questions about this should be directed to your therapist.

Adjustments to Your Orthotics

Usually your orthotics are comfortable within a couple of weeks of breaking them in. You should feel an improvement in your symptoms within about a month. If you notice that you are unable to get used to your orthotics or that your symptoms are not improving, adjustments to the devices may be necessary. Many times, a simple heat adjustment or change in the prescription can be accomplished and your orthotics returned to you in a matter of a day or two. Other times, a more extensive modification is necessary and the orthotics will be sent to the lab. In this case you may be without your devices for a couple of weeks. We strive to minimize the time you are without your devices, but the best orthotics is an effective and comfortable one. Your feedback is vitally important, and we encourage you to call the office and report your progress to your therapist after the first 2 weeks.

PLANTAR FASCIITIS
SUMMARY OVERVIEW

ICD-9

728.71   726.73

APTA Preferred Practice Pattern: **4D, 4E, 4F, 4J**

EXAMINATION
- History and Systems Review
- Tests and Measures
  Systems review per APTA's *Guide to Physical Therapy Practice*
  - Footwear analysis
  - Gait, locomotion, and balance
  - Joint integrity and mobility
  - Orthotics, protective and supportive devices
  - Pain
  - Posture
  - ROM
- Establish Plan of Care

GOALS/OUTCOMES
- Normal gait pattern without assistive devices
- Midfoot stability
- Functional foot and ankle ROM
- Foot and ankle strength to 5/5, especially posterior tibialis and flexor digitorum muscles
- Pain: 2/10 or less without assistive device
- Return to previous functional status for ADLs and vocational, recreational, and sports activities as identified by patient
- Independence in a progressive home exercise program emphasizing function

INTERVENTION
NUMBER OF VISITS 6–11

- Patient Instruction
  - Basic Anatomy and Biomechanics
  - Handouts
  - Functional Considerations
- Direct Interventions
  - Acute Phase: 2–4 Visits
  - Subacute/Chronic Phases: 4–7 Visits
- Functional Carryover

DISCHARGE PLANNING AND PATIENT RESPONSIBILITY
- Criteria for Discharge
  - All rehabilitation goals achieved with the exception of return to previous functional status for recreational and sports activities
  - Demonstrated understanding of role of protective devices, including orthotics
  - Demonstrated understanding of biomechanical factors and training errors
- Circumstances Requiring Additional Visits
  - History of additional lower-extremity pathology
  - Presence of other medical conditions
  - Severe obesity
- Home Program
  - Flexibility
  - Strengthening exercises for toe flexors, posterior tibialis, gastrocnemius/soleus
  - Fitness walking/running/return to sport progression
  - Plyometrics as appropriate
  - Cryotherapy after activity
- Monitoring

PLANTAR FASCIITIS

ICD-9

726.73   Calcaneal spur
728.71   Plantar fascial fibromatosis
APTA Preferred Practice Pattern: 4D, 4E, 4F, 4J

EXAMINATION

History and Systems Review

- History of current condition
  - Onset of injury
  - Pattern of symptoms (edema or discomfort, a.m. vs. p.m.)
  - Current footwear, supports, orthotics
- Past history of current condition
  - Other lower-extremity problems
  - Instability/injury of foot and ankle
- Other tests and measures
  - X-rays
  - Imaging (other)
- Functional status and activity level (current/prior)
- Patient's functional goals

Tests and Measures

Systems review per APTA's *Guide to Physical Therapy Practice*

- Footwear analysis
  - Wear patterns indicating heel whip or excessive pronation
  - Shoe style and structure in relation to biomechanical needs
- Gait, locomotion, and balance
  - Weight-bearing tolerance
  - Degree and rate of pronation in stance phase
  - Assistive devices
  - Toe walking
  - Heel walking
  - Running
  - Hopping
- Joint integrity and mobility
  - Soft-tissue stress test
    - Passive metatarsophalangeal joint extension of all digits with eversion of rearfoot
  - Palpation for tissue integrity/pain
    - Inferior aspect of calcaneal tuberosity
    - Medial aspect of calcaneal tuberosity

- Midfoot
- Longitudinal arch
- Metatarsal heads
- Achilles tendon/triceps suræ
- Orthotics, protective and supportive devices
- Pain
  - Measured on visual analog scale
- Posture
  - Biomechanical screening:
    If the screen is positive, a full biomechanical assessment may be indicated. See *Biomechanical Lower Extremity Dysfunction* guideline.
  - Static stance
    - Relaxed calcaneal posture
    - Arch contour/Feiss line
  - General lower-extremity alignment
  - Specific foot alignment
    - Calcaneal (in subtalar neutral position)
    - Forefoot to rearfoot alignment
- ROM
  - Talocrural dorsiflexion with knee extended and flexed
  - Hallux extension
  - Ratio of inversion to eversion in rearfoot: 2:1
  - Hip rotation in extended position

Establish Plan of Care

- Based on history, tests, and measures

GOALS/OUTCOMES

- Normal gait pattern without assistive devices
- Midfoot stability
- Functional foot and ankle ROM:
  - Dorsiflexion: 10° in subtalar neutral with knee extended, 15° with knee flexed
  - Plantarflexion: >40°
  - Hallux dorsiflexion: >60°
- Foot and ankle strength to 5/5, especially posterior tibialis and flexor digitorum muscles

- Pain: 2/10 or less without assistive device
- Return to previous functional status for ADLs and vocational, recreational, and sports activities as identified by patient
- Independence in a progressive home exercise program emphasizing function

INTERVENTION
NUMBER OF VISITS 6–11

Coordination, Communication, and Documentation
- Provision of services between admission and discharge that facilitate cost-effective and efficient integration or reintegration to home, community, or work
- Documentation of therapeutic intervention is required for each episode of care and serves as the basic foundation for communication
- Coordination and additional communication will depend on the patient's impairment and home/work/ community/leisure situation and requirements. Such services may include:
  - Case management
  - Coordination of care and collaboration with those integral to the patient's rehabilitation program
  - Coordination and monitoring of the delivery of available resources
  - Referrals to other health-care professionals
  - Identification of resources, support groups, or advocacy services
  - Provision of educational or training information
  - Technical assistance
- Specific coordination and communication provisions:
  - Referral for biomechanical orthotics

Patient Instruction

Basic Anatomy and Biomechanics
- Location, attachments, and function of the plantar fascia (Gray. 1995. 891–892)
- The mechanism of injury, the consequences of Achilles tendon and triceps suræ tightness, and foot and ankle weakness
- The importance of midfoot stabilization via:
  - Taping
  - Temporary or permanent custom-molded orthotics as indicated
  - Stable, motion-controlling athletic shoes or oxfords

Handouts
- Contrast baths
- Toe and ankle ROM
- Flexibility exercises for the gastrocnemius/soleus muscle group
- Toe flexor and posterior tibialis strengthening exercises

Functional Considerations
- Walking, running, and activity level appropriate to symptoms, muscle performance, and foot support
- Proper footwear, heel cups, heel lifts, or orthotics if pronation is significant
- Use of cryotherapy and stretching after activity

Direct Interventions

Acute Phase: 2–4 Visits
- Therapeutic exercise and home program
  - Stretching
    - Gastrocnemius/soleus stretching in subtalar neutral
    - Plantar fascia
    - Toe flexors
  - Strengthening
    - Posterior tibialis
    - Toe flexors
    - Gastrocnemius and soleus muscles
  - Gait training for maximal stance stability, weight-bearing as tolerated
- Functional training
  - Rest and cessation of running, jumping, and athletic activities
  - Protection
    - Heel cups
    - Heel pads
    - Cushioned innersole
    - Taping
    - No barefoot walking
    - Orthotics
    - Splinting
  - Cryotherapy: every 2–3 hours for 20–30 minutes per session
- Manual therapy techniques
  - Soft-tissue techniques
    - Deep tissue massage to the plantar fascia, gastrocnemius, and soleus
    - Myofascial release to gastrocnemius, soleus muscles
    - ASTYM treatment

FOOT AND ANKLE | PLANTAR FASCIITIS 71

- ○ Joint mobilization to hypomobile joints
  - ▪ Talocrural
  - ▪ Rearfoot
  - ▪ Midtarsal
  - ▪ Forefoot
  - ▪ Digits
- Electrotherapeutic modalities
  - ○ Iontophoresis
  - ○ Electrical stimulation
- Physical agents and mechanical modalities
  - ○ Phonophoresis
  - ○ Cryotherapy
  - ○ Pulsed ultrasound
- Goals/outcomes
  - ○ Pain: 4/10 or less
  - ○ Foot and ankle ROM:
    - ▪ Dorsiflexion: 5° in subtalar joint neutral with knee extended, 10° with knee flexed
    - ▪ Plantarflexion: 20°
    - ▪ Hallux dorsiflexion: 50°
  - ○ Normal gait pattern using ambulatory aids as needed
  - ○ Foot ankle strength: 4/5

Subacute/Chronic Phases: 4–7 Visits

- Therapeutic exercise and home program
  - ○ Flexibility
    - ▪ Gastrocnemius and soleus muscle and Achilles tendon lengthening
    - ▪ Toe flexors
    - ▪ Plantar fascia
  - ○ Strengthening exercises
    - ▪ Manual resistive exercises
    - ▪ Closed-kinetic chain
  - ○ Toe and heel raises
  - ○ SportCord™ for forward, backward, and sideways lunges
  - ○ Step progression
  - ○ Plyometrics and elastic band exercises
  - ○ Progressive gait training for stance stability and control of excessive pronation
  - ○ Neuromuscular/balance/proprioceptive reeducation
    - ▪ Forward and backward walking, progressing to hopping and jumping
    - ▪ BAPS
  - ○ Cardiovascular conditioning
    - ▪ Stationary bicycle
    - ▪ Treadmill

- ▪ Stair climber
- Functional training
  - ○ Activity level
    - ▪ Graded walking/running activities
    - ▪ Protection as needed with activity
  - ○ Heel pads
  - ○ Heel cups
  - ○ Orthotics or taping
  - ○ Cryotherapy 1–2 times per day or after activity
- Manual therapy techniques
  - ○ Soft-tissue techniques
    - ▪ Deep tissue massage to anterior and medial calcaneal areas
    - ▪ Myofascial release to gastrocnemius, soleus, and plantar fascia
  - ○ Joint mobilization continued to hypomobile joints
  - ○ Assisted stretching to gastrocnemius and soleus using contract/relax techniques
- Therapeutic devices and equipment
  - ○ Functional biomechanics
    - ▪ Integration of specific structural components that may relieve symptoms, including the choice of shoes and custom biomechanical orthotics to control excessive compensatory pronation
- Electrotherapeutic modalities
  - ○ Electrical stimulation
- Physical agents and mechanical modalities
  - ○ Cryotherapy
  - ○ Phonophoresis
- Goals/outcomes
  - ○ Normal gait pattern without assistive devices
  - ○ Pain: 2/10 or less
  - ○ Foot and ankle strength: 5/5
  - ○ Return to previous functional status for ADLs and vocational, recreational, and sports activities as identified by patient
  - ○ Demonstrated compliance with and independence in home exercise program

Functional Carryover

- Instruction is given regarding specific training errors that may exacerbate symptoms
- Counsel patient regarding cross-training options

DISCHARGE PLANNING AND PATIENT RESPONSIBILITY

Criteria for Discharge
- All rehabilitation goals achieved with the exception of return to previous functional status for recreational and sports activities
- Demonstrated understanding of role of protective devices including orthotics
- Demonstrated understanding of biomechanical factors and training errors

Circumstances Requiring Additional Visits
- History of additional lower-extremity pathology
- Presence of other medical conditions
- Severe obesity

Home Program
- Flexibility
  - Achilles tendon/gastrocnemius/soleus
  - Toe flexors
  - Plantar fascia
- Strengthening exercises for toe flexors, posterior tibialis, gastrocnemius/soleus
  - Resistive tubing
  - Closed-kinetic chain exercises
    - Toe raises
    - Step exercises
- Fitness walking/running/return to sport progression
- Plyometrics as appropriate
- Cryotherapy after activity

Monitoring
- Patient is to recheck/call at 2 weeks post-discharge to monitor continued healing and return to function
- If necessary, schedule a 4 week follow-up at clinic to monitor objective parameters and modify home program

REFERENCES

1. American Physical Therapy Association. *Guide To Physical Therapist Practice*. Alexandria, VA: APTA; 1997.
2. Cailliet R. *Foot and Ankle Pain*. 2nd ed. Philadelphia, PA: FA Davis; 1983.
3. Gray G. *Lower Extremity Functional Profile*. Adrian, MI: Wynn Marketing; 1995.
4. Gray H; Williams PL, ed. *Gray's Anatomy*. 38th ed. New York, NY: Churchill Livingstone; 1995.
5. Gross MT. Lower quarter screening for skeletal malalignment: suggestions for orthotics and shoewear. *J Orthop Sports Phys Ther*. 1995;21(6):389-405.
6. Hart A, Hopkins C, Ford B. *ICD-9-CM Expert For Physicians, Volume 1&2*. 7th ed. USA: Ingenix; 2005.
7. Kessler R, Hertling D. *Management of Common Musculoskeletal Disorders: Physical Therapy Principles and Methods*. 2nd ed. Philadelphia, PA: Harper & Row; 1990.
8. Quaschnick, M. The diagnosis and management of plantar fasciitis. *Nurse Pract*. 1996;21(4):50-54, 60-63, 64-65.
9. Rodgers MM. Dynamic foot biomechanics. *J Orthop Sports Phys Ther*. 1995;21(6):306-316.
10. Schepsis A, Leach RE, Gorzyca J. Plantar fasciitis: etiology treatment surgical results and review of literature. *Clin Orthop Rel Res*. May 1991:266.

74   PLANTAR FASCIITIS | FOOT AND ANKLE

POSTERIOR TIBIALIS TENDINITIS (SHIN SPLINTS)
SUMMARY OVERVIEW

ICD-9

726.72

APTA Preferred Practice Pattern: **4D, 4E, 4F, 4J**

EXAMINATION

- History and Systems Review
- Tests and Measures
  - Gait, locomotion, and balance
  - Muscle performance
  - Orthotics, protective and supportive devices
  - Pain
  - Posture
  - ROM
  - Special tests
- Establish Plan of Care

GOALS/OUTCOMES

- Normal gait pattern without assistive device on all surfaces
- Normal foot and ankle ROM
- Ankle and midfoot stabilizer strength to 5/5 on manual muscle test or equivalent to uninvolved leg
- Pain: 2/10 or less
- Return to previous functional status for ADLs and vocational, recreational, and sports activities as identified by patient
- Independence in a progressive home exercise program emphasizing function

INTERVENTION
NUMBER OF VISITS: 5–11

- Patient Instruction
  - Basic Anatomy and Biomechanics
  - Educational Materials
  - Functional Considerations
- Direct Interventions
  - Acute Phase: 1–4 Visits
  - Subacute/Chronic Phases: 4–7 Visits
- Functional Carryover

DISCHARGE PLANNING AND PATIENT RESPONSIBILITY

- Criteria for Discharge
  - Patient has achieved all rehabilitation goals with the exception of return to previous functional status for recreational and sports activities
  - Patient demonstrates understanding of proper footwear, orthotics, and proper training schedule to prevent exacerbation of symptoms
- Circumstances Requiring Additional Visits
  - History of additional lower-extremity pathology
  - Presence of other medical conditions
  - Severe obesity
- Home Program
  - Flexibility exercises
  - Strengthening exercises for toe flexors, posterior tibialis, gastrocnemius, soleus
  - Running/fitness walking/return to sport progression as appropriate
  - Plyometrics as appropriate
  - Cryotherapy after activity
- Monitoring

SUMMARY OVERVIEW | FOOT AND ANKLE | POSTERIOR TIBIALIS TENDINITIS (SHIN SPLINTS)   75

POSTERIOR TIBIALIS TENDINITIS (SHIN SPLINTS)

ICD-9
726.72   Tibialis tendinitis
APTA Preferred Practice Pattern: **4D, 4E, 4F, 4J**

EXAMINATION

History and Systems Review
- History of current condition
  - Sudden change in arch contour
    - Rule out rupture
  - Location of symptoms
  - Aggravating factors
  - Weight-bearing tolerance
  - Accompanying lower-extremity symptoms
- Past history of current condition
  - Prior history of lower-extremity problems
- Other tests and measures
- Functional status and activity level (current/prior)
- Patient's functional goals/patient's goals for therapeutic intervention

Tests and Measures
Systems review per APTA's *Guide to Physical Therapy Practice*
- Gait, locomotion, and balance
  - Weight-bearing tolerance
  - Arch height
  - Assistive devices
  - Excessive or prolonged pronation
- Muscle performance
  - Ankle
    - Emphasis on plantarflexion inversion (tibialis posterior)
  - Heel raise
  - Toe walking
  - Hop on one foot
  - Palpation
    - Tibialis posterior
      a. Muscle belly (medial tibia)
      b. Tendon (posterior and inferior to medial malleolus)
      c. Insertion (navicular and plantarly into midfoot)
- Orthotics, protective and supportive devices
  - Footwear analysis
    - Wear patterns indicating heel whip or excessive pronation

- Shoe style and structure in relation to biomechanical needs
- Pain
  - Measured on visual analog scale
- Posture
  - Biomechanical screening
    If positive, a full biomechanical assessment may be indicated. See *Biomechanical Lower Extremity Dysfunction* guideline.
  - Static stance
    - Relaxed calcaneal posture
    - Single-leg standing
      a. Look for compensatory pronation, degree of hip and/or ankle instability
      b. Arch contour/Feiss line (Navicular drop)
  - General lower-extremity alignment
  - Specific foot alignment
    - Calcaneal posture in subtalar neutral position
    - Forefoot to rearfoot alignment
- ROM
  - Particular attention to dorsiflexion in subtalar neutral with knee extended
- Special tests
  - Tinnel's
    - Rule out Tarsal Tunnel Syndrome
  - Heel raises
    - Observe function of tendon in heel inversion with plantarflexion

Establish Plan of Care
- Based on history, tests, and measures

GOALS/OUTCOMES
- Normal gait pattern without assistive device on all surfaces
- Normal foot and ankle ROM
  - Plantarflexion: 40°
  - Dorsiflexion: 10° in subtalar neutral with knee extended, 15° with knee flexed
  - Ratio of inversion to eversion: 2:1

- Ankle and midfoot stabilizer strength to 5/5 on manual muscle test or equivalent to uninvolved leg
- Pain: 2/10 or less
- Return to previous functional status for ADLs and vocational, recreational, and sports activities as identified by patient
- Independence in a progressive home exercise program emphasizing function

INTERVENTION
NUMBER OF VISITS: 5–11

Coordination, Communication, and Documentation
- Provision of services between admission and discharge that facilitate cost-effective and efficient integration or reintegration to home, community, or work
- Documentation of therapeutic intervention is required for each episode of care and serves as the basic foundation for communication
- Coordination and additional communication will depend on the patient's impairment and home/work/community/leisure situation and requirements. Such services may include:
  - Case management
  - Coordination of care and collaboration with those integral to the patient's rehabilitation program
  - Coordination and monitoring of the delivery of available resources
  - Referrals to other health-care professionals
  - Identification of resources, support groups, or advocacy services
  - Provision of educational or training information
  - Technical assistance
- Specific coordination and communication provisions; referral for:
  - Biomechanical orthotics
  - Biomechanically sound footwear

Patient Instruction

Basic Anatomy and Biomechanics
- Location, attachments, and function of the posterior tibialis tendon and calf muscles
- Pertinent Gray's Anatomy (Gray. 1995. 884–885, 888)
- Review of the history of current condition and/or faulty mechanics

Educational Materials
- Calf stretching
- Contrast baths
- Gait training for improved stance stability
- Ankle stabilizer strengthening exercises

Functional Considerations
- Education regarding proper amount of walking/running as appropriate to the patient's symptoms, muscle performance, and foot support
- Education regarding footwear and need for heel lifts or orthotics if significant stance instability is present
- Use of cryotherapy and stretching after activity
- Stretching and strengthening techniques for the ankle and posterior tibial tendon for complete rehabilitation

Direct Interventions

Acute Phase: 1–4 Visits
- Therapeutic exercise and home program
  - AROM of ankle
  - Gastrocnemius, soleus and Achilles tendon stretching in subtalar neutral
  - Gait training for improved stance stability with graded weight-bearing/assistive devices as appropriate
  - Cardiovascular conditioning via biking, swimming, or upper body ergometer to maintain conditioning level
- Functional training
  - Activity level
    - Rest and cessation of running, jumping, and athletic activities
    - Protection
      a. Orthotics for support of medial arch
      b. Very limited barefoot walking
  - Cryotherapy: Every 2–3 hours for 20 minutes per session
- Manual therapy techniques
  - Soft-tissue techniques
    - Friction massage to posterior tibial muscle or tendon
    - Soft-tissue mobilization to gastrocnemius/soleus
  - Assisted stretching to tight gastrocnemius and soleus, as indicated, using contract/relax techniques
- Electrotherapeutic modalities
  - Iontophoresis
  - Electrical stimulation

FOOT AND ANKLE | POSTERIOR TIBIALIS TENDINITIS (SHIN SPLINTS) 77

- Physical agents and mechanical modalities
  - Cryotherapy
  - Pulsed ultrasound
  - Phonophoresis
- Goals/outcomes
  - Pain: 4/10 or less
  - Full weight-bearing ambulation with orthotics or assistive devices as necessary
  - Foot and ankle ROM:
    - Plantarflexion: 30°
    - Dorsiflexion: 5° in subtalar neutral with knee extended, 10° with knee flexed

Subacute/Chronic Phases: 4–7 Visits
- Therapeutic exercise and home program
  - Flexibility
    - Gastrocnemius and soleus muscles
    - Anterior and posterior tibialis muscles and tendons
    - Toe flexors
    - Plantar fascia
  - Strengthening exercises
    - Closed-kinetic chain
      a. Toe and heel raises
      b. SportCord™ for forward, backward, and sideways lunges
      c. Step progression
      d. Plyometrics
    - Elastic band exercises
    - Manual resistive exercises
  - Neuromuscular/balance/proprioceptive reeducation
    - BAPS
  - Progressive gait training for stance stability
  - Cardiovascular conditioning
    - Stationary bicycle
    - Treadmill
    - Stair climber
- Functional training
  - Activity level
    - Graded walking/running activities
    - Protection as needed with activity
      a. Heel pads
      b. Heel cups
      c. Taping
      d. Orthotics
  - Cryotherapy after activity
- Manual therapy techniques
  - Soft-tissue techniques

- Deep friction massage to the site of the lesion in posterior tibialis
- Myofascial release to the gastrocnemius and soleus
  - Joint mobilization as indicated to restore normal foot and ankle ROM
- Therapeutic devices and equipment
  - Functional biomechanics
    - Integration of specific structural or biomechanical components that may relieve symptoms, including the choice of shoes and custom biomechanical orthotics to control excessive compensatory pronation
- Electrotherapeutic modalities
  - Electrical stimulation
- Physical agents and mechanical modalities
  - Cryotherapy
  - Ultrasound
  - Phonophoresis
- Goals/outcomes
  - Normal gait pattern without assistive device on all surfaces
  - Pain: 2/10 or less
  - Strength: 5/5 on manual muscle test or equivalent to uninvolved leg
  - Return to previous functional status for ADLs and vocational, recreational, and sports activities as identified by patient
  - Normal foot and ankle ROM:
    - Plantarflexion: 40°
    - Dorsiflexion: 10° in subtalar neutral with knee extended, 15° with knee flexed
    - Ratio of inversion to eversion: 2:1

Functional Carryover
- Instruction is given regarding specific training errors that may exacerbate symptoms
- Counsel patient in cross-training options

DISCHARGE PLANNING AND PATIENT RESPONSIBILITY

Criteria for Discharge
- Patient has achieved all rehabilitation goals with the exception of return to previous functional status for recreational and sports activities
- Patient demonstrates understanding of proper footwear, orthotics, and proper training schedule to prevent exacerbation of symptoms

Circumstances Requiring Additional Visits
- History of additional lower-extremity pathology
- Presence of other medical conditions
- Severe obesity

Home Program
- Flexibility exercises
  - Achilles tendon
  - Gastrocnemius
  - Soleus
  - Anterior and posterior tibialis muscles
- Strengthening exercises for toe flexors, posterior tibialis, gastrocnemius, soleus
  - Resistive tubing
  - Heel raises
  - Toe raises
  - Step exercises
- Running/fitness walking/return to sport progression as appropriate
- Plyometrics as appropriate
- Cryotherapy after activity

Monitoring
- Patient will recheck/call at 2 weeks post-discharge to allow monitoring of continued healing and return to function
- If necessary, schedule a 4 week follow-up at clinic to monitor objective parameters and modify home program

REFERENCES

1. American Physical Therapy Association. *Guide To Physical Therapist Practice*. Alexandria, VA: APTA; 1997.
2. Cailliet R. *Foot and Ankle Pain*. 2nd ed. Philadelphia, PA: FA Davis; 1983.
3. Curwin S, Stanish WD. *Tendinitis: Its Etiology and Treatment*. Lexington, MA: DC Heath; 1984.
4. Gray G. *Lower Extremity Functional Profile*. Adrian, MI: Wynn Marketing; 1995.
5. Gray H; Williams PL, ed. *Gray's Anatomy*. 38th ed. New York, NY: Churchill Livingstone; 1995.
6. Gross ML, Davlin L, Evanski P. Effectiveness of orthotic shoe inserts in the long distance runner. *Am J Sports Med*. 1991;19:409-412.
7. Gross MT. Lower quarter screening for skeletal malalignment: suggestions for orthotics and shoewear. *J Orthop Sports Phys Ther*. 1995;21(6):389-405.
8. Hart A, Hopkins C, Ford B. *ICD-9-CM Expert For Physicians, Volume 1&2*. 7th ed. USA: Ingenix; 2005.
9. Kessler R, Hertling D. *Management of Common Musculoskeletal Disorders: Physical Therapy Principles and Methods*. 2nd ed. Philadelphia, PA: Harper & Row; 1990.
10. Magee DJ. *Orthopedic Physical Assessment*. 2nd ed. Philadelphia, PA: WB Saunders; 1987.
11. Rodgers MM. Dynamic foot biomechanics. *J Orthop Sports Phys Ther*. 1995;21(6):306-316.
12. Sammarco GJ. *Rehabilitation of The Foot and Ankle*. St. Louis, MO: Mosby-Yearbook; 1995.
13. Tomaro JE, Butterfield SL. Biomechanical treatment of traumatic foot and ankle injuries with the use of foot orthotics. *J Orthop Sports Phys Ther*. 1995;21(6):373-380.

80   POSTERIOR TIBIALIS TENDINITIS (SHIN SPLINTS) | FOOT AND ANKLE

Knee

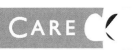

KNEE

Accelerated Anterior Cruciate Ligament Reconstruction	83
Iliotibial Band Syndrome	89
Knee Arthroscopy	95
Knee Contusion	101
Knee Degenerative Joint Disease	105
Knee Enthesopathy	111
Knee Hypomobility/Infrapatellar Contracture Syndrome (IPCS)	117
Knee Sprain/Strain	123
Meniscal Repair	129
Meniscus Tear (Without Surgery)	135
Patellar Tendinitis	141
Patellofemoral Syndrome	147
Posterior Cruciate Ligament Reconstruction	153
Total Knee Replacement—Inpatient	159
Total Knee Replacement—Outpatient	163

82   Knee

ACCELERATED ANTERIOR CRUCIATE LIGAMENT RECONSTRUCTION
SUMMARY OVERVIEW

ICD-9

844.2

APTA Preferred Practice Pattern: **4E, 4J**

EXAMINATION

- History and Systems Review
- Tests and Measures
  Systems review per APTA's *Guide to Physical Therapy Practice*
  - Anthropometric characteristics
  - Gait, locomotion, and balance
  - Joint integrity
  - Muscle performance
  - Pain
  - ROM
- Establish Plan of Care

GOALS/OUTCOMES

- Knee ROM: 0–135°
- Edema: Less than 1 cm joint line girth difference compared to uninvolved knee
- Normal gait pattern without assistive devices on all surfaces
- Strength: 70% of uninvolved leg as measured on one-repetition maximum leg press test or other closed-kinetic chain functional test, such as single-leg squat excursion or lunge distance
- Normal patellar mobility
- Return to previous functional status for ADLs and vocational, recreational, and sports activities as identified by patient
- Independence in a progressive home exercise program emphasizing function

INTERVENTION
NUMBER OF VISITS: 8–17

- Patient Instruction
  - Basic Anatomy and Biomechanics
  - Handouts
  - Functional Considerations
  - Description of Surgical Procedure
- Direct Interventions
  - Phase I: Acute Injury, 1–2 Visits Preoperative
  - Phase II: 1–3 Visits, Weeks 1–2 Postoperative
  - Phase III: 6–9 Visits, Weeks 3–5 Postoperative
  - Phase IV: 1–5 Visits, Weeks 6 Through Discharge Postoperative
- Functional Carryover

DISCHARGE PLANNING AND PATIENT RESPONSIBILITY

- Criteria for Discharge
  - Patient has achieved all rehabilitation goals with the exception of return to full sport and recreational activities
  - Patient demonstrates understanding of exercise progression and proper training schedule to prevent exacerbation of symptoms
- Circumstances Requiring Additional Visits
  - Significant deconditioning prior to surgery
  - Presence of other medical conditions
  - Postoperative complications
  - History of additional lower-extremity pathology
- Home Program
  - As the patient's muscle performance improves, agility workouts can become more vigorous
  - Transition into the *Return to Sport Anterior Cruciate Ligament Reconstruction* guideline as appropriate to achieve previous functional status for recreational and sports activities
  - Encourage the patient to begin Figure 8, backward running, and progress running program as tolerated/desired
- Monitoring

ACCELERATED ANTERIOR CRUCIATE LIGAMENT RECONSTRUCTION

ICD-9
    844.2   Sprain of cruciate ligament of knee
APTA Preferred Practice Pattern: 4E, 4J

EXAMINATION

History and Systems Review
- History of current condition
  - Date and type of surgical procedure
  - Postoperative progression/complications
- Past history of current condition
  - Previous lower-extremity problems
- Past medical/surgical history
- Functional status and activity level (current/prior)
- Social habits
- Social history
- Family history
- Growth and development
- Occupation/employment
- General demographics
- Patient's functional goals

Tests and Measures
Systems review per APTA's *Guide to Physical Therapy Practice*
- Anthropometric characteristics
  - Comparative girth measurement at joint line
- Gait, locomotion, and balance
  - Weight-bearing status
  - Use of brace
- Joint integrity
  - Patellar glides
  - Lachman Test
    This test will provide information about the integrity of the graft. The test is performed with the patient supine and in approximately 15° of knee flexion. An attempt is then made to translate the tibia anteriorly on a fixed femur. A "mushy" endpoint is a positive test.
- Muscle performance
  - Quadriceps recruitment
- Pain
  - Measured on visual analog scale
- ROM
  - Active
  - Passive

Establish Plan of Care
- Based on history, tests, and measures

GOALS/OUTCOMES
- Knee ROM: 0–135°
- Edema: Less than 1 cm joint line girth difference compared to uninvolved knee
- Normal gait pattern without assistive devices on all surfaces
- Strength: 70% of uninvolved leg as measured on one-repetition maximum leg press test or other closed-kinetic chain functional test, such as single-leg squat excursion or lunge distance
- Normal patellar mobility
- Return to previous functional status for ADLs and vocational, recreational, and sports activities as identified by patient
- Independence in a progressive home exercise program emphasizing function

INTERVENTION
NUMBER OF VISITS: 8–17

Coordination, Communication, and Documentation
- Provision of services between admission and discharge that facilitate cost-effective and efficient integration or reintegration to home, community, or work
- Documentation of therapeutic intervention is required for each episode of care and serves as the basic foundation for communication
- Coordination and additional communication will depend on the patient's impairment and home/work/community/leisure situation and requirements. Such services may include:
  - Case management
  - Coordination of care and collaboration with those integral to the patient's rehabilitation program
  - Coordination and monitoring of the delivery of available resources
  - Referrals to other health-care professionals

84   ACCELERATED ANTERIOR CRUCIATE LIGAMENT RECONSTRUCTION | KNEE

o Identification of resources, support groups, or advocacy services
o Provision of educational or training information
o Technical assistance
• Specific coordination and communication provisions:
o Referral for biomechanical orthotics

Patient Instruction

Basic Anatomy and Biomechanics
• Role of anterior cruciate ligament (ACL) in controlling tibial translation
• Importance of muscular muscle performance in decelerating tibial translation (protecting and assisting ACL) in a closed-kinetic chain position
• Pertinent Gray's Anatomy (Gray. 1995. 697–704, 707–708, 869, 876)

Handouts
• Phase-specific home exercise programs
• Home cryotherapy techniques

Functional Considerations
• Weight-bearing status and functional activity restrictions as appropriate to phase
• Use of immobilizer or brace as instructed by physician
• Functional progression regarding stairs or varied terrain

Description of Surgical Procedure
• Review of operative procedure and relation to joint biomechanics, rehabilitation, and function

Direct Interventions

Phase I: Acute Injury, 1–2 Visits Preoperative
Surgery is often postponed for 6 weeks following injury. This should be predominately a home treatment phase.
• Therapeutic exercise and home program
o ROM
▪ Active
▪ Passive
o Assistive ROM using bicycle as tolerated
o Ergometry to maintain cardiovascular fitness
o Strengthening as tolerated by the joint (i.e., no increase of edema/pain is acceptable)
o Self-patellar mobilization

• Manual therapy techniques
o Joint mobilization
▪ Patellar mobilization
• Physical agents and mechanical modalities
o Cryotherapy
• Goals/outcomes
o Achieve ROM: 0–135°
o Resolve edema
o Address patient concerns regarding surgery
o Review postoperative rehabilitation program
o Mental preparation for surgery

Phase II: 1–3 Visits, Weeks 1–2 Postoperative
• Days 1–2
o Therapeutic exercises and home program
▪ Passive flexibility
a. 10-minute session hourly of passive extension with cryo-cuff removed and heel propped on pillows, allowing knee to relax into full extension
b. 90° of flexion, sitting
▪ Active strengthening
a. Quad sets and straight-leg raises
b. Sitting leg extension 90–30°
o Physical agents and mechanical modalities
▪ Cryotherapy, elevation
▪ Instruct/monitor continuous passive motion
• Days 3–14
o Therapeutic exercises and home program
▪ Ambulation with crutches, partial weight bearing, per physician's order
▪ Exercises, as above (Week 2: Some increase in activity allowed, such as part-time return to job/classes using immobilizer)
▪ Prone hangs includable for hyperextension, up to 10 minutes with ankle weight of 2 lbs
▪ Supine wall slide with 2 lb ankle weight
▪ Self-patellar mobilization
• Goals/outcomes
o Obtain full extension relative to uninvolved leg
o Achieve 90° flexion
o Improve quadriceps control
o Minimize edema
o Promote wound healing

KNEE | ACCELERATED ANTERIOR CRUCIATE LIGAMENT RECONSTRUCTION   85

Phase III: 6–9 Visits, Weeks 3–5 Postoperative

- Therapeutic exercise and home program
  - Closed-kinetic chain exercises
    - Vastus medialis oblique (VMO) training
    - Squats
    - Step ups
    - Heel raises
    - Stair climber
    - Stationary bicycle
    - Leg press
    - SportCord™ activities
  - Open kinetic chain exercises for hamstrings
    - Weights
    - Isokinetics
    - Resistive tubing
  - Flexibility
    - Knee ROM
    - Static lower-extremity stretches
  - Gait training
    - Focus on normal pattern with assistive device
  - Neuromuscular/balance/proprioceptive reeducation
    - Gait drills
      a. Backward walking
      b. Balance beam walking
    - BAPS, balance board
    - Balance/reach
      a. Balancing on involved leg, reaching in various directions with uninvolved leg to maximum distance
- Manual therapy techniques
  - Joint mobilization
    - Patellar mobilization
    - Tibiofemoral mobilization as appropriate
- Electrotherapeutic modalities
  - Electrical stimulation until functional VMO recruitment in stance is achieved
- Physical agents and mechanical modalities
  - Cryotherapy
- Goals/outcomes
  - Normal gait pattern without assistive devices
  - ROM: 0–125°
  - Increased exercise tolerance on closed-kinetic chain exercises
  - Normal patellar ROM

Phase IV: 1–5 Visits, Weeks 6 Through Discharge Postoperative

- Therapeutic exercise and home program
  - A conservative running program can be initiated if strength is 70% or better on a one-repetition maximum leg press test as compared to uninvolved leg
  - Perform lateral shuffles, carioca, and rope jumping
  - If department program is continued, devices such as Profitter, slideboard, etc., can be used
  - Resume sport-specific activities
  - Although limited participation can start at 8 weeks, most patients will require an additional 3 or 4 months to fully develop muscle performance and confidence
- Manual therapy techniques
  - None if Phase III ROM goals are achieved
- Therapeutic devices and equipment
  - Functional biomechanics
    - Integration of specific structural or biomechanical components that may enhance the longevity of the surgically repaired ACL, including choice of shoes or custom biomechanical orthotics to control excessive compensatory pronation
- Physical agents and mechanical modalities
  - None
- Goals/outcomes
  - Strength: 70% of uninvolved leg as measured on a one-repetition maximum leg press test or other closed-kinetic chain functional test, such as single-leg squat excursion or lunge distance
  - Return to full recreational and sports activities as previously indicated by patient
  - ROM: 0–135°

Functional Carryover

- Importance of adequate muscle performance prior to resuming high-load or abrupt activities, such as skiing or soccer
- Instruct patient in variety of cross-training options to reduce risk of future overuse injury

DISCHARGE PLANNING AND PATIENT RESPONSIBILITY

Criteria for Discharge
- Patient has achieved all rehabilitation goals with the exception of return to full sport and recreational activities
- Patient demonstrates understanding of exercise progression and proper training schedule to prevent exacerbation of symptoms

Circumstances Requiring Additional Visits
- Significant deconditioning prior to surgery
- Presence of other medical conditions
- Postoperative complications
- History of additional lower-extremity pathology

Home Program
- As the patient's muscle performance improves, agility workouts can become more vigorous
- Transition into the *Return to Sport Anterior Cruciate Ligament Reconstruction* guideline as appropriate to achieve previous functional status for recreational and sports activities
- Encourage the patient to begin Figure 8, backward running, and progress running program as tolerated/desired

Monitoring
- Follow the patient every 4–6 weeks with a leg press test and KT1000 evaluation if possible and/or as desired by the surgeon
- If the transition to the *Return to Sport Anterior Cruciate Ligament Reconstruction* guideline is made, follow-up as indicated per the guideline

REFERENCES

1. American Physical Therapy Association. *Guide to Physical Therapist Practice.* Alexandria, VA: APTA; 1997.
2. Bak K, Jorgensen U, Ekstrand J, Scavenius M. Results of reconstruction of acute ruptures of the anterior cruciate ligament with an iliotibial band autograft. *Knee Surg Sports Traumatol Arthrosc.* 1999;7(2):111-117.
3. Chen CH, Chen WJ, Shih CH. Arthroscopic anterior cruciate ligament reconstruction with quadriceps tendon-patellar bone autograft. *J Trauma.* 1999;46:678-682.
4. Clancy WG Jr, Nelson DA, Reider B, Narechania RG. Anterior cruciate ligament reconstruction using one-third of the patellar ligament, augmented by extra articular tendon transfers. *J Bone Joint Surg Am.* 1982;64:352-359.
5. Fleming BC, Beynnon BD, Renstrom PA. The strain behavior of the anterior cruciate ligament during stair climbing: an in vivo study. *Arthroscopy* 1999;15:185-191.
6. Gray H; Williams PL, ed. *Gray's Anatomy.* 38th ed. New York, NY: Churchill Livingstone; 1995.
7. Hart A, Hopkins C, Ford B. *ICD-9-CM Expert For Physicians, Volume 1&2.* 7th ed. USA: Ingenix; 2005.
8. Mangine RE, Noyes FR, DeMaio M. Minimal projection program: advanced weight-bearing and range of motion after ACL reconstruction—weeks 1-5. *Orthopedics.* 1992;16:504-515.
9. McCarroll JR, Retting AC, Shelbourne KD. Anterior cruciate ligament injuries in the young athlete with open physes. *Am J Sports Med.* 1988;16:44-47.
10. McCarroll JR, Retting AC, Shelbourne KD. Athletes and their anterior cruciate ligament injury. *Surg Rounds Orthop.* 1989;3:29-44.
11. Muneta T, Sekiya I, Ogiuchi T, et al. Effects of aggressive early rehabilitation on the outcome of anterior cruciate ligament reconstruction with multi-strand semitendinosus tendon. *Int Orthop* 1998:22:352-256.
12. Petersen W, Laprell H. Combined injuries of the medial collateral ligament and the anterior cruciate ligament: early ACL reconstruction versus late ACL reconstruction. *Arch Orthop Trauma Surg.* 1999;119:258-62.
13. Petsche TS, Hutchinson MR. Loss of extension after reconstruction of the anterior cruciate ligament. *J Am Acad Orthop Surg.* 1999;7(2):119-127.

14. Shelbourne KD, Davis TJ. Evaluation of knee stability before and after participation in a functional sports agility program during rehabilitation after anterior cruciate ligament reconstruction. *Am J Sports Med.* 1999;27:156-161.

15. Shelbourne KD, Nitz PA. Accelerated rehabilitation after anterior cruciate ligament reconstruction. *Am J Sports Med.* 1990;18:389-417.

16. Shelbourne KD, Patel DV. Treatment of limited motion after anterior cruciate ligament reconstruction. *Knee Surg Sports Traumatol Arthrosc* 1999:7(2):85-92.

17. Shelbourne KD, Whitaker HJ, McCarroll JR. Anterior cruciate ligament injury: evaluation of intraarticular reconstruction of acute tears without repair, two to seven year follow-up of 155 athletes. *Am J Sports Med.* 1990;18:484-489.

18. Shelbourne KD, Wilckens JH. Current concepts in ACL rehabilitation. *Orthop Rev.* 1990;19:957-964.

19. Shelbourne KD, Wilckens JH, Mollabashy A, De Carlo MS. Arthrofibrosis in the acute ACL reconstruction: the effect of timing of reconstruction and rehabilitation protocol. *Am J Sports Med.* 1991;19:332-336.

20. Shelbourne KD, Klootwyk TE, De Carlo MS. Update on accelerated rehabilitation after ACL reconstruction. *J. Orthop Sports Phys Ther.* 1992;15(6):303-308.

21. Shelbourne KD, Baele JR. Treatment of combined anterior cruciate ligament and medial collateral ligament injuries. *Am J. Surg.* 1988;1:56-58.

ILIOTIBIAL BAND SYNDROME
SUMMARY OVERVIEW

ICD-9

844.9

APTA Preferred Practice Pattern: 4D, 4E, 4J

EXAMINATION

- History and Systems Review
- Tests and Measures

  Systems review per APTA's *Guide to Physical Therapy Practice*

  - Gait, locomotion, and balance
  - Joint integrity and mobility
  - Muscle performance
  - Orthotics, protective and supportive devices
  - Pain
  - Posture
  - ROM
- Establish Plan of Care

GOALS/OUTCOMES

- ROM
- Pain: 2/10 or less
- Strength equal to uninvolved side as measured by appropriate closed-kinetic chain functional test, such as lunges, balance/reach distance, or multidirectional unilateral hop test
- Return to previous functional status for ADLs and vocational, recreational, and sports activities as identified by patient
- Resolution of inflammatory process as documented by elimination of tenderness to palpation
- Independence in a progressive home exercise program emphasizing function

INTERVENTION
NUMBER OF VISITS: 5–10

- Patient Instruction
  - Basic Anatomy and Biomechanics
  - Handouts
  - Functional Considerations
- Direct Interventions
  - Acute Phase: 2–4 Visits
  - Subacute Phase: 3–6 Visits
- Functional Carryover

DISCHARGE PLANNING AND PATIENT RESPONSIBILITY

- Criteria for Discharge
  - Patient displays understanding of principles of training to avoid recurrent symptoms
  - Biomechanical factors that may have been instrumental in the onset of the original symptoms have been addressed appropriately
  - All goals/outcomes have been met with the exception that the patient may not achieve full return to previous functional status for recreational and sports activities but shows signs of progression
- Circumstances Requiring Additional Visits
  - History of additional lower-extremity pathology
  - Additional treatments may be needed to work intensely on passive iliotibial band-lengthening procedures if adequate gains are not made in the course of 8 visits
- Home Program
  - Explain stretching and strengthening exercises as described in Subacute Phase
  - Stress importance of adequate warm-up and cool-down, as well as training principles, to reduce risk of future injury
- Monitoring

SUMMARY OVERVIEW | KNEE | ILIOTIBIAL BAND SYNDROME   89

ILIOTIBIAL BAND SYNDROME

ICD-9
844.9   Sprain of unspecified site of knee and leg
APTA Preferred Practice Pattern: 4D, 4E, 4J

EXAMINATION

History and Systems Review
- History of current condition
  - Date of onset and precipitating factors
  - Training patterns
    - Activity
    - Terrain
    - Distance
    - Speed
    - Mileage
    - Cross-training
  - Aggravating factors
- Past history of current condition
  - Previous lower-extremity injury
- Functional status and activity level (current/prior)
- Patient's functional goals

Tests and Measures
Systems review per APTA's *Guide to Physical Therapy Practice*
- Gait, locomotion, and balance
  - Characteristics
    - Walking and running assessed as symptoms permit
    - Excessive or prolonged pronation
    - Presence of heel whip
    - Apparent excessive transverse plane motion at the hip
  - Lunge distance
  - Single-leg squat excursion
  - Balance/reach
- Joint integrity and mobility
- Muscle performance
  - Resisted testing
    - Hip abductors
    - Hamstrings
    - Quadriceps
    - Hip flexors
- Orthotics, protective and supportive devices
  - Footwear
    - Wear patterns
    - Excessive compression of midsole
    - Appropriateness of shoe style (support)
    - Current orthotic support
- Pain
  - Measured on visual analog scale
  - Pain with resisted hip abduction
  - Pain with resisted palpation: Lateral knee, tensor fasciæ latæ, gluteus medius
- Posture
  - Static stance
    - Relaxed calcaneal position
    - Forefoot position
  - General lower-extremity alignment
    - Genu varus/valgus
  - Specific foot alignment
    - Rearfoot varus
    - Forefoot varus/valgus
- ROM
  - Flexibility
    - Iliotibial band
    - Quadriceps
    - Psoas
    - Hamstrings
    - Gluteals
    - Gastroc
    - Soleus

Establish Plan of Care
- Based on history, tests, and measures

GOALS/OUTCOMES
- ROM
  - Thomas test showing leg on the plinth and at least 70° knee flexion
  - Ankle dorsiflexion to at least 10° in subtalar neutral with knee extended and 15° with knee flexed
  - Ober test showing increased vs. initial evaluation adduction
  - Straight-leg raise test improved by 15° vs. initial eval
  - Internal and external hip rotation to at least 40° as measured in 90° hip flexion

- Pain: 2/10 or less
- Strength equal to uninvolved side as measured by appropriate closed-kinetic chain functional test, such as lunges, balance/reach distance, or multidirectional unilateral hop test
- Return to previous functional status for ADLs and vocational, recreational, and sports activities as identified by patient
- Resolution of inflammatory process as documented by elimination of tenderness to palpation
- Independence in a progressive home exercise program emphasizing function

INTERVENTION
Number of Visits: 5–10

Coordination, Communication, and Documentation

- Provision of services between admission and discharge that facilitate cost-effective and efficient integration or reintegration to home, community, or work
- Documentation of therapeutic intervention is required for each episode of care and serves as the basic foundation for communication
- Coordination and additional communication will depend on the patient's impairment and home/work/community/leisure situation and requirements. Such services may include:
  ○ Case management
  ○ Coordination of care and collaboration with those integral to the patient's rehabilitation program
  ○ Coordination and monitoring of the delivery of available resources
  ○ Referrals to other health-care professionals
  ○ Identification of resources, support groups, or advocacy services
  ○ Provision of educational or training information
  ○ Technical assistance
- Specific coordination and communication provisions:
  ○ Referral for biomechanical orthotics

Patient Instruction

Basic Anatomy and Biomechanics
- Integration of the kinetic chain and the relationship of movement in one area to the stress imposed on other areas
- Pertinent Gray's Anatomy (Gray. 1995. 698, 869, 871, 876, 1931)

Handouts
- Home exercise program
  ○ Stretching
    ▪ Hamstrings, especially biceps femoris
    ▪ Quadriceps
    ▪ Iliotibial band/tensor fasciæ latæ
    ▪ Gastrocnemius/soleus
    ▪ Hip flexors
  ○ Strengthening
    ▪ Squats
    ▪ Lunges—anterior, lateral, posterior, rotational
    ▪ Balance/reach
      a. Reaching with arms
      b. Reaching with opposite leg
    ▪ Step up/step down
- Home cryotherapy or contrast baths

Functional Considerations
- Avoidance of aggravating activities during acute phase
- Periodization of training
  ○ Alternating of "hard" and "easy" days
  ○ Importance of active rest
  ○ Changing terrain—soft vs. hard surfaces, slopes, hills, trails, camber of road
  ○ Cross-training options
  ○ Monitoring intensity of workout through log books
  ○ Frequency of competitions
- Footwear
  ○ Proper footwear for type of activity (e.g., no aerobic or cross-training shoes for running)
  ○ Replacing shoes every 6–9 months or 500–700 miles—see *Orthotics: Choosing the Right Shoe* guideline in Foot and Ankle section
  ○ Proper type of footwear for biomechanical needs (e.g., motion control vs. cushioning)
- Cross-training
  ○ Maintain current level of cardiovascular fitness without exacerbation of symptoms

Direct Interventions

Acute Phase: 2–4 Visits

- Therapeutic exercise and home program
  - Stretching
    - Hamstrings
    - Quadriceps
    - Gastrocnemius/soleus
    - Gluteals
    - Iliotibial band
    - Adductors
  - Strengthening
    - Partial squats
    - Strides
    - Lunges
      a. Anterior
      b. Lateral
    - Walking as tolerated
    - Upper body ergometer
  - Neuromuscular/balance/proprioceptive reeducation
    - BAPS
      a. Using handholds as needed, alternating direction and speed of rotation
    - Balance/reach
      a. Rotating and reaching to opposite side with arms at shoulder height or waist height as tolerated
      b. Reaching posteriorly with uninvolved leg
    - Gait drills
      a. Backward walking
      b. Balance beam walking, forward and backward
      c. Cariocas, alternating right and left leads
- Manual therapy techniques
  - Soft-tissue techniques
    - Soft-tissue mobilization to gluteus medius, tensor fasciæ latæ, or iliotibial band as appropriate
    - Friction massage as tolerated
  - Gentle, passive stretching to tight hamstrings, quadriceps, gastrocnemius, soleus, or iliotibial band within pain-free limitations using contract/relax or hold/relax techniques
- Electrotherapeutic modalities
  - Iontophoresis
- Physical agents and mechanical modalities
  - Pulsed or continuous ultrasound as appropriate for reduction of inflammation or deep heating prior to soft-tissue mobilization
  - Cryotherapy
- Goals/outcomes
  - Decrease inflammation as documented by reduction of edema, normalization of skin temperature, or decreased tenderness to palpation
  - Pain: 5/10 or less
  - Improve functional strength and neuromuscular/balance/proprioceptive ability as measured by increased distance on balance and reach tasks or lunges, or by improved coordination on BAPS
  - Flexibility
    - Thomas test showing 10° hip flexion and at least 50° knee flexion
    - Ankle dorsiflexion to at least 5° in subtalar neutral with knee extended and 10° with knee flexed
    - Ober test showing adduction of leg to within 3" of the plinth
    - Straight-leg raise test to at least 60°
    - Internal and external hip rotation to at least 20° as measured in 90° hip flexion

Subacute Phase: 3–6 Visits

- Therapeutic exercise and home program
  - Stretching
    - Sustained static stretching of all lower-extremity muscle groups as in acute stage
    - Dynamic stretching of hamstrings and gluteals
      a. High marching
      b. High kicks
  - Strengthening
    - Squats to 90° knee flexion as tolerated
    - Lunges
      a. Lateral rotation
      b. Posterior
      c. Posterolateral rotation
    - Step up/step down
      a. Progression to jump up/jump down as tolerated using 4", 6", 8", 12" step height as appropriate
    - Leg press
    - Leg extension
    - Leg curl
  - Agility drills
    - Shuttle runs
    - Carioca on stairs
    - Run and cut in all directions
    - Skipping
    - Backward running

92   Iliotibial Band Syndrome | Knee

○ Cardiovascular
 ▪ Stationary cycling: Using moderate resistance to achieve 75% of age-predicted maximum heart rate for 20–30 minutes, incorporating intervals, standing cycling, and unilateral work as appropriate
 ▪ Stair machine: Using multiple approaches and foot positions to enhance muscle performance and proprioception as well as cardiovascular muscle performance
   a. Backward
   b. Sideways
   c. Forward
 ▪ Fitness walking or walking/jogging: Initially only on level ground; progression to hills, uneven terrain, and intervals as appropriate
○ Neuromuscular/balance/proprioceptive reeducation
 ▪ BAPS minimizing handhold, using additional challenges of ball toss/catch, ball dribbling, tennis racquet drills, weight resistance, eyes closed, head movements, and speed or direction changes as appropriate
 ▪ Unilateral stance balance/reach drills
   a. Reaching with one or both hands to uninvolved side at waist height, knee height, or floor level as appropriate
   b. Reaching with uninvolved leg posteriorly toward involved side
• Manual therapy techniques
 ○ Deep soft-tissue mobilization or friction massage to gluteus medius, tensor fasciæ latæ, and iliotibial tract as indicated
 ○ Assisted stretching to all lower-extremity muscles as appropriate, using contract/relax and hold/relax techniques
• Therapeutic devices and equipment
 ○ Functional biomechanics
  ▪ Integration of specific structural or biomechanical components that may relieve symptoms, including the choice of shoes and/or custom biomechanical orthotics to control excessive compensatory pronation
• Physical agents and mechanical modalities
 ○ Cryotherapy as needed after activity
 ○ Deep or superficial thermal modalities as needed prior to manual therapy techniques

• Goals/outcomes
 ○ Resolution of inflammatory process as documented by elimination of tenderness to palpation
 ○ Pain: 0/10 for ADLs, 2/10 or less after activity
 ○ Strength equal to uninvolved side as measured by appropriate closed-kinetic chain functional test, such as lunges, balance/reach distance, or multidirectional unilateral hop test
 ○ Return to previous functional status for ADLs and vocational activities

Functional Carryover
• Importance of proper periodization of training, including intensity, frequency, and duration to avoid return of symptoms
• Importance of proper biomechanical support (i.e., shoes and/or orthotics to minimize excessive stress from inappropriate timing or amount of pronation)

DISCHARGE PLANNING AND PATIENT RESPONSIBILITY

Criteria for Discharge
• Patient displays understanding of principles of training to avoid recurrent symptoms
• Biomechanical factors that may have been instrumental in the onset of the original symptoms have been addressed appropriately
• All goals/outcomes have been met with the exception that the patient may not achieve full return to previous functional status for recreational and sports activities but shows signs of progression

Circumstances Requiring Additional Visits
• History of additional lower-extremity pathology
• Additional treatments may be needed to work intensely on passive iliotibial band-lengthening procedures if adequate gains are not made in the course of several visits

Home Program
• Explain stretching and strengthening exercises as described in Subacute Phase
• Stress importance of adequate warm-up and cool-down, as well as training principles, to reduce risk of future injury

KNEE | ILIOTIBIAL BAND SYNDROME   93

Monitoring

- Follow-up visits scheduled as needed to address any return of symptoms as patient progresses to previous functional level
- If patient was fitted with custom-molded, biomechanical orthotics, follow up with a phone call or visit as appropriate at 2-week and 4-week intervals to assess tolerance and response to device

REFERENCES

1. American Physical Therapy Association. *Guide to Physical Therapist Practice.* Alexandria, VA: APTA; 1997.
2. Donatelli R. *The Biomechanics of The Foot And Ankle.* Philadelphia, PA: FA Davis; 1990.
3. Gould JA, ed. *Orthopedic and Sports Physical Therapy.* St Louis, MO: CV Mosby; 1990.
4. Gray G. *Lower Extremity Functional Profile.* Adrian, MI: Wynn Marketing; 1995.
5. Gray H; Williams PL, ed. *Gray's Anatomy.* 38th ed. New York, NY: Churchill Livingstone; 1995.
6. Gross MT. Lower quarter screening for skeletal malalignment: suggestions for orthotics and shoewear. *J Orthop Sports Phys Ther.* 1995;21(6):389-405.
7. Hart A, Hopkins C, Ford B. *ICD-9-CM Expert For Physicians, Volume 1&2.* 7th ed. USA: Ingenix; 2005.
8. Holmes JC, Pruitt AL, Whalen NJ. Iliotibial band syndrome in cyclists. *Am J Sports Med.* 1993;21:419-424.
9. Hunter-Griffin LY, ed. *Athletic Training And Sports Medicine.* 2nd ed. Park Ridge, IL: American Academy of Orthopedic Surgeons; 1991.
10. Kendall FP, McCreary EK, Provance PG. *Muscles Testing and Function.* 4th ed. Baltimore, MD: Williams & Wilkins; 1993.
11. Muhle C, Ahn JM, Yeh L, et al. Iliotibial band friction syndrome: MR imaging findings in 16 patients and MR arthrographic study of six cadaveric knees. *Radiology.* 1999;212(1);103-110.
12. Nemeth WC, Sanders BL. The lateral synovial recess of the knee: anatomy and role in chronic iliotibial band friction syndrome. *Arthroscopy.* 1996;12:574-580.
13. Orchard JW, Fricker PA, Abud AT, Mason BR. Biomechanics of iliotibial band friction syndrome in runners. *Am J Sports Med.* 1996;24:375-379.
14. Powers CM, Maffucci R, Hampton S. Rearfoot posture in subjects with patellofemoral pain. *J Orthop Sports Phys Ther.* 1995;22(4):155-160.

KNEE ARTHROSCOPY
SUMMARY OVERVIEW

ICD-9

715.96   717.83   717.9   718.86   719.46   836.3   836.6

APTA Preferred Practice Pattern: **4B, 4C, 4D, 4E, 4F, 4G, 4I, 4J, 6B, 7A**

EXAMINATION

- History and Systems Review
- Tests and Measures
  Systems review per APTA's *Guide to Physical Therapy Practice*
  - Anthropometric measurements
  - Assistive and adaptive devices
  - Gait, locomotion, and balance
  - Joint integrity and mobility
  - Muscle performance
  - Pain
  - ROM
- Establish Plan of Care

GOALS/OUTCOMES

- Knee ROM: 0–135°
- Strength: 70% of uninvolved leg on one-repetition maximum leg press test or other closed-kinetic chain functional test, such as single-leg squat excursion or lunge distance. Manual muscle test: 4/5 quads, hams.
- Pain: 2/10 or less
- Normal gait pattern without assistive devices
- Pain-free, unassisted stair negotiation
- Return to previous functional status for ADLs and vocational, recreational, and sports activities as identified by patient
- Independence in a progressive home exercise program emphasizing function

INTERVENTION
NUMBER OF VISITS: 6–14

- Patient Instruction
  - Basic Anatomy and Biomechanics
  - Handouts
  - Functional Considerations
- Direct Interventions
  - Acute Phase: Protection, 1–2 Visits, Home Exercise Program, 3–7 Days
  - Subacute Phase I: Moderate Protection, 2–6 Visits
  - Subacute Phase II: Early Functional, 3–6 Visits
- Functional Carryover

DISCHARGE PLANNING AND PATIENT RESPONSIBILITY

- Criteria for Discharge
  - All subacute goals have been achieved
  - Minimal effusion is present
  - Patient displays competency with home program and progression toward previous functional status for recreational and sports activities
- Circumstances Requiring Additional Visits
  - History of additional lower-extremity pathology
  - Postoperative complications including ligamentous adhesions
  - Presence of other medical conditions
  - Ongoing extensor lag
  - Reflex sympathetic dystrophy as postoperative complication
  - Anticipated return to high-level athletics or heavy work
- Home Program
  - Flexibility exercises
  - Closed-kinetic chain strengthening progression
  - Fitness walking/running/other sports progression as appropriate
- Monitoring

SUMMARY OVERVIEW | KNEE | KNEE ARTHROSCOPY   95

KNEE ARTHROSCOPY

ICD-9

715.96	Osteoarthrosis, unspecified whether generalized or localized, lower leg
717.83	Old disruption of anterior cruciate ligament
717.9	Unspecified internal derangement of knee
718.86	Other joint derangement, not elsewhere classified, lower leg
719.46	Pain in joint, lower leg
836.3	Dislocation of patella, closed
836.6	Other dislocation of knee, open

APTA Preferred Practice Pattern: 4B, 4C, 4D, 4E, 4F, 4G, 4I, 4J, 6B, 7A

EXAMINATION

History and Systems Review

- History of current condition
  - Date of surgery, type of procedure
  - Postoperative rehab/complications
- Past history of current condition
  - Previous lower-extremity injuries
- Functional status and activity level (current/prior)
- Patient's functional goals

Tests and Measures

Systems review per APTA's *Guide to Physical Therapy Practice*

- Anthropometric measurements
  - Comparative girth measurements
- Assistive and adaptive devices
  - Crutch or cane fit
  - Ability to use device
- Gait, locomotion, and balance
  - Excessive or prolonged compensatory pronation
  - Patterns of compensation/limping
  - Weight-bearing status
  - Proprioceptive testing
    - Romberg
- Joint integrity and mobility
  - Patellar orientation relative to femur
  - Assessment of joint hypermobility/hypomobility (classification/grade)

- Muscle performance
  - Manual muscle test
  - Squatting
  - Step ups/step downs
  - Lunge tests in all directions
- Pain
  - Measured on visual analog scale
  - Type/classification
- ROM
  - Hip
  - Knee
  - Ankle

Establish Plan of Care

- Based on history, tests, and measures

GOALS/OUTCOMES

- Knee ROM: 0–135°
- Strength: 70% of uninvolved leg on one-repetition maximum leg press test or other closed-kinetic chain functional test, such as single-leg squat excursion or lunge distance. Manual muscle test: 4/5 quads, hams.
- Pain: 2/10 or less
- Normal gait pattern without assistive devices
- Pain-free, unassisted stair negotiation
- Return to previous functional status for ADLs and vocational, recreational, and sports activities as identified by patient
- Independence in a progressive home exercise program emphasizing function

INTERVENTION
NUMBER OF VISITS: 6–14

Coordination, Communication, and Documentation
- Provision of services between admission and discharge that facilitate cost-effective and efficient integration or reintegration to home, community, or work
- Documentation of therapeutic intervention is required for each episode of care and serves as the basic foundation for communication
- Coordination and additional communication will depend on the patient's impairment and home/work/community/leisure situation and requirements. Such services may include:
  - Case management
  - Coordination of care and collaboration with those integral to the patient's rehabilitation program
  - Coordination and monitoring of the delivery of available resources
  - Referrals to other health-care professionals
  - Identification of resources, support groups, or advocacy services
  - Provision of educational or training information
  - Technical assistance
- Specific coordination and communication provisions:
  - Referral for biomechanical orthotics

Patient Instruction

Basic Anatomy and Biomechanics
- Pertinent Gray's Anatomy (Gray. 1995. 697–708, 869–876)
- Importance of restoring normal lower-extremity muscle performance and patellar ROM for a normal gait pattern
- Biomechanical integration of the kinetic chain, including the importance of excessive or inadequate motion in one area contributing to the stress imposed on another area

Handouts
- Home exercise program
  - Motor performance
  - Flexibility

- Self-mobilization techniques
- Cryotherapy
- Krames Communications (1100 Grundy Lane, San Bruno, CA 94066)
  - *Understanding Arthroscopy*
  - *Knee Arthroscopy*
  - *After Arthroscopy*

Functional Considerations
- Amount of activity or walking appropriate given weight-bearing tolerance
- Proper positioning and positions to avoid during ADLs

Direct Interventions

Acute Phase: Protection, 1–2 Visits, Home Exercise Program, 3–7 Days
- Therapeutic exercise and home program
  - A/AROM and AROM with emphasis on extension
  - PROM
  - Quad sets
  - Straight-leg raises /resistive band exercises as tolerated
  - Ankle pumps
  - Weight shifting as appropriate to weight-bearing status
  - Mini squats as appropriate to weight-bearing status
- Manual therapy techniques
  - Joint mobilization
    - Patellar mobilization
    - Tibiofemoral mobilization
- Electrotherapeutic modalities
  - For pain/edema
- Physical agents and mechanical modalities
  - Cryotherapy, with cryo-cuff if available
- Goals/outcomes
  - ROM: 5–90°
  - Strength: No extensor lag of quadriceps
  - Pain: 3/10 or less
  - Functional activity
    - Ability to ambulate partial weight bearing—full weight bearing with assistive device as needed
    - Negotiate stairs with assistive device

KNEE | KNEE ARTHROSCOPY **97**

Subacute Phase I: Moderate Protection, 2–6 Visits

- Therapeutic exercise and home program
  - VMO sets in sitting
  - Stationary bicycle
  - Calf strengthening on isokinetic machine or resistive band
  - Leg press using light weight
  - Straight-leg raises in standing with resistive band, weight-bearing on both involved and uninvolved leg as appropriate
  - Lower-extremity flexibility exercises
  - Gait drills for neuromuscular/balance/proprioceptive reeducation as indicated by weight-bearing status
    - Backward walking
    - Side steps or carioca as appropriate
- Manual therapy techniques
  - Joint mobilization
    - Oscillatory mobilization for pain relief
    - Patellar mobilization
  - Passive lower-extremity stretching techniques
  - Soft-tissue mobilization, cross-fiber mobilization at incision
- Electrotherapeutic modalities
  - For edema
  - Muscle reeducation if quad control poor/fair using surface EMG
- Physical agents and mechanical modalities
  - Cryotherapy
- Goals/outcomes
  - ROM: 0–120°
  - Strength: Quadriceps motor performance 4-/5 of uninvolved extremity
  - Pain: 2/10 or less
  - Functional activity
    - Full weight bearing, normal gait pattern with assistive device as needed

Subacute Phase II: Early Functional, 3–6 Visits

- Therapeutic exercise and home program
  - VMO training in standing
  - Progressive resistance leg press
  - Standing heel raises
  - Step up/step down
  - Partial lunges in all directions
  - Neuromuscular/balance/proprioceptive reeducation
    - Gait drills
      a. Carioca

b. Balance beam walk, forward and backward
c. Toe walk
d. Heel walk
- Balance/reach activities: Unilateral stance balance on involved leg, reaching uninvolved leg in various directions to maximum distance
- BAPS: With additional challenges from varying directions and speed of rotation, eyes closed, or minimum handhold as appropriate
  - Stationary cycling for cardiovascular conditioning with additional challenges from unilateral cycling, speed, or resistance intervals as appropriate
- Manual therapy techniques
  - Joint mobilization as needed
- Therapeutic devices and equipment
  - Functional biomechanics
    - Integration of specific structural or biomechanical components that may relieve symptoms, including the choice of shoes and/or custom biomechanical orthotics to control excessive compensatory pronation
- Electrotherapeutic modalities
  - For any residual edema
- Physical agents and mechanical modalities
  - Cryotherapy
- Goals/outcomes
  - ROM: 0–135°
  - Strength: 70% of uninvolved leg on leg press or other closed-kinetic chain test, such as single-leg squat excursion or lunge distance
  - Pain: 2/10 or less
  - Functional activity
    - Unassisted, pain-free stair negotiation
    - Normal gait pattern without assistive device
    - Functional status and activity level (current/prior) for ADLs and vocational activities

Functional Carryover

- Educate patient on future knee care
  - Proper squatting technique
  - Managing flare-ups and effusion
  - Consideration of cross-training as a method to decrease articular loading
  - Need to continue maintenance rehabilitation home program
- Proper progression to return to recreational and sports activities, including recommendations on periodization

of intensity, frequency, and duration of training to minimize risk for future injury

DISCHARGE PLANNING AND PATIENT RESPONSIBILITY

Criteria for Discharge
- All subacute goals have been achieved
- Minimal effusion is present
- Patient displays competency with home program and progression toward previous functional status for recreational and sports activities

Circumstances Requiring Additional Visits
- History of additional lower-extremity pathology
- Postoperative complications including ligamentous adhesions
- Presence of other medical conditions
- Ongoing extensor lag
- Reflex sympathetic dystrophy as postoperative complication
- Anticipated return to high-level athletics or heavy work

Home Program
- Flexibility exercises
- Closed-kinetic chain strengthening progression
  - Squats
  - Lunges
    - Straight (anterior/posterior/lateral)
    - Rotational (rotating body to face direction of lunge)
  - Balance/reach
    - Straight, progressing to rotational
  - Step up/step down
    - Progressing height of step and distance from step as appropriate
  - Jumping, hopping, skipping, and cutting

- Fitness walking/running/other sports progression as appropriate

Monitoring
- One visit, depending upon the patient's individual needs for late-stage assessment of functional progression prior to beginning sport-specific activities

REFERENCES

1. American Physical Therapy Association. *Guide to Physical Therapist Practice.* Alexandria, VA: APTA; 1997.
2. Gray G. *Lower Extremity Functional Profile.* Adrian, MI: Wynn Marketing; 1995.
3. Gray H; Williams PL, ed. *Gray's Anatomy.* 38th ed. New York, NY: Churchill Livingstone; 1995.
4. Gross MT. Lower quarter screening for skeletal malalignment: suggestions for orthotics and shoewear. *J Orthop Sports Phys Ther.* 1995;21(6):389-405.
5. Hart A, Hopkins C, Ford B. *ICD-9-CM Expert For Physicians, Volume 1&2.* 7th ed. USA: Ingenix; 2005.
6. Levitt R, Deisinger JA, Remondet Wall J, Ford L, Cassisi JE. EMG feedback-assisted postoperative rehabilitation of minor arthroscopic knee surgeries. *J Sports Med Phys Fitness.* 1995;35:218-223.
7. Matthews P, St-Pierre DM. Recovery of muscle strength following arthroscopic meniscectomy. *J Ortho Sports Phys Ther.* 1997;23(1):18-26.
8. Nelson WE, Henderson RC, Hooker DN, Cross N. Isometric strength following knee arthroscopy. *Orthopedics.* 1996;19:501-504.
9. Wheatley WB, Krome J, Martin DF. Rehabilitation programmes following arthroscopic meniscectomy in athletes. *Sports Med.* 1996;21:447-456.
10. Whitelaw GP, DeMuth KA, Demos HA, Schepsis A, Jacques E. The use of the cryo/cuff versus ice and elastic wrap in the postoperative care of knee arthroscopy patients. *Am J Knee Surg.* 1995;8(1):28-30; discussion, 30-31.

KNEE CONTUSION
SUMMARY OVERVIEW

ICD-9

924.10   924.11

APTA Preferred Practice Pattern: **7B**

EXAMINATION

- History and Systems Review
- Tests and Measures
  Systems review per APTA's *Guide to Physical Therapy Practice*
  - Anthropometric characteristics
  - Assistive and adaptive devices
  - Circulation
  - Gait, locomotion, and balance
  - Integumentary integrity
  - Joint integrity and mobility
  - Muscle performance
  - Orthotics, protective and supportive devices
  - Pain
  - ROM
- Establish Plan of Care

GOALS/OUTCOMES

- Knee ROM: 0–135°
- Strength: 80% of uninvolved leg on one-repetition maximum leg press test or other closed-kinetic chain functional test, such as single-leg squat excursion or lunge distance. Manual muscle test: 4/5 quads, hams.
- Pain: 2/10 or less
- Normal gait pattern without any assistive device
- Pain-free, unassisted stair negotiation
- Return to previous functional status for ADLs and vocational, recreational, and sports activities as identified by patient
- Independence in a progressive home exercise program emphasizing function

INTERVENTION
NUMBER OF VISITS: 5–10

- Patient Instruction
  - Basic Anatomy and Biomechanics
  - Handouts
  - Functional Considerations
- Direct Interventions
  - Acute Phase: 1–4 Visits
  - Subacute Phase: 4–6 Visits
- Functional Carryover

DISCHARGE PLANNING AND PATIENT RESPONSIBILITY

- Criteria for Discharge
  - All subacute goals have been achieved
  - Minimal effusion is present
  - Patient displays competency with home program and progression toward previous functional status for recreational and sports activities
- Circumstances Requiring Additional Visits
  - History of additional lower-extremity pathology
  - Presence of other medical conditions
  - Ongoing extensor lag
  - Anticipated return to high-level athletics or heavy work
  - Severe degenerative changes
- Home Program
  - Flexibility exercises
  - Closed-kinetic chain strengthening progression
  - Fitness walking/running/other sports progression as appropriate
- Monitoring

KNEE CONTUSION

ICD-9

924.10   Contusion of lower leg
924.11   Contusion of knee

APTA Preferred Practice Pattern: **7B**

EXAMINATION

History and Systems Review

- History of current condition
  - Date of injury/onset
- Past history of current condition
  - Previous lower-extremity injury
- Other tests and measures
- Medications
- Past medical/surgical history
- Functional status and activity level (current/prior)
- Patient's functional goals

Tests and Measures

Systems review per APTA's *Guide to Physical Therapy Practice*

- Anthropometric characteristics
  - Comparative girth measurements
- Assistive and adaptive devices
  - Crutch or cane fit
  - Ability to use device
- Circulation (arterial, venous, lymphatic)
- Gait, locomotion, and balance
  - Patterns of compensation/limping
  - Weight-bearing status
  - Proprioceptive testing
- Integumentary integrity
- Joint integrity and mobility
  - Patellar orientation
  - Assessment of joint hypermobility/hypomobility (classification/grade)
- Muscle performance (including strength, power, and endurance)
  - Manual muscle test
  - Functional strength assessment including squatting, step up/step down, lunges, single-leg balance reach
- Orthotics, protective and supportive devices
- Pain
  - Measured on visual analog scale
  - Type and classification

- ROM (including muscle length)
  - Hip
  - Knee
  - Ankle

Establish Plan of Care

- Based on history, tests, and measures

GOALS/OUTCOMES

- Knee ROM: 0–135°
- Strength: 80% of uninvolved leg on one-repetition maximum leg press test or other closed-kinetic chain functional test, such as single-leg squat excursion or lunge distance. Manual muscle test: 4/5 quads, hams.
- Pain: 2/10 or less
- Normal gait pattern without any assistive device
- Pain-free, unassisted stair negotiation
- Return to previous functional status for ADLs and vocational, recreational, and sports activities as identified by patient
- Independence in a progressive home exercise program emphasizing function

INTERVENTION

NUMBER OF VISITS: 5–10

Coordination, Communication, and Documentation

- Provision of services between admission and discharge that facilitate cost-effective and efficient integration or reintegration to home, community, or work
- Documentation of therapeutic intervention is required for each episode of care and serves as the basic foundation for communication
- Coordination and additional communication will depend on the patient's impairment and home/work/community/leisure situation and requirements. Such services may include:
  - Case management
  - Coordination of care and collaboration with those integral to the patient's rehabilitation program

102   KNEE CONTUSION | KNEE

- Coordination and monitoring of the delivery of available resources
- Referrals to other health-care professionals
- Identification of resources, support groups, or advocacy services
- Provision of educational or training information
- Technical assistance
• Specific coordination and communication provisions

Patient Instruction

Basic Anatomy and Biomechanics
• Pertinent Gray's Anatomy (Gray. 1989. 437–447; 526–532)
• Importance or restoring normal lower-extremity muscle performance and patellar ROM for normal gait pattern
• Biomechanical integration of the kinetic chain, including the importance of excessive or inadequate motion in one area contributing to the stress imposed on another area

Handouts
• Commercially available products, such as:
  - Krames Communications (1100 Grundy Lane, San Bruno, CA 94066)
    ▪ *Knee Owner's Manual*
• Home program
  - Motor performance
  - Flexibility
• Cryotherapy
• Self-mobilization techniques

Functional considerations
• Amount of activity or walking appropriate given weight-bearing tolerance and irritability
• Proper positioning and positions to avoid during ADLs (including stairs, kneeling, and squatting)

Direct Interventions

Acute Phase: 1–4 Visits
• Manual therapy techniques as indicated
  - Joint mobilization
    ▪ Patellar mobilization
    ▪ Tibiofemoral mobilization
• Electrotherapeutic modalities
  - For pain/inflammation

• Physical agents and mechanical modalities
  - Cryotherapy, with cryo-cuff if available
• Therapeutic exercise and home program
  - Multi arc quad sets in sitting
  - Stationary bicycle
  - Calf strengthening on isokinetic machine or resistive bands
  - Leg press using light weight (could include Total Gym®/Shuttle)
  - 4-way hip in standing with resistive band weight bearing on both involved and uninvolved leg as appropriate
  - Lower-extremity flexibility exercises
  - Neuromuscular/balance/proprioceptive reeducation
• Goals/outcomes
  - ROM: 0–90°
  - Strength: No extensor lag of quadriceps
  - Pain: 3/10 or less
  - Functional activity
    ▪ Ability to ambulate full weight bearing without limp
    ▪ Negotiate stairs with assistive device

Subacute Phase: 4–6 Visits
• Manual therapy techniques
  - Joint mobilization
    ▪ Oscillatory mobilization for pain relief
    ▪ Patellar mobilization
  - Passive lower-extremity stretching techniques
• Electrotherapeutic modalities
  - For inflammation
  - Muscle reeducation if quad control poor/fair using surface EMG
• Physical agents and mechanical modalities
  - Cryotherapy
• Therapeutic devices and equipment
  - Functional biomechanics
    ▪ Integration of specific structural or biomechanical components that may relieve symptoms, including the choice of shoes and/or custom biomechanical orthotics to control excessive compensatory pronation
• Therapeutic exercise and home program
  - VMO training in standing
  - Progressive resistance leg press
  - Standing heel raises
  - Step up/step down

- Partial lunges in all directions
- Neuromuscular/balance/proprioceptive reeducation
  - Plyometric drills: Could include jumping and hopping activities)
  - Balance/reach activities: Unilateral stance balance on involved leg, reaching uninvolved leg in various directions to maximum distance
  - BAPS: With additional challenges from varying directions and speed of rotation, eyes closed, or minimum handhold as appropriate
- Stationary cycling for cardiovascular conditioning with additional challenges from unilateral cycling, speed, or resistance intervals as appropriate
- Return to running program

Functional Carryover
- Integration of home exercise program into vocational environment
- Completion of ergonomic adjustments to home, automobile, and vocational areas
- Incorporation of proper posture and body mechanics to avoid exacerbation of symptoms
- Recognition/avoidance of activities that increase or exacerbate radiating symptoms

DISCHARGE PLANNING AND PATIENT RESPONSIBILITY

Criteria for Discharge
- All subacute goals have been achieved
- Minimal effusion is present
- Patient displays competency with home program and progression toward previous functional status for recreational and sports activities

Circumstances Requiring Additional Visits
- History of additional lower-extremity pathology
- Presence of other medical conditions
- Ongoing extensor lag
- Anticipated return to high-level athletics or heavy work
- Severe degenerative changes

Home Program
- Flexibility exercises
- Closed-kinetic chain strengthening progression
  - Squats
  - Lunges

- Straight (anterior/posterior/lateral)
- Rotational (rotating body to face direction of lunge)
  - Balance/reach
    - Straight, progressing to rotational
  - Step up/step down
    - Progressing height of step and distance from step as appropriate
  - Jumping, hopping, skipping, and cutting
- Fitness walking/running/other sports progression as appropriate

Monitoring
- One visit, depending on the patient's individual needs for late-stage assessment of functional progression

REFERENCES
1. American Physical Therapy Association. *Guide to Physical Therapist Practice.* Alexandria, VA: APTA; revised 2003
2. Gray G. *Lower Extremity Functional Profile.* Adrian, MI: Wynn Marketing; 1995.
3. Gray H; Williams PL, ed. *Gray's Anatomy.* 37th ed. New York, NY: Churchill Livingstone; 1989.
4. Hart A, Hopkins C, Ford B. *ICD-9-CM Expert For Physicians, Volume 1&2.* 7th ed. USA: Ingenix; 2005.
5. Kessler R, Hertling D. *Management Of Common Musculoskeletal Disorders.* 1st ed. Philadelphia; Harper and Row; 1983.
6. Stratford PW, Spadoni G. The reliability, consistency and clinical application of a numeric pain rating scale. *Physiotherapy Canada.* 2001;53:88-91, 114.
7. Whitelaw GP, DeMuth KA, Demos HA, Schepsis A, Jacques E. The use of the cryo/cuff versus ice and elastic wrap in the postoperative care of knee arthroscopy patients. *Am J Knee Surg.* 1995;8(1):28-30; discussion, 30-31.

KNEE DEGENERATIVE JOINT DISEASE
SUMMARY OVERVIEW

ICD-9

715.96

APTA Preferred Practice Pattern: 4C, 4D, 4F, 4G, 4H, 4I, 4J, 6B

EXAMINATION

- History and Systems Review
- Tests and Measures
  Systems review per APTA's *Guide to Physical Therapy Practice*
  - Aerobic capacity
  - Anthropometric characteristics
  - Gait, locomotion, and balance
  - Joint integrity and mobility
  - Motor performance
  - Pain
  - Posture
  - ROM
- Establish Plan of Care

GOALS/OUTCOMES

- Pain: 2/10 or less
- Pain-free knee ROM of 5–120°, avoiding joint irritation
- Cardiovascular fitness through activities that do not exacerbate joint symptoms, such as swimming, upper-body ergometry, or aqua aerobics
- Functional muscle performance
- Independent, pain-free gait pattern on all surfaces with assistive devices as needed
- Return to previous functional status for ADLs and vocational, recreational, and sports activities as identified by patient
- Independence in a progressive home exercise program emphasizing function

INTERVENTION
NUMBER OF VISITS: 6–14

- Patient Instruction
  - Basic Anatomy and Biomechanics
  - Handouts
  - Functional Considerations
- Direct Interventions
  - Acute Phase: 1–4 Visits
  - Subacute Phase: 5–10 Visits
- Functional Carryover

DISCHARGE PLANNING AND PATIENT RESPONSIBILITY

- Criteria for Discharge
  - All goals/outcomes have been met with possible exceptions listed in guideline
- Circumstances Requiring Additional Visits
  - History of additional lower-extremity pathology
  - Lumbar pathology
  - Severe deconditioning
- Home Program
  - Patient is to continue exercises for strengthening and endurance at least 3 times a week
  - Patient is encouraged to start swimming and aquatic exercise program, if available, and to continue low-resistance cycling
  - Patient is advised to minimize stresses on knee joint by avoiding prolonged flexion, kneeling, and prolonged stooping activities (i.e., gardening, washing kitchen floor, etc.)
  - Patient is cautioned regarding climbing steep hills and steps
- Monitoring

KNEE DEGENERATIVE JOINT DISEASE

ICD-9

    715.96   Osteoarthrosis, unspecified whether generalized or localized, lower leg

APTA Preferred Practice Pattern: 4C, 4D, 4F, 4G, 4H, 4I, 4J, 6B

EXAMINATION

History and Systems Review

- History of current condition
  - Pain/stiffness proportional to activity/rest
- Past history of current condition
  - Previous lower-extremity injuries/surgeries
  - Treatments
- Functional status and activity level (current/prior)
- Patient's functional goals

Tests and Measures

Systems review per APTA's *Guide to Physical Therapy Practice*

- Aerobic capacity
- Anthropometric characteristics
  - Comparative girth measurement at knee joint center
- Gait, locomotion, and balance
  - Characteristics during sitting, standing
    - Stair negotiation
    - Footwear
    - Assistive devices
  - Mirror posturing
  - Balance/reach tests
    - Unilateral stance balance with simultaneous reaching of opposite leg in various directions, comparing distance reached with involved leg vs. uninvolved leg
- Joint integrity and mobility
  - Passive motion tests for flexion/extension to determine status of joint surfaces (such as crepitation)
- Motor performance
  - Squatting
  - Stairs
  - Kneeling
  - Climbing test
    - Standing with one foot on the table, the patient lunges further toward the table to test full range of flexion of the elevated extremity at the hip, knee, and ankle, plus extension of the opposite hip and knee

- Pain
  - Measured on visual analog scale
  - Classification of pain (sharp, dull, episodic, tight)
- Posture
  - Static stance position
  - General lower-extremity alignment
- ROM
  - Active
    - Bilaterally
      a. Hip
      b. Knee
      c. Ankle

Establish Plan of Care

- Based on history, tests, and measures

GOALS/OUTCOMES

- Pain: 2/10 or less
- Pain-free knee ROM of 5–120°, avoiding joint irritation
- Cardiovascular fitness through activities that do not exacerbate joint symptoms, such as swimming, upper-body ergometry, or aqua aerobics
- Functional muscle performance
  - Stair negotiation in a reciprocal fashion
  - Independent transfers to and from sitting
- Independent, pain-free gait pattern on all surfaces with assistive devices as needed
- Return to previous functional status for ADLs and vocational, recreational, and sports activities as identified by patient
- Independence in a progressive home exercise program emphasizing function

INTERVENTION
NUMBER OF VISITS: 6–14

Coordination, Communication, and Documentation

- Provision of services between admission and discharge that facilitate cost-effective and efficient integration or reintegration to home, community, or work
- Documentation of therapeutic intervention is required for each episode of care and serves as the basic foundation for communication
- Coordination and additional communication will depend on the patient's impairment and home/work/community/leisure situation and requirements. Such services may include:
  - Case management
  - Coordination of care and collaboration with those integral to the patient's rehabilitation program
  - Coordination and monitoring of the delivery of available resources
  - Referrals to other health-care professionals
  - Identification of resources, support groups, or advocacy services
  - Provision of educational or training information
  - Technical assistance
- Specific coordination and communication provisions:
  - Referral for biomechanical orthotics

Patient Instruction

Basic Anatomy and Biomechanics
- Pertinent Gray's Anatomy (Gray. 1995. 680–681, 697–704, 707–708, 876, 869)
- Importance of adequate joint ROM, muscle flexibility, and muscle performance in promoting proper gait and reducing excessive force on other areas of the lower quadrant

Handouts
- Home exercise program
  - Flexibility
  - Motor performance
  - Neuromuscular/balance/proprioceptive reeducation
- Home cryotherapy/thermal modalities

Functional Considerations
- Instruction regarding use of assistive devices as indicated
- Techniques to minimize joint loading during ADLs, such as stair techniques, ambulation on uneven terrain
- Sleeping positioning
- Modification of home environment as needed for discharge
- Diet modification instructions

Direct Interventions

Acute Phase: 1–4 Visits
- Therapeutic exercise and home program
  - Pain-free isometrics for quadriceps and hamstrings
  - PROM to AROM: ROM only if active ROM causes too much pain
  - Gentle passive stretching, including gastrocnemius/soleus
  - Aquatic exercises
- Manual therapy techniques
  - Manual assisted exercise
    - PROM in pain-free range
  - Joint mobilization
    - Long-axis distraction for pain relief
    - Patellar mobilization
- Electrotherapeutic modalities
  - Electrical stimulation
- Physical agents and mechanical modalities
  - Cryotherapy
- Goals/outcomes
  - ROM: 10–100°
  - Pain: 5/10 or less
  - Functional activity
    - Pain-free normal gait pattern for ADLs with assistive device as needed
  - Functional muscle performance
    - Independent transfers to and from sitting

Subacute Phase: 5–10 Visits
- Therapeutic exercise and home program
  - Active exercises for lower extremity—progress to strengthening in pain-free range with tubing, free weights, isokinetic, and closed-kinetic chain exercises
  - Aquatic therapy if available
  - Cycling
  - Elliptical trainer

KNEE | KNEE DEGENERATIVE JOINT DISEASE

- Stretching exercises for all muscle groups
- Neuromuscular/balance/proprioceptive reeducation
- BAPS
- Balance/reach
- Gait drills
- Manual therapy techniques
  - Joint mobilization
    - Patellar mobilization
    - Long-axis distraction for stretching and pain relief
    - Tibiofemoral mobilization
- Therapeutic devices and equipment
  - Functional biomechanics
    - Instruction in proper footwear choices to minimize biomechanical stresses from excessive or prolonged compensatory pronation
- Electrotherapeutic modalities
  - Electrical stimulation
- Physical agents and mechanical modalities
  - Ultrasound
  - Superficial thermal modalities for decreasing stiffness and promoting relaxation
- Goals/outcomes
  - ROM: 5–120°
  - Pain: 2/10 or less
  - Functional muscle performance
    - Stair negotiation
    - Retrieving objects from floor level
  - Maintaining cardiovascular fitness through activities that do not exacerbate joint symptoms, such as swimming, upper body ergometry, aquatic aerobics, elliptical trainer

Functional Carryover

- Continue ambulation as tolerated
- Use handrails for stairs if needed
- Use proper gait sequence for stairs
- Use proper body mechanics for ADLs, including lifting, pushing, pulling, and climbing

DISCHARGE PLANNING AND PATIENT RESPONSIBILITY

Criteria for Discharge

- All goals/outcomes have been met except:
  - Patient may not be able to retrieve objects from floor level without assistance
  - Patient may not have returned to previous status for recreational and sports activities

Circumstances Requiring Additional Visits

- History of additional lower-extremity pathology
- Lumbar pathology
- Severe deconditioning

Home Program

- Patient is to continue exercises for strengthening and endurance at least 3 times a week
- Patient is encouraged to start swimming and aquatic exercise program, if available, and to continue low-resistance cycling
- Patient is advised to minimize stresses on knee joint by avoiding prolonged flexion, kneeling, and prolonged stooping activities (i.e., gardening, washing kitchen floor)
- Patient is cautioned regarding climbing steep hills and steps

Monitoring

- Patient is to recheck/call after 2 weeks on home exercise program to ensure progression toward previous functional status for ADLs and vocational, recreational, and sports activity previously indicated

REFERENCES

1. American Physical Therapy Association. *Guide to Physical Therapist Practice.* Alexandria, VA: APTA; 1997.

2. Banwell BF, Gall V. *Physical Therapy Management Of Arthritis.* New York, NY: Churchill Livingston; 1987.

3. Cailliet R. *Knee Pain and Disability.* 2nd ed. Philadelphia, PA: FA Davis; 1983.

4. Deyle G, Henderson N, Matekel R, et al. Effectiveness of manual therapy and exercise in osteoarthritis of the knee. *Ann Intern Med.* 2000;132(3):173-81.

5. Gray G. *Lower Extremity Functional Profile.* Adrian, MI: Wynn Marketing; 1995.

6. Gray H; Williams PL, ed. *Gray's Anatomy.* 38th ed. New York, NY: Churchill Livingstone; 1995.

7. Gross MT. Lower quarter screening for skeletal malalignment: suggestions for orthotics and shoewear. *J Orthop Sports Phys Ther.* 1995;21(6):389-405.

8. Hart A, Hopkins C, Ford B. *ICD-9-CM Expert For Physicians, Volume 1&2.* 7th ed. USA: Ingenix; 2005.

9. Micholivitz SL. *Thermal Agents In Rehabilitation.* 2nd ed. Philadelphia, PA: FA Davis; 1986.

10. Powers CM, Maffucci R. Rearfoot posture in subjects with patellofemoral pain. *J Orthop Sports Phys Ther.* 1995;22(4):155-160.

11. Reid DC. *Sports Injury Assessment and Rehabilitation.* New York, NY: Churchill Livingstone; 1992.

12. Thomas K, Muir K, Doherty M, et al. Home based exercise program for knee pain and knee osteoarthritis: randomized controlled trial. *BMJ.* 2002;325:752.

KNEE ENTHESOPATHY
SUMMARY OVERVIEW

ICD-9

726.6

APTA Preferred Practice Pattern: 4E, 4D, 4I

EXAMINATION
- History and Systems Review
- Tests and Measures
  Systems review per APTA's *Guide to Physical Therapy Practice*
  - Anthropometric characteristics
  - Assistive and adaptive devices
  - Circulation
  - Gait, locomotion, and balance
  - Integumentary integrity
  - Joint integrity and mobility
  - Muscle performance
  - Orthotics, protective and supportive devices
  - Pain
  - Posture
- Establish Plan of Care

GOALS/OUTCOMES
- Knee ROM: 0–135°
- Strength: 70% of uninvolved leg on one-repetition maximum leg press test or other closed-kinetic chain functional test, such as single-leg squat excursion or lunge distance. Manual muscle test: 4/5 quads, hams.
- Pain: 2/10 or less
- Normal gait pattern without any assistive device
- Pain-free, unassisted stair negotiation
- Return to previous functional status for ADLs and vocational, recreational, and sports activities
- Independence in a progressive home exercise program emphasizing function

INTERVENTION
NUMBER OF VISITS: 5–10

- Patient Instruction
  - Basic Anatomy and Biomechanics
  - Handouts
  - Functional Considerations
- Direct Interventions
  - Acute Phase: 2–4 Visits
  - Subacute Phase: 3–6 Visits
- Functional Carryover

DISCHARGE PLANNING AND PATIENT RESPONSIBILITY
- Criteria for Discharge
  - All subacute goals have been achieved
  - Minimal effusion is present
  - Patient displays competency with home program and progression toward previous functional status for recreational and sports activities
- Circumstances Requiring Additional Visits
  - History of additional lower-extremity pathology
  - Presence of other medical conditions
  - Ongoing extensor lag
  - Anticipated return to high-level athletics or heavy work
  - Severe degenerative changes
- Home Program
  - Flexibility exercises
  - Closed-kinetic chain strengthening progression
  - Fitness walking/running/other sports progression as appropriate
- Monitoring

KNEE ENTHESOPATHY

ICD-9
> 726.6   Enthesopathy of knee

APTA Preferred Practice Pattern: 4E, 4D, 4I

EXAMINATION

History and Systems Review
- History of current condition
  - Date of injury/onset
- Past history of current condition
  - Previous lower-extremity injury
- Other tests and measures
- Medications
- Past medical/surgical history
- Functional status and activity level (current/prior)
- Patient's functional goals

Tests and Measures
Systems review per APTA's *Guide to Physical Therapy Practice*
- Anthropometric characteristics
  - Comparative girth measurement
- Assistive and adaptive devices
  - Crutch or cane fit
  - Ability to use device
- Circulation (arterial, venous, lymphatic)
- Gait, locomotion, and balance
  - Patterns of compensation/limping
  - Weight-bearing status
  - Proprioceptive testing
- Integumentary integrity
- Joint integrity and mobility; assess for hypermobilty, hypomobility, crepitis, and instability
  - Patellar orientation and mobility
  - Tibia femoral glides and conjunct rotation at end ranges
  - Proximal and distal tibia fibula glides
- Muscle performance (including strength, power, endurance, and length)
  - Manual muscle test (hip, knee, and ankle)
  - Functional strength assessment including squatting, step up/step down, lunges, single-leg balance reach
- Orthotics, protective and supportive devices
- Pain
  - Measured on visual analog scale

- Type and classification
- Posture
  - Static stance
    - Relaxed calcaneal position
    - Forefoot position
  - General lower-extremity alignment
    - Genu varus/valgus
  - Specific foot alignment
    - Rearfoot varus
    - Forefoot varus/valgus
- ROM (including muscle length)
  - Hip
  - Knee
  - Ankle

Establish Plan of Care
- Based on history, tests, and measures

GOALS/OUTCOMES
- Knee ROM: 0–135°
- Strength: 70% of uninvolved leg on one-repetition maximum leg press test or other closed-kinetic chain functional test, such as single-leg squat excursion or lunge distance. Manual muscle test: 4/5 quads, hams.
- Pain: 2/10 or less
- Normal gait pattern without any assistive device
- Pain-free, unassisted stair negotiation
- Return to previous functional status for ADLs and vocational, recreational, and sports activities as identified by patient
- Independence in a progressive home exercise program emphasizing function

INTERVENTION

NUMBER OF VISITS: 5–10

Coordination, Communication, and Documentation

- Provision of services between admission and discharge that facilitate cost-effective and efficient integration or reintegration to home, community, or work
- Documentation of therapeutic intervention is required for each episode of care and serves as the basic foundation for communication
- Coordination and additional communication will depend on the patient's impairment and home/work/ community/leisure situation and requirements. Such services may include:
  - Case management
  - Coordination of care and collaboration with those integral to the patient's rehabilitation program
  - Coordination and monitoring of the delivery of available resources
  - Referrals to other health-care professionals
  - Identification of resources, support groups, or advocacy services
  - Provision of educational or training information
  - Technical Assistance
- Specific coordination and communication provisions

Patient Instruction

Basic Anatomy and Biomechanics

- Pertinent Gray's Anatomy (Gray. 1989. 437–447; 526–532)
- Importance of restoring normal lower-extremity muscle performance and patellar ROM for normal gait pattern
- Biomechanical integration of the kinetic chain, including the importance of excessive or inadequate motion in one area contributing to the stress imposed on another area

Handouts

- Commercially available products, such as:
  - Krames Communications (1100 Grundy Lane, San Bruno, CA 94066)
    - *Knee Owner's Manual*
- Home program
  - Motor performance
  - Flexibility
- Cryotherapy
- Self-mobilization techniques

Functional Considerations

- Amount of activity or walking appropriate given weight-bearing tolerance and irritability
- Proper positioning and positions to avoid during ADLs (including stairs, kneeling, and squatting)

Direct Interventions

Acute Phase: 2–4 Visits

- Manual therapy techniques as indicated
  - Joint mobilization
    - Patellar mobilization
    - Tibiofemoral mobilization
- Electrotherapeutic modalities
  - For pain/inflammation
- Physical agents and mechanical modalities
  - Cryotherapy, with cryo-cuff if available
- Therapeutic exercise and home program
  - Multi arc quad sets in sitting
  - Stationary bicycle
  - Calf strengthening on isokinetic machine or resistive bands
  - Leg press using light weight (could include Total Gym®/Shuttle)
  - 4-way hip in standing with resistive band weight-bearing on both involved and uninvolved leg as appropriate
  - Lower-extremity flexibility exercises
  - Neuromuscular/balance/proprioceptive reeducation
- Goals/outcomes
  - ROM: 0–90°
  - Strength: no extensor lag of quadriceps
  - Pain: 3/10 or less
  - Functional activity
    - Ability to ambulate full weight bearing without limp
    - Negotiate stairs with assistive device

Subacute Phase: 3–6 Visits

- Manual therapy techniques
  - Joint mobilization
    - Oscillatory mobilization for pain relief
    - Patellar mobilization
  - Passive lower-extremity stretching techniques
  - Soft-tissue mobilization, cross-fiber mobilization
- Electrotherapeutic modalities
  - For inflammation
  - Muscle reeducation if quad control poor/fair using surface EMG

KNEE | KNEE ENTHESOPATHY   113

- Physical agents and mechanical modalities
  - Cryotherapy
- Therapeutic devices and equipment
  - Functional biomechanics
    - Integration of specific structural or biomechanical components that may relieve symptoms, including the choice of shoes and/or custom biomechanical orthotics to control excessive compensatory pronation
- Therapeutic exercise and home program
  - VMO training in standing
  - Progressive resistance leg press
  - Standing heel raises
  - Step up/step down
  - Partial lunges in all directions
  - Neuromuscular/balance/proprioceptive reeducation
    - Plyometric drills: Could include jumping and hopping activities)
    - Balance/reach activities: Unilateral stance balance on involved leg, reaching uninvolved leg in various directions to maximum distance
    - BAPS: With additional challenges from varying directions and speed of rotation, eyes closed, or minimum handhold as appropriate
  - Stationary cycling for cardiovascular conditioning with additional challenges from unilateral cycling, speed, or resistance intervals as appropriate
  - Return to running program

Functional Carryover

- Integration of home exercise program into vocational environment
- Completion of ergonomic adjustments to home, automobile, and vocational areas
- Incorporation of proper posture and body mechanics to avoid exacerbation of symptoms
- Recognition/avoidance of activities that increase or exacerbate radiating symptoms

DISCHARGE PLANNING AND PATIENT RESPONSIBILITY

Criteria for Discharge

- All subacute goals have been achieved
- Minimal effusion is present
- Patient displays competency with home program and progression toward previous functional status for recreational and sports activities

Circumstances Requiring Additional Visits

- History of additional lower-extremity pathology
- Presence of other medical conditions
- Ongoing extensor lag
- Anticipated return to high-level athletics or heavy work
- Severe degenerative changes

Home Program

- Flexibility exercises
- Closed-kinetic chain strengthening progression
  - Squats
  - Lunges
    - Straight (anterior/posterior/lateral)
    - Rotational (rotating body to face direction of lunge)
  - Balance/reach
    - Straight, progressing to rotational
  - Step up/step down
    - Progressing height of step and distance from step as appropriate
  - Jumping, hopping, skipping, cutting
- Fitness walking/running/other sports progression as appropriate

Monitoring

- One visit, depending upon the patient's individual needs for late-stage assessment of functional progression

REFERENCES

1. American Physical Therapy Association. *Guide to Physical Therapist Practice*. Alexandria, VA: APTA; revised 2003.

2. Gray G. *Lower Extremity Functional Profile*. Adrian, MI: Wynn Marketing; 1995.

3. Gray H; Williams PL, ed. *Gray's Anatomy*. 37th ed. New York, NY: Churchill Livingstone; 1989.

4. Hart A, Hopkins C, Ford B. *ICD-9-CM Expert For Physicians, Volume 1&2*. 7th ed. USA: Ingenix; 2005.

5. Kessler R, Hertling D. *Management of Common Musculoskeletal Disorders*. 1st ed. Philadelphia; Harper and Row; 1983

6. Sperryn, PN. ABC of sports medicine: overuse injury in sport. *BMJ*. May 28, 1994;308:1430-32.

7. Stratford PW, Spadoni G. The reliability, consistency and clinical application of a numeric pain rating scale. *Physiotherapy Canada*. 2001;53:88-91, 114.

8. Whitelaw GP, DeMuth KA, Demos HA, Schepsis A, Jacques E. The use of the cryo/cuff versus ice and elastic wrap in the postoperative care of knee arthroscopy patients. *Am J Knee Surg*. 1995;8(1):28-30; discussion, 30-31.

KNEE HYPOMOBILITY/INFRAPATELLAR CONTRACTURE SYNDROME (IPCS)

SUMMARY OVERVIEW

ICD-9

718.56   719.56   844.0

APTA Preferred Practice Pattern: 4A, 4B, 4E, 4H, 4I, 4J

EXAMINATION

- History and Systems Review
- Tests and Measures
  Systems review per APTA's *Guide to Physical Therapy Practice*
  - Gait, locomotion, and balance
  - Joint integrity
  - Muscle performance
  - Pain
  - Special tests
- Establish Plan of Care

GOALS/OUTCOMES

- Pain: 2/10 or less
- Normal patellar passive mobility
- Normal ROM
- Strength: No extensor lag of quadriceps and 70% of uninvolved leg on leg press or other closed-kinetic chain functional test
- Normal gait pattern without assistive devices on all surfaces
- Return to previous functional status for ADLs and vocational and recreational activities as identified by patient
- Independence in a progressive home exercise program emphasizing function

INTERVENTION
NUMBER OF VISITS: 6–14

- Patient Instruction
  - Basic Anatomy and Biomechanics
  - Handouts
  - Functional Considerations
- Direct Interventions
  - Acute Phase: 2–6 Visits
  - Subacute Phase: 4–8 Visits
  - Chronic Phase
- Functional Carryover

DISCHARGE PLANNING AND PATIENT RESPONSIBILITY

- Criteria for Discharge
  - Patient shows good understanding and performance of home exercise program
  - All rehabilitation goals have been achieved with the exception of return to previous functional status for recreational activities
- Circumstances Requiring Additional Visits
  - History of additional lower-extremity pathology
  - Postoperative complications
  - Surgical debridement performed at any stage during treatment will result in additional care
- Home Program
  - Ongoing active and passive stretches for maintaining patellofemoral joint ROM and overall knee ROM, especially extension
  - Comprehensive lower-extremity strengthening
  - Neuromuscular/balance/proprioceptive exercises
  - Flexibility exercises
- Monitoring

KNEE HYPOMOBILITY/INFRAPATELLAR CONTRACTURE SYNDROME (IPCS)

ICD-9
> 718.56 Ankylosis of joint, lower leg
> 719.56 Stiffness of joint, not elsewhere classified, lower leg
> 844.0 Sprain of lateral collateral ligament of knee

APTA Preferred Practice Pattern: 4A, 4B, 4E, 4H, 4I, 4J

The following protocol addresses resultant knee hypomobility from Infrapatellar Contracture Syndrome (IPCS), an unfortunate but not uncommon result of knee surgery, particularly intraarticular ligament reconstruction. This is a unique subgroup of patients. The purpose of this guideline is to enable the clinician to recognize the syndrome and manage it effectively.

EXAMINATION

History and Systems Review
- History of current condition
  - Stiffness and pain
  - Date and type of surgical procedure
  - Postoperative progression and treatment
    - Transitions in weight-bearing status
    - Complications
- Past history of current condition
  - Previous lower-extremity injuries or surgeries
- Functional status and activity level (current/prior)
- Patient's functional goals

Tests and Measures
Systems review per APTA's *Guide to Physical Therapy Practice*
- Gait, locomotion, and balance
  - Antalgic gait
  - Assistive devices
- Joint integrity and mobility
  - Key is loss of knee extension
  - Patellar ROM
  - Usually restricted in all directions, especially in superior glide
  - Passive patellar tilt restricted
    - Lateral border is parallel or actually posterior to transcondylar plane
- Muscle performance
  - Quadricep inhibition
    - Inability to actively perform a quad set

- Pain
  - Measured on visual analog scale
  - Type, classification
- Special tests
  - "Shelf sign" present
    - Induration of infrapatellar tissue extends to distal attachment of patellar tendon and results in abrupt step off, or "shelf"

Establish Plan of Care
- Based on history, tests, and measures

GOALS/OUTCOMES
- Pain: 2/10 or less
- Normal patellar passive mobility
- Normal ROM:
  - Knee: 0–135°
  - Ankle: 10° dorsiflexion in subtalar neutral with knee extended
- Strength: No extensor lag of quadriceps and 70% of uninvolved leg on leg press or other closed-kinetic chain functional test
- Normal gait pattern without assistive devices on all surfaces
- Return to previous functional status for ADLs and vocational and recreational activities as identified by patient
- Independence in a progressive home exercise program emphasizing function

INTERVENTION
NUMBER OF VISITS: 6–14

Coordination, Communication, and Documentation

- Provision of services between admission and discharge that facilitate cost-effective and efficient integration or reintegration to home, community, or work
- Documentation of therapeutic intervention is required for each episode of care and serves as the basic foundation for communication
- Coordination and additional communication will depend on the patient's impairment and home/work/community/leisure situation and requirements. Such services may include:
  - Case management
  - Coordination of care and collaboration with those integral to the patient's rehabilitation program
  - Coordination and monitoring of the delivery of available resources
  - Referrals to other health-care professionals
  - Identification of resources, support groups, or advocacy services
  - Provision of educational or training information
  - Technical assistance
- Specific coordination and communication provisions:
  - Referral back to physician for possible manipulation if no results with treatment

Patient Instruction

Basic Anatomy and Biomechanics
- Pertinent Gray's Anatomy (Gray. 1995. 697–708, 869, 876)
- Explanation of the role of patellar ROM in normal knee function

Handouts
- Commercially available products, such as:
  - Krames Communications (1100 Grundy Lane, San Bruno, CA 94066)
    - *Knee Owner's Manual*
- Home exercise program
  - Quadriceps strengthening
  - Gastrocnemius/soleus stretching
  - Patellar self-mobilization

Functional Considerations
- Amount of activity appropriate for the patient's weight-bearing tolerance and gait pattern and the irritability of injury
- Functional progression regarding stairs, varied terrain, vigor of loading (walking vs. running vs. jumping), and home exercises

Direct Interventions

Acute Phase: 2–6 Visits
- Therapeutic exercise and home program
  - A/PROM for extension
  - Quad sets
  - Hamstring and gastrocnemius stretches
  - Self-mobilization for patellar ROM
- Manual therapy techniques
  - Joint mobilization
    - Patellar mobilization
    - Oscillatory mobilization for pain relief
  - Passive hamstring stretching
- Electrotherapeutic modalities
  - TENS
  - Biofeedback for quad reeducation
- Physical agents and mechanical modalities
  - Biofeedback for quadriceps training/strengthening
  - Pulsed ultrasound to infrapatellar fat pack region
- Goals/outcomes
  - ROM:
    - Knee: 5° knee extension
    - Ankle: 5° dorsiflexion in subtalar neutral with knee extended
  - Strength: No extensor lag of quadriceps
  - Pain: 6/10 or less

Subacute Phase: 4–8 Visits
- Therapeutic exercise and home program
  - Strengthening exercises should be performed in the available range so as not to perpetuate inflammation
  - Progress from open- to closed-kinetic chain exercises in pain-free range
    - Squats
    - Lunges
    - Step up/step down
    - Lower-extremity stretching
    - Neuromuscular/balance/proprioceptive exercises

KNEE | KNEE HYPOMOBILITY/INFRAPATELLAR CONTRACTURE SYNDROME   119

- Manual therapy techniques
  - Joint mobilization
    - Progressive patellar mobilization
    - Progress to Grade III–IV knee mobilization with emphasis on extension
  - Passive lower quadrant stretches as indicated
- Therapeutic devices and equipment
  - Postoperative use of extension splint at night if debridement was performed
- Physical agents and mechanical modalities
  - As in Acute Phase
- Goals/outcomes
  - ROM:
    - Knee: 0–135°
    - Ankle: 10° dorsiflexion in subtalar neutral with knee extended
  - Strength: 70% of uninvolved leg on leg press or other closed-kinetic chain functional test
  - Pain: 2/10 or less
  - Normal patellar ROM
  - Independent gait pattern on all surfaces and stairs
  - Return to previous functional status for ADLs and vocational activities

Chronic Phase

- Patient has history of multiple surgeries, with persistent motion loss in extension and flexion, residual knee arthrosis, or both resulting in moderate to severe impairment
- Vigorous physical therapy may fail to achieve gains in these patients because of the associated arthrosis
- Additional surgery will be reserved for pain control and confined to "salvage" procedures
- Goals/outcomes
  - Attain subacute goals

Functional Carryover

- Patient must incorporate exercises to restore patellar ROM and knee extension into his or her daily routine in Phase I and II
- Specific attention should be paid to low-intensity, long-duration exercises done for short intervals frequently throughout the day
- Future exercises/recreational activities may need to be selected based on low patellofemoral joint loading if residual problems occur, such as cycling rather than running, etc.

DISCHARGE PLANNING AND PATIENT RESPONSIBILITY

Criteria for Discharge

- Patient shows good understanding and performance of home exercise program
- All rehabilitation goals have been achieved with the exception of return to previous functional status for recreational activities

Circumstances Requiring Additional Visits

- History of additional lower-extremity pathology
- Postoperative complications
- Surgical debridement performed at any stage during treatment will result in additional care

Home Program

- Ongoing active and passive stretches for maintaining patellofemoral joint ROM and overall knee ROM, especially extension
- Comprehensive lower-extremity strengthening
- Neuromuscular/balance/proprioceptive exercises
- Flexibility exercises

Monitoring

- Expect phone follow-up by patient at 4–6 weeks to assure progression and continued healing
- Patient is to recheck/call at 6 months and 1 year post-discharge to ensure progression toward previous functional status for ADLs and vocational, sports, and recreational activities

REFERENCES

1. American Physical Therapy Association. *Guide to Physical Therapist Practice*. Alexandria, VA: APTA; 1997.

2. Ellen MI, Jackson HB, DiBiase SJ. Uncommon causes of anterior knee pain: a case report of infrapatellar contracture syndrome. *Am J Phys Med Rehabil.* 1999;78;376-380.

3. Gray H; Williams PL, ed. *Gray's Anatomy.* 38th ed. New York, NY: Churchill Livingstone; 1995.

4. Hart A, Hopkins C, Ford B. *ICD-9-CM Expert For Physicians, Volume 1&2.* 7th ed. USA: Ingenix; 2005.

5. Irrgang JJ, Harner CD. Loss of motion following knee ligament reconstruction. *Sports Med.* 1995;19;150-159.

6. Paulos LE, Rosenberg TD, Drawbert J, Manning J, Abbott P. Infrapatellar contracture syndrome: an unrecognized cause of knee stiffness with patellar entrapment and patella infera. *Am J Sports Med.* 1987;15:331-341.

7. Peacock EE. Some biochemical and biophysical aspects of joint stiffness of the knee: role of collagen synthesis as opposed to altered molecular bonding. *Ann Surg.* 1966;164:1-12.

8. Petshe TS, Hutchinson MR. Loss of extension after reconstruction of the anterior cruciate ligament. *J Am Acad Orthop Surg.* 1999;7(2):119-127.

9. Shelbourne KD, Patel DV, Martini DJ. Classification and management of arthrofibrosis of the knee after anterior cruciate ligament reconstruction. *Am J Sports Med.* 1996;24:857-862.

10. Shelbourne KD, Wilckens JH, Mollabashy A, DeCarlo M. Arthrofibrosis in acute anterior cruciate ligament reconstruction: the effect of timing of reconstruction and rehabilitation. *Am J Sports Med.* 1991;19:332-336.

11. Sprague N, O'Connor R, Fox J. Arthroscopic treatment of postoperative knee fibroarthrosis. *Clin. Orthop.* 1982;166:165-172.

122   KNEE HYPOMOBILITY/INFRAPATELLAR CONTRACTURE SYNDROME | KNEE

KNEE SPRAIN/STRAIN
SUMMARY OVERVIEW

ICD-9

844.0   844.1   844.8   844.9

APTA Preferred Practice Pattern: 4D, 4E, 4J

EXAMINATION

- History and Systems Review
- Tests and Measures
  Systems review per APTA's *Guide to Physical Therapy Practice*
  - Anthropometric characteristics
  - Gait, locomotion, and balance
  - Joint integrity and mobility
  - Motor performance
  - Pain
  - Posture
  - Special tests
- Establish Plan of Care

GOALS/OUTCOMES

- Pain: 2/10 or less
- Edema to less than 1 cm difference on girth measurements
- Full, pain-free ROM of 0–135° or equivalent to uninvolved leg
- Strength: 70% of uninvolved leg on leg press or other closed-kinetic chain test, such as single-leg squat excursion or lunge distance
- Return to previous functional status for ADLs and vocational, recreational, and sports activities as identified by patient
- Normal gait pattern without assistive devices
- Independence in a progressive home exercise program emphasizing function

INTERVENTION
NUMBER OF VISITS: 5–12

- Patient Instruction
  - Basic Anatomy and Biomechanics
  - Handouts
  - Functional Considerations
- Direct Interventions
  - Acute Phase: 1–3 Visits
  - Subacute Phase: 4–9 Visits
- Functional Carryover

DISCHARGE PLANNING AND PATIENT RESPONSIBILITY

- Criteria for Discharge
  - Patient has achieved all subacute goals
  - Patient demonstrates independence in a progressive home exercise program emphasizing function
- Circumstances Requiring Additional Visits
  - Positive stress tests
  - History of additional lower-extremity pathology
  - Difficulty in regaining knee extension may require additional visits for manual therapy procedures
- Home Program
  - Patient should be cautioned in returning to activities involving high-load or abrupt and uncontrolled change in direction for 6–12 months
  - Functional strengthening progression
  - Flexibility
- Monitoring

SUMMARY OVERVIEW | KNEE | KNEE SPRAIN/STRAIN   123

KNEE SPRAIN/STRAIN

ICD-9

844.0	Sprain of lateral collateral ligament of knee
844.1	Sprain of medial collateral ligament of knee
844.8	Sprain of other specified sites of knee and leg
844.9	Sprain of unspecified site of knee and leg

APTA Preferred Practice Pattern: 4D, 4E, 4J

EXAMINATION

History and Systems Review

- History of current condition
  - Date of onset
  - Mechanism of injury
- Past history of current condition
  - Previous injuries/surgeries to lower quarter
- Past medical/surgical history
  - Tuberculosis
  - Gonorrhea
  - Ulcerative colitis
  - Reiter's syndrome
  - Ankylosing spondylitis
  - Gout
- Functional status and activity level (current/prior)
- Patient's functional goals

Tests and Measures

Systems review per APTA's *Guide to Physical Therapy Practice*

- Anthropometric characteristics
  - Leg length in supine, long sitting, and standing
  - Comparative girth measurements
- Gait, locomotion, and balance
  - Assistive devices
  - Stance phase weight-bearing
  - Stride length symmetry
  - Arm swing
  - Pelvic symmetry
  - Excessive or prolonged compensatory pronation
  - Weight shift
  - BAPS as appropriate to degree of sprain
  - Balance/reach test
    - Unilateral stance balance, reaching with opposite leg
    - Unilateral stance balance, reaching with arms

- Joint integrity and mobility
  - Stress tests

    These primarily indicate ligamentous lesions but can implicate all restraining structures; results must correlate with other objective findings. For further detail, consult *Sports Injury Assessment and Rehabilitation* (Reid. 1992. 451–475).

    All tests below are performed with patient supine. Attention is given to: Excessive motion, end feel
    - Medial stress test

      Thigh relaxed, valgus force applied to lateral knee
      a. In full extension
      b. In 30° of flexion
    - Lateral stress test

      As above, varus force to medial knee
      a. In full extension
      b. In 30° of flexion
    - Anterior stress test

      Attempt to pull tibia anteriorly on femoral condyles
      a. Anterior drawer—knee in 80–90° flexion
      b. Lachman—knee in 20–30° flexion
    - Posterior stress test
      a. Posterior drawer: Push tibia posteriorly with knee in 80–90° flexion
      b. Godfrey test: Assure that tibial tuberosities are equally positioned with knee in 80–90° flexion. A posterior cruciate ligament-deficient knee will relax in a "sagged" position (tibial tuberosities posteriorly positioned relative to uninvolved knee).

- Motor performance
  - Squatting
  - Kneeling
  - Climbing
    - Standing with one foot on the table, the patient lunges further toward the table to test full range of flexion of the elevated extremity at the hip, knee, and ankle, plus extension of the opposite hip and knee
  - Hopping
- Pain
  - Measured on visual analog scale
- Posture
  - Static, nonweight-bearing alignment of hip, knee, and subtalar and midtarsal joints
  - Static stance position
    - Genu varus/valgus/recurvatum
- Special tests
  - McMurray
  - Apley
  - Pivot shift
  - Patellar ROM

Establish Plan of Care
- Based on history, tests, and measures

GOALS/OUTCOMES
- Pain: 2/10 or less
- Edema to less than 1 cm difference on girth measurements
- Full, pain-free ROM of 0–135° or equivalent to uninvolved leg
- Strength: 70% of uninvolved leg on leg press or other closed-kinetic chain test, such as single-leg squat excursion or lunge distance
- Return to previous functional status for ADLs and vocational, recreational, and sports activities as identified by patient
- Normal gait pattern without assistive devices
- Independence in a progressive home exercise program emphasizing function

INTERVENTION
NUMBER OF VISITS: 5–12

Coordination, Communication, and Documentation
- Provision of services between admission and discharge that facilitate cost-effective and efficient integration or reintegration to home, community, or work
- Documentation of therapeutic intervention is required for each episode of care and serves as the basic foundation for communication
- Coordination and additional communication will depend on the patient's impairment and home/work/community/leisure situation and requirements. Such services may include:
  - Case management
  - Coordination of care and collaboration with those integral to the patient's rehabilitation program
  - Coordination and monitoring of the delivery of available resources
  - Referrals to other health-care professionals
  - Identification of resources, support groups, or advocacy services
  - Provision of educational or training information
  - Technical assistance

Patient Instruction

Basic Anatomy and Biomechanics
- Location and function of involved structures
- Pertinent Gray's Anatomy (Gray. 1995. 698–704, 707–708, 869, 876)
- History of current condition and importance of protection of healing structures
- Importance of adequate ROM and proper biomechanical alignment of all joints in kinetic chain to reduce stress on involved knee

Handouts
- Home cryotherapy/thermal modalities
- Home exercise program
  - Flexibility
  - Motor performance
  - Gait training with assistive device and immobilizer

KNEE | KNEE SPRAIN/STRAIN   125

Functional Considerations

- Instruction in use of immobilizer
- Education regarding amount of walking appropriate to level of injury

Direct Interventions

Acute Phase: 1–3 Visits

Primary focus: Control inflammation and effusion

- Therapeutic exercise and home program
  Utilization of knee immobilizer until 90° flexion is achieved
  - Stretching in pain-free range
    - Gentle AROM
      a. Heel slides
      b. Supine wall slides
    - Static stretching
      a. Hamstrings
      b. Quadriceps
      c. Gastrocnemius and soleus
      d. Psoas
      e. Gluteals
  - Strengthening (without immobilizer, as tolerated)
    - Isometrics for quadriceps and hamstrings
    - Short arc quads
    - Straight-leg raises; 4-directional as appropriate
  - Aquatic therapy
- Manual therapy techniques
  - Joint mobilization
    - Patellar mobilization
  - Soft-tissue techniques
    - Soft-tissue mobilization
    - Friction massage
- Electrotherapeutic modalities
  - Electrical stimulation
- Physical agents and mechanical modalities
  - Cryotherapy
  - Elevation and compressive bandage/immobilizer
- Goals/outcomes
  - ROM: 5–90°
  - Strength: A minimum of 3/5 on manual muscle test
  - Pain: 4/10 or less
  - Independent, normal gait pattern with crutches, minimal weight-bearing until full pain-free knee extension

Subacute Phase: 4–9 Visits

Primary focus: Control forces; increase ROM, muscle performance, and flexibility

- Therapeutic exercise and home program
  - Strengthening
    - Straight-leg raises with free weights or tubing
    - Vastus medialis oblique strengthening
    - Proprioceptive neuromuscular facilitation
    - Leg press: Bilateral and unilateral
    - Modified squats
    - Heel raises
    - Isokinetic strengthening
    - Hamstring strengthening
  - Cardiovascular
    - Stationary cycling
    - Elliptical
    - Aquatic therapy
    - Treadmill
  - Neuromuscular/balance/proprioceptive reeducation
    - Tilt board/balance board
    - BAPS
    - One-legged standing
  - Continue flexibility program for all muscle groups
- Manual therapy techniques
  - Soft-tissue techniques
    - Friction massage at site of lesion (contraindicated if lesion is at proximal attachment of medial collateral ligament, as Pellagrin-Stein Syndrome may develop)
  - Joint mobilization for normal osteokinematics, including patellar mobilization as needed
- Electrotherapeutic modalities
  - Electrical stimulation as needed for edema
- Physical agents and mechanical modalities
  - Ultrasound
  - Superficial thermal modalities for increased blood flow for the medial collateral ligament
  - Cryotherapy for edema as needed
- Goals/outcomes
  - ROM: Pain-free 0–135°
  - Strength: 70% of uninvolved leg on leg press or other closed-kinetic chain test, such as single-leg squat excursion or lunge distance
  - Pain: 2/10 or less
  - Return to previous functional status for ADLs and vocational activities
  - Unassisted, normal gait pattern

Functional Carryover

- May resume normal activity level as pain subsides and motion returns
- Functional activities
  - Start sport-specific training
  - May need functional bracing depending on level of injury or per physician preference
  - May ambulate full weight bearing when full knee extension against gravity is obtained

DISCHARGE PLANNING AND PATIENT RESPONSIBILITY

Criteria for Discharge

- Patient has achieved all subacute goals
- Patient demonstrates independence in a progressive home exercise program emphasizing function

Circumstances Requiring Additional Visits

- Positive stress tests
- History of additional lower-extremity pathology
- Difficulty in regaining knee extension may require additional visits for manual therapy procedures

Home Program

- Patient should be cautioned in returning to activities involving high-load or abrupt and uncontrolled change in direction for 6–12 months
- Functional strengthening progression
- Flexibility

Monitoring

- Schedule phone calls or follow-up visits as needed to ensure return to previous functional status for recreational and sports activities

REFERENCES

1. American Physical Therapy Association. *Guide to Physical Therapist Practice.* Alexandria, VA: APTA; 1997.
2. Beard DJ, Dodd CA, Trundle HR, Simpson AH. Proprioception enhancement for anterior cruciate deficiency: a randomized trial of two physiotherapy regimes. *J Bone Joint Surg Br.* 1994;76:654-659.
3. Beckrath K, Wooden C, Worrell T, Ingersoll CD, Farr J. Effects of patella taping on patella position and perceived pain. *Med Sci Sports Exerc.* 1993;25:989-992.
4. Gray G. *Lower Extremity Functional Profile.* Adrian, MI: Wynn Marketing; 1995.
5. Gray H; Williams PL, ed. *Gray's Anatomy.* 38th ed. New York, NY: Churchill Livingstone; 1995.
6. Gryzlo SM, Patek RM, Pink M, Perry J. Electromyographic analysis of knee rehabilitation exercises. *J Orthop Sports Phys Ther.* 1994;20(1):36-43.
7. Hart A, Hopkins C, Ford B. *ICD-9-CM Expert For Physicians, Volume 1&2.* 7th ed. USA: Ingenix; 2005.
8. Kannus P, Jarvinen M. Thigh muscle function after partial tear of the medial ligament compartment of the knee. *Med Sci Sports Exerc.* 1991;23:4-9.
9. Kessler RM, Hertling D. Management of common musculoskeletal disorders: physical therapy principles and methods. Philadelphia, PA: JB Lippincott; 1983.
10. Noyes F, Paulos L, Mooar L, Signaer B. Knee sprains and acute knee hemarthrosis. *Phys Ther.* 1980;60(12):1596-1601.
11. Noyes F, Grood E, Butter D, Raterman L. Knee ligament tests. *Phys Ther.* 1980;60:1578-1581.
12. Noyes F, Paulos L, Mooar L, Signaer B. Knee sprains and acute knee hemarthrosis. *Phys Ther.* 1980;60:1596-1601.
13. Nyland J, Brosky T, Currier D, Nitz A, Caborn D. Review of the afferent neural system of the knee and its contribution to motor learning. *J Orthop Sports Phys Ther.* 1994;19(1):2-11.
14. Pickard MA, Venner RM, Ford I, Todd BD. The influence of immediate physiotherapy in the out-patient management of acute knee injuries: a controlled study. *Arch Emerg Med.* 1990;7:249-252.
15. Reid DC. Sports injury assessment and rehabilitation. New York, NY: Churchill Livingstone; 1992.
16. Reider B, Sathy MR, Talkington J, Blyznak N, Kollias S. Treatment of isolated medial collateral ligament injuries in athletes with early functional rehabilitation: a five-year follow-up study. *Am J Sports Med.* 1994;22:470-477.
17. Whitelaw GP Jr, Rullo DJ, Markowitz HD, Marandola MS, DeWaele MJ. A conservative approach to anterior knee pain. *Clin Orthop Rel Res.* 1989;246:234-237.
18. Yack HJ, Collins CE, Whieldon TJ. Comparison of closed and open kinetic chain exercise in the anterior cruciate deficient knee. *Am J Sports Med.* 1993;21:49-54

128   KNEE SPRAIN/STRAIN | KNEE

MENISCAL REPAIR
SUMMARY OVERVIEW

ICD-9

717.0   717.1   717.2   717.3   717.4   717.5   717.9   836.0   836.1
836.2

APTA Preferred Practice Pattern: 4E, 4I, 4J

EXAMINATION

- History and Systems Review
- Tests and Measures
  Systems review per APTA's *Guide to Physical Therapy Practice*
  - Anthropometric characteristics
  - Gait, locomotion, and balance
  - Motor function
  - Pain
  - ROM
- Establish Plan of Care

GOALS/OUTCOMES

- Pain: 2/10 or less
- AROM of involved knee: 0–120° or equivalent to uninvolved leg
- Normal gait pattern without assistive device
- Strength: 70% of uninvolved leg as measured on a closed-kinetic chain test, such as leg press or other functional test
- Return to previous functional status for ADLs and vocational, recreational, and sports activities as identified by patient
- Neuromuscular/balance/proprioceptive ability: 90% of uninvolved leg as measured by single leg stance time on dynamic surface, such as foam or rock board
- Independence in a progressive home exercise program emphasizing function

INTERVENTION
NUMBER OF VISITS: 6–13

- Patient Instruction
  - Basic Anatomy and Biomechanics
  - Handouts
  - Functional Considerations
  - Description of Surgical Procedure
- Direct Interventions
  - Phase I: Maximal Protection, 1–4 Visits, Weeks 1–2
  - Phase II: Moderate Protection, 2–4 Visits, Weeks 3–4
  - Phase III: Light Activity, 1–2 Visits, Weeks 5–12
  - Phase IV: Return to Activity, 2–3 Visits, Weeks 13–24
- Functional Carryover

DISCHARGE PLANNING AND PATIENT RESPONSIBILITY

- Criteria for Discharge
  - Patient has achieved all subacute goals
  - Patient demonstrates independence in a progressive home exercise program emphasizing function
- Circumstances Requiring Additional Visits
  - History of additional lower-extremity pathology
  - Postoperative complications
  - Presence of other medical conditions
  - Anticipated return to high-level athletics or heavy work requirements
- Home Program
  - Patient shows progression toward recreation/sport-specific activities as appropriate
- Monitoring

SUMMARY OVERVIEW | KNEE | MENISCAL REPAIR   129

MENISCAL REPAIR

ICD-9

717.0	Old bucket handle tear of medial meniscus
717.1	Derangement of anterior horn of medial meniscus
717.2	Derangement of posterior horn of medial meniscus
717.3	Other and unspecified derangement of medial meniscus
717.4	Derangement of lateral meniscus
717.5	Derangement of meniscus, not elsewhere classified
717.9	Unspecified internal derangement of knee
836.0	Tear of medial cartilage or meniscus of knee, current
836.1	Tear of lateral cartilage or meniscus of knee, current
836.2	Other tear of cartilage or meniscus of knee, current

APTA Preferred Practice Pattern: 4E, 4I, 4J

EXAMINATION

History and Systems Review
- History of current condition
  - Surgical procedure and date
    - Complications
- Past history of current condition
  - Previous injuries/surgeries to lower extremities
- Functional status and activity level (current/prior)
- Patient's functional goals

Tests and Measures
Systems review per APTA's *Guide to Physical Therapy Practice*

All meniscal tests are contraindicated in the presence of surgical repair.
- Anthropometric characteristics
  - Comparative girth measurement at joint line
- Gait, locomotion, and balance
  - Assistive devices
- Motor function
  - Quad and hamstring tone/inhibition
  - Hip muscle function
- Pain
  - Measured on visual analog scale
  - Type/classification

- ROM
  - Knee A/PROM
  - Patellar PROM
  - Muscle length
    - Psoas
    - Quadriceps
    - Hamstrings
    - Gastroc/soleus
    - Tensor fasciæ latæ/iliotibial band

Establish Plan of Care
- Based on history, tests, and measures

GOALS/OUTCOMES
- Pain: 2/10 or less
- AROM of involved knee: 0–120° or equivalent to uninvolved leg
- Normal gait pattern without assistive device
- Strength: 70% of uninvolved leg as measured on a closed-kinetic chain test, such as leg press or other functional test
- Return to previous functional status for ADLs and vocational, recreational, and sports activities as identified by patient
- Neuromuscular/balance/proprioceptive ability: 90% of uninvolved leg as measured by single leg stance time on dynamic surface, such as foam or rock board
- Independence in a progressive home exercise program emphasizing function

130   MENISCAL REPAIR | KNEE

INTERVENTION

NUMBER OF VISITS: 6–13

Coordination, Communication, and Documentation

- Provision of services between admission and discharge that facilitate cost-effective and efficient integration or reintegration to home, community, or work
- Documentation of therapeutic intervention is required for each episode of care and serves as the basic foundation for communication
- Coordination and additional communication will depend on the patient's impairment and home/work/community/leisure situation and requirements. Such services may include:
  - Case management
  - Coordination of care and collaboration with those integral to the patient's rehabilitation program
  - Coordination and monitoring of the delivery of available resources
  - Referrals to other health-care professionals
  - Identification of resources, support groups, or advocacy services
  - Provision of educational or training information
  - Technical assistance

Patient Instruction

Basic Anatomy and Biomechanics

- Triplanar biomechanical function of the knee and the role of the meniscus as a stabilizer
- Role of proper biomechanical alignment of the foot in function of the knee
- Pertinent Gray's Anatomy (Gray. 1995. 697–708, 869, 876)

Handouts

- Home cryotherapy/thermal modalities
- Home exercise program appropriate to phase of recovery

Functional Considerations

- Use of appropriate ambulatory aides to reduce limping, improve stance stability, and reduce stress on involved extremity

- Instruction regarding stair climbing techniques, gait pattern on uneven terrain, and progression/return to sports
- Instruction regarding proper choice of footwear to minimize excessive or prolonged compensatory pronation and enhance stability

Description of Surgical Procedure

- Review of operative procedure in relation to joint biomechanics, rehabilitation, and function

Direct Interventions

Phase I: Maximal Protection, 1–4 Visits, Weeks 1–2

- Therapeutic exercise and home program
  - AROM as tolerated
  - Submaximal isometrics
    - Quadriceps
    - Hip abductors
    - Hip adductors
    - Hamstrings
    - Hip extensors
  - Gait training, weight bearing as tolerated
- Manual therapy techniques
  - PROM in tolerated range
  - Joint mobilization
    - Patellar mobilization
  - Soft-tissue techniques
    - Gentle scar massage of incisions after 10 days to prevent adhesions
- Electrotherapeutic modalities
  - Electrical stimulation for edema reduction, muscle reeducation, and pain control
- Physical agents and mechanical modalities
  - Cryotherapy
- Goals/outcomes
  - Knee ROM: 0–110°
  - Strength
    - Quadriceps and hamstrings, 4/5 on manual muscle test
    - 0° quad lag
  - Pain: 1/10 or less at rest
  - Functional activity
    - Nonweight-bearing gait pattern with assistive device
    - Independent transfers
    - Stair negotiation with assistive device

KNEE | MENISCAL REPAIR   131

Phase II: Moderate Protection, 2–4 Visits, Weeks 3–4

- Therapeutic exercise and home program
  - Straight-leg raises with free weights or surgical tubing
  - Unilateral leg press with minimal resistance
  - Partial squats
  - Vastus medialis oblique training
  - Stationary bicycle
  - Swimming
- Manual therapy techniques
  - Joint mobilization
    - Tibiofemoral mobilization
    - Patellar mobilization
  - Soft-tissue techniques
    - Scar mobilization
- Electrotherapeutic modalities
  - Electrical stimulation for edema, quad reeducation, pain
- Physical agents and mechanical modalities
  - Cryotherapy
- Goals/outcomes
  - Knee ROM: 0–130°
  - Strength: Quadriceps and hamstrings, 4+/5
  - Pain
    - 0/10 at rest
    - 2/10 or less after light activity
  - Functional activity
    - Full-weight-bearing gait pattern
    - Progression in neuromuscular/balance/proprioceptive training

Phase III: Light Activity, 1–2 Visits, Weeks 5–12

- Therapeutic exercise and home program
  - Flexibility exercises for all lower-extremity muscle groups
    - Gastrocnemius/soleus
    - Quadriceps
    - Hamstrings
    - Gluteals
    - Psoas
  - Strengthening
    - Isotonic progressive resistive exercises
    - Functional exercises
      a. Squats
      b. Lunges
      c. Step up/step down
    - Endurance training on cycle

- Walking (if ROM is within normal limits)
  - Neuromuscular/balance/proprioceptive reeducation
    - BAPS
    - Balance/reach
      a. Unilateral stance balancing with simultaneous reaching of uninvolved leg in all directions
      b. Unilateral stance balancing with simultaneous reaching of one or both arms in all directions
- Manual therapy techniques
- Goals/outcomes
  - Strength: 70% of uninvolved leg as measured on a closed-kinetic chain test, such as leg press or other functional test
  - Neuromuscular/balance/proprioception: 70% of uninvolved leg as measured by single leg stance time

Phase IV: Return to Activity, 2–3 Visits, Weeks 13–24

- Therapeutic exercise and home program
  - Minimal motor performance maintenance program is 3 times per week
  - If running is a desired activity, then jog/walk program is initiated and increased up to 1½ miles over a three-week period
  - If sprinting is a desired goal, an orderly progression is followed
  - Once sprinting is tolerated, then cutting and twisting movements can be added in the form of carioca, Figure 8, circle running, and cutting
- Goals/outcomes
  - Pain-free active ROM: 0–135° or equivalent to uninvolved leg
  - Pain
    - 0/10 for ADLs
    - 2/10 or less with activity
  - Strength: 90% of uninvolved leg as measured on a closed-kinetic chain test, such as leg press or other functional test
  - Normal gait pattern without assistive device
  - Return to previous functional status for ADLs and vocational activities

Functional Carryover

- Emphasize maintenance as a prophylactic against further joint damage
- Guide the patient into cross-training activities for aerobic conditioning vs. a steady regimen of running

DISCHARGE PLANNING AND PATIENT RESPONSIBILITY

Criteria for Discharge
- Patient has achieved all subacute goals
- Patient demonstrates independence in a progressive home exercise program emphasizing function

Circumstances Requiring Additional Visits
- History of additional lower-extremity pathology
- Postoperative complications
- Presence of other medical conditions
- Anticipated return to high-level athletics or heavy work requirements

Home Program
- Patient shows progression toward recreation/sport-specific activities as appropriate

Monitoring
- Patient is to recheck/call at 2 weeks post-discharge to ensure progression toward previous functional status for ADLs and vocational, recreational, and sports activities

REFERENCES

1. American Physical Therapy Association. *Guide to Physical Therapist Practice.* Alexandria, VA: APTA; 1997.
2. Barber FA, Click SD. Meniscus repair rehabilitation with concurrent ACL reconstruction. *Arthroscopy.* 1997;13:433-437.
3. Barber FA, Stone RG. Meniscal repair: an arthroscopic technique. *J Bone Joint Surg.* 1985;67(8):39-41.
4. Gray H; Williams PL, ed. *Gray's Anatomy.* 38th ed. New York, NY: Churchill Livingstone; 1995.
5. Hart A, Hopkins C, Ford B. *ICD-9-CM Expert For Physicians, Volume 1&2.* 7th ed. USA: Ingenix; 2005.
6. Kohn D, Aagaard H, Verdonk R, Dienst M, Seil R. Postoperative follow-up and rehabilitation after meniscus replacement. *Scand J Med Sci Sports.* 1999;9(3):177-180.
7. Marianni PP, Santori N, Adriani E, Mastantuono M. Accelerated rehabilitation after arthroscopic meniscal repair: a clinical and MRI evaluation. *Arthroscopy.* 1996;12:680-686.
8. Shelborune KD, Patel DV, Adsit WS, Porter DA. Rehabilitation after meniscal repair. *Clin Sports Med.* 1996;15:595-612.

MENISCUS TEAR (WITHOUT SURGERY)
SUMMARY OVERVIEW

ICD-9

717.0   717.1   717.2   717.3   717.4   717.5   717.9   836.0   836.1
836.2

APTA Preferred Practice Pattern: 4I, 4D, 4H

EXAMINATION

- History and Systems Review
- Tests and Measures
  Systems review per APTA's *Guide to Physical Therapy Practice*
  - Anthropometric characteristics
  - Gait, locomotion, and balance
  - Joint integrity and mobility
  - Ligamentous stability tests
  - Motor function
  - Muscle length
  - Orthotics, protective and supportive devices
  - Pain
  - Palpation
  - ROM
- Establish Plan of Care

GOALS/OUTCOMES

- Pain: 2/10 or less
- Knee AROM: 0–135° or equal to non-involved
- Normal gait pattern without assistive device
- Strength: 85% of uninvolved leg as measured on a closed-kinetic chain test, such as leg press or other functional test, no extensor lag
- Neuromuscular/balance/proprioceptive ability: 90% of uninvolved leg as measured by single leg stance time
- Return to previous functional status for ADLs and vocational, recreational, and sports activities as identified by patient
- Independence in a progressive home exercise program emphasizing function

INTERVENTION
NUMBER OF VISITS: 5–12

- Patient Instruction
  - Basic Anatomy and Biomechanics
  - Handouts
  - Functional Considerations
- Direct Interventions
  - Acute Phase: 3–6 Visits
  - Subacute Phase: 2–6 Visits
- Functional Carryover

DISCHARGE PLANNING AND PATIENT RESPONSIBILITY

- Criteria for Discharge
  - Patient has achieved all subacute goals
  - Patient demonstrates independence in a progressive home exercise program emphasizing function
- Circumstances Requiring Additional Visits
  - Severe degenerative changes
  - History of other pathology
  - Presence of other medical conditions
  - Cognitive limitations
  - Anticipated return to high-level athletics or heavy work requirements
- Home Program
  - Patient instructed in progression toward recreation/ sport-specific activities as appropriate given time of sports season
  - Patient instructed in progressive return to full ADLs and/or vocational duties
- Monitoring

MENISCUS TEAR (WITHOUT SURGERY)

ICD-9

717.0	Old bucket handle tear of medial meniscus
717.1	Derangement of anterior horn of medial meniscus
717.2	Derangement of posterior horn of medial meniscus
717.3	Other and unspecified derangement of medial meniscus
717.4	Derangement of lateral meniscus
717.5	Derangement of meniscus, not elsewhere classified
717.9	Unspecified internal derangement of knee
836.0	Tear of medial cartilage or meniscus of knee, current
836.1	Tear of lateral cartilage or meniscus of knee, current
836.2	Other tear of cartilage or meniscus of knee, current

APTA Preferred Practice Pattern: 4I, 4D, 4H

EXAMINATION

History and Systems Review

- History of current condition
- Past history of current condition
- Other tests and measures
- Medications
- Past medical/surgical history
- Functional status and activity level (current/prior)
- Patient's functional goals

Tests and Measures

Systems review per APTA's *Guide to Physical Therapy Practice*

- Anthropometric characteristics
  - Girth at joint line, 5–6" superior and inferior to joint line
  - Observation of edema or joint effusion
  - Muscle atrophy
- Gait, locomotion, and balance
  - Assistive devices
  - Star test for balance
- Joint integrity and mobility
  - Patellar tracking and stability
  - McMurray's test
- Ligamentous stability tests: ACL, PCL, LCL, MCL
- Motor function (motor control and motor learning)
  - Quad and hamstring tone and inhibition
  - Muscle performance (including strength, power, and endurance)
  - Hip rotators and abductors, calf

- Muscle length
  - Psoas, quadriceps, hamstrings, gastrocsoleus, ITB
- Orthotics, protective and supportive devices
  - Braces, foot orthotics
- Pain
  - Measured on visual analog
- Palpation including joint line and MCL
- ROM
  - Knee A/PROM
  - Patellar PROM
  - Ankle dorsiflexion

Establish Plan of Care

- Based on history, tests, and measures

GOALS/OUTCOMES

- Pain: 2/10 or less
- Knee AROM: 0–135° or equal to non-involved
- Normal gait pattern without assistive device
- Strength: 85% of uninvolved leg as measured on a closed-kinetic chain test, such as leg press or other functional test, no extensor lag
- Neuromuscular/balance/proprioceptive ability: 90% of uninvolved leg as measured by single leg stance time
- Return to previous functional status for ADLs and vocational, recreational, and sports activities as identified by patient
- Independence in a progressive home exercise program emphasizing function

INTERVENTION
NUMBER OF VISITS: 5–12

Coordination, Communication, and Documentation

- Provision of services between admission and discharge that facilitate cost-effective and efficient integration or reintegration to home, community, or work
- Documentation of therapeutic intervention is required for each episode of care and serves as the basic foundation for communication
- Coordination and additional communication will depend on the patient's impairment and home/work/community/leisure situation and requirements. Such services may include:
  - Case management
  - Coordination of care and collaboration with those integral to the patient's rehabilitation program
  - Coordination and monitoring of the delivery of available resources
  - Referrals to other health-care professionals
  - Identification of resources, support groups, or advocacy services
  - Provision of educational or training information
  - Technical assistance
- Specific coordination and communication provisions
  - Communication of athlete's return to participation status with school certified athletic trainer, coach, or athletic director

Patient Instruction

Basic anatomy and biomechanics

- Use skeletal model to assist in description of anatomy and function of meniscus and ligaments of the knee joint.

Handouts

- Home program: VHI home program instructions
- Precautions to avoid reinjury, joint protection guidelines
- Guidelines for application of heat, tape, brace, orthotics
- Pertinent clinical information

Functional considerations

- Posture (sitting, standing, sleeping, driving)
- Assistive devices (crutches, canes, walkers, collars, tape, etc.)
- Precautions
- Alteration of ADLs
- Body mechanic instruction for lifting, pushing, pulling, etc.
- Training recommendations (cross training, periodization, etc.)

Direct Interventions

Acute Phase: 3–6 Visits

- Therapeutic exercise and home program
  - AROM as tolerated
  - Gait training, weight bearing as tolerated
  - Straight-leg raises with free weights or surgical tubing
  - Unilateral leg press with minimal resistance
  - Partial squats
  - Vastus medialis oblique training
  - Stationary bicycle
  - Swimming or other aquatic therapy
- Manual therapy techniques
  - PROM in tolerated range
  - Joint mobilization
    - Mobilizations with movements for flexion and/or extension loss
  - Soft-tissue techniques
    - Edema reduction for joint effusion or peripatellar edema
- Electrotherapeutic modalities
  - Electrical stimulation for edema reduction, muscle reeducation, and pain control
- Physical agents and mechanical modalities
  - Cryotherapy
- Goals/outcomes
  - Knee ROM: 0–125°
  - Strength
    - Quadriceps and hamstrings: 4/5 on manual muscle test
    - 0° quad lag
  - Pain: 3/10 or less at rest
  - Functional activity
    - Partial to full weight-bearing gait pattern
    - Stair negotiation with handrail

KNEE | MENISCUS TEAR (WITHOUT SURGERY) 137

Subacute Phase: 2–6 Visits

- Therapeutic exercise and home program
  - Flexibility exercises for all lower-extremity muscle groups
    - Gastrocnemius/soleus
    - Quadriceps
    - Hamstrings
    - ITB
    - Psoas
  - Strengthening
    - Functional exercises
      a. Squats
      b. Lunges
      c. Step up/step down
    - Endurance training on cycle, elliptical machine
    - Walking
  - Neuromuscular/balance/proprioceptive reeducation
    - BAPS, Fitter
    - Balance/reach
      a. Unilateral stance balancing with simultaneous reaching of uninvolved leg in all directions
      b. Unilateral stance balancing with simultaneous reaching of one or both arms in all directions, incorporate ocular and vestibular component via head turning and eye closure
  - If running is a desired activity, then jog/walk program is initiated and increased up to 1½ miles over a 3-week period
  - If sprinting is a desired goal, an orderly progression is followed
  - Once sprinting is tolerated, then cutting and twisting movements can be added in the form of carioca, Figure 8, circle running, and cutting
- Manual therapy techniques
- Goals/outcomes
  - Pain-free active ROM: 0–135° or equivalent to uninvolved leg
  - Pain
    - 0/10 for ADLs
    - 2/10 or less with activity
  - Strength: 90% of uninvolved leg as measured on a closed-kinetic chain test, such as leg press or other functional test
  - Normal gait pattern without assistive device

- Return to previous functional status for ADLs and vocational activities
  - Neuromuscular/balance/proprioception: 90% of uninvolved leg as measured by single leg stance time

Functional Carryover

- Guide the patient into cross-training activities for aerobic conditioning vs. a steady regimen of running
- Integration of home exercise program into vocational environment
- Completion of ergonomic adjustments to home, automobile, and vocational areas
- Incorporation of proper posture and body mechanics to avoid exacerbation of symptoms
- Recognition/avoidance of activities that increase or exacerbate radiating symptoms

DISCHARGE PLANNING AND PATIENT RESPONSIBILITY

Criteria for Discharge

- Patient has achieved all subacute goals
- Patient demonstrates independence in a progressive home exercise program emphasizing function

Circumstances Requiring Additional Visits

- Severe degenerative changes
- History of other pathology
- Presence of other medical conditions
- Cognitive limitations
- Anticipated return to high-level athletics or heavy work requirements

Home Program

- Patient instructed in progression toward recreation/sport-specific activities as appropriate given time of sports season
- Patient instructed in progressive return to full ADLs and/or vocational duties

Monitoring

- Patient is to recheck/call at two weeks post-discharge to ensure progression toward previous functional status for ADLs and vocational, recreational, and sports activities

REFERENCES

1. American Physical Therapy Association. *Guide to Physical Therapist Practice.* Alexandria, VA: APTA; revised 2003.

2. Musnick, D, Pierce, M. *Conditioning For Outdoor Fitness.* The Mountaineers: Seattle, WA; 1999.

3. Hart A, Hopkins C, Ford B. *ICD-9-CM Expert For Physicians, Volume 1&2.* 7th ed. USA: Ingenix; 2005.

4. Heckman, TP, Barber-Westin, SD, Noyes, FR. Meniscal repair and transplantation: indications, techniques, rehabilitation and clinical outcome. *J Orthop Sports Phys Ther.* 2006;36(10):795-814.

PATELLAR TENDINITIS
SUMMARY OVERVIEW

ICD-9

726.64

APTA Preferred Practice Pattern: **4D, 4E, 4F, 4J**

EXAMINATION

- History and Systems Review
- Tests and Measures
  Systems review per APTA's *Guide to Physical Therapy Practice*
  - Gait, locomotion, and balance
  - Muscle performance
  - Orthotics, protective and supportive equipment
  - Pain
  - Posture
  - ROM
- Establish Plan of Care

GOALS/OUTCOMES

- Pain: 0/10 at rest and 3/10 or less after activity
- Pain-free active knee ROM: 0–135°
- Quadriceps strength: 5/5 on manual muscle test or 70% of uninvolved leg on leg press or other closed-kinetic chain test, such as single-leg squat excursion or lunge distance
- Return to previous functional status for ADLs and vocational, recreational, and sports activities as identified by patient
- Independence in a progressive home exercise program emphasizing function

INTERVENTION
NUMBER OF VISITS: 5–10

- Patient Instruction
  - Basic Anatomy and Biomechanics
  - Handouts
  - Functional Considerations
- Direct Interventions
  - Acute Phase: 1–4 Visits
  - Subacute Phase: 4–6 Visits
- Functional Carryover

DISCHARGE PLANNING AND PATIENT RESPONSIBILITY

- Criteria for Discharge
  - All rehabilitation goals have been met
  - Patient demonstrates tolerance to eccentric loading program
  - Patient demonstrates independence in home program
- Circumstances Requiring Additional Visits
  - History of additional lower-extremity pathology
- Home Program
  - Stress importance of adequate warm-up, stretching, appropriate playing surface, and cryotherapy
  - Address jumping/landing technique if relevant and correct to reduce excessive transverse and frontal plane motion at the foot/ankle and knee
  - Advise patient regarding self-friction massage
- Monitoring

SUMMARY OVERVIEW | KNEE | PATELLAR TENDINITIS   141

PATELLAR TENDINITIS

ICD-9
726.64   Patellar tendinitis
APTA Preferred Practice Pattern: **4D, 4E, 4F, 4J**

EXAMINATION

History and Systems Review
- History of current condition
  - Onset
  - Current functional limitations
  - Aggravating factors
- Past history of current condition
  - Previous knee or leg injuries
- Other tests and measures
  - Review of diagnostic reports
    - Radiographic
      a. Rule out Osgood-Schlatters and Sinding-Larsen-Johansson disease, especially in adolescent patients
- Functional status and activity level (current/prior)
  - Recent increase in activity frequency or intensity
- Patient's functional goals

Tests and Measures
Systems review per APTA's *Guide to Physical Therapy Practice*
- Gait, locomotion, and balance
  - Gait analysis
    - Excessive, prolonged, or late compensatory pronation
    - Contribution of footwear to poor biomechanical alignment
    - Utilization of knee extension in gait
- Muscle performance
  - Palpation
    - Point tenderness in substance of tendon: 65% of cases are at inferior patellar pole
  - Tensile loading: One or both tests will elicit pain
    - Passive stretch of extensor mechanism
    - Active contraction of extensor mechanism while on stretch
  - Hip abduction and external rotation strength assessment
  - Functional tests
    - Jumping activity

  a. Will usually demonstrate a position of genu valgum and internal rotation on takeoff and landing
    - Squatting
    - Stair descent
- Orthotics, protective and supportive equipment
  - Footwear analysis
    - Wear pattern indicating heel whip or excessive pronation
    - Shoe style and structure relative to biomechanical needs
- Pain
  - Measured on visual analog scale
- Posture
  - Static stance
    - Relaxed calcaneal position
  - General lower-extremity alignment
    - Genu varus/valgus
  - Specific foot alignment
    - Forefoot varus/valgus
    - Rearfoot varus
- ROM
  - Especially full extension

Establish Plan of Care
- Based on history, tests, and measures

GOALS/OUTCOMES
- Pain: 0/10 at rest and 3/10 or less after activity
- Pain-free active knee ROM: 0–135°
- Quadriceps strength: 5/5 on manual muscle test or 70% of uninvolved leg on leg press or other closed-kinetic chain test, such as single-leg squat excursion or lunge distance
- Return to previous functional status for ADLs and vocational, recreational, and sports activities as identified by patient
- Independence in a progressive home exercise program emphasizing function

INTERVENTION
NUMBER OF VISITS: 5–10

Coordination, Communication, and Documentation

- Provision of services between admission and discharge that facilitate cost-effective and efficient integration or reintegration to home, community, or work
- Documentation of therapeutic intervention is required for each episode of care and serves as the basic foundation for communication
- Coordination and additional communication will depend on the patient's impairment and home/work/community/leisure situation and requirements. Such services may include:
  - Case management
  - Coordination of care and collaboration with those integral to the patient's rehabilitation program
  - Coordination and monitoring of the delivery of available resources
  - Referrals to other health-care professionals
  - Identification of resources, support groups, or advocacy services
  - Provision of educational or training information
  - Technical assistance
- Specific coordination and communication provisions:
  - Referral for biomechanical orthotics

Patient Instruction

Basic Anatomy and Biomechanics

- Importance of adequate joint ROM, muscle flexibility, and muscle performance
- Biomechanical link between excessive or prolonged pronation and increased patellar loading
- Pertinent Gray's Anatomy (Gray. 1995. 692, 698–704, 707–708, 869)

Handouts

- Home exercise program
  - Stretching
    - Hamstrings
    - Quadriceps
    - Gastrocnemius and soleus
  - Strengthening of anterior tibial musculature
  - Closed-kinetic chain exercise progression

Functional Considerations

- Techniques to decrease loading, such as stair techniques and use of appropriate support devices
- Footwear choices to minimize or control excessive or prolonged pronation as indicated

Direct Interventions

Acute Phase: 1–4 Visits

- Therapeutic exercise and home program
  - Eccentric/concentric program for anterior tibial musculature
    - Patient starts in full plantarflexion, therapist passively stretches further into plantarflexion, then provides resistance first for concentric then for eccentric dorsiflexion
    - Therapist may instruct patient to do this using opposite foot or resistive tubing for resistance
  - Stretching
    - Hamstrings
    - Quadriceps
    - Gastrocnemius and soleus
- Manual therapy techniques
  - Joint mobilization
    - Patellar mobilization
  - Soft-tissue techniques
    - Soft-tissue mobilization
    - Friction massage
- Therapeutic devices and equipment
  - Trial of patellar compression strap and/or taping
- Electrotherapeutic modalities
  - Iontophoresis
- Physical agents and mechanical modalities
  - Cryotherapy
  - Pulsed ultrasound/phonophoresis
- Goals/outcomes
  - Full knee ROM: 0–120°
  - Pain
    - 0/10 at rest
    - 5/10 or less with activity
  - Functional activity
    - Pain-free ADLs
    - Full-weight-bearing, normal gait pattern with assistive device as necessary

KNEE | PATELLAR TENDINITIS 143

Subacute Phase: 4–6 Visits

- Therapeutic exercise and home program
  - Self-stretching as indicated
    - Quadriceps
    - Hamstrings
    - Gastrocnemius/soleus
    - Hip flexors
  - Symptoms permitting (pain 0/10 at rest, 5/10 or less if active), progressive eccentric loading program at levels below the forces required to elicit pain
    - Warm up with cycling, step machine, or hot packs for 10 minutes
    - Static or hold/relax quadriceps stretch: 3 repetitions with 30-second stretch
    - Specific exercises: 3 sets of 10–30 repetitions as appropriate, based on clinical judgment (exercises are listed from low load to high load)
      a. Resistive band, leg press, shuttle, etc., at light resistance
      b. Short arc standing squats: 20–40°
      c. Standing squats to 90°
      d. Step up/step down 4–8" as tolerated
      e. Partial to full lunges (body weight only)
      f. Plyometrics: Bounding, box jumps, etc.
- Manual therapy techniques
  - Joint mobilization
    - Patellar mobilization
  - Soft-tissue techniques
    - Soft-tissue mobilization
    - Friction massage
  - Assisted stretching to quadriceps and hamstrings as indicated using contract/relax techniques
- Physical agents and mechanical modalities
  - Superficial thermal therapy
  - Continuous ultrasound
  - Cryotherapy
- Goals/outcomes
  - Quadriceps strength of 5/5 on manual muscle test or muscle performance of 70% of uninvolved leg on leg press or other closed-kinetic chain functional test, such as single-leg squat excursion or lunge distance
  - Pain analog: 0/10 at rest; 1–3/10 after activity
  - Functional activity: Running and stairs pain-free, pain within 1–3/10 range after jumping or start/stop activities

Functional Carryover

- Early phase avoidance of high-load activities
- Self-taping
- Emphasis on proper periodization of training, including frequency, duration, and intensity of exercise, as well as on protocol for returning to previous level of activity

DISCHARGE PLANNING AND PATIENT RESPONSIBILITY

Criteria for Discharge

- All rehabilitation goals have been met
- Patient demonstrates tolerance to eccentric loading program
- Patient demonstrates independence in home program

Circumstances Requiring Additional Visits

- History of additional lower-extremity pathology

Home Program

- Stress importance of adequate warm-up, stretching, appropriate playing surface, and cryotherapy
- Address jumping/landing technique if relevant and correct to reduce excessive transverse and frontal plane motion at the foot/ankle and knee
- Advise patient regarding self-friction massage

Monitoring

- Phone follow-up by patient at 4–6 weeks to ensure progression toward previous functional status for ADLs and vocational, recreational, and sports activities
- Clinic visit may be required to progress home exercises to next level or toward more sport-specific activities

REFERENCES

1. American Physical Therapy Association. *Guide to Physical Therapist Practice.* Alexandria, VA: APTA; 1997.

2. Curwin S, Stanish WD. *Tendinitis: Its Etiology and Treatment.* Lexington, MA: Callamore Press; 1984.

3. Gray G. *Lower Extremity Functional Profile.* Adrian, MI: Wynn Marketing; 1995.

4. Gray H; Williams PL, ed. *Gray's Anatomy.* 38th ed. New York, NY: Churchill Livingstone; 1995.

5. Gross MT. Lower quarter screening for skeletal malalignment: suggestions for orthotics and shoewear. *J Orthop Sports Phys Ther.* 1995:21(6):389-405.

6. Hart A, Hopkins C, Ford B. *ICD-9-CM Expert For Physicians, Volume 1&2.* 7th ed. USA: Ingenix; 2005.

7. Powers CM, Maffucci R, Hampton S. Rearfoot posture in subjects with patellofemoral pain. *J Orthop Sports Phys Ther.* 1995;22:155-160.

8. Reid DC. *Sports Injury Assessment and Rehabilitation.* New York, NY: Churchill Livingstone; 1993:401-409.

146   PATELLAR TENDINITIS | KNEE

PATELLOFEMORAL SYNDROME
SUMMARY OVERVIEW

ICD-9

717.7   717.9   726.64   733.92   755.64   822.0   822.1   836.3   836.4   836.59

APTA Preferred Practice Pattern: 4A, 4D, 4E, 4F, 4G, 4H, 4I, 4J

EXAMINATION

- History and Systems Review
- Tests and Measures
  Systems review per APTA's *Guide to Physical Therapy Practice*
  - Gait, locomotion, and balance
  - Joint integrity and mobility
  - Muscle performance
  - Orthotic, protective, or supportive devices
  - Pain
  - Postural assessment
  - ROM
- Establish Plan of Care

GOALS/OUTCOMES

- Knee ROM: 0–135°
- Flexibility
- Vastus medialis oblique contraction palpable or readable on EMG device at 0°, 45°, and 90° of knee flexion
- Pain: 2/10 or less
- Strength: 70% of uninvolved leg on leg press or other closed-kinetic chain test, such as single-leg squat excursion or lunge distance without taping
- Pain-free gait pattern and stair negotiation without taping
- Return to previous functional status for ADLs and vocational, recreational, and sports activities as identified by patient
- Independence in progressive program emphasizing closed-kinetic chain functional exercise

INTERVENTION
NUMBER OF VISITS: 5–12

- Patient Instruction
  - Basic Anatomy and Biomechanics
  - Handouts
  - Functional Considerations
  - Description of Surgical Procedures
- Direct Interventions
  - Acute Phase: 2–4 Visits
  - Subacute Phase: 3–8 Visits
- Functional Carryover

DISCHARGE PLANNING AND PATIENT RESPONSIBILITY

- Criteria for Discharge
  - Patient demonstrates independence in taping techniques
  - Patient has achieved all rehabilitation goals except return to previous functional status for recreational and sports activities
- Circumstances Requiring Additional Visits
  - History of additional lower-extremity pathology
  - Diagnosis secondary-surgical intervention
- Home Program
  - Emphasize ongoing maintenance as key
  - Consider patellar brace for people who cannot wean from tape within 2 months of starting program. This should be used for 6–12 months.
- Monitoring

SUMMARY OVERVIEW | KNEE | PATELLOFEMORAL SYNDROME   147

PATELLOFEMORAL SYNDROME

ICD-9

717.7	Chondromalacia of patella
717.9	Unspecified internal derangement of knee
726.64	Patellar tendinitis
733.92	Chondromalacia
755.64	Congenital deformity of knee (joint)
822.0	Closed fracture of patella
822.1	Open fracture of patella
836.3	Dislocation of patella, closed
836.4	Dislocation of patella, open
836.59	Other dislocation of knee, closed

APTA Preferred Practice Pattern: **4A, 4D, 4E, 4F, 4G, 4H, 4I, 4J**

EXAMINATION

History and Systems Review

- History of current condition
  - Onset
  - Location of pain
  - Aggravating factors
- Past history of current condition
  - Previous lower-extremity injury
- Functional status and activity level (current/prior)
- Patient's functional goals

Tests and Measures

Systems review per APTA's *Guide to Physical Therapy Practice*

- Gait, locomotion, and balance
  - Heel whip
  - Circumduction
  - Excessive or prolonged compensatory pronation in ambulation
  - Contribution of footwear to poor biomechanical alignment
  - Walking
  - Squatting
    - Single leg, double leg
  - Step up/step down
- Joint integrity and mobility
  - Patellar orientation relative to femur
    - Glide component
      a. Patellar tracking in sagittal plane
    - Tilt component
      a. Medial/lateral borders level to frontal plane

- Rotational component
  a. Long axis of femur and patella parallel
- Anterioposterior component
  a. Superior/inferior poles level in frontal plane
- Muscle performance
  - Palpable vastus medialis oblique (VMO) contraction at:
    - 0° knee flexion
    - 45° knee flexion
    - 90° knee flexion
  - Quadriceps motor performance
    - Open kinetic chain
      a. Manual muscle test
    - Closed-kinetic chain
      a. Leg press or squat
- Orthotic, protective, or supportive devices
- Pain
  - Measured on visual analog scale
  - Pain with prolonged sitting (*movie sign*)
- Postural assessment
  - Static stance
    - Relaxed calcaneal position
  - Lower extremity alignment
    - Genu varus/vargus
    - Tibial torsion
  - Specific foot alignment
    - Forefoot varus/valgus
    - Rearfoot varus
    - Halux valgus with callus on first metatarsal
- ROM:
  - Flexibility
  - Hamstrings

- Gastrocnemius
- Soleus
- Iliotibial band/tensor fasciæ latæ
- Quadriceps
- Iliopsoas

Establish Plan of Care

- Based on history, tests, and measures

GOALS/OUTCOMES

- Knee ROM: 0–135°
- Flexibility
  - Negative Ely test for proper quadriceps and iliopsoas flexibility
  - Thomas test showing full hip extension and knee flexion to at least 70°
  - Straight leg raise to at least 80°
  - Ober test showing adduction to plinth level
  - Active ankle dorsiflexion in subtalar neutral to 10° with knee extended, 15° with knee flexed
- VMO contraction palpable or readable on EMG device at 0°, 45°, and 90° of knee flexion
- Pain: 2/10 or less
- Strength: 70% of uninvolved leg on leg press or other closed-kinetic chain test, such as single-leg squat excursion or lunge distance without taping
- Pain-free gait pattern and stair negotiation without taping
- Return to previous functional status for ADLs and vocational, recreational, and sports activities as identified by patient
- Independence in progressive program emphasizing closed-kinetic chain functional exercise

INTERVENTION
NUMBER OF VISITS: 5–12

Coordination, Communication, and Documentation

- Provision of services between admission and discharge that facilitate cost-effective and efficient integration or reintegration to home, community, or work
- Documentation of therapeutic intervention is required for each episode of care and serves as the basic foundation for communication
- Coordination and additional communication will depend on the patient's impairment and home/work/

community/leisure situation and requirements. Such services may include:
  - Case management
  - Coordination of care and collaboration with those integral to the patient's rehabilitation program
  - Coordination and monitoring of the delivery of available resources
  - Referrals to other health-care professionals
  - Identification of resources, support groups, or advocacy services
  - Provision of educational or training information
  - Technical assistance
- Specific coordination and communication provisions:
  - Referral for biomechanical orthotics

Patient Instruction

Basic Anatomy and Biomechanics

- Pertinent Anatomical References (Gray. 1995. 697–704, 707–708, 869), (Hollinshead. 1985. 459–463), (Netter. 1989. 476–481)
- Lower-extremity biomechanical dysfunction and its role in the onset and exacerbation of patellofemoral syndrome, including: Excessive and prolonged pronation, genu valgum, and major muscle group flexibility

Handouts

- Taping techniques
- Self mobilization
- Home exercise program
  - Flexibility
  - Strengthening
    - Terminal extension exercises
      a. Quadsets
      b. Short arc quads
      c. Straight leg raises
    - Closed-kinetic chain exercises
      a. Modified step ups
      b. Modified lunges
      c. Modified squats
    - Backward walking/running

Functional Considerations

- Avoidance of excessive patellar loading positions or postures, such as:
  - Full squatting

KNEE | PATELLOFEMORAL SYNDROME **149**

- Kneeling
- Cycling with a low seat or big gears
- Open kinetic chain knee extension under load beyond 30°
- Cryotherapy to control edema
- Recommendations for types of footwear that help control excessive pronation, such as lace-up oxfords or athletic shoes whenever possible
- Gait training

Description of Surgical Procedures
- Lateral retinacular release and patellar realignment are the significant procedures
- Review of operative procedure and relation to biomechanics, rehabilitation, and function

Direct Interventions

Acute Phase: 2–4 Visits
Pertains to moderate to severe inflammation or recent subluxation/dislocation
- Therapeutic exercise
  - Gluteus medius strengthening to de-emphasize vastus lateralis and tensor fasciæ latæ in gait
  - Foot inverter strengthening to counter excessive pronation
  - Gait training
  - Self-stretching of all tight lower-extremity musculature found in evaluation
    - Hamstrings
    - Gastrocnemius
    - Soleus
    - Iliotibial band
    - Psoas
    - Quadriceps
  - VMO sets as soon as possible, utilizing EMG biofeedback if available
  - Side steps with knees locked and feet internally rotated
  - Plantar flexion/inversion exercises
- Manual therapy techniques
  - Joint mobilization
    - Oscillatory mobilization for pain
  - Passive lateral retinacular stretching as tolerated
- Therapeutic devices and equipment
  - Application of patellar taping
    - Daily use

- Improve tracking and VMO activity/control (see "Patellar Taping Techniques for Glide Rotation")
- Physical agents and mechanical modalities
  - Cryotherapy
  - Electrical stimulation
  - Application of patellar taping daily use
  - Improve tracking and VMO activity/control
- Goals/outcomes
  - Knee ROM: Full 0–120°
  - Motor performance: 50–70% of uninvolved leg on leg press test when taped
  - Pain: 0/10 when taped
  - Pain-free, normal gait pattern and stair negotiation when taped
  - VMO contraction palpable or readable on EMG device at 0°, 45°, and 90° of knee flexion
  - Flexibility
    - Thomas test showing 10° hip flexion and knee flexion to at least 50°
    - Straight-leg raise to at least 60°
    - Ober test showing adduction to within 3" of the level of the plinth
    - Ankle dorsiflexion in subtalar joint neutral with knee extended, 10° with knee flexed

Subacute Phase: 3–8 Visits
This phase may be entirely home exercise program, with biweekly rechecks. Some patients could be seen in-department for up to 6 visits.
- Therapeutic exercise
  - Progress VMO sets to standing
  - Partial squats: Progress to one-leg squats
  - Step up/step down
  - Lunges in all directions
  - Foot inverter strengthening
  - Appropriate stretches as in acute phase
  - Leg press/shuttle
  - Pain-free aerobic conditioning
  - Neuromuscular/balance/proprioceptive reeducation
    - Gait drills
      a. Backward walking
      b. SportCord™ activities
      c. Balance beam walking
    - BAPS, balance board
    - Balance/reach, balancing on involved leg, reaching in various directions with uninvolved leg to maximum distance

- Manual therapy techniques
  - Vigorous passive stretching of lateral structures, (i.e., iliotibial band and lateral retinaculum)
- Physical agents and mechanical modalities
  - Cryotherapy following exercises
- Functional biomechanics
  - Integration of specific structural or biomechanical components that may relieve symptoms, including the choice of shoes and/or custom biomechanical orthotics to control excessive compensatory pronation
  - Cycling: Instruction on proper seat height for individual, emphasizing approximately 24° angle at knee with foot in 6 o'clock position
- Goals/outcomes
  - ROM: 0–135°
  - Pain: 0/10 on some limited activities, but likely will need tape for minimum of two weeks to remain pain-free
  - Functional activities
    - Pain-free gait pattern without taping
    - Pain-free stair negotiation without taping

Functional Carryover
- Instruction regarding gradual tapering off of taping as appropriate
- Instruction regarding proper periodization of training, including frequency, intensity, and duration
- Emphasis on continuation of home exercise program

DISCHARGE PLANNING AND PATIENT RESPONSIBILITY

Criteria for Discharge
- Patient demonstrates independence in taping techniques
- Patient has achieved all rehabilitation goals except return to previous functional status for recreational and sports activities

Circumstances Requiring Additional Visits
- History of additional lower-extremity pathology
- Diagnosis secondary to surgical intervention

Home Program
- Emphasize ongoing maintenance as key
  - VMO training
  - Flexibility
  - Muscle performance
- Consider patellar brace for people who cannot wean from tape within 2 months of starting program. This should be used for 6–12 months.

Monitoring
- Patient is to recheck/call at 4–6 weeks post-discharge to assess progression toward full, pain-free ADLs and vocational, recreational, and sports activities

KNEE | PATELLOFEMORAL SYNDROME

REFERENCES

1. Arrol B, Ellis-Pegler E, Edwards A, Sutchcliffe G. Patelloferoral pain syndrome: a critical review of the clinical trials on nonoperative therapy. *Am J Sports Med.* 1997;25:207-212.

2. American Physical Therapy Association. *Guide to Physical Therapist Practice.* Alexandria, VA: APTA; 1997.

3. Brown DE, Alexander AH, Lichtman DM. The Elmslie-Trillat procedure: evaluation in patellar dislocation and subluxation. *Am J Sports Med.* 1984;12:104-109.

4. Eng JJ. Evaluation of soft foot orthotics in the treatment of patellofemoral pain syndrome. *Phys Ther.* 1993;73:62-68.

5. Flynn TW. Patellofemoral joint compressive forces in forward and backward running. *J Orthop Sports Med.* 1995;21:277-282.

6. Gilleard W. The effect of patellar taping on the onset of vastus medialis obliquus and vastus lateralis muscle activity in persons with patellofemoral pain. *Phys Ther.* 1998;78:25-32.

7. Gould JA. *Orthopedic and Sports Physical Therapy.* 2nd ed. St Louis, MO: CV Mosby; 1990.

8. Gray G. *Lower Extremity Functional Profile.* Adrian, MI: Wynn Marketing; 1995.

9. Gray H; Williams PL, ed. *Gray's Anatomy.* 38th ed. New York, NY: Churchill Livingstone; 1995.

10. Gross MT. Lower quarter screening for skeletal malalignment: suggestions for orthotics and shoewear. *J Orthop Sports Phys Ther.* 1995;21(6):389-405.

11. Hart A, Hopkins C, Ford B. *ICD-9-CM Expert For Physicians, Volume 1&2.* 7th ed. USA: Ingenix; 2005.

12. Hollinshead WH. *Cornelius Rosse Textbook Of Anatomy.* Philadelphia, PA: Harper & Row; 1985.

13. LaPrade J, Culham E, Brower B. Comparison of five isometric exercises in the recruitment of the vastus medialis oblique in persons with and without patellofemoral pain syndrome. *J Orthop Sports Phys Ther.* 1998;27(3):197-204.

14. McConnell M. *McConnell Patellofemoral Treatment Plan.* McConnell Seminars, PO Box 9400, Marina Del Rey, CA 90295. Dec. 1991. Course Notes

15. Netter FH. *Atlas of Human Anatomy.* Summit, NJ: CIBA-GEIGY Corporation; 1989.

16. Osborne AH, Fulford PC. Lateral release for Chondromalacia patella. *J Bone Joint Surg Br.* 1982;64:202-205.

17. Powers CM, Maffucci R, Hampton S. Rearfoot posture in subjects with patellofemoral pain. *J Orthop Sports Phys Ther.* 1995;22(4):155-160.

18. Puniello M. Iliotibial band tightness and medial patellar glide in patients with patellofemoral dysfunction. *J Orthop Sports Phys Ther.* 1993;17(3):144-148.

19. Reid DC. *Sports Injury Assessment and Rehabilitation.* New York, NY: Churchill Livingstone; 1992:345-436.

POSTERIOR CRUCIATE LIGAMENT RECONSTRUCTION
SUMMARY OVERVIEW

ICD-9

717.84

APTA Preferred Practice Pattern: **4E, 4J**

EXAMINATION

- History and Systems Review
- Tests and Measures
  Systems review per APTA's *Guide to Physical Therapy Practice*
  - Anthropometric characteristics
  - Gait, locomotion, and balance
  - Integumentary integrity
  - Pain
  - ROM
  - Special tests
- Establish Plan of Care

GOALS/OUTCOMES

- Joint line girth measurements equal to uninvolved extremity
- Strength: 90% of uninvolved leg as measured on manual muscle test, closed-kinetic chain functional test, or isokinetic test for quadriceps and hamstrings
- Neuromuscular/balance/proprioception: 90% of uninvolved leg on single leg hop distance
- Pain-free AROM: 0–135°, strive for symmetrical hyperextension if applicable
- Return to previous functional status for ADLs and vocational, recreational, and sports activities as identified by patient
- Prevention of further progression of active articular changes of patellofemoral and medial tibiofemoral joint
- Independence in a progressive home exercise program emphasizing function

INTERVENTION
NUMBER OF VISITS: 8–29

- Patient Instruction
  - Basic Anatomy and Biomechanics
  - Handouts
  - Functional Considerations
- Direct Interventions
  - Phase I: 1–4 Visits, Weeks 1–3
  - Phase II: 1–3 Visits, Weeks 4–6
  - Phase III: 1–6 Visits, Weeks 7–12
  - Phase IV: 3–10 Visits, Months 4–6
  - Phase V: 1–4 Visits, Months 7–12
  - Phase VI: 1–2 Visits, 12 Months Postoperative
- Functional Carryover

DISCHARGE PLANNING AND PATIENT RESPONSIBILITY

- Criteria for Discharge
  - Patient has achieved all rehabilitation goals except return to previous functional status for recreation and sports activities
  - Patient has demonstrated understanding of exercise progression and proper training schedule to prevent exacerbation of symptoms
- Circumstances Requiring Additional Visits
  - History of additional lower-extremity pathology
  - Postoperative complications
  - Presence of other medical conditions
  - Significant deconditioning prior to surgery
  - Inability to achieve flexion AROM due to fibrosis secondary to range limits during protective phases
- Home Program
  - Patient is to wear sports brace for first 12 months after returning to sports
  - Continuation of strengthening and flexibility exercises is strongly recommended in individuals wishing to return to vigorous sport or recreational activity
- Monitoring

SUMMARY OVERVIEW | KNEE | POSTERIOR CRUCIATE LIGAMENT RECONSTRUCTION   153

POSTERIOR CRUCIATE LIGAMENT RECONSTRUCTION

ICD-9
    717.84   Old disruption of posterior cruciate ligament
APTA Preferred Practice Pattern: 4E, 4J

EXAMINATION

History and Systems Review
- History of current condition
  - Date and type of surgical procedure
  - Postoperative progression/complication
- Past history of current condition
  - Prior history of lower-extremity injury
- Functional status and activity level (current/prior)
- Patient's functional goals

Tests and Measures
Systems review per APTA's *Guide to Physical Therapy Practice*
- Anthropometric characteristics
  - Edema
  - Comparative girth measurements at knee joint level, above and below
- Gait, locomotion, and balance
  - Assistive devices
  - Weight-bearing status
- Integumentary integrity
  - Skin color
  - Surgical incision
- Pain
  - Measured on visual analog scale
  - Type, classification
- ROM
  - Knee A/PROM
  - Patellar PROM
  - Muscle length
    - Psoas
    - Quadriceps
    - Hamstrings
    - Gastroc/soleus
    - Tensor fasciæ latæ/iliotibial band
- Special tests
  - No special tests for postoperative posterior cruciate ligament (PCL) as maximal protection is essential; however, presence of posterior tibial sag is an indicator of graft instability in lieu of stress test

Establish Plan of Care
- Based on history, tests, and measures

GOALS/OUTCOMES
- Joint line girth measurements equal to uninvolved extremity
- Strength: 90% of uninvolved leg as measured on manual muscle test, closed-kinetic chain functional test, or isokinetic test for quadriceps and hamstrings
- Neuromuscular/balance/proprioception: 90% of uninvolved leg on single leg hop distance
- Pain-free AROM: 0–135°, strive for symmetrical hyperextension if applicable
- Return to previous functional status for ADLs and vocational, recreational, and sports activities as identified by patient
- Prevention of further progression of active articular changes of patellofemoral and medial tibiofemoral joint
- Independence in a progressive home exercise program emphasizing function

INTERVENTION
Number of Visits: 8–29

Coordination, Communication, and Documentation
- Provision of services between admission and discharge that facilitate cost-effective and efficient integration or reintegration to home, community, or work
- Documentation of therapeutic intervention is required for each episode of care and serves as the basic foundation for communication
- Coordination and additional communication will depend on the patient's impairment and home/work/community/leisure situation and requirements. Such services may include:
  - Case management
  - Coordination of care and collaboration with those integral to the patient's rehabilitation program
  - Coordination and monitoring of the delivery of available resources

154   POSTERIOR CRUCIATE LIGAMENT RECONSTRUCTION | KNEE

○ Referrals to other health-care professionals
○ Identification of resources, support groups, or advocacy services
○ Provision of educational or training information
○ Technical assistance
• Specific coordination and communication provisions:
○ Referral for biomechanical orthotics

Patient Instruction

Basic Anatomy and Biomechanics
• Pertinent Gray's Anatomy (Gray. 1995. 697–704, 707–708, 869, 876)
• Biomechanical function of the posterior cruciate ligament in triplanar stability of the knee, and the importance of adequate muscle performance and flexibility in proper kinematics

Handouts
• Home cryotherapy/thermal modalities or contrast bath for edema reduction
• Phase-specific home exercise program

Functional Considerations
• Proper application and use of brace as indicated
• Instruction in stair techniques, ambulation on uneven terrain, and proper progression of activities as appropriate to phase of recovery

Direct Interventions

Phase I: 1–4 Visits, Weeks 1–3
The initial week is chiefly bed rest, elevation, PROM three times a day, and cryotherapy only. The brace is locked at 20° for first 5 weeks (or according to physician preference) and unlocked for PROM exercises only.
• Therapeutic exercise and home program
○ ROM per physician's preference (out of brace). The remaining exercises are done with the brace locked at 20° flexion:
▪ Isometrics co-contraction
a. Set quadriceps, then set hamstrings
▪ Leg raises
▪ Hip isotonic (no extension)
▪ Cycling with uninvolved leg
▪ Upper body ergometer
▪ Gait training—non-weight-bearing

• Manual therapy techniques
○ Joint mobilization
▪ Patellar mobilization
• Electrotherapeutic modalities
○ Electromagnetic stimulation to quad at 20°
○ Interferential for edema as indicated
• Physical agents and mechanical modalities
○ Cryotherapy as needed
• Goals/outcomes
○ Independent, nonweight-bearing ambulation with crutches (or per physician's protocol)
○ ROM: 0–40°
○ Decreased edema
○ Pain: 5/10 or less

Phase II: 1–3 Visits, Weeks 4–6
In general, a ROM brace is worn for the first phase, and then transition occurs to a sports brace as indicated by the physician.
• Therapeutic exercise and home program
○ PROM: 0–85°
○ Continue co-contraction to 0° extension
○ Continue leg raises and hip isotonic (no extension)
○ Continue cycling with uninvolved leg
○ Upper body ergometer
○ May start swimming with brace in 10° flexion
○ May start shallow water exercises
▪ Hip abduction
▪ Hip adduction
▪ Hip flexion and extension
▪ Toe raises and mini squats
▪ Water walking, forward/backward
• Manual therapy techniques
○ Patellar mobilization
○ Soft-tissue mobilization/cross fiber mobilization at incision
• Physical agents and mechanical modalities
○ Continue with electrical stimulation for quadriceps
○ Cryotherapy/elevation for edema and pain control
• Goals/outcomes
○ Pain-free active ROM: 0–85°
○ 50% weight-bearing with crutches and brace locked at 10° extension and 70° flexion (at 6th week)
○ Pain: 4/10 or less

Phase III: 1–6 Visits, Weeks 7–12

- Therapeutic exercise and home program
  - Progress weight bearing in gait
    - Start 75% weight-bearing (with or without brace)
  - Continue co-contraction at 0° of extension
  - Continue with leg raises, hip isotonic without extension, with knee at 10–70°
  - Begin Profitter with knee at 0–70° At Week 9:
    a. Begin balance coordination exercises with brace at 0–90°
    b. Begin cycling (stationary) out of brace, full revolutions
- Manual therapy techniques
  - Patellar mobilization as needed
- Physical agents and mechanical modalities
  - As needed for pain control or edema reduction
- Goals/outcomes
  - ROM: 0–125°
  - Full weight-bearing, no brace
  - Complete resolution of edema
  - Pain: 2/10 or less
  - Return to previous functional status for ADLs and vocational activities

Phase IV: 3–10 Visits, Months 4–6

Aerobic conditioning and functional activities are increasingly emphasized.

- Therapeutic exercise and home program
  All aerobic activities with sports brace at 10–90°
  - Begin level ground outdoor cycling
  - Walking full weight-bearing
  - Continue swimming as tolerated
  - Cross-country ski machine
  - Rowing
  - Running/jogging at 6th month
  - Isotonic strengthening
    - Mini squats
    - Short arc quads (SAQ)
    - Power training via leg press, squats, toe raises (low repetitions, brace 0–90°). Not recommended if serious articular cartilage damage is present. See surgical report.
  - Isokinetics (0–90°)
    - Anterior shear pad placed on distal tibia
    - Seated position for flexion/extension
    - Start with high speeds, 180° per second and higher
    - Flexion limit controlled by brace or machine

- Functional biomechanics
  Integration of specific structural components that may enhance the longevity of the surgically repaired PCL, including choice of shoes or custom biomechanical orthotics to control excessive compensatory pronation
- Goals/outcomes
  - ROM: 0–135°
  - Pain: 1/10 or less
  - Strength: 50% of uninvolved leg
    - 180°/sec. isokinetic test
    - Manual muscle test
    - Closed-kinetic chain functional test
  - Neuromuscular/balance/proprioception: To 80% of uninvolved leg for single leg stance duration

Phase V: 1–4 Visits, Months 7–12

- Therapeutic exercise and home program
  - Continue aerobic and functional activity level as tolerated—limited flexion
  - Patient may start seated hill climbing on outdoor cycle; may progress to standing hill climbing at 9th month
  - Continue aerobic activities with brace at 10°—full flexion range
    - Swimming
    - Walking, running/jogging
    - Stair machine
    - Cross-country ski machine
    - Rowing
  - Continue mini squats/leg press/toe raises with brace at 10° of full flexion range
  - Continue SAQ (0–40°)
  - Continue isokinetics
    - Quadriceps only
  - Continue power training
    - Start hamstring curls (0–90°)
    - Start full range (low repetitions) of leg press, squats, and toe raises
- Goals/outcomes
  - Strength of quadriceps and hamstring muscles to achieve 90% of uninvolved leg as measured with manual muscle testing or appropriate closed-kinetic chain test
  - Neuromuscular/balance/proprioception and power to achieve hop distance of 90% of uninvolved leg
  - Full, pain-free AROM 0–135°

Phase VI: 1–2 Visits, 12 Months Postoperative

- Return to sports at 12 months postoperative minimum

Functional Carryover

- Importance of adequate muscle performance prior to resuming high-load or abrupt activities, such as skiing or soccer
- Instruct patient in variety of cross-training options to reduce risk of future overuse injury

DISCHARGE PLANNING AND PATIENT RESPONSIBILITY

Criteria for Discharge

- Patient has achieved all rehabilitation goals except return to previous functional status for recreation and sports activities
- Patient has demonstrated understanding of exercise progression and proper training schedule to prevent exacerbation of symptoms

Circumstances Requiring Additional Visits

- History of additional lower-extremity pathology
- Postoperative complications
- Presence of other medical conditions
- Significant deconditioning prior to surgery
- Inability to achieve flexion AROM due to fibrosis secondary to range limits during protective phases

Home Program

- Patient is to wear sports brace for first 12 months after returning to sports
- Continuation of strengthening and flexibility exercises is strongly recommended in individuals wishing to return to vigorous sport or recreational activity

Monitoring

- Patient is to recheck/call at 2 weeks post-discharge to ensure progression to previous functional status for recreational and sports activities

REFERENCE

1. American Physical Therapy Association. *Guide to Physical Therapist Practice.* Alexandria, VA: APTA; 1997.
2. Anderson JK, Noyes FR. Principles of posterior cruciate ligament reconstruction. *Orthopedics* 1995;18:493-500.
3. Bianchi M. Acute tears of the posterior cruciate ligament: clinical study and results of operative treatment in 27 cases. *Am J Sports Med.* 1983;11:308-314.
4. Engle RP, Meade TD, Canner GC. Rehabilitation of posterior cruciate ligament injuries: In: *Rehabilitation of the Knee: A Problem Solving Approach.* Philadelphia, PA: FA Davis; 1993:304-329.
5. Gray H; Williams PL, ed. *Gray's Anatomy.* 38th ed. New York, NY: Churchill Livingstone; 1995.
6. Hart A, Hopkins C, Ford B. *ICD-9-CM Expert For Physicians, Volume 1&2.* 7th ed. USA: Ingenix; 2005.
7. Kim SJ, Kim HK, Kim HJ. Arthroscopic posterior cruciate reconstruction using a one-incision technique. *Clin Orthop Rel Res.* February 1999:155-166.
8. Reid DC. *Sports Injury Assessment and Rehabilitation.* New York, NY: Churchill Livingston; 1992.
9. Rosenberg T. *Clinical Protocol For Rehabilitation Following PCL Reconstruction Utilizing Allograft.* 5848 S 300 E, Salt Lake City, UT, 84107.
10. St Pierre P, Miller SD. Posterior cruciate ligament injuries. *Clin Sports Med.* 1999;18:199-211,vii.
11. Wilk KE. Rehabilitation of isolated and combined posterior cruciate ligament injuries. *Clin Sports Med.* 1994;13:649-677.
12. Zavatsky AB, Beard DJ, O'Conner JJ. Cruciate ligament loading during isometric muscle contractions: a theoretical basis for rehab. *Am J Sports Med.* 1994;22:418-423.

TOTAL KNEE REPLACEMENT—INPATIENT
SUMMARY OVERVIEW

ICD-9

    V43.65

APTA Preferred Practice Pattern: 4I

EXAMINATION

- History and Systems Review
- Tests and Measures
  Systems review per APTA's *Guide to Physical Therapy Practice*
  - Anthropometric characteristics
  - Arousal, attention, and cognition
  - Gait, locomotion, and balance
  - Integumentary integrity
  - Muscle performance
  - Pain
  - ROM
  - Self-care and home management
  - Ventilation, respiration, and circulation
- Establish Plan of Care

GOALS/OUTCOMES

- Independent/supervised functional level for indicated tasks
- Active assistive ROM: 5–90°
- Demonstrated functional straight leg raise without extensor lag

INTERVENTION
NUMBER OF VISITS: 4–10 (2–5 DAYS DURING ACUTE HOSPITALIZATION)

- Patient Instruction
  - Basic Anatomy and Biomechanics
  - Handouts
  - Functional Considerations
- Direct Interventions
  - Acute Phase (2–5 days During Acute Hospitalization): 4–10 Visits
- Functional Carryover

DISCHARGE PLANNING AND PATIENT RESPONSIBILITY

- Criteria for Discharge
  - Understands and demonstrates knee limitations as dictated by surgical procedure
  - Maintains good posture and body mechanics
  - Short term rehabilitation goals (acute hospital) have been achieved
  - Initiated progression toward previous functional status for ADLs
- Circumstances Requiring Additional Visits
  - Cognitive limitations
  - Comorbidities effecting ability to recover or progress
  - Postoperative complications (deep vein thrombosis, infections)
  - Multiple barriers to discharge (stairs, limited weight bearing, safety impairment)
- Home Program
  - Referral to home health or outpatient physical therapy is recommended
  - Continue inpatient exercise program 2–3 times daily
  - Advance ambulation 1–2 minutes daily if no increase in pain level
- Monitoring

SUMMARY OVERVIEW | KNEE | TOTAL KNEE REPLACEMENT—INPATIENT   159

TOTAL KNEE REPLACEMENT—INPATIENT

ICD-9
    V43.65   Knee joint replacement
APTA Preferred Practice Pattern: 4I

EXAMINATION

History and Systems Review
- History of current condition
  - Surgical procedure/date
  - Surgical report
    - Total knee arthroplasty surgical approach
    - Post operative weight-bearing status (physician prescribed)
  - Complications
  - Chart review
    - Health history
    - Advanced directive
    - Supplements (i.e. IV lines, oxygen needs, catheter)
- Medications
- Past medical/surgical history
  - Comorbidities
- Functional status and activity level
  - Prior functional status
    - Assistive devices
    - History of falls
- Living environment
  - Barriers to discharge
    - Support system
    - Stairs
- Patient's functional goals

Tests and Measures
Systems review per APTA's *Guide to Physical Therapy Practice*
- Anthropometric characteristics
  - Palpation of key landmarks
  - Height
  - Edema/knee girth
- Arousal, attention, and cognition
  - Orientation
  - Motivational level
  - Cognitive status in relation to compliance with postoperative limitations
  - Safety
    - Observation of knee precautions
    - Safety judgement

- Gait, locomotion, and balance
  - Gait analysis
    - Weight-bearing tolerance/maintenance of weight-bearing status
    - Appropriate use of assistive device
    - Stride length
    - Physiologic response to activity
  - Balance assessment
    - Fall risk
  - Use of knee immobilizer and effects on gait
- Integumentary integrity
  - Sensation
  - Bleeding
- Muscle performance
  - Quality of movement
    - Ability to straight leg raise without extensor lag
  - Strength
    - Manual muscle test of uninvolved extremities, involved ankle dorsi/plantar flexors
    - Functional strength of involved extremity, hip, and knee
- Pain
  - Pain and soreness with joint movement, 0/10
- ROM
  - Functional ROM of uninvolved extremities
    - Lumbar, hips, knees, ankles, shoulders, elbows, wrists, and hands
  - Goniometric measure of involved knee flexion and extension in supine
- Self-care and home management
  - Ability to transfer
    - Toilet transfers
    - Bed mobility
      a. Therapeutic devices and equipment
  - Use of immobilizer
- Ventilation, respiration, and circulation
  - Pedal pulse
  - Signs and symptoms of deep vein thrombosis

Establish Plan of Care
- Based on history, tests, and measures

GOALS/OUTCOMES
- Independent/supervised functional level for:
  - Transfers in and out of bed, on and off a commode, up and down from an appropriate chair (tall/elevated)
  - Gait training at a household level with the appropriate assistive device
  - Stair climbing one or more step(s), consistent with their home environment, with appropriate assistive device, with and without handrail
  - Performance of home exercise program, 5–10 repetitions each, 2–3 times a day
  - Adherence to total knee arthroplasty precautions and correctly incorporating them into any of the above situations, including maintaining weight-bearing status
- Active assistive ROM: 5–90°
- Demonstrated functional straight leg raise without extensor lag

INTERVENTION
NUMBER OF VISITS: 4–10 (2–5 DAYS DURING ACUTE HOSPITALIZATION)

Coordination, Communication, and Documentation
- Provision of services between admission and discharge that facilitate cost-effective and efficient integration or reintegration to home, community, or work
- Documentation of therapeutic intervention is required for each episode of care and serves as the basic foundation for communication
- Coordination and additional communication will depend on the patient's impairment and home/work/community/leisure situation and requirements. Such services may include:
  - Case management
  - Coordination of care and collaboration with those integral to the patient's rehabilitation program
  - Coordination and monitoring of the delivery of available resources
  - Referrals to other health-care professionals
  - Identification of resources, support groups, or advocacy services
  - Provision of educational or training information
  - Technical assistance

- Specific coordination and communication provisions:
  - Set up of controlled passive motion machine (if prescribed)
  - Occupational therapy for adaptive equipment and ADLs carryover

Patient Instruction

Basic Anatomy and Biomechanics
- Krames Communications (1100 Grundy Lane, San Bruno, CA 94066)
  - *After Total Knee Replacement*
- Pertinent Gray's Anatomy (Gray. 1995. 680–681, 683, 697–704, 707–709, 869, 876)

Handouts
- Total knee precautions
  - No twisting
- Use of controlled passive motion machine (if prescribed by physician)
- Use of athrombic pumps (if prescribed by physician)
- ROM and weight-bearing limitations, dependent upon surgical procedure
- Home exercise program
  - Ankle pumps
  - Quad sets
  - Gluteal sets
  - Heel slides
  - Short-arc quads
  - Hamstring sets
  - Straight-leg raises
  - Sitting knee flexion and extension

Functional Considerations
- Modification of home environment for safety
  - Remove throw rugs
  - Add pillows to low chairs frequented
  - Handrails as needed (bathroom, shower, stairs)
  - Rearranging furniture as needed (allowing room for assistive device)

Direct Interventions

Acute Phase (2–5 days During Acute Hospitalization): 4–10 Visits
- Therapeutic exercise and home program
  - Resistive exercise to the uninvolved extremities

- Active, active/assisted knee flexion and extension to the postoperative limb
- Ankle pumps, quad sets, gluteal sets, hamstring sets, heel slides, and short-arc quads and straight leg raising of the postoperative limb with patient in bed
- Sitting knee extension
- Standing knee flexion of the postoperative limb
- Functional training
  - Transfer training
    - In and out of bed
    - From bed to and from chair
    - To and from commode or elevated toilet seat
  - Gait training
    - Instruction in weight-bearing status
    - Gait instruction with assistive device
      a. Level surface
      b. Stair training
- Manual therapy techniques
  - Patellar mobilization
- Electrotherapeutic modalities
  - Functional electrical stimulation to quadriceps femoris
- Physical agents and mechanical modalities
  - Apply athrombic pumps (discontinue when client ambulatory)
  - Use of ice and elevation, cryo-cuff

Functional Carryover

- Independence in gait pattern with assistive device at a household level

DISCHARGE PLANNING AND PATIENT RESPONSIBILITY

Criteria for Discharge

- Understands and demonstrates knee limitations as dictated by surgical procedure
- Maintains good posture and body mechanics
- Short term rehabilitation goals (acute hospital) have been achieved
- Initiated progression toward previous functional status for ADLs

Circumstances Requiring Additional Visits

- Cognitive limitations
- Comorbidities effecting ability to recover or progress

- Postoperative complications (deep vein thrombosis, infections)
- Multiple barriers to discharge (stairs, limited weight bearing, safety impairment)

Home Program

- Referral to home health or outpatient physical therapy is recommended
- Continue inpatient exercise program 2–3 times daily
- Advance ambulation 1–2 minutes daily if no increase in pain level

Monitoring

- Ideally, rehabilitation is complete when the operative knee ROM and strength are 90–100% of the non-operative and the patient has resumed all functional and some recreational activities without pain
- Patient not referred for outpatient or home health services should call after 2–3 weeks to ensure ongoing progress toward functional rehabilitation goals

REFERENCE

1. American Physical Therapy Association. *Guide to Physical Therapist Practice*. Alexandria, VA: APTA; 1997.
2. D'Lima DD, Colwell CW Jr, Morris BA, Hardwick ME, Kozin F. The effect of preoperative exercise on total knee replacement outcomes. *Clin Orthop Rel Res*. May 1996:174-182.
3. Gotlin RS, Hershkowitz S, Juris PM, et al. Electrical stimulation effect on extensor lag and length of hospital stay after total knee arthroplasty. *Arch Phys Med Rehab*. 1994;75:957-959.
4. Gray H; Williams PL, ed. *Gray's Anatomy*. 38th ed. New York, NY: Churchill Livingstone; 1995.
5. Hart A, Hopkins C, Ford B. *ICD-9-CM Expert For Physicians, Volume 1&2*. 7th ed. USA: Ingenix; 2005.
6. Lewek M, Stevens J, Snyder-Mackler L. The use of electrical stimulation to increase quadriceps femoris muscle force in an elderly patient following a total knee arthroplasty. *Phys Ther*. September 2001;81(9):1565-1571.
7. Mizner RL, Stevens JE, Snyder-Mackler L. Voluntary activation and decreased force production of the quadriceps femoris muscle after total knee arthroplasty. *Phys Ther*. April 2003;83(4):359-365.

TOTAL KNEE REPLACEMENT—OUTPATIENT
SUMMARY OVERVIEW

ICD-9

V43.65

APTA Preferred Practice Pattern: 4I

EXAMINATION

- History and Systems Review
- Tests and Measures
  Systems review per APTA's *Guide to Physical Therapy Practice*
  - Aerobic capacity
  - Anthropometric characteristics
  - Arousal, attention, cognition
  - Gait, locomotion, and balance
  - Integumentary integrity
  - Pain
  - ROM
  - Self-care and home management
- Establish Plan of Care

GOALS/OUTCOMES

- AROM of knee: 5–115°
- Lower extremity muscle strength to 5-/5 on manual muscle tests or equal to uninvolved limb
- Independent, pain-free gait pattern with assistive device as needed over all surfaces
- Return to previous functional status for ADLs and vocational and recreational activities as identified by patient
- Ability to perform double leg squat to 90° knee joint angle without hand hold
- Pain: 2/10 or less
- Improved neuromuscular/balance/proprioceptive ability to achieve single leg stance time of 80% of uninvolved leg
- Independence in a progressive home exercise program emphasizing function

INTERVENTION
NUMBER OF VISITS: 7–22

- Patient Instruction
  - Basic Anatomy and Biomechanics
  - Handouts
  - Functional Considerations
  - Description of Surgical Procedure
- Direct Interventions
  - Acute Phase: 1–4 Visits, Weeks 1–2
  - Subacute Phase I: 3–6 Visits, Weeks 3–6
  - Subacute Phase II: 3–12 Visits, Weeks 7–12
- Functional Carryover

DISCHARGE PLANNING AND PATIENT RESPONSIBILITY

- Criteria for Discharge
  - Patient has achieved all rehabilitation goals except previous functional status for recreational activities
  - Patient maintains good posture and body mechanics
- Circumstances Requiring Additional Visits
  - History of other lower-extremity pathology
  - Presence of other medical conditions
  - Postoperative complications
  - Cognitive limitations
- Home Program
  - Strengthening exercises: 3 times a week
  - Cardiovascular training and flexibility (daily)
- Monitoring

TOTAL KNEE REPLACEMENT—OUTPATIENT

ICD-9
   V43.65   Knee joint replacement
APTA Preferred Practice Pattern: 4I

EXAMINATION

History and Systems Review
- History of current condition
  ○ Date of surgery, type of procedure
  ○ Postoperative rehabilitation progression or complications
  ○ Weight-bearing status
- Past history of current condition
  ○ Previous lower-extremity injuries or surgery and treatments
- Functional status and activity level (current/prior)
- Patient's functional goals

Tests and Measures
Systems review per APTA's *Guide to Physical Therapy Practice*
- Aerobic capacity
- Anthropometric characteristics
  ○ Girth measurements
- Arousal, attention, cognition
  ○ Compliance with postoperative limitations
- Gait, locomotion, and balance
  ○ Gait characteristics
    ▪ Swing phase, stance phase
    ▪ Stair negotiation
  ○ Antalgic gait
  ○ Use of assistive devices
  ○ Stride length
  ○ Weight-bearing tolerance
  ○ Adequate extension in stance phase
  ○ Weight shift
  ○ Balance/reach functional tests
  ○ Static/dynamic balance
- Integumentary integrity
  ○ Skin color, sensation, scar tissue, etc.
- Pain
  ○ Measured on visual analog scale
  ○ Classification
- ROM
  ○ Hip

○ Knee; also PROM
○ Foot/ankle
- Self-care and home management
  ○ Transfer status to all surfaces

Establish Plan of Care
- Based on history, tests, and measures

GOALS/OUTCOMES
- AROM of knee: 5–115°
- Lower extremity muscle strength to 5-/5 on manual muscle tests or equal to uninvolved limb
- Independent, pain-free gait pattern with assistive device as needed over all surfaces
- Return to previous functional status for ADLs and vocational and recreational activities as identified by patient
- Ability to perform double leg squat to 90° knee joint angle without hand hold
- Pain: 2/10 or less
- Improved neuromuscular/balance/proprioceptive ability to achieve single leg stance time of 80% of uninvolved leg
- Independence in a progressive home exercise program emphasizing function

INTERVENTION
NUMBER OF VISITS: 7–22

Coordination, Communication, and Documentation
- Provision of services between admission and discharge that facilitate cost-effective and efficient integration or reintegration to home, community, or work
- Documentation of therapeutic intervention is required for each episode of care and serves as the basic foundation for communication
- Coordination and additional communication will depend on the patient's impairment and home/work/

community/leisure situation and requirements. Such services may include:

- ○ Case management
- ○ Coordination of care and collaboration with those integral to the patient's rehabilitation program
- ○ Coordination and monitoring of the delivery of available resources
- ○ Referrals to other health-care professionals
- ○ Identification of resources, support groups, or advocacy services
- ○ Provision of educational or training information
- ○ Technical assistance

Patient Instruction

Basic Anatomy and Biomechanics

- Pertinent Gray's Anatomy (Gray. 1995. 697–709, 869, 876)
- Krames Communications (1100 Grundy Lane, San Bruno, CA 94066)
  - ○ *Total Knee Replacement*
  - ○ *After Total Knee Replacement*

Handouts

- Home cryotherapy/thermal modalities
- Use of continuous passive motion machine as indicated
- Transfers and use of other assistive devices as indicated
- Precautions
  - ○ Avoid twisting, jumping, forced movements

Functional Considerations

- Weight-bearing status and progression
- Stair technique, uneven terrain, and transfers as appropriate
- Avoidance of sleeping with pillows under the knees or in sitting position
- Modification of home environment for discharge, such as raised toilet seat, shower rails

Description of Surgical Procedure

- Review of operative procedure and relation to joint biomechanics, rehabilitation, and function

Direct Interventions

Acute Phase: 1–4 Visits, Weeks 1–2

- Therapeutic exercise and home program
  - ○ Isometrics (quadriceps, hamstrings, gluteals)
  - ○ Active-assisted to active straight-leg raises
  - ○ Ankle pumps
  - ○ Terminal knee extensions
  - ○ Quad sets
  - ○ Stretching/PROM
    - ▪ Gastrocnemius/soleus
    - ▪ Quadriceps
    - ▪ Hamstrings
  - ○ Heel slides and ROM exercises
  - ○ Stationary cycling
  - ○ Gait training, partial weight bearing or full weight bearing per physician instruction
- Functional training
  - ○ Bed mobility and transfers training
  - ○ Self-care
- Manual therapy techniques
  - ○ Joint mobilization
    - ▪ Patellar mobilization
  - ○ Soft-tissue technique
    - ▪ Soft-tissue mobilization to enhance soft-tissue extensibility and stretching
    - ▪ Scar mobilization
- Electrotherapeutic modalities
  - ○ Electrical stimulation
- Physical agents and mechanical modalities
  May be used to manage pain and to assist in muscle reeducation
  - ○ Cryotherapy
  - ○ Compression therapies
  - ○ Continuous passive motion as ordered 5 hours per day, patient to increase flexion 5–10° daily
- Goals/outcomes
  - ○ Functional activities
    - ▪ Independence in bed transfers without trapeze
    - ▪ Independence in gait with assistive device on level surfaces and stairs
    - ▪ Independent ADLs
  - ○ AROM: 5–90° of involved knee
  - ○ Motor performance: 3/5 on manual muscle test
  - ○ Pain: 5/10 or less

Subacute Phase I: 3–6 Visits, Weeks 3–6

- Therapeutic exercise and home program
  - ROM/stretching
  - Continue exercises from Acute Phase I
  - Isotonic with ankle weights and/or resistive bands
    - Knee extension
    - Knee flexion
    - Hip, four-way straight-leg raise
  - Submaximal isokinetics
  - Closed-kinetic chain exercise in pain-free range
    - Partial lunges
    - Modified leg press
    - Heel raises
    - Wall slide
    - Partial squats
  - Balance and coordination training
    - Balance and reach
    - Backward walking
    - BAPS
    - Heel/toe walking
    - Side stepping
    - Mini trampoline
    - Single-limb weight-bearing on involved extremity
  - Aquatic exercises (deep water jog, squats, straight-leg exercises, step-up exercises)
  - Proprioceptive neuromuscular facilitation
  - Aerobic endurance
    - Cycling
    - Upper body ergometer
  - Gait training
    - Progression to ambulation with a cane as tolerated
- Manual therapy techniques
  - Joint mobilization
    - Patellar mobilization as appropriate
  - Soft-tissue mobilization
- Physical agents and mechanical modalities
  - Continued as in Acute Phase I
- Goals/outcomes
  - Independence with transfers to all surfaces
  - AROM: 5–110°
  - Strength: 4/5 on manual muscle test
  - Pain: 3/10 or less

Subacute Phase II: 3–12 Visits, Weeks 7–12

- Therapeutic exercise and home program
  - Emphasis on remaining muscle performance and ROM deficits

- Self-stretching exercises in weight-bearing position on chair or stool
- Step up/step down to assist in ascending and descending stairs
- Decrease utilization of assistive devices in gait
- Emphasis upon functional return, such as golf, bowling, stairs, driving
- Gait training with cane on stairs and uneven surfaces
- Manual therapy techniques
  - Joint mobilization
    - Patellar mobilization as indicated
- Physical agents and mechanical modalities
  - Cryotherapy
  - Thermal modalities
- Goals/outcomes
  - Functional activities
    - Independent, pain-free ADLs
    - Independent, normal gait pattern with cane over all surfaces
    - Return to previous functional status for vocational activities
  - AROM: 5–115°
  - Strength: 5-/5 on manual muscle tests of lower extremity or equal to uninvolved leg
  - Pain: 2/10 or less
  - Improved neuromuscular/balance/proprioceptive ability to achieve single leg stance time of 80% of uninvolved leg

Functional Carryover

- Review of precautions: Avoid pillows under involved knee or prolonged time in recliner
- Modification of home for discharge, such as raised toilet seat
- Functional activities to enhance rehabilitation
  - Using stairs for strengthening
  - Walking program to accomplish errands and improve cardiovascular condition, etc.
- Tapering off of assistive devices as appropriate
- Guidance in return to recreation and sports activities as indicated

DISCHARGE PLANNING AND PATIENT RESPONSIBILITY

Criteria for Discharge

- Patient has achieved all rehabilitation goals except previous functional status for recreational activities
- Patient maintains good posture and body mechanics

Circumstances Requiring Additional Visits

- History of other lower-extremity pathology
- Presence of other medical conditions
- Postoperative complications
- Cognitive limitations

Home Program

- Strengthening exercises: 3 times a week
- Cardiovascular training and flexibility (daily)

Monitoring

- Optimally, rehabilitation is complete when there is no functional difference between the surgical and the non-surgical knees
- Patient is to recheck/call at 2–4 weeks post discharge to ensure progression towards previous functional status for vocational, recreational, and sports activities

REFERENCE

1. American Physical Therapy Association. *Guide to Physical Therapist Practice*. Alexandria, VA: APTA; 1997.
2. Berman AT, Zarro VJ, Bosacco SJ, et al. Quantitative gait analysis after unilateral or bilateral total knee replacement. *J Bone Joint Surg Am*. 1987;69:1340-1345.
3. Brimer MA. New clinical consideration in total knee replacement rehabilitation. *Clin Manage Phys Ther*. 1987;7(1):6-9.
4. Gateley-Jameson K, Barrow D, Bass D, et al. Cementless total knee replacement. *Clin Manage Phys Ther*. 1988;8(6):21-23.
5. Gray, G. *Lower Extremity Functional Profile*. Adrian, MI: Wynn Marketing; 1995.
6. Gray H; Williams PL, ed. *Gray's Anatomy*. 38th ed. New York, NY: Churchill Livingstone; 1995.
7. Hart A, Hopkins C, Ford B. *ICD-9-CM Expert for Physicians, Volume 1&2*. 7th ed. USA: Ingenix; 2005.
8. Kendall FP, McCreary EK, Provance PG. *Muscles Testing and Function*. Baltimore, MD: Williams and Wilkins; 1993.
9. Kroll MA, Otis JC, Sculco TP, et al. The relationship of stride characteristics to pain before and after total knee arthroplasty. *Clin Orthop Rel Res*. 1989;239:191-195.
10. Laskin RS, Rieger MA. The surgical technique for performing a total knee arthroplasty. *Orthop Clin North Am*. 1989;20:31-48.
11. Mangine RE. *Physical Therapy of the Knee*. New York, NY: Churchill Livingston; 1988:210-219.
12. Richardson JK, Iglarsh ZA. *Clinical Orthopedic Physical Therapy*. Philadelphia, PA: WB Saunders; 1994.
13. Sandler Goldstein T. *Geriatric Orthopaedics Rehabilitative Management of Common Problems*. Gaithersburg, MD: Aspen Publishers; 1991:93-99.
14. Smidt GL, Albright JP, Deusinger RH. Pre- and postoperative functional changes in total knee patients. *J Orthop Sports Phys Ther*. 1984;6(1):25-29.

168   TOTAL KNEE REPLACEMENT—OUTPATIENT | KNEE

Hip

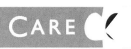

HIP

Hip Degenerative Joint Disease	171
Hip Fracture/Total Hip Replacement—Outpatient	177
Hip Fracture/Total Hip Replacement—Inpatient	183
Hip Soft Tissue Pain	187
Hip Sprain/Strain	193

170   HIP

HIP DEGENERATIVE JOINT DISEASE
SUMMARY OVERVIEW

ICD-9

715.35

APTA Preferred Practice Pattern: **4A, 4F, 4H, 6B**

EXAMINATION

- History and Systems Review
- Tests and Measures
  Systems review per APTA's *Guide to Physical Therapy Practice*
  - Gait, locomotion, and balance
  - Joint integrity and mobility
  - Pain
  - Posture
  - ROM
  - Special tests
- Establish Plan of Care

GOALS/OUTCOMES

- ROM of the lower extremity to allow functional activities
- Pain: 2/10 or less
- Strength of lower-extremity muscles: 4/5 on manual muscle tests or equivalent to uninvolved extremity on closed-kinetic chain functional tests
- Normal gait pattern with assistive devices as needed
- Return to previous functional status for ADLs and vocational and recreational activities as identified by patient
- Independence in a progressive home exercise program emphasizing function

INTERVENTION
NUMBER OF VISITS: 4–16

- Patient Instruction
  - Basic Anatomy and Biomechanics
  - Handouts
  - Functional Considerations
- Direct Interventions
  - Acute Phase: 2–6 Visits
  - Subacute Phase: 2–10 Visits
- Functional Carryover

DISCHARGE PLANNING AND PATIENT RESPONSIBILITY

- Criteria for Discharge
  - All rehabilitation goals achieved with the exception of previous functional status for recreational and sports activities
- Circumstances Requiring Additional Visits
  - History of additional lower-extremity/lumbar pathology
  - Presence of other medical conditions
  - Severe deconditioning
- Home Program
  - Closed-kinetic chain functional exercises
  - Flexibility exercises
  - Functional progression for return to recreational and sports activities
- Monitoring

SUMMARY OVERVIEW | HIP | HIP DEGENERATIVE JOINT DISEASE   171

HIP DEGENERATIVE JOINT DISEASE

ICD-9
> 715.35   Osteoarthrosis, localized, not specified whether primary or secondary, pelvic region and thigh

APTA Preferred Practice Pattern: **4A, 4F, 4H, 6B**

EXAMINATION

History and Systems Review

- History of current condition
  - Mechanism of injury/onset
  - Date of injury/onset
- Past history of current condition
  - Prior treatment
  - Recent injuries to hip
  - Childhood disorders:
    - Congenital dysplasia
    - Slipped capital epiphysis
    - Legg-Calve-Perthes disease
  - Previous lower-extremity injury/surgery
- Other tests and measures
  - Diagnostic testing
- Past medical/surgical history
  - Tuberculosis
  - Ankylosing spondylitis
  - Rheumatoid arthritis
- Functional status and activity level (current/prior)
  - Ambulatory aides
  - Use of adaptive devices or equipment
- Patient's functional goals

Tests and Measures

Systems review per APTA's *Guide to Physical Therapy Practice*

- Gait, locomotion, and balance
  - Trendelenburg
  - Pelvic symmetry
  - Stance phase weight-bearing
  - Stride length symmetry
  - Arm swing
  - Excessive or prolonged compensatory pronation
  - Use of assistive devices
  - Weight shift
  - Balance/reach test

- Unilateral stance on involved extremity, reach in various directions with uninvolved extremity to assess both proprioception and muscle performance in various muscles depending on direction of reach; compare distance reached to similar reaches in unilateral stance on uninvolved extremity.
- Unilateral stance on involved extremity, reach in various directions with one or both arms to assess proprioception and trunk/lower-extremity muscle performance; compare distance reached with similar reaches in unilateral stance on uninvolved extremity.
  - BAPS
- Joint integrity and mobility
  - Passive motion tests to determine status of joint surface
    - Hip scouring test
      a. Test evaluates posterior and lateral hip joint capsule and may elicit a grating sensation or sound in osteoarthritic hips
      b. Knee flexion is combined with hip flexion and adduction with the patient in supine position
      c. A posterolateral force is applied through the joint as the femur is rotated in the acetabulum
- Pain
  - Measured on visual analog scale
- Posture
  If positive, a full biomechanical assessment may be indicated. See *Biomechanical Lower Extremity Dysfunction* guideline.
  - Static, non-weight-bearing alignment of hip, knee, subtalar, and midtarsal joint
  - Static, weight-bearing alignment
  - Leg length in supine, long sitting, and pelvic level in weight-bearing
    - False and true
- ROM
  - AROM
    - Hip
    - Knee

172   HIP DEGENERATIVE JOINT DISEASE | HIP

- Foot/ankle
- Trunk
  - Muscle length
    - Thomas test
    - Ober test
    - Straight-leg raise
    - Gastrocnemius and soleus
    - Patrick/FABRE test
      a. Positive if pain is reproduced directly in hip joint
      b. Inguinal pain implicates hip joint pathology or muscular restrictions
- Special tests
  - Climbing test
    - Standing with one foot on the table, the patient lunges further toward the table to test full range of flexion of the elevated extremity at the hip, knee, and ankle, and extension of the opposite hip and knee
  - Squatting
    - To assess functional ability to retrieve objects from floor
  - Sitting, bending forward to touch floor

Establish Plan of Care

- Based on history, tests, and measures

GOALS/OUTCOMES

- ROM of the lower extremity to allow functional activities:
  - Hip:
    - Flexion: 125°
    - Extension: 0°
    - Internal rotation in neutral: 20°
    - External rotation in neutral: 30°
  - Knee: 5–120°
  - Ankle: Dorsiflexion: 8° in subtalar neutral with knee extended
- Pain: 2/10 or less
- Strength of lower-extremity muscles: 4/5 on manual muscle tests or equivalent to uninvolved extremity on closed-kinetic chain functional tests
- Normal gait pattern with assistive devices as needed
- Return to previous functional status for ADLs and vocational and recreational activities as identified by patient
- Independence in a progressive home exercise program emphasizing function

INTERVENTION
NUMBER OF VISITS: 4–16

Coordination, Communication, and Documentation

- Provision of services between admission and discharge that facilitate cost-effective and efficient integration or reintegration to home, community, or work
- Documentation of therapeutic intervention is required for each episode of care and serves as the basic foundation for communication
- Coordination and additional communication will depend on the patient's impairment and home/work/community/leisure situation and requirements. Such services may include:
  - Case management
  - Coordination of care and collaboration with those integral to the patient's rehabilitation program
  - Coordination and monitoring of the delivery of available resources
  - Referrals to other health-care professionals
  - Identification of resources, support groups, or advocacy services
  - Provision of educational or training information
  - Technical assistance
- Specific coordination and communication provisions:
  - Referral for biomechanical orthotics

Patient Instruction

Basic Anatomy and Biomechanics

- Importance of adequate ROM of all joints in kinetic chain (back, knee, ankle) to reduce stress on involved hip
- Role of excessive or prolonged compensatory pronation in exacerbation or onset of hip pain
- Pertinent Gray's Anatomy (Gray. 1995. 681, 684–689, 869, 876–877)

Handouts

- Home exercise program
  - Closed-kinetic chain exercises
  - Open-chain hip strength exercises with posterior and lateral hip strength emphasis
  - Flexibility exercises
- Home cryotherapy or superficial thermal modalities for pain control

HIP | HIP DEGENERATIVE JOINT DISEASE   173

Functional Considerations

- Awareness of the relationship of joint pain to immobility
- Use of appropriate ambulatory aides to reduce limping, improve stance stability, and reduce stress on involved extremity
- Stair climbing techniques, ambulation on uneven terrain, and progression toward recreational activities
- Proper choice of footwear to minimize excessive or prolonged compensatory pronation and enhance stability

Direct Interventions

Acute Phase: 2–6 Visits

- Therapeutic exercise and home program
  - Flexibility exercise within pain-free range for lower extremity
  - Open- and closed-kinetic chain strengthening exercise without exacerbation of pain
    - Partial squats
    - Resistive band resisted hip exercises
    - Weight shifting
    - Gait drills
    - Upper extremity
    - Aquatic exercises
- Manual therapy techniques
  - Soft-tissue techniques
    - Myofascial release
    - Soft-tissue mobilization
  - Joint mobilization
    - Grade I–II oscillations for pain relief
  - ROM/pain-free stretching
- Physical agents and mechanical modalities
  - Thermal/cryotherapy
  - Ultrasound
- Goals/outcomes
  - Pain: 5/10 or less
  - Normal gait pattern with ambulatory devices as needed, for limited distance
  - Stairs
  - Pain-free ROM to achieve:
    - Hip:
      a. Flexion: 100°
      b. Extension: 0°
      c. Internal rotation in neutral: 10°
      d. External rotation in neutral: 15°

- Functional motor performance
  - Independent transfers to and from sitting

Subacute Phase: 2–10 Visits

- Therapeutic exercise and home program
  - Cardiovascular conditioning
    - Bicycle
    - Aquatic activity
    - Treadmill
    - Elliptical trainer
  - Free weights
  - Closed-kinetic chain exercise
  - Open-chain hip strengthening exercise
  - Progression of flexibility exercises
  - Neuromuscular/balance/proprioceptive reeducation
    - Gait drills
    - BAPS/balance board
- Manual therapy techniques
  - Joint mobilization
    - Grade I–II oscillations for pain relief
    - Progressive grades as tolerated to increase pain-free ROM
  - Passive stretches
  - Manual resistive activities
- Therapeutic devices and equipment
  - Functional biomechanics
    - Integration of specific structural or biomechanical components that may relieve symptoms, including the choice of shoes and/or custom biomechanical orthotics to control excessive compensatory pronation
- Physical agents and mechanical modalities
  - Thermal/cryotherapy
- Goals/outcomes
  - Pain
    - 2/10 or less with daily activity
    - 4/10 or less after exercise
  - ROM of the lower extremity to allow functional activities
  - Strength of lower-extremity muscles of 4/5 on manual muscle test or equivalent to uninvolved extremity on closed-kinetic chain functional tests
  - Normal gait pattern with assistive device as needed
  - Return to previous functional status for ADLs and vocational activities

174   HIP DEGENERATIVE JOINT DISEASE | HIP

Functional Carryover

- Instruction in use of or tapering off of ambulatory aides as appropriate
- In an arthritic hip, it may take months of daily stretching to achieve full functional hip ROM
- Instruction in return to recreational activities with emphasis on proper progression of intensity, frequency, and duration
- Instruction in proper choice of footwear to minimize biomechanical factors that may be contributing to or exacerbating current symptoms
- Pacing daily function to avoid exacerbation of symptoms

DISCHARGE PLANNING AND PATIENT RESPONSIBILITY

Criteria for Discharge

- All rehabilitation goals achieved with the exception of previous functional status for recreational and sports activities

Circumstances Requiring Additional Visits

- History of additional lower-extremity/lumbar pathology
- Presence of other medical conditions
- Severe deconditioning

Home Program

- Closed-kinetic chain functional exercises
  - Squats
  - Weight shift
  - Lunges (anterior, lateral, posterior)
  - Balance/reach
  - Gait drills
- Flexibility exercises
  - Hamstrings
  - Quadriceps
  - Gastrocnemius/soleus
  - Piriformis
  - Hip flexors
  - Low back
  - Iliotibial band
  - "Butterfly" sitting (external rotation and abduction)
  - Side sitting (internal rotation)
- Functional progression for return to recreational and sports activities

Monitoring

- Patient to call at 4–6 weeks post-discharge to ensure progression toward expected return to function
- Schedule follow-up clinic visit in 4 weeks as needed to address persistent symptoms or difficulty returning to full function

HIP | HIP DEGENERATIVE JOINT DISEASE   175

REFERENCES

1. American Physical Therapy Association. *Guide to Physical Therapist Practice*. Alexandria, VA: APTA; 1997.

2. Gerard J, Kleinfield SL. *Orthopaedic Testing: A Rational Approach To Diagnosis*. New York, NY: Churchill Livingstone; 1993.

3. Gray G. *Lower Extremity Functional Profile*. Adrian, MI: Wynn Marketing; 1995.

4. Gray H; Williams PL, ed. *Gray's Anatomy*. 38th ed. New York, NY: Churchill Livingstone; 1995.

5. Hart A, Hopkins C, Ford B. *ICD-9-CM Expert For Physicians, Volume 1&2*. 7th ed. USA: Ingenix; 2005.

6. Hertling D, Kessler R. *Management of Common Musculoskeletal Disorders: Physical Therapy Principles and Methods*. 3rd ed. Philadelphia, PA: Lippincott-Raven Publishers; 1996.

7. Hoeksma HL, Dekker J, Ronday H, et al. Comparison of manual therapy and exercise therapy in osteoarthritis of the hip: a randomized clinical trial. *Arthritis Rheum*. 2004;51(5):722-9.

8. Hoppenfeld S. *Physical Examination Of The Spine And Extremities*. New York, NY: Appleton-Century-Crofts; 1976.

9. Jenkins DB. *Hollinshead's Functional Anatomy of The Limbs and Back*. 6th ed. Philadelphia, PA: WB Saunders; 1991.

10. Kendall FP, McCreary EK, Provance, PG. *Muscles: Testing and Function*. 4th ed. Baltimore, MD: Williams & Wilkins; 1993.

11. Magee DJ. *Orthopedic Physical Assessment*. 3rd ed. Philadelphia, PA: WB Saunders; 1997.

12. O'Sullivan SB, Schmitz TJ. *Physical Rehabilitation: Assessment And Treatment*. 3rd ed. Philadelphia, PA: FA Davis; 1994.

13. Porter-Hoke A. North American Institute of Orthopaedic Manual Therapy Course Notes: Level 1 and 2. Eugene, OR: NAIOMT, Inc; 1993.

14. Richardson JK, Iglarsh AZ. *Clinical Orthopedic Physical Therapy*. Philadelphia, PA: WB Saunders; 1994.

HIP FRACTURE/TOTAL HIP REPLACEMENT—OUTPATIENT
SUMMARY OVERVIEW

ICD-9

719.55   728.9   808.0   820.00   820.01   820.2   820.8   821.00   V43.60
V43.64   V43.69

APTA Preferred Practice Pattern: **4A, 4C, 4D, 4F, 4G, 4H, 4I, 4J, 7A**

EXAMINATION

- History and Systems Review
- Tests and Measures
  Systems review per APTA's *Guide to Physical Therapy Practice*
  - Arousal, attention, cognition
  - Gait, locomotion, and balance
  - Integumentary integrity
  - Muscle performance
  - Pain
  - Posture
  - ROM
- Establish Plan of Care

GOALS/OUTCOMES

- Pain: 2/10 or less
- Normal gait pattern, FWB (as allowed by surgical protocol)
- AROM of the involved hip within total hip precautions or postoperative limitations
- Neuromuscular/balance/proprioceptive reeducation to achieve 80% of uninvolved leg as measured by single leg stance time
- Strength: 4/5 or greater on lower-extremity manual muscle test or 80% of uninvolved leg
- Return to independent functional ADLs, including getting in/out of bed, going up/down stairs, shopping, cooking, housework, driving, bathing, and dressing
- Independence in a progressive home exercise program emphasizing function

INTERVENTION
NUMBER OF VISITS: 7–14

- Patient Instruction
  - Basic Anatomy and Biomechanics
  - Handouts
  - Functional Considerations
- Direct Intervention
  - Acute Phase: 3–7 Visits Over 4 Weeks
  - Subacute Phase: 4–7 Visits Over 4 Week
- Functional Carryover

DISCHARGE PLANNING AND PATIENT RESPONSIBILITY

- Criteria for Discharge
  - Patient understands and demonstrates hip limitations as dictated by surgical procedure
  - Patient maintains good posture and body mechanics
  - All rehabilitation goals have been achieved
  - Patient has initiated progression toward previous functional status for vocational and recreational activities
- Circumstances Requiring Additional Visits
  - History of additional lower-extremity/lumbar pathology
  - Presence of other medical conditions
  - Postoperative complications
  - Preoperative contractures
- Home Program
  - Flexibility exercises
  - Motor performance
  - Gait drills
- Monitoring

SUMMARY OVERVIEW | HIP | HIP FRACTURE/TOTAL HIP REPLACEMENT—OUTPATIENT   177

HIP FRACTURE/TOTAL HIP REPLACEMENT—OUTPATIENT

ICD-9

719.55	Stiffness of joint, not elsewhere classified, pelvic region and thigh
728.9	Unspecified disorder of muscle, ligament, and fascia
808.0	Closed fracture of acetabulum
820.00	Closed fracture of unspecified intracapsular section of neck of femur
820.01	Closed fracture of epiphysis (separation) (upper) of neck of femur
820.2	Closed pertrochanteric fracture of neck of femur
820.8	Closed fracture of unspecified part of neck of femur
821.00	Closed fracture of unspecified part of femur
V43.60	Unspecified joint replacement
V43.64	Hip joint replacement
V43.69	Other joint replacement

APTA Preferred Practice Pattern: 4A, 4C, 4D, 4F, 4G, 4H, 4I, 4J, 7A

EXAMINATION

History and Systems Review

- History of current condition
  - Mechanism of injury and date
  - Surgical procedure and date
  - Postoperative progression/complications
- Past history of current condition
  - Prior treatment
  - History of injuries/falls
- Functional status and activity level (current/prior)
  - Weight-bearing status
  - ADLs status
    - Consider referral to occupational therapy for adaptive devices
- Health status self report
  - General health
  - Role function
  - Psychosocial issues
- Patient's functional goals

Tests and Measures

Systems review per APTA's *Guide to Physical Therapy Practice*

- Arousal, attention, cognition
  - Cognitive status in relation to compliance with postoperative limitations
- Gait, locomotion, and balance
  - Weight-bearing tolerance
  - Appropriate use of assistive device
  - Stride length

- Integumentary integrity
  - Surgical incision
- Muscle performance
  - Strength testing
    - Hip abductors, tensor fasciæ latæ vs. gluteus medius
    - Upper extremity
  - Palpation of muscles and tendons
- Pain
  - Measured on visual analog scale
- Posture
  - True vs. apparent leg length discrepancy assessment
    - Pelvic tilt
    - Adductor contracture
    - Hip capsule tightness
    - Asymmetrical static or dynamic foot position
    - Hip flexion contracture
    - Palpation of key landmarks
- ROM
  - Active/passive
    - Lumbar
    - Hip
    - Knee
    - Ankle
      a. Within hip precautions or postoperative limitations

Establish Plan of Care

- Based on history, tests, and measures

GOALS/OUTCOMES

- Pain: 2/10 or less
- Normal gait pattern, full weight bearing (as allowed by surgical protocol)
- AROM of the involved hip within total hip precautions or postoperative limitations
- Neuromuscular/balance/proprioceptive reeducation to achieve 80% of uninvolved leg as measured by single leg stance time
- Strength: 4/5 or greater on lower-extremity manual muscle test or 80% of uninvolved leg
- Return to independent functional ADLs, including getting in/out of bed, going up/down stairs, shopping, cooking, housework, driving, bathing, and dressing
- Independence in a progressive home exercise program emphasizing function

INTERVENTION
NUMBER OF VISITS: 7–14

Coordination, Communication, and Documentation

- Provision of services between admission and discharge that facilitate cost-effective and efficient integration or reintegration to home, community, or work
- Documentation of therapeutic intervention is required for each episode of care and serves as the basic foundation for communication
- Coordination and additional communication will depend on the patient's impairment and home/work/community/leisure situation and requirements. Such services may include:
  ○ Case management
  ○ Coordination of care and collaboration with those integral to the patient's rehabilitation program
  ○ Coordination and monitoring of the delivery of available resources
  ○ Referrals to other health-care professionals
  ○ Identification of resources, support groups, or advocacy services
  ○ Provision of educational or training information
  ○ Technical assistance
- Specific coordination and communication provisions:
  ○ Referral to orthotics if abduction brace required (high rise or recurrent dislocation)

Patient Instruction

Basic Anatomy and Biomechanics

- Krames Communications (1100 Grundy Lane, San Bruno, CA 94066)
  ○ *Total Hip Replacement*
  ○ *After Total Hip Replacement*
- Pertinent Gray's Anatomy (Gray. 1995. 681, 684–691, 875–876)
- Personal instruction concerning:
  ○ ROM and weight-bearing limitations, dependent upon surgical procedure
  ○ Total hip precautions
    ▪ No hip flexion past 90°
    ▪ No hip adduction
    ▪ No internal rotation past neutral

Handouts

- Home exercise program
- List of precautions specific to surgical procedure

Functional Considerations

- Incorporation of precautions into ADLs
  ○ Addition of pillow to low chair
  ○ Bed mobility
- Decreased speed of movement
- Modification of home environment for safety
  ○ Rearrange furniture
  ○ Remove throw rugs
  ○ Add handrail on stairs

Direct Intervention

Acute Phase: 3–7 Visits Over 4 Week

- Therapeutic exercise and home program
  ○ Flexibility exercises within limitations of total hip precautions
    ▪ Psoas
    ▪ Quadriceps
    ▪ Gastrocnemius
    ▪ Soleus
    ▪ Hamstrings
  ○ Lower-extremity strengthening
    ▪ Open-kinetic chain
      a. Heel slides
      b. Hip abduction in supine
      c. Gluteal sets

HIP | HIP FRACTURE/TOTAL HIP REPLACEMENT—OUTPATIENT

d. Quad sets

e. Ankle pumps

- Closed-kinetic chain
  a. Weight shifting
  b. Modified squats
  c. Modified lunges (anterior, lateral)
  d. Step up/step down
  o Upper extremity strengthening
  o Aquatic exercises
  o Pelvic leveling
  o Neuromuscular/balance/proprioceptive reeducation
  - BAPS
  - Biased stance balance/reach
    a. Reach arms forward at shoulder height and waist height
  o Cardiovascular conditioning
  - Upper body ergometry
- Functional training
  o ADLs training
  - Gait training on level surfaces and stairs with assistive device
  - Transfers to all surfaces when allowed
- Manual therapy techniques
  o Soft-tissue techniques
  - Soft-tissue mobilization of posterolateral hip
  - Scar mobilization
  o Contract/relax techniques
  o Passive stretching of lateral hip, knee, lumbar spine within precautions
- Physical agents and mechanical modalities
  o Superficial thermal modalities
  o Cryotherapy
  o Ultrasound (diagnosis/status dependent)
- Goals/outcomes
  o Pain: 5/10 or less
  o Hip ROM: 70–90° flexion
  o Neuromuscular/balance/proprioceptive reeducation to achieve 50% of uninvolved leg as measured by single leg stance time
  o Strength: 3/5 on lower-extremity manual muscle test
  o Functional activities
  - Independent transfers
  - Independent stair negotiation with assistive device
  - Normal gait pattern with assistive device on level surfaces

Subacute Phase: 4–7 Visits Over 4 Weeks

- Therapeutic exercise and home program
  o Flexibility within limitations of total hip precautions
  o Strengthening to appropriate muscle groups
  - Progress lower-extremity exercise
  - Closed-kinetic chain
    a. Modified squat
    b. Modified lunges (anterior, lateral)
    c. Step up/step down
  o Aquatic exercises
  o Pelvic leveling
  o Neuromuscular/balance/proprioceptive reeducation
  - BAPS
  - SportCord™ resisted forward/backward walking, side stepping
  - Single-leg balance/reach exercises
    a. Reach arms forward
    b. Reach opposite leg forward
    c. Reach opposite leg laterally
  o Cardiovascular conditioning
  - Upper body ergometer
  - Elliptical trainer
  - Walking as appropriate
  - Other low-impact forms of conditioning as appropriate to individual
- Functional training
  o ADLs training
  - Gait training on all surfaces
  - Stair negotiation without assistive devices
- Manual therapy techniques
  o Soft-tissue techniques
  - Soft-tissue mobilization of lateral hip
  - Scar mobilization
  o Contract/relax
  o Passive stretching of lateral hip, knee, lumbar spine within precautions
  o Joint mobilization
  - As needed to restore functional joint ROM of the thoracic and lumbar spines and the lower extremity
- Physical agents and mechanical modalities
  o Superficial thermal modalities
  o Cryotherapy
  o Ultrasound
- Goals/outcomes
  o Pain: 2/10 or less
  o Hip ROM: 90° flexion

180   HIP FRACTURE/TOTAL HIP REPLACEMENT—OUTPATIENT | HIP

- Neuromuscular/balance/proprioceptive reeducation to achieve 80% of uninvolved leg as measured by single leg stance time
- Lower-extremity strength: 4/5
- Functional activity
  - Independent stair negotiation without assistive device
  - Pain-free ADLs
  - Independent, normal gait pattern without assistive device

Functional Carryover
- Patient should be independent in gait pattern and dressing with assistive devices
- Address sexual activity if patient has questions or concerns

DISCHARGE PLANNING AND PATIENT RESPONSIBILITY

Criteria for Discharge
- Patient understands and demonstrates hip limitations as dictated by surgical procedure
- Patient maintains good posture and body mechanics
- All rehabilitation goals have been achieved
- Patient has initiated progression toward previous functional status for vocational and recreational activities

Circumstances Requiring Additional Visits
- History of additional lower-extremity/lumbar pathology
- Presence of other medical conditions
- Postoperative complications
- Preoperative contractures

Home Program
- Flexibility exercises
- Motor performance
- Gait drills

Monitoring
- Patient is to recheck/call at 2 and 8 weeks post-discharge
- Schedule follow-up appointment at 1–2 months to ensure progression toward previous functional status for ADLs and vocational and recreational activities as identified by patient

REFERENCES

1. American Physical Therapy Association. *Guide to Physical Therapist Practice.* Alexandria, VA: APTA; 1997.
2. Bhave A, Mont M, Tennis S, et al. Functional problems and treatment solutions after total hip and knee joint arthroplasty. *J Bone Joint Surg Am.* 2005;87(2).
3. Gerard J, Kleinfeld SL. *Orthopaedic Testing, A Rational Approach To Diagnosis.* New York, NY: Churchill Livingstone; 1993.
4. Gray G. *Lower Extremity Functional Profile.* Adrian, MI: Wynn Marketing; 1995.
5. Gray H; Williams PL, ed. *Gray's Anatomy.* 38th ed. New York, NY: Churchill Livingstone; 1995.
6. Hart A, Hopkins C, Ford B. *ICD-9-CM Expert For Physicians, Volume 1&2.* 7th ed. USA: Ingenix; 2005.
7. Hertling D, Kessler R. *Management of Common Musculoskeletal Disorders: Physical Therapy Principles and Methods.* 3rd ed. Philadelphia, PA: Lippincott-Raven Publishers; 1996.
8. Hoppenfeld S. *Physical Examination of The Spine and Extremities.* New York, NY: Appleton-Century-Crofts; 1976.
9. Ito T, Nakayama Y, Tanaka H, et al. Distraction arthroplasty of the hip by bicentric femoral head prosthesis. *Clin Orthop Rel Res.* 1990;255:186-193.
10. Jenkins DB. *Hollinshead's Functional Anatomy of The Limbs and Back.* 6th ed. Philadelphia, PA: WB Saunders; 1991.
11. Kendall FP, McCreary EK, Provance PG. *Muscles: Testing and Function.* 4th ed. Baltimore, MD: Williams & Wilkins; 1993.
12. Magee DJ. *Orthopedic Physical Assessment.* 3rd ed. Philadelphia, PA: WB Saunders; 1997.
13. Morscher EW. Cementless total hip arthroplasty. *Clin Orthop Rel Res.* 1983;181:76-91.
14. Poker-Hoke A. North American Institute of Orthopaedic Manual Therapy Course Notes: Level 1 and 2. Eugene, OR: NAIOMT, Inc; 1993.
15. Richardson JK, Iglarsh AZ. *Clinical Orthopedic Physical Therapy.* Philadelphia, PA: WB Saunders; 1994.
16. Smidt WR, Clark CR, Smidt GL. Short-term strength and pain changes in total hip arthroplasty patients. *J Orthop Sports Phys Ther.* 1990;12(1):16-23.

182   Hip Fracture/Total Hip Replacement—Outpatient | Hip

HIP FRACTURE/TOTAL HIP REPLACEMENT—INPATIENT
SUMMARY OVERVIEW

ICD-9

719.55   728.9   808.0   820.00   820.01   820.2   820.8   821.00   V43.60
V43.64   V43.69

APTA Preferred Practice Pattern: 4A, 4C, 4D, 4F, 4G, 4H, 4I, 4J, 7A

EXAMINATION

- History and Systems Review
- Tests and Measures
  Systems review per APTA's *Guide to Physical Therapy Practice*
  - Arousal, attention, and cognition
  - Gait, locomotion, and balance
  - Integumentary integrity
  - Joint integrity and mobility
  - Muscle performance
  - Orthotics, protective and supportive devices
  - Pain
  - ROM
  - Self-care and home management
  - Ventilation, respiration, and circulation
- Establish Plan of Care

GOALS/OUTCOMES

- The client will achieve an independent/supervised functional level as detailed in guideline

INTERVENTION
NUMBER OF VISITS: 4–10 (2–5 DAYS DURING ACUTE HOSPITALIZATION)

- Patient Instruction
  - Basic Anatomy and Biomechanics
  - Handouts
  - Functional Considerations
- Direct Interventions
  - Acute Hospitalization: 4–10 Visits, 2–5 Days
- Functional Carryover

DISCHARGE PLANNING AND PATIENT RESPONSIBILITY

- Criteria for Discharge
  - Patient understands and demonstrates hip limitations as dictated by surgical procedure
  - Patient maintains good posture and body mechanics
  - Short-term rehabilitation goals (acute hospital) have been achieved
  - Patient has initiated progression toward previous functional status for ADLs
- Circumstances Requiring Additional Visits
  - Cognitive limitations
  - Comorbidities affecting ability to recover or progress
  - Postoperative complications (deep vein thrombosis, infection)
  - Inability to maintain weight-bearing status or hip precautions
  - Excessive barriers to discharge (multiple flights of stairs, abduction splint)
- Home Program
  - Referral to home health or outpatient physical therapy services is recommended
  - Continue inpatient exercise program independently 2–3 times daily
  - Advance ambulation 1–2 minutes daily as pain and activity tolerance allow, until functional at a community level (or prior level of function)
- Monitoring

SUMMARY OVERVIEW | HIP | HIP FRACTURE/TOTAL HIP REPLACEMENT—INPATIENT   183

HIP FRACTURE/TOTAL HIP REPLACEMENT—INPATIENT

ICD-9

719.55	Stiffness of joint, not elsewhere classified, pelvic region and thigh
728.9	Unspecified disorder of muscle, ligament, and fascia
808.0	Closed fracture of acetabulum
820.00	Closed fracture of unspecified intracapsular section of neck of femur
820.01	Closed fracture of epiphysis (separation) (upper) of neck of femur
820.2	Closed pertrochanteric fracture of neck of femur
820.8	Closed fracture of unspecified part of neck of femur
821.00	Closed fracture of unspecified part of femur
V43.60	Unspecified joint replacement
V43.64	Hip joint replacement
V43.69	Other joint replacement

APTA Preferred Practice Pattern: 4A, 4C, 4D, 4F, 4G, 4H, 4I, 4J, 7A

EXAMINATION

History and Systems Review
- History of current condition
  - Surgical procedure/date
    - Surgical report
    - Total hip arthroplasty surgical approach
    - Postoperative weight-bearing status
  - Complications
  - Chart review
    - Hemoglobin and hematocrit
    - Advanced directives
    - Supplements (i.e. oxygen, IV, catheter)
- Past medical/surgical history
  - Comorbidities
- Functional status and activity level (current/prior)
  - Assistive devices
  - History of falls
- Living environment
  - Support system
  - Stairs
- Patient's functional goals

Tests and Measures
Systems review per APTA's *Guide to Physical Therapy Practice*
- Arousal, attention, and cognition
  - Orientation
  - Motivational level
  - Cognitive status in relation to compliance with postoperative limitations and safety judgement
- Gait, locomotion, and balance
  - Gait analysis
    - Weight-bearing tolerance/maintenance of weight-bearing status
    - Appropriate use of assistive device
    - Stride length
  - Physiologic response to activity
  - Balance assessment
    - Fall risk
  - Total hip replacement precaution during movement
- Integumentary integrity
  - Sensation
  - Bleeding
- Joint integrity and mobility
  - Quality of movement
  - Palpation of key landmarks
  - Edema
- Muscle performance
  - Strength
    - Manual muscle test of uninvolved extremities, involved ankle dorsi/plantar flexors, quadriceps
    - Functional strength of involved extremity, hip extensors (sit to stand, FWB, WBAT only)
- Orthotics, protective and supportive devices
  - Use of abduction pillow or immobilizer
- Pain
  - Pain and soreness with joint movement, 0–10
- ROM
  - Functional ROM of uninvolved extremities
    - Lumbar, hips, knees, ankles, shoulders, elbows, wrists, and hands

○ Goniometric measure of involved knee flexion and extension in supine, up to total hip replacement limitations (0–90°)
- Self-care and home management
  ○ Ability to transfer
    ▪ Toilet transfers
    ▪ Bed mobility
- Ventilation, respiration, and circulation
  ○ Pedal pulse
  ○ Signs and symptoms of deep vein thrombosis

Establish Plan of Care
- Based on history, tests, and measures

GOALS/OUTCOMES
- The client will achieve an independent/supervised functional level for:
  ○ Transfers in and out of bed, on and off a commode, up and down from an appropriate chair (tall/elevated)
  ○ Gait training at a household level with the appropriate assistive device
  ○ Stair climbing one or more steps, consistent with their home environment, with appropriate assistive device with and without handrail
  ○ Performance of home exercise program, 5–10 repetitions each, 2–3 times a day
  ○ Adherence to Total Hip Arthroplasty precautions and correctly incorporating them into any of the above situations, including maintaining weight-bearing status, avoiding hip adduction, flexion more than 90°, and internal rotation

INTERVENTION
Number of Visits: 4–10 (2–5 days during acute hospitalization)

Coordination, Communication, and Documentation
- Provision of services between admission and discharge that facilitate cost-effective and efficient integration or reintegration to home, community, or work
- Documentation of therapeutic intervention is required for each episode of care and serves as the basic foundation for communication
- Coordination and additional communication will depend on the patient's impairment and home/work/

community/leisure situation and requirements. Such services may include:
  ○ Case management
  ○ Coordination of care and collaboration with those integral to the patient's rehabilitation program
  ○ Coordination and monitoring of the delivery of available resources
  ○ Referrals to other health-care professionals
  ○ Identification of resources, support groups, or advocacy services
  ○ Provision of educational or training information
  ○ Technical assistance
- Specific coordination and communication provisions:
  ○ Occupational therapy for adaptive equipment (reacher, sock aid) and ADLs carryover
  ○ Orthotist if abduction brace required (recurrent dislocation or high risk for dislocation)
  ○ Discharge planner

Patient Instruction

Basic Anatomy and Biomechanics
- Krames Communications (1100 Grundy Lane, San Bruno, CA 94066)
  ○ *After Total Hip Replacement*
- Pertinent Gray's Anatomy (Gray. 1995. 681, 684–691, 875–876)

Handouts
- Total hip precautions
  ○ No hip flexion past 90°
  ○ No hip adduction
  ○ No hip internal rotation past neutral
- ROM and weight-bearing limitations, dependent upon surgical procedure
- Home exercise program
  ○ Ankle pumps
  ○ Quad sets
  ○ Gluteal sets
  ○ Heel slides
  ○ Short-arc quads
  ○ Hamstring sets
  ○ Hip abduction

Functional Considerations
- Modification of home environment for safety
  ○ Remove throw rugs

- Add pillows to low chairs
- Handrails as needed (bathroom, shower, stairs)
- Rearrange furniture as needed (allowing room for assistive device)
- Address sexual activity if patient has questions or concerns

Direct Interventions

Acute Hospitalization: 4–10 Visits, 2–5 Days
- Therapeutic exercise and home program
  - Resistive exercise to the uninvolved extremities
  - Active, assistive hip flexion to the post operative limb
  - Ankle pumps, quad sets, gluteal sets, hamstring sets, heel slides, and short-arc quads of the postoperative limb with patient in bed
  - Sitting knee extension
  - Standing hip extension of the postoperative limb
- Functional training
  - Transfer training
    - In and out of bed
    - From bed to and from chair
    - To and from commode or elevated toilet seat
  - Gait training
    - Instruction in weight-bearing status
    - Gait instruction with assistive device
      a. Level surface
      b. Stair training
    - Progress assistive device as appropriate (pick up walker, pick up walker with casters, crutches)
- Therapeutic devices and equipment
  - Place abduction pillow or immobilizer
- Physical agents and mechanical modalities
  - Apply athrombic pumps (discontinue when client ambulatory)

Functional Carryover
- Patient should be independent in gait pattern with assistive device at a household level

DISCHARGE PLANNING AND PATIENT RESPONSIBILITY

Criteria for Discharge
- Patient understands and demonstrates hip limitations as dictated by surgical procedure
- Patient maintains good posture and body mechanics
- Short term rehabilitation goals (acute hospital) have been achieved

- Patient has initiated progression toward previous functional status for ADLs

Circumstances Requiring Additional Visits
- Cognitive limitations
- Comorbidities affecting ability to recover or progress
- Postoperative complications (deep vein thrombosis, infection)
- Inability to maintain weight-bearing status or hip precautions
- Excessive barriers to discharge (multiple flights of stairs, abduction splint)

Home Program
- Referral to home health or outpatient physical therapy services is recommended
- Continue inpatient exercise program independently 2–3 times daily
- Advance ambulation 1–2 minutes daily as pain and activity tolerance allow, until functional at a community level (or prior level of function)

Monitoring
- Patients should be rechecked after 8–12 weeks upon lifting of weight-bearing restrictions
- Ideally, rehabilitation is complete when the patient is ambulating independently without assistive device or limitation from their prior level of function

REFERENCES
1. American Academy of Orthopaedic Surgeons. *Total Hip Replacement Exercise Guide.* 2000.
2. American Physical Therapy Association. *Guide to Physical Therapist Practice.* Alexandria, VA: APTA; 1997.
3. Gray H; Williams PL, ed. *Gray's Anatomy.* 38th ed. New York, NY: Churchill Livingstone; 1995.
4. Hart A, Hopkins C, Ford B. *ICD-9-CM Expert For Physicians, Volume 1&2.* 7th ed. USA: Ingenix; 2005.
5. Krotenberg R, Stitik T, Johnston MV. Incidence of dislocation following hip arthroplasty for patients in the rehabilitation setting. *J Phys Med Rehab.* 1995;74:444-447.
6. Weingarten S, Riedinger MS, Sandhu M. Can practice guidelines safely reduce hospital length of stay? Results from a multicenter interventional study. *Am J Med.* 1998;105:33-40.

HIP SOFT TISSUE PAIN
SUMMARY OVERVIEW

ICD-9

724.3   726.5   843.9

APTA Preferred Practice Pattern: 4E, 4F, 4J

EXAMINATION

- History and Systems Review
- Tests and Measures
  Systems review per APTA's *Guide to Physical Therapy Practice*
  - Gait, locomotion, and balance
  - Joint integrity
  - Muscle performance
  - Pain
  - Posture
  - ROM
  - Special tests
- Establish Plan of Care

GOALS/OUTCOMES

- Pain-free ROM of the hip, knee, ankle, and foot as compared to the uninvolved extremity
- Pain: 2/10 or less
- Strength of lower-extremity muscles of 4/5 on manual muscle tests or equivalent to uninvolved extremity on closed-kinetic chain functional tests
- Pain-free, normal gait pattern without assistive devices on all surfaces
- Return to previous functional status for ADLs and vocational, recreational, and sports activities as identified by patient
- Independence in a progressive home exercise program emphasizing function

INTERVENTION
NUMBER OF VISITS: 5–10

- Patient Instruction
  - Basic Anatomy and Biomechanics
  - Handouts
  - Functional Considerations
- Direct Interventions
  - Acute Phase: 2–4 Visits
  - Subacute Phase: 3–6 Visits
- Functional Carryover

DISCHARGE PLANNING AND PATIENT RESPONSIBILITY

- Criteria for Discharge
  - All rehabilitation goals achieved with possible exceptions listed in guideline
- Circumstances Requiring Additional Visits
  - Severe degenerative changes
  - History of additional lower-extremity/lumbar pathology
  - Presence of other medical conditions
  - Hip contracture (previous prolonged bed rest)
- Home Program
  - Closed-kinetic chain functional exercises
  - Flexibility exercises
  - Functional progression for return to recreational and sports activities
- Monitoring

SUMMARY OVERVIEW | HIP | HIP SOFT TISSUE PAIN

HIP SOFT TISSUE PAIN

ICD-9

724.3	Sciatica
726.5	Enthesopathy of hip region
843.9	Sprain of unspecified site of hip and thigh

APTA Preferred Practice Pattern: 4E, 4F, 4J

EXAMINATION

History and Systems Review

- History of current condition
  - Mechanics of injury/onset
  - Date of injury/onset
- Past history of current condition
  - Childhood disorders, such as:
    - Congenital dysplasia
    - Slipped capital epiphysis
    - Legg-Calvé-Perthes disease
  - Back pain/surgery
  - Knee surgery
  - Ankle sprain
- Other tests and measures
- Past medical/surgical history
  - System pathology
    - Tuberculosis
    - Ankylosing spondylitis
    - Rheumatoid arthritis
- Functional status and activity level (current/prior)
  - Ambulatory aides
  - Occupational activities
  - Recreational activities
- Patient's functional goals

Tests and Measures

Systems review per APTA's *Guide to Physical Therapy Practice*

- Gait, locomotion, and balance
  - Stance phase weight-bearing
  - Stairs
  - Stride length symmetry
  - Arm swing
  - Pelvic symmetry
  - Excessive or prolonged compensatory pronation
  - Weight shift
  - Balance/reach test

- Unilateral stance on involved extremity, reach in various directions with uninvolved extremity to assess both proprioception and muscle performance in various muscles depending on direction of reach; compare distance reached to similar reaches in unilateral stance on uninvolved extremity
- Unilateral stance on involved extremity, reach in various directions with one or both arms to assess proprioception and trunk/lower-extremity muscle performance; compare distance reached with similar reaches in unilateral stance on uninvolved extremity
  - BAPS
- Joint integrity
  - Posterior glide
- Muscle performance
  - Manual muscle testing at hip muscles
- Pain
  - Measured on visual analog scale
- Posture
  If positive, a full biomechanical assessment may be indicated; see *Biomechanical Lower Extremity Dysfunction* guideline.
  - Static, nonweight-bearing alignment of hip, knee, subtalar, and midtarsal joint
  - Static, weight-bearing alignment
  - Leg length in supine, long sitting, and pelvic level in weight-bearing
- ROM
  - Active/passive ROM and muscle performance
    - Hip
    - Knee
    - Foot/ankle
    - Trunk
  - Passive overpressure
  - Muscle length
    - Thomas test
    - Ober test

188 HIP SOFT TISSUE PAIN | HIP

- Straight-leg raise
- Patrick/FABRE test
- Gastrocnemius and Soleus
- Piriformis test
- Special tests
  - Rule out referral from other areas
    - Lumbar consult *Low Back General Pain* guideline
      a. Positive results during Patrick/FABRE or straight-leg raise
      b. Referred pain during flexibility and special tests
      c. Pelvic and spine asymmetries during biomechanical screening
    - Knee
    - Foot/ankle
  - Closed pack, prone, extension abduction, and internal rotation (capsular pattern)
  - Climbing test
    - Standing with one foot up on the table, the patient lunges further toward the table to test full range of flexion of the elevated extremity at the hip, knee, and ankle, as well as extension of the opposite hip and knee
  - Hip scouring test
    - Test evaluates posterior and lateral hip joint capsule and may elicit a grating sensation or sound in osteoarthritic hips
    - Knee flexion is combined with hip flexion and adduction with the patient in supine position
    - A posterolateral force is applied through the joint as the femur is rotated in the acetabulum
    - Fulcrum test: Sitting distal thigh downward pressure (runner's stress fracture) (Boyd. 1997. 486)
  - Squatting

Establish Plan of Care

- Based on history, tests, and measures

GOALS/OUTCOMES

- Pain-free ROM of the hip, knee, ankle, and foot as compared to the uninvolved extremity. Normal ROM:
  - Hip:
    - Flexion: 125°
    - Extension: 0°
    - Internal rotation in neutral: 40°
    - External rotation in neutral: 50°
  - Knee:
    - Flexion: 135°
    - Extension: 0°
  - Ankle:
    - Plantarflexion: 40°
    - Dorsiflexion: 10° in subtalar neutral with knee extended
- Pain: 2/10 or less
- Strength of lower-extremity muscles of 4/5 on manual muscle tests or equivalent to uninvolved extremity on closed-kinetic chain functional tests
- Pain-free, normal gait pattern without assistive devices on all surfaces
- Return to previous functional status for ADLs and vocational, recreational, and sports activities as identified by patient
- Independence in a progressive home exercise program emphasizing function

INTERVENTION
NUMBER OF VISITS: 5–10

Coordination, Communication, and Documentation

- Provision of services between admission and discharge that facilitate cost-effective and efficient integration or reintegration to home, community, or work
- Documentation of therapeutic intervention is required for each episode of care and serves as the basic foundation for communication
- Coordination and additional communication will depend on the patient's impairment and home/work/community/leisure situation and requirements. Such services may include:
  - Case management
  - Coordination of care and collaboration with those integral to the patient's rehabilitation program
  - Coordination and monitoring of the delivery of available resources
  - Referrals to other health-care professionals
  - Identification of resources, support groups, or advocacy services
  - Provision of educational or training information
  - Technical assistance
- Specific coordination and communication provisions:
  - Referral for biomechanical orthotics

HIP | HIP SOFT TISSUE PAIN   189

Patient Instruction

Basic Anatomy and Biomechanics
- Importance of adequate ROM of all joints in kinetic chain (back, knee, ankle) to reduce stress on involved hip
- Role of excessive or prolonged compensatory pronation in exacerbation or onset of hip pain and overuse/irritation of the bursæ and tendons
- Pertinent Gray's Anatomy (Gray. 1995. 684–689, 869–879)

Handouts
- Home exercise program
  - Motor performance exercises
  - Flexibility exercises
- Home cryotherapy or thermal modalities for pain control

Functional Considerations
- Use of appropriate ambulatory aides to reduce limping, improve stance stability, and reduce stress on involved extremity
- Stair climbing techniques, ambulation on uneven terrain, and progression/return to sports
- Proper choice of footwear to minimize excessive or prolonged compensatory pronation and enhance stability

Direct Interventions

Acute Phase: 2–4 Visits
- Therapeutic exercise and home program
  - Flexibility exercise within pain-free range
    - Hamstrings
    - Quadriceps
    - Gastrocnemius/soleus
    - Piriformis
    - Hip flexors
    - Hip internal rotators/external rotators
    - Adductors
    - Iliotibial band
    - Low back
  - Closed-kinetic chain strengthening exercise without exacerbation of pain
    - Squats
    - Weight shift
    - Lunges (anterior, lateral, posterior)
    - Balance/reach
    - Gait drills
    - Step up/step down
  - Open-kinetic chain exercise
    - Pain-free ROM
    - Strengthening exercises with emphasis on gluteus maximus, medius and adductors, and any other weak hip/knee muscles
- Manual therapy techniques (as appropriate per differential assessment)
  - Soft-tissue techniques
    - Myofascial release
    - Friction massage
    - Soft-tissue mobilization
  - Joint mobilization and traction
  - Compression and distraction oscillation technique
  - Passive ROM/pain-free stretching
    - As identified in evaluation
- Electrotherapeutic modalities
  - Iontophoresis
  - Electrical stimulation
- Physical agents and mechanical modalities
  - Thermal modalities/cryotherapy
  - Ultrasound (as appropriate given differential diagnosis)
  - Phonophoresis
- Goals/outcomes
  - Pain: 5/10 or less
  - Normal gait pattern with ambulatory aides as needed
  - Pain-free ROM:
    - Hip:
      a. Flexion: 100°
      b. Extension: 0°
      c. Internal rotation in neutral: 20°
      d. External rotation in neutral: 30°
    - Knee:
      a. Flexion: 110°
      b. Extension: 0°
    - Ankle:
      a. Dorsiflexion: 10°
      b. Plantarflexion: 40°
  - Strength: 4/5 on manual muscle test or 70% of involved extremity on closed-kinetic chain functional tests

Subacute Phase: 3–6 Visits
- Therapeutic exercise and home program
  - Cardiovascular conditioning
    - Bicycle
    - Ski machine
    - Treadmill
  - Free weights
  - Closed-kinetic chain exercise and home program
    - Squats
    - Lunges
    - Step up/step down
    - Pulleys and tubing for home (4-way hip exercises)
  - Progression of flexibility exercises
  - Neuromuscular/balance/proprioceptive reeducation
    - Gait drills
    - BAPS/balance board
- Manual therapy techniques
  - Joint mobilization as needed
  - Manual resistive activities
    - Proprioceptive neuromuscular facilitation patterns
  - Soft-tissue techniques
    - Friction massage
    - Soft-tissue mobilization
  - Passive stretches
- Therapeutic devices and equipment
  - Integration of specific structural or biomechanical components that may relieve symptoms, including the choice of shoes and/or custom biomechanical orthotics to control excessive compensatory pronation
- Electrotherapeutic modalities
  - Iontophoresis
- Physical agents and mechanical modalities
  - Thermal modalities/cryotherapy
  - Phonophoresis
- Goals/outcomes
  - Pain: 2/10 or less
  - Full ROM of hip, knee, ankle/foot as compared to uninvolved extremity
  - Strength of lower-extremity muscles of 4/5 on manual muscle test or equivalent to uninvolved extremity on closed-kinetic chain functional tests
  - Pain-free, normal gait pattern without assistive device
  - Return to previous functional status for ADLs and vocational activities

Functional Carryover
- Instruction in progression for return to maximum vocational, recreational, and sports activities with emphasis placed on proper periodization of intensity, frequency, duration, and cross-training activities

DISCHARGE PLANNING AND PATIENT RESPONSIBILITY

Criteria for Discharge
- All rehabilitation goals achieved except:
  - Functional status and activity level (current/prior) for recreational and sports activities
  - Patient may be discharged at functional hip ROM vs. full range

Circumstances Requiring Additional Visits
- Severe degenerative changes
- History of additional lower-extremity/lumbar pathology
- Presence of other medical conditions
- Hip contracture (previous prolonged bed rest)

Home Program
- Closed-kinetic chain functional exercises
- Flexibility exercises
- Functional progression for return to recreational and sports activities

Monitoring
- Patient to call at 4–6 weeks post-discharge to ensure progression toward expected return to function
- Schedule follow-up clinic visit in 4 weeks as needed to address persistent symptoms or difficulty returning to full function

REFERENCES

1. American Physical Therapy Association. *Guide to Physical Therapist Practice.* Alexandria, VA: APTA; 1997.

2. Boyd KT, Peirce NP, Batt ME. Common hip injuries in sport. *Sports Med.* 1997;25:273-288.

3. Butcher JD, Salzman KL, Lillegard WA. Lower extremity bursitis. *Am Fam Physician.* 1996;53:2317-2324.

4. Gerard J, Kleinfield SL. *Orthopaedic Testing: A Rational Approach To Diagnosis.* New York, NY: Churchill Livingstone; 1993.

5. Gray G. *Lower Extremity Functional Profile.* Adrian, MI: Wynn Marketing; 1995.

6. Gray H; Williams PL, ed. *Gray's Anatomy.* 38th ed. New York, NY: Churchill Livingstone; 1995.

7. Hart A, Hopkins C, Ford B. *ICD-9-CM Expert For Physicians, Volume 1&2.* 7th ed. USA: Ingenix; 2005.

8. Hertling D, Kessler R. *Management of Common Musculoskeletal Disorders: Physical Therapy Principles and Methods.* 3rd ed. Philadelphia, PA: Lippincott-Raven Publishers; 1996.

9. Hoppenfeld S. *Physical Examination of The Spine and Extremities.* New York, NY: Appleton-Century-Crofts; 1976.

10. Jenkins DB. *Hollinshead's Functional Anatomy of The Limbs and Back.* 6th ed. Philadelphia, PA: WB Saunders; 1991.

11. Kendall FP, McCreary EK, Provance PG. *Muscles: Testing and Function.* 4th ed. Baltimore, MD: Williams & Wilkins; 1993.

12. Magee DJ. *Orthopedic Physical Assessment.* 3rd ed. Philadelphia, PA: WB Saunders; 1997.

13. Porter-Hoke A. North American Institute of Orthopaedic Manual Therapy Course Notes: Level 1 and 2. Eugene, OR: NAIOMT, Inc; 1993.

14. Richardson JK, Iglarsh AZ. *Clinical Orthopedic Physical Therapy.* Philadelphia, PA: WB Saunders; 1994.

HIP SPRAIN/STRAIN
SUMMARY OVERVIEW

ICD-9

843.0   843.8   843.9   844.9

APTA Preferred Practice Pattern: 4E, 4F, 4J

EXAMINATION

- History and Systems Review
- Tests and Measures
  Systems review per APTA's *Guide to Physical Therapy Practice*
  - Gait, locomotion, and balance
  - Muscle performance
  - Pain
  - Posture
  - ROM
  - Special tests
- Establish Plan of Care

GOALS/OUTCOMES

- Pain-free ROM of the hip, knee, ankle, and foot as compared to the uninvolved extremity
- Pain: 2/10 or less
- Strength of lower-extremity muscles of 4/5 on manual muscle tests or equivalent to uninvolved extremity on closed-kinetic chain functional tests
- Pain-free, normal gait pattern without assistive devices on all surfaces
- Return to previous functional status for ADLs and vocational, recreational, and sports activities as identified by patient
- Independence in a progressive home exercise program emphasizing function

INTERVENTION
NUMBER OF VISITS: 5–10

- Patient Instruction
  - Basic Anatomy and Biomechanics
  - Handouts
  - Functional Considerations
- Direct Interventions
  - Acute Phase: 2–4 Visits
  - Subacute Phase: 3–6 Visits
- Functional Carryover

DISCHARGE PLANNING AND PATIENT RESPONSIBILITY

- Criteria for Discharge
  - All rehabilitation goals achieved except as indicated in guidelines
- Circumstances Requiring Additional Visits
  - Severe degenerative changes
  - History of additional lower-extremity/lumbar pathology
  - Presence of other medical conditions
- Home Program
  - Closed-kinetic chain functional exercises
  - Flexibility exercises
  - Functional progression for return to recreational and sports activities
- Monitoring

SUMMARY OVERVIEW | HIP | HIP SPRAIN/STRAIN   193

HIP SPRAIN/STRAIN

ICD-9

843.0	Iliofemoral (ligament) sprain
843.8	Sprain of other specified sites of hip and thigh
843.9	Sprain of unspecified site of hip and thigh
844.9	Sprain of unspecified site of knee and leg

APTA Preferred Practice Pattern: **4E, 4F, 4J**

EXAMINATION

History and Systems Review

- History of current condition
  - Mechanics of injury/onset
  - Date of injury/onset
- Past history of current condition
  - Previous history of lumbar or lower-extremity injury or surgery
- Functional status and activity level (current/prior)
  - Ambulatory aides
  - Occupational activities
  - Recreational activities
- Patient's functional goals

Tests and Measures

Systems review per APTA's *Guide to Physical Therapy Practice*

- Gait, locomotion, and balance
  - Stance—phase weight-bearing
  - Stride—length symmetry
  - Stairs—eccentric control
  - Squatting
  - Pelvic symmetry
  - Balance/reach tests
    - Unilateral stance on involved extremity, reach in various directions with uninvolved extremity to assess both proprioception and muscle performance in various muscles depending on direction of reach; compare distance reached to similar reaches in unilateral stance on uninvolved extremity
    - Unilateral stance on involved extremity, reach in various directions with one or both arms to assess proprioception and trunk/lower-extremity muscle performance; compare distance reached with similar reaches in unilateral stance on uninvolved extremity

- Muscle performance
  - Manual muscle testing at the hip, knee, and ankle
- Pain
  - Measured on visual analog scale
- Posture
  If positive for dysfunction, a full biomechanical assessment may be indicated; see *Biomechanical Lower Extremity Dysfunction* Guideline.
  - Static, nonweight-bearing alignment of hip, knee, subtalar, and midtarsal joint
  - Static, weight-bearing alignment
  - Leg length in supine, long sitting, and pelvic level in weight-bearing
- ROM
  - Active/passive ROM and muscle performance
    - Hip
    - Knee
    - Foot/ankle
    - Trunk
  - Passive overpressure
  - Muscle length
    - Thomas test
    - Ober test
    - Straight-leg raise
    - Patrick/FABRE test
    - Gastrocnemius and Soleus
    - Piriformis test
- Special tests
  - Rule out referral from other areas
    - Lumbar—See *Low Back General Pain* guideline
      a. Positive results during Patrick/FABRE or straight-leg raise
      b. Referred pain during flexibility and special tests
      c. Pelvic and spine asymmetries during biomechanical screening
    - Knee
    - Foot/ankle

194   HIP SPRAIN/STRAIN | HIP

- ○ Joint integrity
  - ▪ Passive mobility/capsular assessment: Scour test, Closed pack position etc.
- ○ Climbing test: Standing with one foot up on the table, the patient lunges further toward the table to test full range of flexion of the elevated extremity at the hip, knee, and ankle, as well as extension of the opposite hip and knee

Establish Plan of Care

- Based on history, tests, and measures

GOALS/OUTCOMES

- Pain-free ROM of the hip, knee, ankle, and foot as compared to the uninvolved extremity
  Normal ROM:
  - ○ Hip:
    - ▪ Flexion: 125°
    - ▪ Extension: 0°
    - ▪ Internal rotation in neutral: 40°
    - ▪ External rotation in neutral: 50°
  - ○ Knee:
    - ▪ Flexion: 135°
    - ▪ Extension: 0°
  - ○ Ankle:
    - ▪ Plantarflexion: 40°
    - ▪ Dorsiflexion: 10° in subtalar neutral with knee extended
- Pain: 2/10 or less
- Strength of lower-extremity muscles of 4/5 on manual muscle tests or equivalent to uninvolved extremity on closed-kinetic chain functional tests
- Pain-free, normal gait pattern without assistive devices on all surfaces
- Return to previous functional status for ADLs and vocational, recreational, and sports activities as identified by patient
- Independence in a progressive home exercise program emphasizing function

INTERVENTION
NUMBER OF VISITS: 5–10

Coordination, Communication, and Documentation

- Provision of services between admission and discharge that facilitate cost-effective and efficient integration or reintegration to home, community, or work
- Documentation of therapeutic intervention is required for each episode of care and serves as the basic foundation for communication
- Coordination and additional communication will depend on the patient's impairment and home/work/community/leisure situation and requirements. Such services may include:
  - ○ Case management
  - ○ Coordination of care and collaboration with those integral to the patient's rehabilitation program
  - ○ Coordination and monitoring of the delivery of available resources
  - ○ Referrals to other health-care professionals
  - ○ Identification of resources, support groups, or advocacy services
  - ○ Provision of educational or training information
  - ○ Technical assistance

Patient Instruction

Basic Anatomy and Biomechanics

- Relationship of movement in one area to the stress imposed on other areas

Handouts

- Home exercise program
  - ○ Flexibility exercises
  - ○ Strengthening activities
  - ○ Functional activities
- Home cryotherapy or thermal modalities for pain control

Functional Considerations

- Use of appropriate ambulatory aides to reduce limping, improve stance stability, and reduce stress on involved extremity
- Stair climbing techniques, ambulation on uneven terrain, and progression/return to sports
- Proper choice of footwear to promote lower-extremity stability and comfort

HIP | HIP SPRAIN/STRAIN   195

Direct Interventions

Acute Phase: 2–4 Visits

- Therapeutic exercise and home program
  - Flexibility exercise within pain-free range
    - Hamstrings
    - Quadriceps
    - Gastrocnemius/soleus
    - Piriformis
    - Hip flexors
    - Hip internal rotators/external rotators
    - Adductors
    - Iliotibial band
    - Low back
  - Closed-kinetic chain strengthening exercise without exacerbation of pain
    - Squats
    - Weight shift
    - Lunges (anterior, lateral, posterior)
    - Balance/reach
    - Gait drills
    - Step up/step down
  - Open-kinetic chain exercise
    - Pain-free ROM
    - Strengthening exercises with emphasis on gluteus maximus, medius and adductors, and any other weak hip/knee muscles
- Manual therapy techniques (as appropriate per differential assessment)
  - Soft-tissue techniques
    - Myofascial release
    - Friction massage
    - Soft-tissue mobilization
  - Joint mobilization and traction
  - Compression and distraction oscillation technique
  - Passive ROM/pain-free stretching as identified in evaluation
- Electrotherapeutic modalities
  - TENS/IFC
- Physical agents and mechanical modalities
  - Thermal modalities/cryotherapy
  - Ultrasound (as appropriate given differential diagnosis)
  - Phonophoresis
- Goals/outcomes
  - Pain: 5/10 or less
  - Normal gait pattern with ambulatory aides as needed

- Pain-free ROM:
  - Hip:
    a. Flexion: 100°
    b. Extension: 0°
    c. Internal rotation in neutral: 20°
    d. External rotation in neutral: 30°
  - Knee:
    a. Flexion: 110°
    b. Extension: 0°
  - Ankle:
    a. Dorsiflexion: 10°
    b. Plantarflexion: 40°
- Strength: 4/5 on manual muscle test or 70% of involved extremity on closed-kinetic chain functional tests

Subacute Phase: 3–6 Visits

- Therapeutic exercise and home program
  - Cardiovascular conditioning
    - Bicycle
    - Ski machine
    - Treadmill
  - Free weights
  - Closed-kinetic chain exercise and home program
    - Squats
    - Lunges
    - Step up/step down
    - Pulleys and tubing for home (4-way hip exercises)
  - Progression of flexibility exercises
  - Neuromuscular/balance/proprioceptive reeducation
    - Gait drills
    - BAPS/balance board
- Manual therapy techniques
  - Joint mobilization as needed
  - Manual resistive activities
    - Proprioceptive neuromuscular facilitation patterns
  - Soft-tissue techniques
    - Friction massage
    - Soft-tissue mobilization
  - Passive stretches
- Electrotherapeutic modalities
  - TENS/IFC
- Physical agents and mechanical modalities
  - Thermal modalities/cryotherapy

- Goals/outcomes
  - Pain: 2/10 or less
  - Full ROM of hip, knee, ankle/foot as compared to uninvolved extremity
  - Strength of lower-extremity muscles of 4/5 on manual muscle test or equivalent to uninvolved extremity on closed-kinetic chain functional tests
  - Pain-free, normal gait pattern without assistive device
  - Return to previous functional status for ADLs and vocational activities

Functional Carryover

- Instruction in progression for return to maximum vocational, recreational, and sports activities with emphasis placed on proper periodization of intensity, frequency, duration, and cross-training activities

DISCHARGE PLANNING AND PATIENT RESPONSIBILITY

Criteria for Discharge

- All rehabilitation goals achieved except:
  - Functional status and activity level (current/prior) for recreational and sports activities
  - Patient may be discharged at functional hip ROM/ strength as required for ADLs or work vs. full range/ strength when appropriate

Circumstances Requiring Additional Visits

- Severe degenerative changes
- History of additional lower-extremity/lumbar pathology
- Presence of other medical conditions

Home Program

- Closed-kinetic chain functional exercises
- Flexibility exercises
- Functional progression for return to recreational and sports activities

Monitoring

- Patient to call at 4–6 weeks post-discharge to ensure progression toward expected return to function
- Schedule follow-up clinic visit in 4 weeks as needed to address persistent symptoms or difficulty returning to full function

REFERENCES

1. Gray H; Williams PL, ed. *Gray's Anatomy*. 38th ed. New York, NY: Churchill Livingstone; 1995.
2. Hart A, Hopkins C, Ford B. *ICD-9-CM Expert For Physicians, Volume 1&2*. 7th ed. USA: Ingenix; 2005.
3. Magee DJ. *Orthopedic Physical Assessment*. 3rd ed. Philadelphia, PA: WB Saunders; 1997.
4. Sahrmann SA, *Diagnosis and Treatment of Movement Impairment Syndromes*. St. Louis, MO: Mosby, Inc. 2002.

198   HIP SPRAIN/STRAIN | HIP

Lumbar Spine

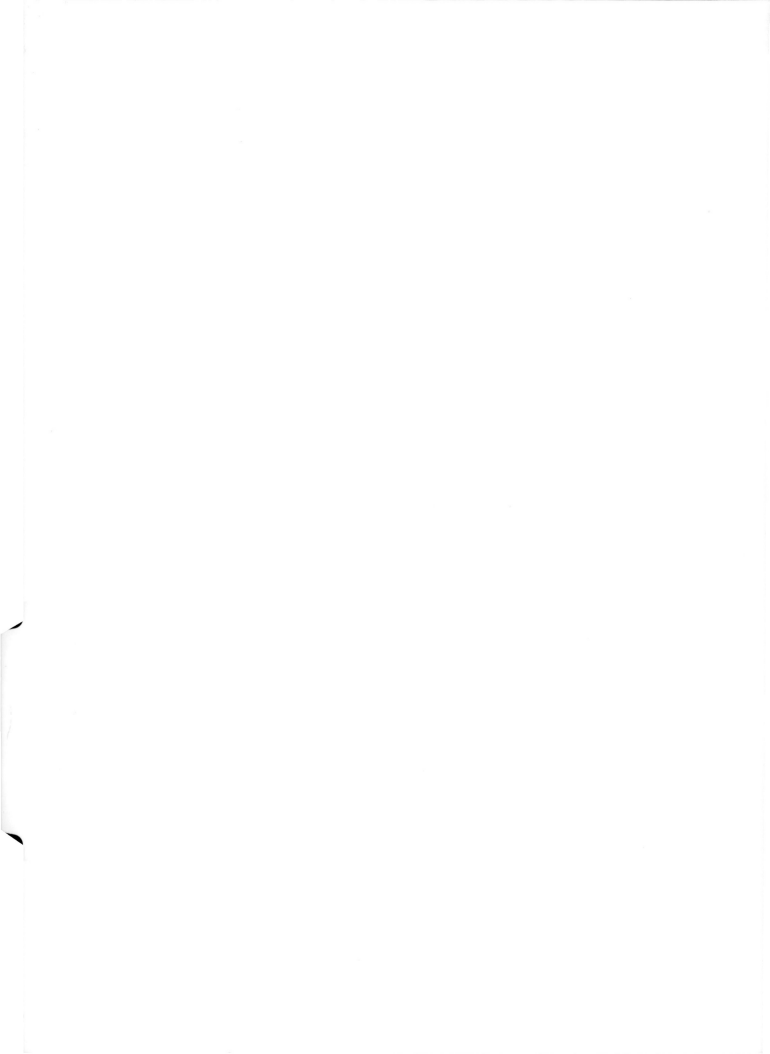

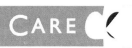

LUMBAR SPINE

Ankylosing Spondylitis	201
Low Back General Pain	209
Lumbar Disc Pathology	219
Lumbar Fracture	227
Lumbar Spondylolysis with Myelopathy	235
Lumbar Surgery—Inpatient	243
Pelvic Floor Dysfunction	249
Postoperative Rehabilitation of The Lumbar Spine	255
Postural Dysfunction	263
Sacroiliac Dysfunction	271
Spinal Stenosis	279
Spondylolisthesis	285

200　Lumbar Spine

ANKYLOSING SPONDYLITIS
SUMMARY OVERVIEW

ICD-9
  720.0
APTA Preferred Practice Pattern: **4F, 4G**

EXAMINATION
- History and Systems Review
- Tests and Measures
  Systems review per APTA's *Guide to Physical Therapy Practice*
  - Aerobic capacity and endurance
  - Anthropometric characteristics
  - Gait, locomotion, and balance
  - Integumentary integrity
  - Joint integrity and mobility
  - Muscle performance
  - Pain
  - Posture
  - ROM
  - Reflex integrity
  - Sensory integrity
  - Special tests
- Establish Plan of Care

GOALS/OUTCOMES
- Patient displays understanding of proper posture and body mechanics
- Pain-free lumbar ROM: A minimum of 80% of AMA guides
- Pain: 2/10 or less
- Strength: 4/5 on manual muscle tests
- Functional ranges
- Return to previous functional status for ADLs and vocational, recreational, and sports activities as identified by patient
- Independence in a progressive home exercise program emphasizing function and maintenance of flexibility
- Increase or maintain aerobic capacity and endurance capabilities
- Maintain erect posture to prevent deformity in the event the disease process continues and the spine fuses
- Establish a cardiovascular and recreational program that the patient can tolerate
- Maintain functional ROM of extremities, especially hips and shoulders
- Independent ADLs with necessary modification of environment, postures, and body mechanics

- Decrease in Bath group scores: BASDAI (Bath Ankylosing Spondylitis Disease Activity Index), BASFI (Bath Ankylosing Spondylitis Functional Index)

INTERVENTION
NUMBER OF VISITS: 7–14

- Patient Instruction
  - Basic Anatomy and Biomechanics
  - Handouts
  - Functional Considerations
- Direct Interventions
  - Acute Phase: 3–6 Visits
  - Subacute Phase: 4–8 Visits
- Functional Carryover

DISCHARGE PLANNING AND PATIENT RESPONSIBILITY
- Criteria for Discharge
  - Patient demonstrates appropriate knowledge and understanding of diagnosis pathology and prognosis and knows how to modify his or her exercise and general activities appropriate to this stage of the disease
  - All goals/outcomes have been achieved
  - Patient demonstrates independent and consistent ability to perform exercises as prescribed by the therapist
- Circumstances Requiring Additional Visits
  - Persistent functional strength deficit or 4/5 on manual muscle test
  - History of previous injury or surgery to related area
  - Persistent radicular symptoms or neurological deficit
  - Severe deconditioning
  - Special occupational needs requiring extensive fitness/ strengthening
  - Patient unable to maintain upright posture
  - Inability to perform normal breathing pattern
  - History of total hip replacement
- Home Program
  - Flexibility exercises
  - Functional strengthening exercises
  - Cardiovascular conditioning
- Monitoring

SUMMARY OVERVIEW | LUMBAR SPINE | ANKYLOSING SPONDYLITIS   201

ANKYLOSING SPONDYLITIS

ICD-9

720.0   Ankylosing spondylitis

APTA Preferred Practice Pattern: **4F, 4G**

EXAMINATION

History And Systems Review

- History of current condition
  - Mechanism of injury/onset
  - Date of onset/diagnosis
  - Usually not painful; therefore, may not be primary diagnosis for referral
  - Location, nature, and behavior of symptoms
    - May start within sacroiliac joint
  - General fatigue/malaise, weight loss, depression, or extremity edema
  - Morning stiffness
  - Aggravating/relieving factors
    - Pain with vigorous activity, prolonged static postures, or rest
  - Presence of cauda equina symptoms
  - Generalized disease symptoms
    - Loss of weight
    - Anemia
    - Pyrexia
  - Patterns of exacerbation and remission
- Past history of current condition
  - Hospitalization
  - Surgical intervention
  - Lower extremity problems
  - Bracing, injection
- Other tests and measures
  - Radiological tests of the pelvis show sacroilitis, fusion of sacroiliac joints. Radiologic tests of the lumbar spine show ossification of the anterior longitudinal ligament and fusion of the facet joints, longitudinal calcification of vertebral bodies, patchy at first, later continuous (bamboo effect).
  - CT will show bony fusions, eroded laminae and spinous processes
  - MRI may be needed to document atlantoaxial subluxation, cauda equina may be inflammatory or compressive
  - Lab tests:
    - Raised erythrocytes
    - Elevated sedimentation rate

- HLA-B27 antigen is positive 90–95% of the time, but is not always present
- Past medical/surgical history
  - Inquire regarding areas of possible systemic pathology, such as:
    - Appendix
    - Abdominal
    - Pancreas
    - Large intestine
    - Kidney
    - Genital/urinary
      a. Bladder
      b. Ureter
      c. Prostate gland
      d. Cervix
      e. Uterus
    - Iritis
    - Cardiac
    - Respiratory
    - Central nervous system disorders
    - Psoriasis
    - Irritable bowel symptoms
- Functional status and activity level (current/prior)
- Patient's functional goals

Tests and Measures

Systems review per APTA's *Guide to Physical Therapy Practice*

- Aerobic capacity and endurance
  - Decreased aerobic capacity and endurance
- Anthropometric characteristics
  - Leg length discrepancy
    - Supine
    - Weight-bearing
- Gait, locomotion, and balance
  - Asymmetrical gait pattern
    - Arm swing
    - Hip transverse plane motion
    - Knee extension in stance phase
    - Knee flexion in swing phase
    - Early heel off
    - Excessive pronation

202   ANKYLOSING SPONDYLITIS | LUMBAR SPINE

- Cervical spine
- Hips
- Integumentary integrity
  - Skin
    - Color change associated with systemic disease
    - Scars
- Joint integrity and mobility
  - Palpation of tendons and ligaments
  - PSIS compression
    - Sitting
    - Prone
  - Costovertebral joints during respiration
  - Atlantoaxia and atlantooccipital joints
  - Longitudinal ligaments
  - Central posterior to anterior glides
    In prone position, with posterior to anterior pressure on spinous or transverse processes
  - Flexion/ extension
  - Side bend
  - Rotation
  - Stress tests
    It is recommended that stress tests be performed at those segments that are hypomobile or that the therapist intends to mobilize to end range (Grades III–V)
    - Joint rigidity of spine or involved extremities with any passive anatomical or accessory movements; different in feel from muscular stiffness
    - No muscle guarding or spasm with spring test
  - Passive intervertebral motion T10–S1
  - Sacroiliac
  - Loss of spring to costovertebral joints
- Muscle performance
  - Resisted testing
  - Key muscle test
    To determine possible palsy, utilize a combination of resistance and repetition (5–10)
    - Hip flexion (L2)
    - Quadriceps (L3)
    - Tibialis anterior (L4)
    - Extensor hallicus longus (L5)
    - Peroneals (S1)
    - Gastrocnemius (S1)
  - Abdominals
  - Spinal extensors
  - Hip extensors
  - Check cervical key muscles
  - Palpation of muscles

- Pain
  - Measured on visual analog scale
- Posture (anterior, posterior, side)
  - Boney landmarks
  - Scoliosis, sway/flat back
  - Flexing posture of spine with loss of normal kypholordotic curves
  - Spinal rigidity observations
  - Enthesopathies may present in weight-bearing postures
- ROM
  - Active
    - Flexion
    - Extension
    - Right and left side bend
  - Overpressure (passive)
  - Spinal rigidity or lack of spinal ROM
    - Solid, unyielding quality of movement vs. loss of soft-tissue elasticity
    - Longitudinal ligaments calcify, as do capsules of facets and costovertebral joints
- Reflex integrity
  - Upper and lower extremities
    - Clonus
    - Babinski
- Sensory integrity
  - Sensation, C2 to S1
- Special tests
  - PSIS symmetry
    - PSIS change in distance sitting to prone
  - Compression overload
  - Cervical spine
  - Chest expansion
  - Chin to chest distance
  - Occiput to wall distance
  - Hips
  - Sacroiliac
  - Patrick/FABRE
    - Patient is supine in FABRE position
    - Inguinal pain implicates hip joint pathology or muscular restrictions
    - To stress the sacroiliac joint, place one hand on the flexed knee and the other on the opposite ASIS and press down
  - Dural tension tests

Establish Plan of Care
- Based on history, tests, and measures

GOALS/OUTCOMES

- Patient displays understanding of proper posture and body mechanics as evidenced by pain-free performance of ADLs and vocational activities
- Pain-free lumbar ROM: A minimum of 80% of AMA guides

	Normal	*80%*
Flexion	60°	50°
Extension	25°	20°
Side bend	25°	20°
Rotation	30°	25°

- Pain: 2/10 or less
- Strength: 4/5 on manual muscle tests
  - Abdominals
  - Spinal extensor
  - Gluteals

  Or specific functional motor performance, such as
  - Squat to 90°
  - Retrieve object from floor
  - Perform work task (weight- and repetition-specific)
- Functional ranges
  - Hip
    - Flexion: 125°
    - Extension: 0°
    - Internal rotation: 20°
    - External rotation: 30°
  - Knee
    - Flexion: 120°
    - Extension: 5°
  - Cervical
    - Flexion: 50°
    - Extension: 60°
    - Rotation: 65°
    - Side bend: 35°
- Return to previous functional status for ADLs and vocational, recreational, and sports activities as defined by patient
- Independence in a progressive home exercise program emphasizing function and maintenance of flexibility
- Increase or maintain aerobic capacity and endurance capabilities
- Maintain erect posture to prevent deformity in the event the disease process continues and the spine fuses
- Establish a cardiovascular and recreational program that the patient can tolerate
- Maintain functional ROM of extremities, especially hips and shoulders

- Independent ADLs with necessary modification of environment, postures, and body mechanics
- Decrease in Bath group scores: BASDAI (The Bath Ankylosing Spondylitis Disease Activity Index), BASFI (The Bath Ankylosing Spondylitis Functional Index)

INTERVENTION
NUMBER OF VISITS: 7–14

Coordination, Communication, and Documentation

- Provision of services between admission and discharge that facilitate cost-effective and efficient integration or reintegration to home, community, or work
- Documentation of therapeutic intervention is required for each episode of care and serves as the basic foundation for communication
- Coordination and additional communication will depend on the patient's impairment and home/work/ community/leisure situation and requirements. Such services may include:
  - Case management
  - Coordination of care and collaboration with those integral to the patient's rehabilitation program
  - Coordination and monitoring of the delivery of available resources
  - Referrals to other health-care professionals
  - Identification of resources, support groups, or advocacy services
  - Provision of educational or training information
  - Technical assistance

Patient Instruction

Basic Anatomy and Biomechanics
- Anatomy of lumbar spine
- Pertinent Gray's Anatomy (Gray. 1995. 510–516, 522–528, 534–537, 809–813, 819–827)
- Biomechanics of lumbar spine and relationship of symptoms to:
  - Mechanisms of injury
  - Segmental mobility dysfunction
  - Muscle weakness or imbalance
  - Postural or lower extremity biomechanical effects
- Educate patient regarding basic anatomy, pathology, and prognosis of ankylosing spondylitis

204   ANKYLOSING SPONDYLITIS | LUMBAR SPINE

Handouts

- Patient education
- Specific home program
- Commercially available products, such as:
  - Krames Communications (1100 Grundy Lane, San Bruno, CA 94066)
    - *Back Basics*
    - *Back to Basics*
    - *Back Owner's Manual*
    - *Back Tips for People Who Sit*
    - *Poor Posture Hurts*
    - *Your Back Is Always Working*
  - McKenzie (PO Box 93, Waikanae, New Zealand)
    - *Treat Your Own Back*
  - Saunders (4250 Norex Drive, Chaska, MN 55318)
    - *For Your Back*
  - Consider purchase of Ankylosing Spondylitis Society educational materials including pamphlets/videos, from:
    Spondylitis Association of America
    PO Box 5872
    Sherman Oaks, CA 91413
    (800) 777-8189,
    or
    National Arthritis Foundation
    1314 Spring Street, NW
    Atlanta, GA 30309
    (404) 872-7100

Functional Considerations

- Avoidance of activities or positions that cause pain
- Recognition of symptoms of systemic disease
- Utilization of proper body mechanics
- Understand the need for hip, upper extremity, and shoulder flexibility

Direct Interventions

Acute Phase: 3–6 Visits

- Therapeutic exercise and home program
  - Stretching exercises to maintain erect posture
    - Pectoral
    - Hamstrings
    - Psoas
    - Latissimus dorsi
    - Abdominals
  - Instruction in diaphragmatic breathing and chest expansion exercises
  - Instruction in ROM/strengthening exercise as appropriate to stage of disease
    - Cat and camel
    - Press-up
    - Spinal rotation
    - Deep neck flexors (if no cranovertebral instability)
    - Transverse abdominis, pelvic floor, multifidi
- Manual therapy techniques
  - Soft-tissue techniques
    - Soft-tissue mobilization
    - Trigger-point techniques
    - Muscle energy techniques
  - Passive stretching
  - Joint mobilization, especially to thoracic spine and costovertebral joints
- Electrotherapeutic modalities
- Physical agents and mechanical modalities
  - Ultrasound·
  - Cryotherapy/thermal modalities
- Goals/outcomes
  - Pain: 2/10 or less
  - Restore or maintain erect posture
  - ROM:
    - Lumbar inclinometer 40–60° total flexion/extension ROM maintained
    - Bilateral straight-leg raise of 70° or higher
  - Ability to perform 10–15 repetitions of home exercise program for maintaining and increasing flexibility
  - Modification of ADLs for management of the disease process

Subacute Phase: 4–8 Visits

- Therapeutic exercise and home program
  - Stretch remaining tight muscle groups
  - Breathing exercises to maintain aerobic capacity and endurance
  - Strengthening of extremities, abdominals, and back extensors
    - Therapeutic ball
    - Squats
    - Lunges
    - Proprioceptive neuromuscular facilitation
    - Spinal stabilization
      a. Deep neck flexors, transverse abdominis, multifidi, pelvic floor

- Cardiovascular conditioning—any activity tolerated by patient, such as:
  - Walking
  - Swimming/aquatic therapy
  - Cross-country ski machine
  - Upper or lower body cycling
- Manual therapy techniques
  - Continue effective soft-tissue techniques
  - Joint mobilization
  - Passive stretching
- Physical agents and mechanical modalities
  Continue effective modalities as in Acute Phase with increased emphasis on use as needed at home.
- Goals/outcomes
  - Establish a regular home flexibility program and a tolerable cardiovascular conditioning program
  - Functional activity
    - Return to part-time or regular work schedule and home ADLs
    - Stand or sit for one hour uninterrupted
    - Walk at slow speeds for minimum of 15 minutes
  - Strength: Maintain at least a manual muscle test grade of:
    - 4/5 for the extremities
    - 4-/5 for the abdominal and back extensors
  - Maintain proper position and flexibility until disease process goes into remission
    - Greater than 60° total inclinometer lumbar flexion/extension ROM
    - Bilateral straight leg raise greater than or equal to 80°
  - Pain: 2/10 or less

Functional Carryover

- Ergonomic evaluation: Proper sitting, standing, and lying postures
- Task-oriented exercises specifically related to work, home, and recreation
  - Contact sports or sports with significant joint loading or jarring should typically be avoided
  - Many patients do well with a variety of forms of activity such as swimming, cross-country skiing, walking, and cycling
  - Postural awareness and appropriate warm-up should be conducted with any exercise activity. Basketball, volleyball, and tennis are sometimes tolerated, since they combine movements with stretching and intermittent jumping.

DISCHARGE PLANNING AND PATIENT RESPONSIBILITY

Criteria for Discharge

- Patient demonstrates appropriate knowledge and understanding of diagnosis pathology and prognosis and knows how to modify his or her exercise and general activities appropriate to this stage of the disease
- All goals/outcomes have been achieved
- Patient demonstrates independent and consistent ability to perform exercises as prescribed by the therapist

Circumstances Requiring Additional Visits

- Persistent functional strength deficit or 4/5 on manual muscle test
- History of previous injury or surgery to related area
- Persistent radicular symptoms or neurological deficit
- Severe deconditioning
- Special occupational needs requiring extensive fitness/strengthening
- Patient unable to maintain upright posture
- Inability to perform normal breathing pattern
- History of total hip replacement

Home Program

- Flexibility exercises
  - Rib cage
  - Spine
  - Upper extremity
  - Lower extremity
- Functional strengthening exercises
  - Squats
  - Lunges
  - Abdominal stabilization
  - Spinal extensors
- Cardiovascular conditioning

Monitoring

- Instruct patient to call for advice should progression halt or a negative trend occur
- Recheck in 2–4 weeks if any symptoms persist or patient is unable to perform all ADLs
- Be sure that patient has information and access where appropriate to support groups, resources, and references

REFERENCES

1. American Physical Therapy Association. *Guide to Physical Therapist Practice*. Alexandria, VA: APTA; 1997.

2. Bakker C, Hidding A, van der Linden S, van Doorslaer E. Cost effectiveness of group physical therapy compared to individualized therapy for ankylosing spondylitis. a randomized controlled trial. *J Rheumatol*. 1994;21:264-268.

3. Bakker C, Rutten-van Mölken M, Hidding A, et al. Patient utilities in ankylosing spondylitis and the association with other outcome measures. *J Rheumatol*. 1994;21:1298-1304.

4. Bakker C, van der Linden S, van Santen-Hoeufft M, Bolwijn P, Hidding A. Problem elicitation to assess patient priorities in ankylosing spondylitis and fibromyalgia. *J Rheumatol*. 1995;22:1304-1310.

5. Carbon RJ, Macey MG, McCarthy DA, et al. The effect of 30 minute cycle ergometry on ankylosing spondylitis. *Br J Rheumatol*. 1996;35:167-177.

6. Garrett S, Jenkinson T, Kennedy LG, et al. A new approach to defining disease status in ankylosing spondylitis: the Bath ankylosing spondylitis disease activity index. *J Rheumatol*. 1994;12:2286-91.

7. Gray H; Williams PL, ed. *Gray's Anatomy*, 38th ed. New York, NY: Churchill Livingstone; 1995.

8. Hart A, Hopkins C, Ford B. *ICD-9-CM Expert For Physicians, Volume 1&2*. 7th ed. USA: Ingenix; 2005.

9. Hidding A, van der Linden S, Gielen X, et al. Continuation of group physical therapy is necessary in ankylosing spondylitis: results of a randomized controlled trial. *Arthritis Care Res*. 1994;7:90-96.

10. Hidding A, van der Linden S, Boers M, et al. Is group physical therapy superior to individualized therapy in ankylosing spondylitis? A randomized controlled trial. *Arthritis Care Res*. 1993;6:117-125.

11. Hidding A, van der Linden S. Factors related to change in global health after group physical therapy in ankylosing spondylitis. *Clin Rheumatol*. 1995;14:347-351.

12. Hidding A, van der Linden S, de Witte L. Therapeutic effects of individual physical therapy in ankylosing spondylitis related to duration of disease. *Clin Rheumatol*. 1993;12:334-340.

13. Ince G, Sarpael T, Durgun B, Erdogan S. Effects of a multimodal exercise program for people with ankylosing spondylitis. *Phys Ther*. 2006; 86: 924-35.

14. Lubrano E, Helliwell P, Moreno P, et al. The assessment of knowledge in ankylosing spondylitis patients by a self-administered questionnaire. *Br J Rheumatol*. 1998;37:437-441.

15. McKenzie R. *Treat Your Own Back*. 6th ed. Waikanae, New Zealand: Spinal Publications; 1985.

16. Russell P, Unsworth A, Haslock I. The effect of exercise on ankylosing spondylitis: a preliminary study. *Br J Rheumatol*. 1993;32:498-506.

17. Saunders HD. *Self-help Manual For Your Back*. Chaska, MN: The Saunders Group, Inc; 1992.

18. Viitanen JV. Thoracolumbar rotation in ankylosing spondylitis: a new noninvasive measurement method. *Spine*. 1993;18: 880-883.

19. Viitanen JV, Kautiainen H, Kokko ML, et al. Age and spine mobility in ankylosing spondylitis. *Scand J Rheumatol*. 1995;24:314-315.

LOW BACK GENERAL PAIN
SUMMARY OVERVIEW

ICD-9

715.90   715.95   715.98   721.3   721.4   724.2   724.5   724.8   724.9

729.1   739.3   846.0   847.2

APTA Preferred Practice Pattern: 4B, 4C, 4D, 4E, 4F, 4G, 4H, 4I, 4J, 5F, 6B

EXAMINATION

- History and Systems Review
- Tests and Measures
  Systems review per APTA's *Guide to Physical Therapy Practice*
  - Anthropometric characteristics
  - Circulation
  - Gait, locomotion, and balance
  - Joint integrity and mobility
  - Muscle performance
  - Pain
  - Palpation
  - Posture
  - ROM
  - Reflex integrity
  - Sensory integrity
  - Special tests
- Establish Plan of Care

GOALS/OUTCOMES

- Patient displays understanding of proper posture and body mechanics as evidenced by pain-free performance of ADLs and vocational activities
- Pain: 2/10 or less with proper body mechanics and posture
- ROM (pain-free)
- Strength: 4/5 on manual muscle test
- Squat to 90°
- Retrieve object from floor
- Perform work task (weight and repetition-specific)
- Functional lower-extremity ROM
- Avoidance of movements causing a reoccurence of symptoms
- Return to previous functional status for ADLs and vocational, recreational, and sports activities as identified by patient
- Independence in a progressive home exercise program emphasizing function

INTERVENTION
NUMBER OF VISITS: 5–12

- Patient Instruction
  - Basic Anatomy and Biomechanics
  - Handouts
  - Functional Considerations
- Direct Interventions
  - Acute Phase: 3–6 Visits
  - Subacute Phase: 2–6 Visits
- Functional Carryover

DISCHARGE PLANNING AND PATIENT RESPONSIBILITY

- Criteria for Discharge
  - Patient demonstrates ability to perform exercises in mechanically correct fashion and is compliant with exercise program as instructed
  - Patient demonstrates appropriate posture and body mechanics during functional activities
  - All rehabilitation goals/outcomes have been achieved with the exception of previous level for recreational and sports activities
- Circumstances Requiring Additional Visits
  - Persistent functional motor performance deficit or 3/5 on manual muscle test
  - History of previous injury or surgery to related area
  - Persistent radicular symptoms or neurological deficit
  - Severe deconditioning
  - Special occupational needs requiring extensive fitness/ strengthening
  - Multiple injury sites including lower extremity
  - Severe traumatic injury with persistent functional/ occupational deficits
- Home Program
  - Flexibility
  - Strength/stabilization
  - Cardiovascular conditioning
- Monitoring

SUMMARY OVERVIEW | LUMBAR SPINE | LOW BACK GENERAL PAIN   209

LOW BACK GENERAL PAIN

ICD-9

715.90	Osteoarthrosis, unspecified whether generalized or localized, site unspecified
715.95	Osteoarthrosis, unspecified whether generalized or localized, pelvic region and thigh
715.98	Osteoarthrosis, unspecified whether generalized or localized, other specified sites
721.3	Lumbosacral spondylosis without myelopathy
721.4	Thoracic or lumbar spondylosis with myelopathy
724.2	Lumbago
724.5	Backache, unspecified
724.8	Other symptoms referable to back
724.9	Other unspecified back disorders
729.1	Myalgia and myositis, unspecified
739.3	Nonallopathic lesions, not elsewhere classified, lumbar region
846.0	Lumbosacral (joint) (ligament) sprain
847.2	Lumbar sprain

APTA Preferred Practice Pattern: 4B, 4C, 4D, 4E, 4F, 4G, 4H, 4I, 4J, 5F, 6B

EXAMINATION

History and Systems Review
- History of current condition
  - Mechanism of injury/onset
  - Date of injury/onset
  - Presence of cauda equina symptoms
  - Location, nature, and behavior of symptoms
    - Radiating symptoms
    - Aggravating/relieving factors
- Past history of current condition
  - Hospitalization
  - Surgical intervention
  - Lower-extremity problems
  - Bracing injections, etc.
  - Corset use
- Past medical/surgical history
  - Systemic pathology
    - Appendix
    - Abdominal
    - Pancreas
    - Large intestine
    - Kidney
    - Genital/urinary
      a. Bladder
      b. Ureter
      c. Prostate gland
      d. Cervix
      e. Uterus

- Functional status and activity level (current/prior)
- Patient's functional goals
- Age of patient
- Patient occupation
- Medications

Tests and Measures
Systems review per APTA's *Guide to Physical Therapy Practice*
- Anthropometric characteristics
  - Leg length discrepancy
    - Supine
    - Weight-bearing
- Circulation (femoral, poplietus, dorsalis pedius pulses)
- Gait, locomotion, and balance
  - Asymmetrical gait pattern
    - Arm swing
    - Hip transverse plane motion
    - Knee extension in stance phase
    - Knee flexion in swing phase
    - Early heel off
    - Excessive pronation
  - Lumbar-sacroiliac weight bearing: Mobility
  - Balance
  - Transitional movements: Sit/stand
  - Presence of drop foot

210   LOW BACK GENERAL PAIN | LUMBAR SPINE

- Joint integrity and mobility
  - Central posterior to anterior glides
    In prone position, with posterior to anterior pressure on spinous or transverse processes
  - Stress tests
    It is recommended that stress tests be performed at those segments that are hypermobile or hypomobile or that the therapist intends to mobilize to end range (Grades III–V)
    - Passive invertebral motion T10–S1
    - Flexion/extension
    - Side bend
    - Rotation
    - Torsion
- Muscle performance
  - Resistive
    - Active, if acute
    - Endrange, if chronic
  - Key muscle test
    To determine possible palsy, utilize a combination of resistance and repetition
    - Hip flexion (L2)
    - Quadriceps (L3)
    - Tibialis anterior (L4)
    - Extensor hallicus longus (L5)
    - Peroneals (S1)
    - Gastrocnemius (S1)
  - Abdominals
  - Spinal extensors
  - Hip extensors
  - Inner unit
- Pain
  - Measured on visual analog scale
- Palpation (tenderness, altered temp, muscle spasm)
- Posture
  - Anterior, posterior, side
  - Bony landmarks
  - Scoliosis, sway back, flat back
  - Pelvic asymmetry
  - Palpation, including key landmarks
  - Muscle symmetry—any presence of hypertrophy or wasting
- ROM
  - Active
    - Flexion
    - Extension
    - Side bend

- Rotation
  - Overpressure (passive)
  - Lower-extremity joint scan—quick test (squat down, bounce 2–3x, and then stand)
- Reflex integrity
  - Reflex testing
    - Patellar tendon (L3)
    - Achilles tendon (S1)
  - Rule out upper motor neuron lesion
    - Clonus
    - Babinski
- Sensory integrity
  - Sensory assessment (T12–S2)
- Special tests
  - Dural tension tests
    Positive for dural inflammation if lower-extremity symptoms are reproduced
    - Slump test
      a. During each phase of the test, note the response of symptoms
      b. Patient is sitting erect
      c. Patient slumps into flexion with the thoracic and lumbar spine
      d. Maintain slump and add cervical flexion
      e. Maintaining spinal flexion, perform unilateral knee extension, followed by ankle dorsiflexion
      f. Maintaining spinal flexion, perform bilateral knee extension, followed by bilateral dorsiflexion
    - Straight-leg raise test
      a. During each phase of the test, note the response of symptoms
      b. The test is positive with the reproduction of lower-extremity radiating symptoms in the range of 30–60° of hip flexion
      c. Patient supine
      d. Passively raise the leg with the knee extended and the hip in neutral
      e. At the point of reproduction of lower-extremity radiating symptoms, drop down minimally and add ankle dorsiflexion
      f. Full tension is achieved with the addition of cervical flexion
    - Ely's test (femoral nerve stretch)
      a. During each phase, note the response of symptoms

LUMBAR SPINE | LOW BACK GENERAL PAIN   211

b. The test is positive with reproduction of anterior lower-extremity radiating symptoms, which usually occurs at approximately 90° of knee flexion
c. Patient is prone
d. Flex knee
e. Maintain the knee flexion, stabilize the pelvis, and extend the hip
○ Compression overload
▪ In supine position with hips and knees flexed to end range
▪ Apply overpressure to lower extremities in superior direction
○ Climbing test
▪ Standing with one foot on the table, the patient lunges further toward the table to test full range of flexion of the elevated extremity at the hip, knee, and ankle, and extension of the opposite hip and knee
○ Patrick/FABRE
▪ Patient is supine in FABRE position
▪ Inguinal pain implicates hip joint pathology or muscular restrictions
▪ To stress the sacroiliac joint, place one hand on the flexed knee and the other on the opposite ASIS and press down
○ Traction
○ Sacroiliac testing (gapping, compression, rotation/torsion)
○ Muscle length (Thomas, Obers, straight-leg raise, Rectus)

Establish Plan of Care
• Based on history, tests, and measures

GOALS/OUTCOMES
• Patient displays understanding of proper posture and body mechanics as evidenced by pain-free performance of ADLs and vocational activities
• Pain: 2/10 or less with proper body mechanics and posture
• ROM (pain-free)
  ○ Lumbar: A minimum of 80% of AMA guides

	Normal	80%
Flexion	60°	50°
Extension	25°	20°
Side bend	25°	20°
Rotation	30°	25°

• Strength: 4/5 on manual muscle test
  ○ Abdominal
  ○ Spinal extensor
  ○ Gluteals
  Or specific functional motor performance, such as
  ○ Squat to 90°
  ○ Retrieve object from floor
  ○ Perform work task (weight and repetition-specific)
• Functional lower-extremity ROM
  ○ Hip
    ▪ Flexion: 125°
    ▪ Extension: 0°
    ▪ Internal rotation: 20°
    ▪ External rotation: 30°
  ○ Knee
    ▪ Flexion: 120°
    ▪ Extension: 5°
  ○ Ankle
    ▪ Dorsiflexion: 8° in subtalar neutral with knee extended
• Avoidance of movements causing a reoccurrence of symptoms
• Return to previous functional status for ADLs and vocational, recreational, and sports activities as identified by patient
• Independence in a progressive home exercise program emphasizing function

INTERVENTION
NUMBER OF VISITS: 5–12

Coordination, Communication, and Documentation
• Provision of services between admission and discharge that facilitate cost-effective and efficient integration or reintegration to home, community, or work
• Documentation of therapeutic intervention is required for each episode of care and serves as the basic foundation for communication
• Coordination and additional communication will depend on the patient's impairment and home/work/community/leisure situation and requirements. Such services may include:
  ○ Case management
  ○ Coordination of care and collaboration with those integral to the patient's rehabilitation program
  ○ Coordination and monitoring of the delivery of available resources

- Referrals to other health-care professionals
- Identification of resources, support groups, or advocacy services
- Provision of educational or training information
- Technical assistance

Patient Instruction

Basic Anatomy and Biomechanics
- Anatomy of lumbar spine
- Pertinent Gray's Anatomy (Gray. 1995. 510–516, 526–528, 534–537, 809–813, 819–827)
- Biomechanics of lumbar spine and relationship of symptoms to:
  - Mechanisms of injury
  - Segmental mobility dysfunction
  - Muscle weakness or imbalance
  - Postural or lower-extremity biomechanical effects

Handouts
- Patient education
- Specific home program
- Commercially available products, such as:
  - Krames Communications (1100 Grundy Lane, San Bruno, CA 94066)
    - *Back Basics*
    - *Back to Basics*
    - *Back Owner's Manual*
    - *Back Tips for People Who Sit*
    - *Poor Posture Hurts*
    - *Your Back Is Always Working*
  - McKenzie (PO Box 93, Waikanae, New Zealand)
    - *Treat Your Own Back*
  - Saunders (4250 Norex Drive, Chaska, MN 55318)
    - *For Your Back*

Functional Considerations
- Review of aggravating positions and activities
- Instruction on positioning for relief of symptoms
- Instruction in posture and body mechanics for various activities
  - Sleeping
  - Sitting/driving
  - Walking/standing
  - Lifting/pushing/pulling/carrying
  - Specific ADLs or vocational tasks

Direct Interventions

Acute Phase: 3–6 Visits
- Therapeutic exercise and home program
  - Positional distraction
  - Home use of thermal modalities/cryotherapy
  - Oscillatory motion
    - Cat and camel
    - Knee to chest
    - Prone propping
    - Lower trunk rotation
  - Initiate spinal stabilization
    - Inner unit
    - Bracing: Co-contraction of trunk musculature
    - Pelvic tilt for abdominal strengthening/pelvic neutral
    - Functional activities
      a. Bed mobility
      b. Sit to stand
      c. Supine to sit
  - Initiate walking program
  - Aquatic therapy
- Manual therapy techniques
  - Soft-tissue techniques
    - Soft-tissue mobilization
    - Trigger-point techniques
    - Strain/counterstrain
    - Myofascial release
    - Muscle energy techniques
    - Friction massage
  - Joint mobilization
    - Grades I–II with intent of pain relief
    - Specific traction at involved segment performed in a position of comfort
    - Grades III–V to hypomobile segments above and below involved segment
  - Assisted ROM and stretching to hips and lower extremities
  - General manual traction or positional distraction
- Electrotherapeutic modalities
- Physical agents and mechanical modalities
  - Cryotherapy/thermal modalities
  - Ultrasound
  - Mechanical traction
- Goals/outcomes
  - Pain: 5/10 or less
  - Voluntary trunk co-contraction in supine, sitting, and standing
  - Ambulation for 10 minutes

Subacute Phase: 2–6 Visits

- Therapeutic exercise and home program
  - Progress trunk ROM
  - Trunk and lower-extremity stretching to restore flexibility in influential muscle groups
    - Ankle plantar flexors
    - Knee flexors and extensors
    - Hip flexors and extensors
    - Hip rotators
    - Spinal flexors and extensors
  - Cardiovascular conditioning
    - Treadmill/walking program
    - Forward
    - Backward
    - Upper or lower body ergometry
    - Swimming/aquatic therapy
    - Ski machine
    - Cycling
  - Progressive strengthening program
    - Abdominals
    - Trunk extensors
    - Lower extremities
  - Neuromuscular/balance/proprioceptive reeducation
    - Quadruped opposite arm/leg lift
    - Unilateral stance balancing, reaching one or both arms in various directions to maximum distance, avoiding use of other leg for counterbalance
      a. Anterior reach: Stimulates hamstrings, soleus, gastrocnemius, and hip/back extensors (depending on height of reach)
      b. Posterior overhead reach: Stimulates abdominals
      c. Lateral rotational reach: Stimulates hip abductors and lateral trunk stabilizers
    - Unilateral stance balancing, reaching opposite leg in various directions to maximum distance
      a. Anterior reach: Stimulates quadriceps, soleus
      b. Posterior reach: Stimulates gluteals, quadriceps, hip/back extensors
      c. Rotational reach to side: Stimulates gluteals, quadriceps, trunk stabilizers, hip abductors, abdominals
  - Functional closed-kinetic chain activities with spinal stabilization
    - Kneeling
    - Squatting
    - Sit to stand
    - Multidirectional lunges
    - Step up/step down
    - Task-oriented exercise dependent on home, work, recreation, and athletic activities
  - Exercises for specific postural conditions
    - Lordotic back
      a. Strengthen abdominals to control pelvic positioning
      b. Stretch lumbar extensors and hip flexors
      c. Mobilize hip into extension
    - Flat back
      a. Stretch into lumbar extension
      b. Strengthen lumbar and hip extensors
      c. Stretch abdominal and hip musculature as necessary
      d. Mobilize lumbar spine into extension
    - Hypermobile back or segment
      a. Strengthen trunk musculature within controlled ROM to promote spinal stabilization
      b. Stretch musculature as necessary
      c. Mobilize hypomobilities above and below involved segment
    - Deconditioned back
      a. Cardiovascular conditioning
      b. Strength/stabilization
      c. Flexibility
  - Task oriented exercises specifically related to work, home, and recreation
- Manual therapy techniques
  - Continue effective soft-tissue techniques
  - Joint mobilization to lumbar and thoracic spine and hips
    - Progressive Grades III–V joint mobilization to hypomobile joints
    - Progress graded specific traction to irritable joints
  - Manually resisted intensive back program (Brown. 1970)
- Physical agents and mechanical modalities
  Continue effective modalities as in Acute Phase with increased emphasis on use as needed at home

- Goals/outcomes
  - Pain: 2/10 or less with ADLs, 0/10 at rest
  - Strength: 4/5 on manual muscle test for abdominals, spinal extensors, and gluteals or achieve predetermined functional motor performance parameter
  - Functional lower-extremity ROM

Functional Carryover

- Incorporation of home exercise program into ADLs and vocational activities
- Importance of utilizing proper body mechanics and lifting techniques to avoid reinjury or exacerbation of symptoms
- Ergonomic modification of work site, including chair, desk height, and computer placement
- Use of cervical or lumbar support for proper postural alignment during work, driving, and ADLs

DISCHARGE PLANNING AND PATIENT RESPONSIBILITY

Criteria for Discharge

- Patient demonstrates ability to perform exercises in mechanically correct fashion and is compliant with exercise program as instructed
- Patient demonstrates appropriate posture and body mechanics during functional activities
- All rehabilitation goals/outcomes have been achieved with the exception of previous level for recreational and sports activities

Circumstances Requiring Additional Visits

- Persistent functional motor performance deficit or 3/5 on manual muscle test
- History of previous injury or surgery to related area
- Persistent radicular symptoms or neurological deficit
- Severe deconditioning
- Special occupational needs requiring extensive fitness/strengthening
- Multiple injury sites including lower extremity
- Severe traumatic injury with persistent functional/occupational deficits

Home Program

- Flexibility
- Strength/stabilization
- Cardiovascular conditioning

Monitoring

- Instruct patient to call for advice should progression halt or a negative trend occur
- Patient is to recheck/call at 2–4 weeks post-discharge to ensure progression toward achieving all goals/outcomes
- Schedule clinic follow-up as needed if symptoms return or patient is unable to achieve previous status for recreational and sports activities

REFERENCES

1. Abenhaim L, Rossignol M, Gobeille D, et al. The prognostic consequences in the making of the initial medical diagnosis of work-related back injuries. *Spine.* April 1, 1995;20(7):791-795.
2. American Physical Therapy Association. *Guide to Physical Therapist Practice.* Alexandria VA: APTA;1997.
3. Beurskens AJ, de Vet HC, Köke AJ, et al. Efficacy of traction for non-specific low back pain: a randomized clinical trial. *Lancet.* December 16, 1995;436(8990):1596-1600.
4. Binkley J, Finch E, Hall J, Black T, Gowland C. Diagnostic classification of patients with low back pain: report on a survey of physical therapy experts. *Phys Ther.* Mar 1993;73(3):138-155.
5. Brown I. Intensive exercise for the low back. *J Am Phys Ther Assoc.* 1970;50(4):487-498.
6. Bullock-Saxton JE, Janda V, Bullock MI. Reflex activation of gluteal muscles in walking: an approach to restoration of muscle function for patients with low-back pain. *Spine.* 1993; 18(6):704-708.
7. Cartas O, Nordin M, Frankel VH, Malgady R, Sheikhzadeh A. Quantification of trunk muscle performance in standing, semistanding and sitting postures in healthy men. *Spine.* 1993;18(5):603-609.
8. Cavanaugh JM. Neural mechanisms of lumbar pain. *Spine.* 1995;20(16):1804-1809.
9. Chan CW, Goldman S, Ilstrup DM, Kunselman AR, O'Neill PI. The pain drawing and Waddell's nonorganic physical signs in chronic low-back pain. *Spine.* 1993; 18(13):1717-1722.
10. Colliton J. Managing back pain during pregnancy. *Medscape Womens Health.* January 2, 1997(1):2.

11. Criscitiello AA, Fredrickson BE. Thoracolumbar spine injuries. *Orthoped.* October 20, 1997(10):939-944.

12. Dettori JR, Bullock SH, Sutlive TG, Franklin RJ, Patience T. The effects of spinal flexion and extension exercises and their associated postures in patients with acute low back pain. *Spine.* 1995;20(21):2303-2312.

13. Deyo RA et al. A controlled trial of transcutaneous electrical nerve stimulation (TENS) and exercise for chronic low back pain. *N Engl J Med.* June 7, 1990;322(23):1627-1634.

14. DiFabio RP, Boissonnault W. Physical therapy and health-related outcomes for patients with common orthopedic disorders. *J Orthop Sports Phys Ther.* March 1998;27(3):219-230.

15. Ehrmann-Feldman D, Rossignol M, Abenhaim L, Gobeille D. Physician referral to physical therapy in a cohort of workers compensated for low back pain. *Phys Ther.* February 1996;76(2):150-157.

16. Franklin ME, Chenier TC, Brauninger L, Cook H, Harris S. Effect of positive heel inclination on posture. *J Orthop Sports Phys Ther.* 1995;21(2):94-99.

17. Gajdosik RL, Albert CR, Mitman JJ. Influence of hamstring length on the standing position and flexion range of motion of the pelvic angle, lumbar angle, and thoracic angle. *J Orthop Sports Phys Ther.* 1994;20(4):214-219.

18. Gam AN, Johannsen F. Ultrasound therapy in musculoskeletal disorders: a meta-analysis. *Pain.* October 1995;63(1):85-91.

19. Garfin SR, Rydevik B, Lind B, Massie J. Spinal nerve root compression. *Spine.* 1995; 20(16):1810-1820.

20. Gill C, Sanford J, Binkley J, Stratford P, Finch E. Low back pain: program description and outcome in a case series. *J Orthop Sports Phys Ther.* 1994;20(1):11-16.

21. Gray H; Williams PL, ed. *Gray's Anatomy.* 38th ed. New York, NY: Churchill Livingstone; 1995.

22. Haldeman S, Rubenstein SM. Cauda equina syndrome in patients undergoing manipulation of the lumbar spine. *Spine.* 1992;17(12):1469-1473.

23. Haldeman S. Diagnostic tests for the evaluation of back and neck pain. *Neurol Clin.* February 1996;14(1):103-117.

24. Haldeman S. Low back pain: current physiologic concepts. *Neurol Clin.* February 1999;17(1):1-15.

25. Hart A, Hopkins C, Ford B. *ICD-9-CM Expert For Physicians, Volume 1&2.* 7th ed. USA: Ingenix; 2005.

26. Heliövaara M, Mäkelä M, Knekt P, Impivaara O, Aromaa A. Determinants of sciatica and low back pain. *Spine.* June 1991;16(6):608-614.

27. Hides JA, Richardson CA, Jull GA. Multifidus muscle recovery is not automatic after resolution of acute, first-episode low back pain. *Spine.* December 1, 1996;21(23):2763-2769.

28. Holmes JA, Damaser MS, Lehman SL. Erector spinae activation and movement dynamics about the lumbar spine in lordotic and kyphotic squat-lifting. *Spine.* 1992; 17(3):327-334.

29. Indahl A, Belund L, Reikaraas O. Good prognosis for low back pain when left untampered. A randomized clinical trial. *Spine.* February 15, 1995;20(4):473-477.

30. Indahl A, Kaigle A, Reikeras O, Holm S. Electromyographic response of the porcine multifidus musculature after nerve stimulation. *Spine.* 1995;20(24):2652-2658.

31. Infante-Rivard C, Lortie M. Prognostic factors for return to work after a first compensated episode of back pain. *Occup Enviorn Med.* July 1996;53(7):488-494.

32. Ito M, Tadano S, Kaneda K. A biomechanical definition of spinal segmental instability taking personal and disc level differences into account. *Spine.* 1993;18(15):2295-2304.

33. Johannsen F, Remvig L, Kryger P, et al. Exercises for chronic low back pain: a clinical trial. *J Orthop Sports Phys Ther.* 1995;22(2):52-59.

34. Khalil TM, Asfour SS, Martinez LM, et al. Stretching in the rehabilitation of low-back pain patients. *Spine.* 1992;17(3):311-317.

35. Khodadadeh S, Eisenstein SM. Gait analysis of patients with low back pain before and after surgery. *Spine.* 1993;18(11):1451-1455.

36. Koury MJ, Scarpelli E. A manual therapy approach to evaluation and treatment of a patient with a chronic lumbar nerve root irritation. *Phys Ther.* June 1994;74(6):548-560.

37. Kuukkanen T, Malkia E. Muscular performance after a 3 month progressive physical exercise program and 9 month follow-up in subjects with low back pain. A controlled study. *Scand J Med Sci Sports.* April 1996;6(2):112-121.

38. Lee D. *The Pelvic Girdle.* New York, Churchill Livingstone. 1999:81-143.

39. Lee JL, Ooi Y, Nakamura K. Measurement of muscle strength of the trunk and the lower extremities in

subjects with history of low back pain. *Spine.* 1995; 20(18):1994-1996.

40. Magnusson ML, Bishop JB, Hasselquist L, et al. Range of motion and motion patterns in patients with low back pain before and after rehabilitation. *Spine.* December 1, 1998;23(23):2631-2639.

41. Mandell PJ, Weitz E, Bernstein JI, et al. Isokinetic trunk strength and lifting strength measures: differences and similarities between low-back injured and noninjured workers. *Spine.* 1992;18(16):2491-2501.

42. McGavin JC. Scientific application of sports medicine principles for acute low back problems. *J Ortho Sports Phys Ther.* August 1997;26(2):105-108.

43. McGill SM. Low back exercises: evidence for improving exercise regimens. *Phys Ther.* July 1998;78(7):754-765.

44. Prescher A. Anatomy and pathology of the aging spine. *Eur J Radiol.* July 1998;27(3):181-195.

45. Rainville J, Ahern DK, Phalen L, Childs LA, Sutherland R. The association of pain with physical activities in chronic low back pain. *Spine.* 1992;17(9):1060-1064.

46. Richardson C, Jull G, Hodges P, Hide S. *Therapeutic Exercises For Spinal Segmental Stabilization In Low Back Pain.* New York, Churchill Livingstone. 1999.

47. Riddle DL. Classification and low back pain: a review of the literature and critical analysis of selected systems. *Phys Ther.* July 1998;78(7):708-737.

48. Risch SV, Norvell NK, Pollock ML, et al. Lumbar motor performance in chronic low back pain patients: physiologic and psychological benefits. *Spine.* 1993; 18(2):232-238.

49. Rissanin A, Kalimo H, Alaranta H. Effect of intensive training on the isokinetic strength and structure of lumbar muscles in patients with chronic low back pain. *Spine.* 1995;20(3):333-340.

50. Roach KE, Brown M, Ricker E, Altenburger P, Tompkins J. The use of patient symptoms to screen for serious back problems. *J Orthop Sports Phys Ther.* 1995; 21(1):2-6.

51. Saal JS. The role of inflammation in lumbar pain. *Spine.* 1995;20(16):1821-1827.

52. Smidt GL, O'Dwyer KD, Lin S, Blanpied PR. The effect of trunk resistive exercise on muscle strength in postmenopausal women. *J Orthop Sports Phys Ther.* 1991;13(6):300-309.

53. Smith SA, Massie JB, Chesnut R, Garfin SR. Straight leg raising: anatomical effects on the spinal nerve root without and with fusion. *Spine.* 1993;18(8):992-999.

54. Sufka A et al. Centralization of low back pain and perceived functional outcome. *J Orthop Sports Phys Ther.* 1998 Mar;27(3):205-212.

55. Swenson R. Differential diagnosis: a reasonable clinical approach. *Neuro Clin.* February 1999;17(1):43-63.

56. Takemasa R, Yamamoto H, Tani T. Trunk muscle strength in and effect of trunk muscle exercises for patients with chronic low back pain. The differences in patients with and without organic lumbar lesions. *Spine.* December 1, 1995;20(23):2522-2530.

57. Tokuhashi Y, Matsuzaki H, Sano S. Evaluation of clinical lumbar instability using the treadmill. *Spine.* 1993; 18(5):2321-2324.

58. Trafimow JH, Schipplein OD, Novak GJ, Andersson GBJ. The effects of quadriceps fatigue on the technique of lifting. *Spine.* 1993;18(3):364-367.

59. Van Tulder MW, Koes BW, Bouter LM. Conservative treatment of acute and chronic nonspecific low back pain. A systematic review of randomized controlled trials of the most common interventions. *Spine.* September 15, 1997;22(18):2128-2156.

60. Vleeming A, Mooney V, Dorman T, Snyders C, Stoeckart R. *Movement, Stability And Low Back Pain.* New York, Churchill Livingstone. 1997.

61. Waddell G, Feder G, Lewis M. Systematic review of bed rest and advice to stay active for acute low back pain. *Br J Gen Pract.* October 1997;47(423):647-652.

62. Walsh MJ. Evaluation of orthopedic testing of the low back for nonspecific lower back pain. *J Manipulative Physiol Ther.* May 1998;21(4):232-236.

63. Wheeler AH, Hanley EN. Spine update nonoperative treatment for low back pain: rest to restoration. *Spine.* 1995;20(3):375-378.

64. Wheeler AH. Diagnosis and management of low back pain and sciatica. *Am Fam Physician.* October 1995;52(5):1333-1341, 1347-1348.

218   LOW BACK GENERAL PAIN | LUMBAR SPINE

LUMBAR DISC PATHOLOGY
SUMMARY OVERVIEW

ICD-9

722.10   722.2   722.52   722.6   722.93   724.3   724.4   953.2

APTA Preferred Practice Pattern: **4A, 4B, 4E, 4F, 4G, 4J**

EXAMINATION

- History and Systems Review
- Tests and Measures
  Systems review per APTA's *Guide to Physical Therapy Practice*
  - Anthropometric characteristics
  - Gait, locomotion, and balance
  - Joint integrity and mobility
  - Muscle performance
  - Pain
  - Postural assessment
  - ROM
  - Circulation
  - Palpation
  - Reflex integrity
  - Sensory integrity
  - Special tests
- Establish Plan of Care

GOALS/OUTCOMES

- Patient displays understanding of proper posture and body mechanics
- Pain: 2/10 or less with activity
- Pain-free lumbar ROM: A minimum of 80% of AMA guides
- Strength: 4/5 on manual muscle test for back extensors, gluteals, abdominals
- Functional lower-extremity ROM
- Avoidance of movements causing a reoccurrence of symptoms
- Return to previous functional status for ADLs and vocational, recreational, and sports activities as identified by patient
- Independence in a progressive home exercise program emphasizing function
- Alleviation of radicular symptoms

INTERVENTION
NUMBER OF VISITS: 6–12

- Patient Instruction
  - Basic Anatomy and Biomechanics
  - Handouts
  - Functional Considerations
- Direct Interventions
  - Acute Phase: 2–6 Visits
  - Subacute Phase: 4–6 Visits
- Functional Carryover

DISCHARGE PLANNING AND PATIENT RESPONSIBILITY

- Criteria for Discharge
  - Demonstration of proper body mechanics
  - Increased lumbar mobility without neurological signs
  - All goals/outcomes achieved with exceptions specified in guideline
- Circumstances Requiring Additional Visits
  - Persistent functional strength deficit or 3/5 on manual muscle test
  - History of previous injury/surgery to related area
  - Persistent radicular symptoms or neurological deficit
  - Severe deconditioning
  - Special occupational needs requiring extensive fitness/ strengthening
  - Postoperative complications
  - Surgery is indicated, however patient is not a surgical candidate due to risk factors
  - Persistent functional/occupational deficits
- Home Program
  - Flexibility exercises to assist maintenance of postural balance
  - Stabilization and strengthening exercise
  - Cardiovascular conditioning program
  - Use of modalities for occasional flare-ups
  - Proper body mechanics and posture for specific activities
- Monitoring

LUMBAR DISC PATHOLOGY

ICD-9

722.10	Displacement of lumbar intervertebral disc without myelopathy
722.2	Displacement of intervertebral disc, site unspecified, without myelopathy
722.52	Degeneration of lumbar or lumbosacral intervertebral disc
722.6	Degeneration of intervertebral disc, site unspecified
722.93	Other and unspecified disc disorder, lumbar region
724.3	Sciatica
724.4	Thoracic or lumbosacral neuritis or radiculitis, unspecified
953.2	Injury to lumbar nerve root

APTA Preferred Practice Pattern: 4A, 4B, 4E, 4F, 4G, 4J

EXAMINATION

History and Systems Review
- History of current condition
  - Mechanism of injury/onset
  - Date of injury/onset
  - Location, nature, and behavior of symptoms
    - Radiating pain in lower extremities
    - Aggravating/relieving factors
      a. Increased symptoms with forward bending or sitting
      b. Symptoms with coughing, sneezing, or bowel movements
  - Presence of cauda equina symptoms
- Past history of current condition
  - Hospitalization
  - Surgical intervention
  - Lower-extremity problems
  - Bracing injections, etc.
  - Pregnancy/childbirth
    - C-section
- Past medical/surgical history
  - Systemic pathology
    - Appendix
    - Abdominal
    - Pancreas
    - Large intestine
    - Kidney
    - Genital/urinary
      a. Bladder
      b. Ureter
      c. Prostate gland
      d. Cervix
      e. Uterus

  - Iritis
  - Cardiac
  - Respiratory
  - Central nervous system disorders
  - Psoriasis
  - Irritable bowel symptoms
- Functional status and activity level (current/prior)
- Patient's functional goals
- Medications
- Patient's occupation
- Age of patient

Tests and Measures
Systems review per APTA's *Guide to Physical Therapy Practice*
- Anthropometric characteristics
  - Leg length discrepancy
    - Supine
    - Weight-bearing
- Gait, locomotion, and balance
  - Asymmetrical gait pattern
    - Arm swing
    - Hip transverse plane motion
    - Knee extension in stance phase
    - Knee flexion in swing phase
    - Early heel off
  - Lumbar-sacroiliac weight bearing: Mobility
  - Balance
  - Transitional movements: Sit to stand
  - Drop foot
  - Excessive or prolonged compensatory pronation

220   LUMBAR DISC PATHOLOGY | LUMBAR SPINE

- Joint integrity and mobility
  - Central posterior to anterior glides
    In prone position, with posterior to anterior pressure on spinous or transverse process
  - Passive intervertebral motion (T10–S2)
  - Flexion/extension
  - Side bend
  - Rotation
  - Stress tests
    It is recommended that stress tests be performed at those segments that are hypomobile and that the therapist intends to mobilize to end range (Grades III–V)
- Muscle performance
  - Resisted testing
  - Key muscle tests, L2–S1
    To determine possible palsy, utilize a combination of resistance and repetition (5–10)
    - Hip flexion (L2)
    - Quadriceps (L3)
    - Tibialis anterior (L4)
    - Extensor hallicus longus (L5)
    - Peroneals (S1)
    - Gastrocnemius (S1)
  - Abdominals
  - Spinal extensors
  - Hip extensor
  - Inner unit, number seconds able to hold
- Pain
  - Measured on visual analog scale
- Postural assessment
  - Anterior, posterior, side
    - Bony landmarks
    - Scoliosis (sway back, flat back)
    - Pelvic asymmetry
      a. Hip rotation—anterior/posterior
    - Flat lumbar spine
    - Antalgic scoliosis/lateral shift
    - Increased lordosis
  - Palpation, including key landmarks
  - Muscle symmetry: Any presence of hypertrophy or wasting
- ROM
  - Generalized loss of motion
  - Active
    - Flexion
      a. Painful extension and loss of flexion

- Extension
- Side bend
  a. Gross limitation of side flexion to one side
- Rotation
  - Overpressure (Passive)
  - Lower-extremity joint scan—quick test
- Circulation (femoral, poplietus, dorsalis pedius pulses)
- Palpation (tenderness, altered temp, muscle spasm)
- Reflex integrity
  - Reflex testing
    - Knee extension (L3)
    - Achilles tendon (S1)
    - Rule out upper motor neuron lesion
      a. Clonis
      b. Babinski
- Sensory integrity
  - Sensory assessment (T12–S2)
- Special tests
  - Dural tension tests (see description under "Special tests" in *Low Back General Pain* guideline)
    - Slump test, straight-leg raise, prone knee bend, Lasegue's test
  - Compression overload
    - In supine position with hips and knees flexed to end range, standing, apply overpressure to lower extremities in superior direction
  - Patrick/FABRE
    - Patient is supine in FABRE position
    - Inguinal pain implicates hip joint pathology or muscular restrictions
    - To stress the sacroiliac joint, place one hand on the flexed knee and the other on the opposite anterior superior iliac spine and press down.
  - Sacroiliac testing (gapping, compression, rotation/torsion)
  - Muscle length (Thomas, Obers, straight-leg raise, Retus)
  - Traction
    - Standing
    - Supine

Establish Plan of Care
- Based on history, tests, and measures

GOALS/OUTCOMES

- Patient displays understanding of proper posture and body mechanics as evidenced by performance of ADLs and vocational activities without an increase in symptoms
- Pain: 2/10 or less with activity
- Pain-free lumbar ROM: A minimum of 80% of AMA guides

	Normal	80%
Flexion	60°	50°
Extension	25°	20°
Side bend	25°	20°

- Strength: 4/5 on manual muscle test for back extensors, gluteals, abdominals
  - Abdominals
  - Spinal extensor
  - Gluteals
  - Inner unit (able to hold for 10 seconds for 10 repetitions)

  Or specific functional strength, such as
  - Squat to 90°
  - Retrieve object from floor
  - Perform work task (weight- and repetition-specific)
- Functional lower-extremity ROM
  - Hip
    - Flexion: 125°
    - Extension: 0°
    - Internal rotation: 20°
    - External rotation: 30°
  - Knee
    - Flexion: 120°
    - Extension: 5°
  - Ankle
    - Dorsiflexion: 8° in subtalar neutral with knee extended
- Avoidance of movements causing a reoccurrence of symptoms
- Return to previous functional status for ADLs and vocational, recreational, and sports activities as identified by patient
- Independence in a progressive home exercise program emphasizing function
- Alleviation of radicular symptoms

INTERVENTION

NUMBER OF VISITS: 6–12

Coordination, Communication, and Documentation

- Provision of services between admission and discharge that facilitate cost-effective and efficient integration or reintegration to home, community, or work
- Documentation of therapeutic intervention is required for each episode of care and serves as the basic foundation for communication
- Coordination and additional communication will depend on the patient's impairment and home/work/community/leisure situation and requirements. Such services may include:
  - Case management
  - Coordination of care and collaboration with those integral to the patient's rehabilitation program
  - Coordination and monitoring of the delivery of available resources
  - Referrals to other health-care professionals
  - Identification of resources, support groups, or advocacy services
  - Provision of educational or training information
  - Technical assistance

Patient Instruction

Basic Anatomy and Biomechanics

- Anatomy of lumbar spine
- Biomechanics of lumbar spine in relation to:
  - Stress on disc
  - Mechanism of injury
  - Segmental mobility dysfunction
  - Muscle weakness or imbalance
  - Postural or lower-extremity biomechanical dysfunction
- Pertinent Gray's Anatomy (Gray. 1995. 510–516, 526–528, 534–537, 809–813, 819–827)

Handouts

- Specific home program—Patient must be an active participant and do the home program

- Commercially available products, such as:
  - Krames Communications (1100 Grundy Lane, San Bruno, CA 94066)
    - *Back Owner's Manual*
    - *Poor Posture Hurts*
  - McKenzie (PO Box 93, Waikanae, New Zealand)
    - *Treat Your Own Back*
  - Saunders (4250 Norex Drive, Chaska, MN 55318)
    - *For Your Back*

Functional Considerations
- Posture awareness in relation to activity; importance of avoiding prolonged flexion and emphasizing extension
  - Sitting/driving
  - Walking
  - Lifting/pushing/pulling/carrying
- Use of corset or lumbar support
- Sleeping posture progression
  - Supine with knees flexed
  - Supine with knees extended
  - Fetal position
- Idea of *centralization* of symptoms vs. aggravation of radiating signs and symptoms
  - A sudden change or progression of neurological signs necessitates consultation with physician

Direct Interventions

Acute Phase: 2–6 Visits
- Therapeutic exercise and home program
  - Initiate lumbar stabilization
    - Identify patient's optimal spinal position to decrease symptoms (*neutral spine*)
  - Instruction in ADLs limitations, bed mobility, and avoidance of sitting
  - Prone lying with pillows progressing to prone on elbows
  - Walking program progression
  - Aquatic therapy
  - Extensor strengthening
    - Backward walking
    - Sit to stand
    - Modified squats
    - Modified lunges
  - Initiate spinal and lower-extremity flexibility in pain-free positions

- Manual therapy techniques
  - Soft-tissue techniques
    - Myofacial release
    - Strain/counterstrain
    - Soft-tissue mobilization
    - Trigger-point techniques
  - Joint mobilization
    - Grade I or II with intent of pain relief
    - Specific traction at involved segment performed in a position of comfort
    - Grades III–V to hypomobile segments above and below involved segment
  - Assisted passive stretching techniques
    - Trunk
    - Hips
    - Lower extremities
    - Dural stretching
- Electrotherapeutic modalities
- Physical agents and mechanical modalities
  - Cryotherapy/thermal modalities
  - Ultrasound
  - Mechanical traction (intermittent)
    - In position of comfort/relief
- Goals/outcomes
  - Pain: Reduced with activities and rest
  - Prone lying 30 minutes, maintaining centralization of symptoms
  - Ambulation for 10 minutes on level surface
  - Lumbar ROM: 60% of AMA guides
    - Flexion: 35°
    - Extension: 15°
    - Side bend: 15°

Subacute Phase: 4–6 Visits
- Therapeutic exercise and home program
  - Progress from prone on flexed elbows to extended elbow press-up
  - Progress lumbar stabilization as appropriate
  - Spinal extensor strengthening
  - Closed-kinetic chain activities with spinal stabilization
    - Squats
    - Multidirectional lunges
    - Kneeling
    - Step up/step down
  - Lower-extremity stretching
    - Quadriceps

LUMBAR SPINE | LUMBAR DISC PATHOLOGY   223

- Hamstrings
- Gastrocnemius
- Hip extensors
- Hip flexors
- Hip rotators
- Dural stretches
  - Cardiovascular conditioning program
    - Upper body ergometry
    - Walking program/treadmill
    - Cycling
    - Swimming
  - Neuromuscular/balance/proprioceptive reeducation
    - Quadruped opposite arm/leg lift
    - Unilateral stance balancing, reaching one or both arms in various directions to maximum distance, avoiding use of other leg for counterbalance
      a. Anterior reach: Stimulates hamstrings, soleus, gastrocnemius, and hip/back extensors (depending on height of reach)
      b. Posterior overhead reach: Stimulates abdominals
      c. Lateral rotational reach: Stimulates hip abductors and lateral trunk stabilizers
    - Unilateral stance balancing, reaching opposite leg in various directions to maximum distance
      a. Anterior reach: Stimulates quadriceps, soleus
      b. Posterior reach: Stimulates gluteals, quadriceps, hip/back extensors
      c. Rotational reach to side: Stimulates gluteals, quadriceps, trunk stabilizers, hip abductors, abdominals
- Manual therapy techniques
  - Soft-tissue techniques
    - Soft-tissue mobilization
    - Trigger-point techniques
    - Myofascial release
    - Strain/counterstrain
  - Joint mobilization
  - Specific traction at the involved segment, progressing from a position of comfort to restoration of normal segmental mobility
    - Grades III–V to hypomobile segments in the thoracic and lumbar spine

- Physical agents and mechanical modalities
  - Continue effective modalities as in Acute Phase with increased emphasis on use as needed at home
- Goals/outcomes
  - Pain: Less with extended walking, rated 0–2/10
  - Absence of symptoms during rest in all positions
  - Strength: 4/5 on manual muscle test for abdominals, hip musculature, or spinal extensors
    - Abdominal
    - Spinal extensor
    - Gluteals

  Or specific functional motor performance, such as
    - Squat to 90°
    - Retrieve object from floor
    - Perform work task (weight- and repetition-specific)
  - Pain-free activity when patient is using proper body mechanics
  - Functional lower-extremity ROM
  - Pain-free lumbar AROM: 80% of AMA guides

Functional Carryover

- Integration of home exercise program into ADLs and vocational activities
- Importance of utilizing proper body mechanics and lifting techniques to avoid reinjury or exacerbation of symptoms
- Completion of ergonomic adjustments to home, automobile, and vocational environments

DISCHARGE PLANNING AND PATIENT RESPONSIBILITY

Criteria for Discharge

- Demonstration of proper body mechanics
- Increased lumbar mobility without neurological signs
- All goals/outcomes achieved with the possible exception of:
  - Return to previous vocational activity may be delayed depending upon physical demands
  - Return to previous recreational/sports activities

Circumstances Requiring Additional Visits

- Persistent functional strength deficit or 3/5 on manual muscle test
- History of previous injury/surgery to related area
- Persistent radicular symptoms or neurological deficit
- Severe deconditioning
- Special occupational needs requiring extensive fitness/strengthening
- Postoperative complications
- Surgery is indicated, however patient is not a surgical candidate due to risk factors
- Persistent functional/occupational deficits

Home Program

- Flexibility exercises to assist maintenance of postural balance
- Stabilization and strengthening exercise
- Cardiovascular conditioning program
- Use of modalities for occasional flare-ups
- Proper body mechanics and posture for specific activities, such as:
  - Sitting
  - Lifting

Monitoring

- Instruct patient to call for advice should progression halt or a negative trend occur
- Patient is to recheck/call at 2 weeks post-discharge to ensure progression toward achieving all goals/outcomes
- Schedule clinic follow-up as needed if symptoms return or patient is unable to achieve previous status for recreational/sports activities
- Return to physician

REFERENCE

1. Acherman SJ, Steinberg EP, Bryan RN, BenDebba M, Long DM. Persistent low back pain in patients suspected of having herniated nucleus pulposus: radiologic predictors of functional outcome—implications for treatment selection. *Radiology.* 1997;203:815-822.

2. American Physical Therapy Association. *Guide to Physical Therapist Practice.* Alexandria, VA: APTA; 1997.

3. Buckwalter JA. Spine update aging and degeneration of the human intervertebral disc. *Spine.* 1995;20:1307-1314.

4. Carragee EJ, Helms E, O'Sullivan GS. Are postoperative activity restrictions necessary after posterior lumbar discectomy? A prospective study of outcomes in 50 consecutive cases. *Spine.* 1996;21:1893-1897.

5. Cassidy JD, Loback D, Yong-Hing K, Tchang S. Lumbar facet joint asymmetry: intervertebral disc herniation. *Spine.* 1992;17:570-574.

6. Cyriax J. Refresher course for general practitioners: the treatment of lumbar disk lesions. *J Orthop Sports Phys Ther.* 1990;12(4):163-168.

7. DiFabio RP, Mackey G, Golte JB. Physical therapy outcomes for patients receiving worker's compensation following treatment for herniated lumbar disc and mechanical low back pain syndrome. *J Orthop Sports Phys Ther.* 1996;23(3):180-187.

8. Gray H; Williams PL, ed. *Gray's Anatomy.* 38th ed. New York, NY: Churchill Livingstone; 1995.

9. Hart A, Hopkins C, Ford B. *ICD-9-CM Expert For Physicians, Volume 1&2.* 7th ed. USA: Ingenix; 2005.

10. Hoffman RM, Wheeler KJ, Deyo RA. Surgery for herniated lumbar discs: a literature synthesis. *J Gen. Intern Med.* 1993;8:487-496.

11. Lee D. *The Pelvic Girdle.* New York, NY: Churchill Livingstone; 1999:81-143.

12. Maigne J, Rime B, Deligne B. Computed tomographic follow-up study of forty-eight cases of nonoperatively treated lumbar intervertebral disc herniation. *Spine.* 1992;17:1071-1074.

13. Manniche C. Assessment and exercise in low back pain: with special reference to the management of pain and disability following first time lumbar disc surgery. *Dan Med Bull.* 1995;42:301-313.

14. Manniche C, Skall HF, Braendholt L, et al. Clinical trial of postoperative dynamic back exercises after first lumbar discectomy. *Spine*. 1993;18:92-97.

15. Manniche C, Asmussen K, Lauritsen B, et al. Intensive dynamic back exercises with or without hyperextension in chronic back pain after surgery for lumbar disc protrusion: a clinical trial. *Spine*. 1993;18:560-567.

16. Nadler SF, Campagnolo DI, Tomaio AC, Stitik TP. High lumbar disc: diagnostic and treatment dilemma. *Am J Phys Med Rehabil*. 1998;77:538-544.

17. Richardson C, Jull G, Hodges P, Hide S. *Therapeutic Exercises For Spinal Segmental Stabilization In Low Back Pain*. New York, NY: Churchill Livingstone; 1999.

18. Roberts S, Eisenstein SM, Menage J, Evans EH, Ashton IK. Mechanoreceptors in intervertebral discs: morphology, distribution, and neuropeptides. *Spine*. 1995;20:2645-2651.

19. Saunders HD. *Self Help Manual For Your Back*. Chaska, MN; The Saunders Group, Inc; 1992.

20. Saunders HD. Use of spinal traction in the treatment of neck and back conditions. *Clin Orthop Rel Res*. 1983;179:31-38.

21. Slotman GJ, Stein SC. Laminectomy compared with laparoscopic discectomy and outpatient laparoscopic discectomy for herniated L5-S1 intervertebral disks. *J Laparoendosc Adv Surg Tech A*. 1998;8:261-267.

22. van der Heijden GJ, Beurskens AJ, Koes BW, et al. The efficacy of traction for back and neck pain: a systematic, blinded review of randomized clinical trial methods. *Phys Ther*. 1995;75:93-104.

23. Vleeming A, Mooney V, Dorman T, Snyders C, Stoeckart R. *Movement, Stability and Low Back Pain*. New York, NY: Churchill Livingstone; 1997.

24. Vucetic N, DeBri E, Svensson O. Clinical history in lumbar disc herniation: a prospective study in 160 patients. *Acta Orthop Scand*. 1997;68:116-120.

LUMBAR FRACTURE
SUMMARY OVERVIEW

ICD-9

733.13   805.4   805.8

APTA Preferred Practice Pattern: **4D, 4H, 4J**

EXAMINATION

- History and Systems Review
- Tests and Measures

  Systems review per APTA's *Guide to Physical Therapy Practice*
  - Anthropometric characteristics
  - Gait, locomotion, and balance
  - Integumentary integrity
  - Joint integrity and mobility
  - Muscle performance
  - Pain
  - Posture
  - ROM
  - Reflex integrity
  - Sensory integrity
  - Special tests
- Establish Plan of Care

GOALS/OUTCOMES

- Patient displays understanding of proper posture and body mechanics
- Normal healing of fracture site
- Proper body mechanics and postural awareness
- Pain: 2/10 or less
- Pain-free lumbar ROM: A minimum of 80% of AMA guides
- Strength: 4/5 on manual muscle test for back extensors, gluteals, abdominals
- Functional lower-extremity ROM
- Avoidance of movements causing a reoccurrence of symptoms
- Return to previous functional status for ADLs and vocational, recreational, and sports activities as identified by patient
- Independence in a progressive home exercise program emphasizing function

INTERVENTION
NUMBER OF VISITS: 6–12

- Patient Instruction
  - Basic Anatomy and Biomechanics
  - Handouts
  - Functional Considerations
- Direct Interventions
  - Acute Phase: 3–6 Visits
  - Subacute Phase: 3–6 Visits
- Functional Carryover

DISCHARGE PLANNING AND PATIENT RESPONSIBILITY

- Criteria for Discharge
  - All goals/outcomes have been met with the possible exception of return to sport/recreational activities
  - Patient demonstrates independent and consistent ability to perform exercises as prescribed by the therapist
  - Patient is versed in the expectations of continued improvement and decreasing symptoms with continuation of their home program
  - Patient demonstrates appropriate posture and body mechanics during functional activities
- Circumstances Requiring Additional Visits
  - Persistent functional motor performance deficit or 3/5 on manual muscle test
  - History of previous injury/surgery to related area
  - Persistent radicular symptoms or neurological deficit
  - Severe deconditioning
  - Special occupational needs requiring extensive fitness/strengthening
  - Postoperative complications/infection
  - Severe postoperative scarring
  - Instability at fracture/surgical site
  - Multiple fracture/injury sites
  - Arthritic conditions
  - Hip dysfunction
- Home Program
  - Flexibility
  - Functional strengthening/stabilization
  - Cardiovascular conditioning
- Monitoring

LUMBAR FRACTURE

ICD-9
733.13	Pathologic fracture of vertebrae
805.4	Closed fracture of lumbar vertebra without mention of spinal cord injury
805.8	Closed fracture of unspecified part of vertebral column without mention of spinal cord injury

APTA Preferred Practice Pattern: 4D, 4H, 4J

EXAMINATION

History and Systems Review
- History of current condition
  - Mechanism of injury/onset
  - Date of injury/onset
  - Location, nature, and behavior of symptoms
    - Radiating symptoms
    - Aggravating/relieving factors
  - Presence of cauda equina symptoms
- Past history of current condition
  - Hospitalization
  - Lower-extremity problems
  - Bracing injections, etc.
  - Surgical intervention—past surgeries
- Other tests and measures
  - Current radiologic results
  - Exact location/area of fracture, type of fracture, and amount of healing that has taken place
- Past medical/surgical history
  - Systemic pathology
    - Appendix
    - Abdominal
    - Pancreas
    - Large intestine
    - Kidney
    - Genital/urinary
      a. Bladder
      b. Ureter
      c. Prostate gland
      d. Cervix
      e. Uterus
- Functional status and activity level (current/prior)
- Patient's functional goals
- Age
- Occupation
- Current medications

Tests and Measures
Systems review per APTA's *Guide to Physical Therapy Practice*
- Anthropometric characteristics
  - Leg length discrepancy
    - Supine
    - Weight-bearing
- Gait, locomotion, and balance
  - Asymmetrical gait pattern
    - Arm swing
    - Hip transverse plane motion
    - Knee extension in stance phase
    - Knee flexion in swing phase
    - Early heel off
    - Excessive pronation
  - Lumbar-sacroiliac weight bearing: Mobility
  - Balance
  - Transitional movements: Sit/stand
- Integumentary integrity
  - Skin
    - Color change
    - Temperature change
    - Scars
- Joint integrity and mobility
  - Central posterior to anterior glides (as appropriate surrounding fracture site)
    In prone position, with posterior to anterior pressure on spinous or transverse processes
  - Flexion/extension
  - Side bend
  - Rotation
  - Stress tests (only with fully healed fracture)
    It is recommended that stress tests be performed at those segments that are hypomobile or that the therapist intends to mobilize to end range (Grades III–V)
  - Passive intervertebral motion T10–S1
    - Prone
      a. Central posterior to anterior glides: T12–L5

228   LUMBAR FRACTURE | LUMBAR SPINE

b. Rotation: T12–L5

c. Side bend: T12–L5

- Sidelying

  a. Flexion

  b. Extension

  c. Side bend

  d. Rotation

○ Palpation

- Fracture site
- Spinous processes
- Transverse processes
- Posterior superior iliac spine
- Supraspinous ligament
- Paraspinal musculature
- Quadratus lumborum
- Gluteal musculature

• Muscle performance

○ Resisted testing

○ Key muscle tests

To determine possible palsy, utilize a combination of resistance and repetition

- Hip flexion (L2)
- Quadriceps (L3)
- Tibialis anterior (L4)
- Extensor hallicus longus (L5)
- Peroneals (S1)
- Gastrocnemius (S1)

○ Abdominals

○ Spinal extensors

○ Hip extensor

○ Inner unit

○ Palpation

○ Muscle tone

- Atrophy
- Hypertrophy
- Spasm

• Pain

○ Measured on visual analog scale

• Posture

○ Anterior, posterior, side

○ Bony landmarks

○ Scoliosis, sway back, flat back

○ Pelvic asymmetry

○ Neck and shoulder symmetry

- Thoracic curvature
- Scoliotic curvature
- Lower-extremity alignment

○ Lumbar curvature

○ Soft-tissue observation

• ROM

○ Active (as appropriate pending bracing and physician restriction on motion)

- Flexion
- Extension
- Side bend
- Rotation

○ Overpressure (passive)

○ Resisted (neutral if active)

○ Lower-extremity joint scan—quick test

• Reflex integrity

○ Reflex testing

- Patellar tendon (L3)
- Achilles tendon (S1)

○ Rule out upper motor neuron lesion

- Clonus
- Babinski

• Sensory integrity

○ Sensory assessment (T12–S2)

• Special tests

○ Dural tests (see description under "Special Tests" in *Low Back General Pain* guideline)

○ Compression overload (only with fully healed fracture)

- In supine position with hips and knees flexed to end range
- Apply overpressure to lower extremities in superior direction

○ Patrick/FABRE

- Patient is supine in FABRE position
- Inguinal pain implicates hip joint pathology or muscular restrictions
- To stress the sacroiliac joint, place one hand on the flexed knee and the other on the opposite ASIS and press down

○ Traction

○ Muscle length (Thomas, Obers, straight-leg raise, Rectus)

Establish Plan of Care

• Based on history, tests, and measures

LUMBAR SPINE | LUMBAR FRACTURE   229

GOALS/OUTCOMES

- Patient displays understanding of proper posture and body mechanics as evidenced by pain-free performance of ADLs and vocational activities
- Normal healing of fracture site
- Proper body mechanics and postural awareness as evidenced by symptom-free tolerance of postural requirements during normal ADLs and vocational activities
- Pain: 2/10 or less
- Pain-free lumbar ROM: A minimum of 80% of AMA guides

	Normal	*80%*
Flexion	60°	50°
Extension	25°	20°
Side bend	25°	20°
Rotation	30°	25°

- Strength: 4/5 on manual muscle test for back extensors, gluteals, abdominals
  - Abdominals
  - Spinal extensor
  - Gluteals
  - Inner unit (able to hold for 10 seconds for 10 repetitions)

  Or specific functional motor performance, such as
  - Squat to 90°
  - Retrieve object from floor
  - Perform work task (weight- and repetition-specific)
- Functional lower-extremity ROM
  - Hip
    - Flexion: 125°
    - Extension: 0°
    - Internal rotation: 20°
    - External rotation: 30°
  - Knee
    - Flexion: 120°
    - Extension: 5°
  - Ankle
    - Dorsiflexion: 8° in subtalar neutral with knee extended
- Avoidance of movements causing a reoccurrence of symptoms
- Return to previous functional status for ADLs and vocational, recreational, and sports activities as identified by patient
- Independence in a progressive home exercise program emphasizing function

INTERVENTION
NUMBER OF VISITS: 6–12

Coordination, Communication, and Documentation

- Provision of services between admission and discharge that facilitate cost-effective and efficient integration or reintegration to home, community, or work
- Documentation of therapeutic intervention is required for each episode of care and serves as the basic foundation for communication
- Coordination and additional communication will depend on the patient's impairment and home/work/community/leisure situation and requirements. Such services may include:
  - Case management
  - Coordination of care and collaboration with those integral to the patient's rehabilitation program
  - Coordination and monitoring of the delivery of available resources
  - Referrals to other health-care professionals
  - Identification of resources, support groups, or advocacy services
  - Provision of educational or training information
  - Technical assistance

Patient Instruction

Basic Anatomy and Biomechanics
- Anatomy of lumbar spine
- Biomechanics of lumbar spine and relationship of symptoms to:
  - Mechanisms of injury
  - Segmental mobility dysfunction
  - Muscle weakness or imbalance
  - Postural or lower-extremity biomechanical effects
- Pertinent Gray's Anatomy (Gray. 1995. 510–516, 526–528, 534–537, 809–813,819–827)

Handouts
- Patient education, precautions
- Specific home program
- Commercially available products, such as:
  - Krames Communications (1100 Grundy Lane, San Bruno, CA 94066)
    - *Back Basics*
    - *Back Owner's Manual*

230   LUMBAR FRACTURE | LUMBAR SPINE

- *Back Tips for People Who Sit*
- *Poor Posture Hurts*
- *Your Back Is Always Working*
- Specific home program

Functional Considerations
- Specific avoidance of activities causing pain
  - Instruction on positioning for relief of symptoms
  - Review of aggravating positions and activities
- Instruction in posture and proper body mechanics for various activities ADLs
  - Sitting/driving
  - Standing/walking
  - Sleeping
  - Lifting/pushing/pulling/carrying
  - Specific ADLs or vocational tasks
- Role of cardiovascular conditioning exercises in fracture healing

Direct Interventions

Acute Phase: 3–6 Visits
- Therapeutic exercise and home program
  - Flexibility (within pain-free ROM)
    - Pectorals
    - Quadriceps, hip flexors
    - Hamstrings
    - Gluteals, hip rotators
    - Gastrocnemius/soleus
    - Thoracic/Lumbar paraspinals
  - Pelvic clock/bracing exercises for establishment of pain-free position during exercises neutral spine—initiate lumbar stabilization
  - Walking
    - Forward
    - Backward
  - Swimming or aquatic activities
- Manual therapy techniques
  - Soft-tissue techniques
    - Soft-tissue mobilization
    - Trigger-point techniques
    - Muscle energy techniques
    - Strain/counterstrain
  - Passive stretching
    - Hips
    - Lower extremities
    - Trunk

- Proprioceptive neuromuscular facilitation
- Joint mobilization
  - Grade I only at fracture site until healed
  - Grades III–V to specific hypomobilities above and below fracture site with maximal protection of healing segment
- Therapeutic devices and equipment
  - Immobilization with corsets if necessary to protect fracture site
- Electrotherapeutic modalities
- Physical agents and mechanical modalities
  - Cryotherapy/thermal modalities
- Goals/outcomes
  - Pain: 5/10 or less
  - Improve posture awareness as evidenced by pain-free performance of basic ADLs and home exercises
  - Protect fracture while healing occurs
  - Pain-free active lumbar ROM of at least
    - Flexion: 25°
    - Extension: 10°
    - Side bend: 10°
    - Rotation: 25°
  - Initiate cardiovascular conditioning program

Subacute Phase: 3–6 Visits
- Therapeutic exercise and home program
  - Progressive strengthening program
    - Abdominals
    - Back and hip extensors
    - Gluteals
    - Lower extremity
  - Cardiovascular conditioning
    - Upper body ergometry
    - Walking program/treadmill
    - Ski machine
    - Aquatic therapy/swimming
  - Neuromuscular/balance/proprioceptive reeducation
    - Quadruped opposite arm/leg lift
    - Unilateral stance balancing, reaching one or both arms in various directions to maximum distance, avoiding use of other leg for counterbalance
      a. Anterior reach: Stimulates hamstrings, soleus, gastrocnemius, and hip/back extensors (depending on height of reach)
      b. Posterior overhead reach: Stimulates abdominals
      c. Lateral rotational reach: Stimulates hip abductors and lateral trunk stabilizers

- Unilateral stance balancing, reaching opposite leg in various directions to maximum distance
    a. Anterior reach: Stimulates quadriceps, soleus
    b. Posterior reach: Stimulates gluteals, quadriceps, hip/back extensors
    c. Rotational reach to side: Stimulates gluteals, quadriceps, trunk stabilizers, hip abductors, abdominals
  ○ Functional closed chain activities with spinal stabilization
- Manual therapy techniques
  ○ Continue effective soft-tissue techniques
  ○ Joint mobilization
    ▪ Progress grade of mobilization as indicated at healed fracture site
    ▪ Continue specific mobilization of proximal and distal hypomobilities including the hip
  ○ Assisted stretching to remaining shortened postural muscles
- Physical agents and mechanical modalities
  Continue effective modalities as in Acute Phase with increased emphasis on use as needed at home
- Goals/outcomes
  ○ Pain: 2/10 or less with ADL, 0/10 at rest
  ○ Functional lower-extremity ROM
  ○ Lumbar AROM: Achieve a minimum of 80% of AMA guides
    ▪ Flexion: 48°
    ▪ Extension: 20°
    ▪ Lateral flexion: 20°
    ▪ Rotation: 5°
  ○ Strength: 4/5 on manual muscle test for abdominal and hip/spinal extensors or achieve predetermined functional motor performance parameter
  ○ Return to previous functional status for ADLs and vocational activities

Functional Carryover

- Ergonomic modification of work site, including chair, desk height, and computer placement
- Use of cervical or lumbar support for proper postural alignment during work, driving, and ADLs
- Utilization of proper body mechanics and lifting techniques to avoid re-injury or exacerbation of symptoms
- Incorporation of home exercise program into ADLs/vocational activities
- Gradual return to impact/contact activities

DISCHARGE PLANNING AND PATIENT RESPONSIBILITY

Criteria for Discharge

- All goals/outcomes have been met with the possible exception of return to sport/recreational activities
- Patient demonstrates independent and consistent ability to perform exercises as prescribed by the therapist
- Patient is versed in the expectations of continued improvement and decreasing symptoms with continuation of their home program
- Patient demonstrates appropriate posture and body mechanics during functional activities

Circumstances Requiring Additional Visits

- Persistent functional motor performance deficit or 3/5 on manual muscle test
- History of previous injury/surgery to related area
- Persistent radicular symptoms or neurological deficit
- Severe deconditioning
- Special occupational needs requiring extensive fitness/strengthening
- Postoperative complications/infection
- Severe postoperative scarring
- Instability at fracture/surgical site
- Multiple fracture/injury sites
- Arthritic conditions
- Hip dysfunction

Home Program

- Flexibility
  ○ Spinal
  ○ Hips
  ○ Lower extremity
- Functional strengthening/stabilization
  ○ Squats/multidirectional lunges with bracing
  ○ Abdominal and extensor strengthening with therapeutic ball
  ○ Bracing with controlled resisted rotation and upper extremity diagonals
- Cardiovascular conditioning

Monitoring

- Patient is instructed to call for advice if a negative trend occurs

REFERENCE

1. American Physical Therapy Association. *Guide to Physical Therapist Practice*. Alexandria, VA: APTA; 1997.

2. Cantor JB, Lebwohl NH, Garvey T, Eismont FJ. Nonoperative management of stable thoracolumbar burst fractures with early ambulation and bracing. *Spine*. 1993;18:971-976.

3. Domenicucci M, Preite R, Ramieri A, et al. Thoracolumbar fractures without neurosurgical involvement: surgical of conservative treatment?. *J Neurosurg. Sci*. 1996;40:1-10.

4. Gray H; Williams PL, ed. *Gray's Anatomy*. 38th ed. New York, NY: Churchill Livingstone; 1995.

5. Hart A, Hopkins C, Ford B. *ICD-9-CM Expert For Physicians, Volume 1&2*. 7th ed. USA: Ingenix; 2005.

6. Lee D. *The Pelvic Girdle*. New York, NY: Churchill Livingstone; 1999:81-143.

7. Louis CA, Gauthier VY, Louis RP. Posterior approach with Louis plates for fracture of the thoracolumbar and lumbar spine with and without neurologic deficits. *Spine*. 1998;23:2030-2039.

8. Miles JW, Barrett GR. Rib fractures in athletes. *Sports Med*. 1991;12:66-69.

9. Mirza SK, Chapman JR, Anderson PA. Functional outcome of thoracolumbar burst fractures managed with hyperextension casting or bracing and early mobilization. *Spine*. 1996;21:2170-2175.

10. Oner FC, van der Rijt RR, Ramos LM, Dhert WJ, Vervout AJ. Changes in the disc space after fractures of the thoracolumbar spine. *J Bone Joint Surg*. 1998;80:833-839.

11. Reid DC. *Sports Injury Assessment and Rehabilitation*. New York, NY: Churchill Livingston; 1992.

12. Richardson C, Jull G, Hodges P, Hide S. *Therapeutic Exercises For Spinal Segmental Stabilization In Low Back Pain*. New York, NY: Churchill Livingstone; 1999.

13. Vanichkachorn JS, Vaccaro AR. Nonoperative treatment of thoracolumbar fractures. *Orthopedics*. 1997;20;948-953.

14. Vleeming A, Mooney V, Dorman T, Snyders C, Stoeckart R. Movement, stability and low back pain. New York, NY: Churchill Livingstone; 1997.

15. Zindrick MR. The role of transpedicular fixation systems for stabilization of the lumbar spine. *Orthop Clin North Am*. 1991;22:333-344.

234   LUMBAR FRACTURE | LUMBAR SPINE

LUMBAR SPONDYLOLYSIS WITH MYELOPATHY
SUMMARY OVERVIEW

ICD9:

    721.4   721.91   722.73

APTA Preferred Practice Pattern: **4F, 4I, 5H**

EXAMINATION

- History and Systems review
- Tests and Measures
  Systems review per APTA's *Guide to Physical Therapy Practice*
  - Anthropometric characteristics
  - Gait, locomotion, and balance
  - Joint integrity and mobility
  - Muscle performance
  - Pain
  - Postural assessment
  - ROM
  - Reflex integrity
  - Sensory integrity
  - Special tests
- Establish Plan of Care

GOALS/OUTCOMES

- Patient displays understanding of proper posture and body mechanics
- Pain: 2/10 or less with activity
- Pain-free lumbar ROM: A minimum of 80% of AMA guides
- Strength: 4/5 or better on manual muscle test
- Functional lower-extremity ROM
- Avoidance of movements causing a reoccurrence of symptoms
- Return to previous functional status for ADLs and vocational, recreational, and sports activities as identified by patient
- Independence in a progressive home exercise program emphasizing function
- Alleviation of radicular symptoms

INTERVENTION
NUMBER OF VISITS: 6–13

- Patient Instruction
  - Basic Anatomy and Biomechanics
  - Handouts
  - Functional Considerations
- Direct Interventions
  - Acute Phase 3–5 Visits
  - Subacute Phase: 3–8 Visits
- Functional Carryover

DISCHARGE PLANNING AND PATIENT RESPONSIBILITY

- Criteria for Discharge
  - Demonstration of proper body mechanics
  - Increased lumbar mobility without neurological signs
  - All goals/outcomes achieved with the possible exceptions listed in the guideline
- Circumstances Requiring Additional Visits
  - Persistent functional strength deficit or 3/5 on manual muscle test
  - History of previous injury/surgery to related area
  - Persistent radicular symptoms or neurological deficit
  - Severe deconditioning
  - Special occupational needs requiring extensive fitness/strengthening
  - Postoperative complications
  - Surgery is indicated, however patient is not a surgical candidate due to risk factors
  - Persistent functional/occupational deficits
- Home Program
  - Flexibility exercises to assist maintenance of postural balance
  - Stabilization and strengthening exercise
  - Cardiovascular conditioning program
  - Use of modalities for occasional flare-ups
  - Proper body mechanics and posture for specific activities
- Monitoring

SUMMARY OVERVIEW | LUMBAR SPINE | LUMBAR SPONDYLOLYSIS WITH MYELOPATHY   235

LUMBAR SPONDYLOLYSIS WITH MYELOPATHY

ICD9:

721.4	Thoracic or lumbar spondylosis with myelopathy
721.91	Spondylosis of unspecified site, with myelopathy
722.73	Intervertebral disc disorder with myelopathy, lumbar region

APTA Preferred Practice Pattern: 4F, 4I, 5H

EXAMINATION

History and Systems review

- History of current condition
  - Age
  - Medications
  - Mechanism of injury/onset
  - Date of injury/onset
  - Presence of cauda equine symptoms
  - Location, nature, and behavior of symptoms
    - Radiating pain in lower extremities
    - Aggravating/relieving factors
    - Pain worse in morning or evening
    - Paresthesia
    - Perceived weakness/decreased strength
- Past history of current condition
  - Hospitalization
  - Surgical intervention
  - Lower-extremity problems
  - Bracing, injections, etc.
  - Systemic pathology
    - Appendix
    - Abdominal
    - Pancreas
    - Large intestine
    - Kidney
    - Genital/urinary (bladder, uteter, prostate, cervix, uterus)
    - Iritis
    - Cardiac
    - Respiratory
    - Central nervous system disorders
    - Psoriasis
    - Irritable bowel symptoms
- Functional status and activity level
  - Occupation
- Patient's functional goals

Tests and Measures

Systems review per APTA's *Guide to Physical Therapy Practice*

- Anthropometric characteristics
  - Leg length discrepancy
    - Supine
    - Weight-bearing
- Gait, locomotion, and balance
  - Asymmetrical gait pattern
    - Arm swing
    - Hip transverse plane motion
    - Knee extension in stance phase
    - Knee flexion in swing phase
    - Early heel off
  - Lumbar-sacroiliac weight bearing: mobility
  - Balance: Double/single legs, eyes open/closed
  - Transitional movements: Sit/stand
  - Drop foot
  - Excessive or prolonged compensatory pronation
- Joint integrity and mobility
  - Central posterior to anterior glides
  - Passive intervertebral motions (T10–S2)
  - Flexion/extension
  - Side bend
  - Rotation
  - Stress tests—it is recommended that stress tests be performed at those segments that are hypomobile and that the therapist intends to mobilize to end range (Grades III–V)
- Muscle Performance
  - Resisted testing
  - Key muscle tests: L2–S1. To determine possible palsy, utilize a combination of resistance and repetition (5–10)
    - Hip flexion (L2)
    - Quadriceps (L3)
    - Tibialis anterior (L4)
    - Extensor hallicus longus (L5)
    - Fibularis, a.k.a. peroneals (S1)
    - Gastrocnemius (S1)

236　LUMBAR SPONDYLOLYSIS WITH MYELOPATHY | LUMBAR SPINE

- Abdominals
- Spinal extensors
- Hip Extensor
- Inner unit, number of seconds able to hold
- Pain
  - Measured on visual analog scale
- Postural assessment
  - Anterior, posterior, lateral views
    - Bony landmarks
    - Scoliosis, sway back, flat back
    - Pelvic asymmetry
    - Hip rotation—anterior/posterior
    - Antalgic scoliosis/lateral shift
  - Palpation, including key landmarks
  - Muscle symmetry—presence of hypertrophy, spasm, or wasting
- ROM
  - Generalized loss of motion
  - Active
    - Flexion
    - Extension
    - Side bending
    - Rotation
  - Overpressure
  - Combined Motions
  - Lower-extremity joint scan—quick test (squat down, bounce 2–3 times, return to standing)
- Reflex integrity
  - Knee extension (L3)
  - Achilles tendon (S1)
  - Rule out upper motor neuron lesion
    - Clonus
    - Babinski
- Sensory integrity
  - Sensory assessment (T12–S2)
- Special tests
  - Dural tension tests (see description under "Special Tests" in *Low Back General Pain* guideline)
    - Slump test
    - Straight-leg raise
    - Lasegue's test
    - Prone knee bend
  - Compression overload—supine position with hips and knees flexed to end range, apply overpressure to lower extremities in cranial direction
  - Patrick/FABRE
    - Patient is supine in FABRE position

- Inguinal pain implicated hip joint pathology or muscular restrictions
- Stress the sacroiliac joint, place one hand on the flexed knee and the other on the opposite ASIS and press down
  - Traction
    - Standing
    - Supine
  - Sacroiliac testing
    - Gapping
    - Compression
    - Rotation/torsion
  - Muscle length
    - Thomas
    - Obers
    - Straight-leg raise
  - Circulation
    - Femoral pulse
    - Popliteus pulse
    - Doraslis pedius pulse

Establish Plan of Care

- Based on history, tests, and measures

GOALS/OUTCOMES

- Patient displays understanding of proper posture and body mechanics as evidenced by performance of ADLs and vocational activities without an increase in symptoms
- Pain: 2/10 or less with activity
- Pain-free lumbar ROM: A minimum of 80% of AMA guides

	Normal	80%
Flexion	60°	50°
Extension	25°	20°
Side Bend	25°	20°
Rotation	30°	25°

- Strength: 4/5 or better on manual muscle test
  - Abdominals
  - Spinal extensor
  - Gluteals
  - Inner unit (able to hold for 10 seconds for 10 reps)
  - Or specific functional strength, such as
  - Squat to 90°
  - Retrieve object from floor
  - Perform work task (weight- and repetition-specific)

- Functional lower-extremity ROM
  - Hip
    - Flexion: 125°
    - Extension: 0°
    - Internal rotation: 20°
    - External rotation: 30°
  - Knee
    - Flexion: 120°
    - Extension: 0°
  - Ankle
    - Dorsiflexion: 8° in subtalar neutral with knee extended
- Avoidance of movements causing a reoccurrence of symptoms
- Return to previous functional status for ADLs and vocational, recreational, and sports activities as identified by patient
- Independence in a progressive home exercise program emphasizing function
- Alleviation of radicular symptoms

INTERVENTION
NUMBER OF VISITS: 6–13

Coordination, Communication, and Documentation
- Provision of services between admission and discharge that facilitate cost-effective and efficient integration or reintegration to home, community, or work
- Documentation of therapeutic intervention is required for each episode of care and serves as the basic foundation for communication
- Coordination and additional communication will depend on the patient's impairment and home/work/community/leisure situation and requirements. Such services may include:
  - Case management
  - Coordination of care and collaboration with those integral to the patient's rehabilitation program
  - Coordination and monitoring of the delivery of available resources
  - Referrals to other health-care professionals
  - Identification of resources, support groups, or advocacy services
  - Provision of educational or training information
  - Technical assistance

Patient Instruction

Basic Anatomy and Biomechanics
- Anatomy of lumbar spine
- Biomechanics of lumbar spine in relation to:
  - Stress on disc
  - Mechanism of injury
  - Segmental mobility dysfunction
  - Muscle weakness or imbalance
  - Postural or lower-extremity biomechanical dysfunction
- Pertinent Gray's Anatomy (Gray. 1995. 510–516, 526–528, 534–537, 809–813, 819–827)

Handouts
- Specific home program—Patient must be an active participant and do the home program
- Commercially available products, such as:
  - Krames Communications (1100 Grundy Lane, San Bruno, CA 94066)
    - *Back Owner's Manual*
    - *Poor Posture Hurts*
    - *Back basics*
    - *Back to basics*
    - *Back tips for people who sit*
    - *Your back is always hurting*
  - McKenzie (PO Box 93, Waikanae, New Zealand)
    - *Treat Your Own Back*
  - Saunders (4250 Norex Drive, Chaska, MN 55318)
    - *For Your Back*

Functional Considerations
- Posture awareness in relation to activity
  - Sitting/driving
  - Walking
  - Lifting/pushing/pulling/carrying
  - Sleeping
  - Specific job tasks
- Instruction on position of comfort
- Review aggravating positions
- Instruction of posture and body mechanics for various positions
- Use of corset or lumbar support

Direct Interventions

Acute Phase 3–5 Visits

- Therapeutic exercise and home program
  - Initiate lumbar stabilization
    - Pelvic floor
    - Transverse abdominus
    - Multifidus
  - Identify patient's optimal spinal position to decrease symptoms ("neutral spine")
  - Instruction in ADLs limitations, bed mobility, and avoidance of sitting
  - Walking program progression
  - Aquatic therapy
  - Initiate spinal and lower-extremity flexibility in pain-free positions
- Manual therapy techniques
  - Soft-tissue techniques
    - Myofacial release
    - Strain/counterstrain
    - Soft-tissue mobilization
    - Trigger-point techniques
  - Joint mobilization
    - Grade I or II with intent of pain relief
    - Specific traction at involved segment performed in a position of comfort
    - Grades III–V to hypomobile segments above and below involved segment
  - Assisted passive stretching techniques
    - Trunk
    - Hips
    - Lower extremities
    - Dural stretching
- Electrotherapeutic modalities
- Physical agents and mechanical modalities
  - Cryotherapy/thermal modalities
  - Ultrasound
  - Mechanical traction (intermittent)
  - In position of comfort/relief
- Goals/outcomes
  - Pain: Reduced with activities and rest
  - Prone lying 30 minutes, maintaining centralization of symptoms
  - Ambulation for 10 minutes on level surface
  - Lumbar ROM: 60% of AMA guides
    - Flexion: 35°
    - Extension: 15°
    - Side bend: 15°

Subacute Phase: 3–8 Visits

- Therapeutic exercise and home program
  - Progress lumbar stabilization as appropriate
  - Spinal extensor strengthening
  - Closed-kinetic chain activities with spinal stabilization
    - Squats
    - Multidirectional lunges
    - Kneeling
    - Step up/step down
- Lower-extremity stretching
  - Quadriceps
  - Hamstrings
  - Gastrocnemius
  - Hip extensors
  - Hip flexors
  - Hip rotators
  - Dural stretches
- Cardiovascular conditioning program
  - Upper body ergometry
  - Walking program/treadmill
  - Cycling
  - Swimming
- Neuromuscular/balance/proprioceptive reeducation
  - Quadruped opposite arm/leg lift
  - Unilateral stance balancing, reaching one or both arms in various directions to maximum distance, avoiding use of other leg for counterbalance
    - Anterior reach: Stimulates hamstrings, soleus, gastrocnemius, and hip/back extensors (depending on height of reach)
    - Posterior overhead reach: Stimulates abdominals
    - Lateral rotational reach: Stimulates hip abductors and lateral trunk stabilizers
  - Unilateral stance balancing, reaching opposite leg in various directions to maximum distance
    - Anterior reach: Stimulates quadriceps, soleus
    - Posterior reach: Stimulates gluteals, quadriceps, hip/back extensors
    - Rotational reach to side: Stimulates gluteals, quadriceps, trunk stabilizers, hip abductors, abdominals

- Manual therapy techniques
  - Soft-tissue techniques
    - Soft-tissue mobilization
    - Trigger-point techniques
    - Myofascial release
    - Strain/counterstrain
  - Joint mobilization
    - Specific traction at the involved segment, progressing from a position of comfort to restoration of normal segmental mobility
    - Grades III–V to hypomobile segments in the thoracic and lumbar spine
- Physical agents and mechanical modalities
  Continue effective modalities as in Acute Phase with increased emphasis on use as needed at home
- Goals/outcomes
  - Pain: less with extended walking, rated 0–2/10
  - Absence of symptoms during rest in all positions
  - Strength: 4/5 on manual muscle test for abdominals, hip musculature, or spinal extensors
    - Abdominal
    - Spinal extensor
    - Gluteals
    Or specific functional motor performance, such as
    - Squat to 90°
    - Retrieve object from floor
    - Perform work task (weight- and repetition-specific)
  - Pain-free activities when patient is using proper body mechanics
  - Functional lower-extremity ROM
  - Pain-free lumbar AROM: 80% of AMA guides

Functional Carryover

- Integration of home exercise program into ADLs and vocational activities
- Importance of utilizing proper body mechanics and lifting techniques to avoid reinjury or exacerbation of symptoms
- Completion of ergonomic adjustments to home, automobile, and vocational environments

DISCHARGE PLANNING AND PATIENT RESPONSIBILITY

Criteria for Discharge

- Demonstration of proper body mechanics
- Increased lumbar mobility without neurological signs
- All goals/outcomes achieved with the possible exception of:
  - Return to previous vocational activity may be delayed depending upon physical demands
  - Return to previous recreational/sports activities

Circumstances Requiring Additional Visits

- Persistent functional strength deficit or 3/5 on manual muscle test
- History of previous injury/surgery to related area
- Persistent radicular symptoms or neurological deficit
- Severe deconditioning
- Special occupational needs requiring extensive fitness/strengthening
- Postoperative complications
- Surgery is indicated, however patient is not a surgical candidate due to risk factors
- Persistent functional/occupational deficits

Home Program

- Flexibility exercises to assist maintenance of postural balance
- Stabilization and strengthening exercise
- Cardiovascular conditioning program
- Use of modalities for occasional flare-ups
- Proper body mechanics and posture for specific activities, such as:
  - Sitting
  - Lifting

Monitoring

- Instruct patient to call for advice should progression halt or a negative trend occur
- Patient is to recheck/call at 2 weeks post-discharge to ensure progression toward achieving all goals/outcomes
- Schedule clinic follow-up as needed if symptoms return or patient is unable to achieve previous status for recreational/sports activities
- Return to physician

REFERENCES

1. American Physical Therapy Association. *Guide to Physical Therapist Practice.* 2nd ed. Alexandria VA; 2001.

2. Atlas S, Deyo R. Evaluating and managing acute low back pain in the primary care setting. *J Gen Intern Ned.* 2001;16:120-131.

3. Briggs AM, Greig AM, Wark JD, Fazzalari NL, Bennell KL. A review of anatomical and mechanical factors affecting vertebral body integrity. *Int J Med Sci.* 2004;1(3):170-180.

4. Brown I. Intensive exercise for the low back. *J Am Phys Ther Assoc.* 1970;50(4):487-498.

5. Gray H; Williams PL, ed. *Gray's Anatomy.* 38th ed. New York, NY: Churchill Livingstone; 1995.

6. Hart A, Hopkins C, Ford B. *ICD-9-CM Expert For Physicians, Volume 1&2.* 7th ed. USA: Ingenix; 2005.

7. Heck J, Sparano J. A classification system for the assessment of lumbar pain in athletes. *J Athl Train.* 2000;35(2):204-211.

8. Magee D. *Orthopedic Physical Assessment.* Pennsylvania, Saunders. 2002:467-559.

9. Ralston S, Weir M. Suspecting lumbar spondylolysis in adolescent low back pain. *Clin Pediatr (Phila).* May 1998;37,5:287-293.

10. Resnik L, Dobrzykowski E. Guide to outcomes measurement for patients with low back pain syndromes. *J Orthop Sports Phys Ther.* 2003;22:307-318.

11. van den Hoogen HJ, Koes BW, Devillé W, van Eijk JT, Bouter LM. The inter-observer reproducibility of Lasègue's sign in patients with low back pain in general practice. *Br J Gen Pract.* 1996;46:727-730.

12. Waddell G, Main CJ, Morris EW, et al. Normality and reliability in the clinical assessment of backache. *Br Med J (Clin Res Ed).* 1982;284:1519-1523

LUMBAR SURGERY—INPATIENT
SUMMARY OVERVIEW

ICD-9

722.80   722.83   737.12   737.22   V45.4

APTA Preferred Practice Pattern: **4B, 4G, 4H, 4J**

EXAMINATION

- History and Systems Review
- Tests and Measures
  Systems review per APTA's *Guide to Physical Therapy Practice*
  - Arousal, attention, cognition
  - Gait, locomotion, and balance
  - Muscle performance
  - Orthotic, protective, supportive devices
  - Pain
  - ROM
  - Self-care and home management
  - Sensory integrity
- Establish Plan of Care

GOALS/OUTCOMES

- The client will achieve an independent/supervised functional level
- Pain: Less than 2/10 with activity or at rest

INTERVENTION
NUMBER OF VISITS: 2–4 (1–2 DAYS DURING ACUTE HOSPITALIZATION)

- Patient Instruction
  - Basic Anatomy and Biomechanics
  - Handouts
  - Functional Considerations
- Direct Interventions
  - Acute Hospitalization (1–2 days)
- Functional Carryover

DISCHARGE PLANNING AND PATIENT RESPONSIBILITIES

- Criteria for Discharge
  - Client understands and demonstrates lami precautions
  - Client maintains good posture and body mechanics
  - Short term rehabilitation goals (Acute Hospitalization) have been achieved
  - Patient has initiated progress toward previous functional status for ADLs
- Circumstances Requiring Additional Visits
  - Excessive pain
  - Unresolved foot drop or other radicular symptoms of lower extremity with strength < 3/5
  - Post operative cognitive changes or other complications
- Home Program
  - Home exercise program (for laminectomy and microdiscectomy only)
- Monitoring

SUMMARY OVERVIEW | LUMBAR SPINE | LUMBAR SURGERY—INPATIENT   243

LUMBAR SURGERY—INPATIENT

ICD-9

722.80	Postlaminectomy syndrome, unspecified region
722.83	Postlaminectomy syndrome, lumbar region
737.12	Kyphosis, postlaminectomy
737.22	Other postsurgical lordosis
V45.4	Postprocedural arthrodesis status

APTA Preferred Practice Pattern: **4B, 4G, 4H, 4J**

EXAMINATION

History and Systems Review

- History of current condition
  - Surgical procedure
    - Laminectomy vs. microdiscectomy vs. lumbar fusion
    - Bracing or corset required
    - Complications
- Functional status and activity level (current/prior)
- Living environment
  - Barriers to discharge
    - Support system
    - Stairs
- Patient's functional goals

Tests and Measures

Systems review per APTA's *Guide to Physical Therapy Practice*

- Arousal, attention, cognition
  - Orientation
  - Motivation level
  - Cognitive status in relation to compliance with postoperative limitations
  - Observation of laminectomy precautions
  - Safety judgement
- Gait, locomotion, and balance
  - Gait analysis
    - Appropriate use of assistive device (if needed)
    - Stride length
  - Balance assessment
    - Fall risk
- Muscle performance
  - Manual muscle tests of lower extremities: Hip flexion, quadriceps, hamstrings, ankle dorsi/plantar flexors, extensor hallicus longus

- Orthotic, protective, supportive devices
  - Use of corset or abdominal binder as per physician
- Pain
  - Pain at surgical site
  - Pain in involved extremity (dermatomal distribution)
- ROM
  - Functional ROM of lower extremities
- Self-care and home management
  - Ability to transfer
    - Bed mobility with log rolling
    - Toilet transfers
- Sensory integrity

Establish Plan of Care

- Based on history, tests, and measures

GOALS/OUTCOMES

- The client will achieve an independent/supervised functional level for:
  - Transfers in and out of bed, on and off toilet, on and off chair
  - Gait training at a household to limited community level, as per the client's prior functional level with an appropriate assistive device as needed
  - Stair climbing one or more steps, consistent with their home environment, with appropriate assistive device or handrail
  - Performance of home exercise program, 2–3 times a day
  - Adherence to laminectomy precautions and incorporating them into the above activities, including no bending or twisting of waist
- Pain: Less than 2/10 with activity or at rest

244   LUMBAR SURGERY—INPATIENT | LUMBAR SPINE

INTERVENTION

NUMBER OF VISITS: 2–4 (1–2 DAYS DURING ACUTE HOSPITALIZATION)

Coordination, Communication, and Documentation

- Provision of services between admission and discharge that facilitate cost-effective and efficient integration or reintegration to home, community, or work
- Documentation of therapeutic intervention is required for each episode of care and serves as the basic foundation for communication
- Coordination and additional communication will depend on the patient's impairment and home/work/community/leisure situation and requirements. Such services may include:
  ○ Case management
  ○ Coordination of care and collaboration with those integral to the patient's rehabilitation program
  ○ Coordination and monitoring of the delivery of available resources
  ○ Referrals to other health-care professionals
  ○ Identification of resources, support groups, or advocacy services
  ○ Provision of educational or training information
  ○ Technical assistance
- Specific coordination and communication provisions:
  ○ Referral to work hardening for return to work

Patient Instruction

Basic Anatomy and Biomechanics

- Commercially available products, such as:
  ○ Krames Communications (1100 Grundy Lane, San Bruno, CA 94066)
    ▪ *Spinal Surgery for Your Lower Back*
    ▪ *The Post-Op Back Book*

Handouts

- Laminectomy precautions
  ○ No bending over at waist
  ○ No twisting waist
  ○ Avoid sitting longer than 15–30 minutes (as per physician)
  ○ No lifting more than 5–10 lbs
- Home Exercise program (for laminectomy and microdiscectomy only)

Functional Considerations

- Modification of home environment for safety
  ○ Removal of throw rugs
  ○ Use of pillows in chairs/bed for appropriate support
  ○ Handrails as needed
  ○ Hand-held shower as needed
  ○ Rearranging furniture as needed (if using assistive device)
- Address sexual activity if patient has questions or concerns

Direct Interventions

Acute Hospitalization (1–2 days)

- Therapeutic exercise and home program
  ○ Single knee to chest, double knee to chest, hamstring stretch, abdominal curls, pelvic tilts, ankle pumps (for laminectomy and microdiscectomy only)
- Functional training
  ○ Transfer training
    ▪ Log rolling in bed
    ▪ Bed to and from chair
    ▪ Toilet transfers
  ○ Gait training
    ▪ Gait instruction with assistive or orthotic device as needed
      a. Level surface
      b. Stair training
- Therapeutic devices and equipment
  ○ Instruction donning/doffing corset/brace if applicable
- Physical agents and mechanical modalities
  ○ Apply antithrombic pumps (discontinue when patient is ambulatory)

Functional Carryover

- Patient is able to ambulate and transfer independently
- Patient should demonstrate safe posture and body mechanics with routine activities
- Instruct patient in independently donning and doffing brace

LUMBAR SPINE | LUMBAR SURGERY—INPATIENT   245

DISCHARGE PLANNING AND PATIENT RESPONSIBILITIES

Criteria for Discharge
- Client understands and demonstrates laminectomy precautions
- Client maintains good posture and body mechanics
- Short term rehabilitation goals (Acute Hospitalization) have been achieved
- Patient has initiated progress toward previous functional status for ADLs

Circumstances Requiring Additional Visits
- Excessive pain
- Unresolved foot drop or other radicular symptoms of lower extremity with strength < 3/5
- Post operative cognitive changes or other complications

Home Program
- Home exercise program (for laminectomy and microdiscectomy only)
  - Single knee to chest
  - Double knee to chest
  - Hamstring stretch
  - Abdominal curls
  - Pelvic tilts
  - Ankle pumps

Monitoring
- Patient will follow-up with physical therapist or physician in 2 weeks to monitor progress toward functional goals

REFERENCES

1. American Physical Therapy Association. *Guide to Physical Therapist Practice*. Alexandria, VA: APTA; 1997.
2. Atlas SJ, Deyo RA, Keller RB, et al. The Maine lumbar spine study, part III: 1-year outcomes of surgical and nonsurgical management of lumbar spinal stenosis. *Spine*. 1996;21:1787-1795.
3. Brown I. Intensive exercise for the low back. *J Am Phys Ther Assoc*. 1970;50(4):487-498.
4. Connolly PJ, Grob D. Bracing of patients after fusion for degenerative problems of the lumbar spine—yes or no? *Spine*. 1998;23:1426-1428.
5. Deen HG, Zimmerman RS, Lyons MK, et al. Use of the exercise treadmill to measure baseline functional status and surgical outcome in patients with severe lumbar spinal stenosis. *Spine*. 1998;23:244-248.
6. Ferreira PH, Ferreira ML, Hodges PW. Changes in recruitment of the abdominal muscles in people with low back pain: ultrasound measurement of muscle activity. *Spine*. 2004;29:2560-6
7. Gluck NI. Passive care and active rehabilitation in a patient with failed back surgery syndrome. *J Manipulative Physiol Ther*. 1996;19:41-47.
8. Gray H; Williams PL, ed. *Gray's Anatomy*. 38th ed. New York, NY: Churchill Livingstone; 1995.
9. Hart A, Hopkins C, Ford B. *ICD-9-CM Expert For Physicians, Volume 1&2*. 7th ed. USA: Ingenix; 2005.
10. Herno A, Airaksinen O, Sarri T. Long-term results of surgical treatment of lumbar spinal stenosis. *Spine*. 1993;18:1471-1474.
11. Hides J, Wilson S, Stanton W, et al. An MRI investigation into the function of the transversus abdominis muscle during "drawing-in" of the abdominal wall. *Spine* 2006;31:175-8.
12. Hodges PW, Richardson CA. Altered trunk recruitment in people with low back pain with upper limb movement at different speeds. *Arch Phys Med Rehabil*. 1999; 80: 1005-12.
13. Hu RW, Jaglal S, Axcell T, Anderson G. A population based study of reoperations after back surgery. *Spine*. 1997;22:2265-2270.
14. Katz JN, Lipson SJ, Chang LC, et al. Seven-to-10-year outcome of decompressive surgery for degenerative lumbar spinal stenosis. *Spine*. 1996;21:92-98.
15. Kuslich SD, Ulstrom CL, Griffith SL, Ahern JW, Dowdle JD. The Bagby and Kuslich method of lumbar interbody fusion: history, techniques, and 2-year

follow-up results of a united states prospective, multicenter trial. *Spine.* 1998;23:1267-1278.

16. Manniche C. Assessment and exercise in low back pain: with special reference to the management of pain and disability following first time lumbar disc surgery. *Dan Med Bull.* 1995;42:301-313.

17. Manniche C, Skall HF, Braendholt L, et al. Clinical trial of postoperative dynamic back exercises after first lumbar discectomy. *Spine.* 1993;18:92-97.

18. Manniche C, Asmussen K, Lauritsen B, et al. Intensive dynamic back exercises with or without hyperextension in chronic back pain after surgery for lumbar disc protrusion: a clinical trial. *Spine.* 1993;18:560-567.

19. Moseley GL, Hodges PW, Gandevia SC. Deep and superficial fibers of the lumbar multifidus muscle are differentially active during voluntary arm movements. *Spine.* 2002;27:29-36.

20. Richardson CA, Snijders CJ, Hides JA, et al. The relation between the transversus abdominis muscles, sacroiliac joint mechanics, and low back pain. *Spine.* 2002;27:399-405.

21. Slotman GJ, Stein SC. Laminectomy compared with laparoscopic discectomy and outpatient laparoscopic discectomy for herniated L5-S1 intervertebral disks. *J Laparoendosc Adv Surg Technol A.* 1998;8:261-267.

22. Timm KE. A randomized-control study of active and passive treatments for chronic low back pain following L5 laminectomy. *J Orthop Sports Med.* 1994;20:276-286.

23. Urquhart DM, Hodges PW. Differential activity of regions of the transversus abdominis during trunk rotation. *Eur Spine J.* 2005;14:393-400.

24. Waddell G, Reilly S, Torsney B, et al. Assessment of the outcome of low back surgery. *J Bone Joint Surg.* 1988;70:723-727.

25. Weiner BK, Fraser RD. Spine update: lumbar interbody cages. *Spine.* 1998;23:634-640.

26. Zdelblick TA. A prospective, randomized study of lumbar fusion: preliminary results. *Spine.* 1993;18:983-991.

27. Zindrick MR. The role of transpedicular fixation systems for stabilization of the lumbar spine. *Orthop Clin North Am.* 1991;22:333-344.

248   LUMBAR SURGERY—INPATIENT | LUMBAR SPINE

PELVIC FLOOR DYSFUNCTION
SUMMARY OVERVIEW

ICD-9

569.42	596.59	564.8	595.1	618.8	625.0	625.1	625.6	625.8
625.9	696.5	719.45	724.79	787.6	788.3	788.4	788.6	

APTA Preferred Practice Pattern: 4A, 4B, 4C, 4D, 4E, 4F, 4G, 4H, 7A, 7C, 7D

EXAMINATION

- History and Systems Review
- Tests and Measures
  Systems review per APTA's *Guide to Physical Therapy Practice*
  - Assistive and adaptive devices
  - Gait, locomotion, and balance
  - Integumentary integrity
  - Joint integrity and mobility
  - Motor function
  - Muscle performance
  - Pain
  - Posture
  - ROM
  - Reflex integrity
  - Sensory integrity
  - Self-care and home management
- Establish Plan of Care

GOALS/OUTCOMES

- Full participation in home/community/occupational activities, not limited by voiding concerns
- Resting tone of pelvic floor muscles normalized
- Pain free as evidenced by biofeedback and pain-free intercourse
- Contraction of pelvic floor muscles grade 4/5 with 10-second hold and 10 quick flick contraction
- Voiding pattern every 3- to 4-hour interval during the day and less than once at night with normal fluid intake
- Able to perform techniques to defer urgency and identify bladder irritants in diet
- Frequency and severity of leakage is reduced by 50%
- Ability to independently perform activities related to self-care, toileting, and home management
- Independent of transfer, gait, and locomotion for toileting

INTERVENTION
NUMBER OF VISITS: 5–12

- Patient Instruction
  - Basic Anatomy and Biomechanics
  - Handouts
- Direct Interventions
  - Treatment Phase: 5–12 Visits
- Functional Carryover

DISCHARGE PLANNING AND PATIENT RESPONSIBILITY

- Criteria for Discharge
  - Patient has reached all goals with exception of voiding schedule of every 3–4 hours but has understanding of progressing schedule independently
  - Ability to use home unit for biofeedback or electrical stimulation
- Circumstances Requiring Additional Visits
  - Decreased pelvic floor contraction and incoordination of pelvic floor contraction/relaxation
  - History of previous injury or surgery to related area
- Home Program
  - Aerobic conditioning
  - Strengthening/relaxation of pelvic floor muscles
  - Biofeedback or electrical stimulation as appropriate
  - Strengthening and stretching of appropriate hip and abdominal muscles
- Monitoring

SUMMARY OVERVIEW | LUMBAR SPINE | PELVIC FLOOR DYSFUNCTION   249

PELVIC FLOOR DYSFUNCTION

ICD-9

569.42	Anal or rectal pain
596.59	Other functional disorder of bladder
564.8	Other specified functional disorders of intestine
595.1	Chronic interstitial cystitis
618.8	Other specified genital prolapse
625.0	Dyspareunia
625.1	Vaginismus
625.6	Stress incontinence, female
625.8	Other specified symptoms associated with female genital organs
625.9	Unspecified symptom associated with female genital organs
696.5	Other and unspecified pityriasis
719.45	Pain in joint, pelvic region and thigh
724.79	Other disorders of coccyx
787.6	Incontinence of feces
788.3	Urinary incontinence
788.4	Frequency of urination and polyuria
788.6	Other abnormality of urination

APTA Preferred Practice Pattern: 4A, 4B, 4C, 4D, 4E, 4F, 4G, 4H, 7A, 7C, 7D

EXAMINATION

History and Systems Review

- History of current condition
  - Mechanism of injury/onset
  - Date of injury/onset
  - Nature of symptoms
    - Aggravating/relieving factors
  - Incontinence
    - Severity and frequency
    - Position with leakage
    - Protection
    - Urge characteristics
  - Current therapeutic interventions—physician's plan of care
  - Onset and pattern of symptoms—bladder diary, pain scales
- Other tests and measures
  - Urine cultures, urodynamics, cystourethrograph, videouradynamics, cystoscope, manometry, pudenal nerve, conduction studies
- Medications
- Past medical/surgical history
  - Appendix
  - Abdominal
  - Pancreas
  - Large intestine
  - Diuretics, antidepressants, opiods, antihistamine, estrogen, calcium channel blockers
  - Diabetes
  - Fecal incontinence, constipation, hemorrhoids
  - Menopausal state, dysmenorrhea, pelvic inflammatory disease, prolapse, endometriosis
  - Integumentary skin lesion
  - Multiple sclerosis, Parkinson's, spina bifida, spinal cord injury, cerebral vascular accident, closed head injury
  - Pregnancy/OB-GYN
    - C-section
    - Traumatic deliveries
    - Gravid/parity
    - Complications
    - Prolonged pushing
  - Sexual abuse
  - Kidney
  - Genital/urinary
    - Bladder
    - Ureter
    - Prostate gland
    - Cervix
    - Uterus
  - Sexually transmitted disease

- Functional status and activity level: current/prior
- Social habits
  - Current exercise status
    - Fitness
    - Kegel exercise
  - Avoidance of community work/activities due to embarrassment
- Social history
  - Family and caregiver resources—functional incontinence
  - Social interactions, social activities, and support systems
  - Demands of job or child care: prolonged sitting, standing, lifting
- Living environment
  - Assistive devices available at home, work, bathroom
- Patient's functional goals

Tests and Measures

Systems review per APTA's *Guide to Physical Therapy Practice*

- Assistive and adaptive devices
  - Ability to use and care for device
  - Safety
  - Barriers
- Gait, locomotion, and balance
  - With or without assistive device
- Integumentary integrity
  - Skin color
    - Irritation, dryness, lack of estrogen
  - Exposed abdominal structures—prolapse of bladder, rectum, uterus with and without bearing down
  - Hemorrhoids
  - Symmetry of tissue, abdominal and perineum
  - Scar tissue
  - Epistiotomy
  - Abdominal surgery
- Joint integrity and mobility
  - Dynamic and static position of sacroiliac, pubic, and hip joints
  - Nature and quality of movement
  - Joint hypermobility and hypomobility
    - Lumbar spine
    - Sacroiliac joint
    - Overpressure
  - Pain and soreness
  - Soft-tissue edema, inflammation, or restriction

- Motor function
  - Performance
  - Preferred postures, including toilet position
- Muscle performance
  - Functional muscle motor performance, power and endurance—stop test, provocation test
  - Muscle strength, power, and endurance using manual muscle tests or dynamometry—digital exam or dynamometry (perineal perionometry) of pelvic floor muscles isolated from large muscle groups
  - Symmetry of contraction: anterior wall vs. posterior wall
    - Ability to lift with pelvic diaphragm
    - Ability to move clitoris downward
    - Clock exam
  - Muscle tone of vaginal wall
    - Hypotonic, hypertonic
  - Ability to relax muscle groups
  - Pain and soreness and trigger-points
  - Electromyography
- Pain
  - Measured on visual analog scale
  - Review of daily activity log: Bladder diary, pain charts, exercise log
  - Pain, behavior, and reaction during specific movements
  - Muscle soreness
  - Pain and soreness with joint movement
  - Pain perception
  - Pain with palpation
- Posture
  - Resting posture
  - Pelvic alignment
  - Alignment with lower-extremity landmarks
  - Lumbar scan
- ROM
  - Lower-extremity muscles that have direct impact on pelvic floor muscles
  - Functional ROM
  - Multi-segmental movement
  - Muscle, joint, or soft-tissue characteristics
- Reflex integrity
  - Normal reflexes: Anal wink, bulbocavernous reflex, cough
- Sensory integrity
  - Deep sensation
  - Superficial sensations

LUMBAR SPINE | PELVIC FLOOR DYSFUNCTION   251

- Self-care and home management (including ADLs)
  - Adaptive skills
  - Environment and tasks
  - Ability to transfer
  - Safety: Review of daily activities log (bladder diary)

Establish Plan of Care

- Based on history, tests, and measures

GOALS/OUTCOMES

- Full participation in home/community/occupational activities, not limited by voiding concerns
- Resting tone of pelvic floor muscles normalized
- Pain free as evidenced by biofeedback and pain-free intercourse
- Contraction of pelvic floor muscles grade 4/5 with 10-second hold and 10 quick flick contraction
- Voiding pattern every 3- to 4-hour interval during the day and less than once at night with normal fluid intake
- Able to perform techniques to defer urgency and identify bladder irritants in diet
- Frequency and severity of leakage is reduced by 50%
- Ability to independently perform activities related to self-care, toileting, and home management
- Independent of transfer, gait, and locomotion for toileting

INTERVENTION
NUMBER OF VISITS: 5–12

Coordination, Communication, and Documentation

- Provision of services between admission and discharge that facilitate cost-effective and efficient integration or reintegration to home, community, or work
- Documentation of therapeutic intervention is required for each episode of care and serves as the basic foundation for communication
- Coordination and additional communication will depend on the patient's impairment and home/work/community/leisure situation and requirements. Such services may include:
  - Case management
  - Coordination of care and collaboration with those integral to the patient's rehabilitation program
  - Coordination and monitoring of the delivery of available resources
  - Referrals to other health-care professionals
  - Identification of resources, support groups, or advocacy services
  - Provision of educational or training information
  - Technical assistance
- Specific coordination and communication provisions:
  - Consult with urologists and gynecologists
  - Social worker/case manager

Patient Instruction

Basic Anatomy and Biomechanics

- Anatomy of the pelvis, pelvic floor musculature, urogenital organs, and abdominal wall
- Biomechanics of pelvis as it relates to the pelvic floor muscles
- Nervous system control of urinary system
- Pertinent Gray's Anatomy (Gray. 1995. 829–835, 1813–1847)
- Additional resource/support group information on diagnosis and treatment
- American Foundation for Urologic Disease, 1120 North Charles Street, Baltimore, MD 21201, (301) 727-2908
- American Physical Therapy Association Section on Women's Health, PO Box 327, Alexandria, VA 22313, (800) 999-2782
- Interstitial Cystitis Association, PO Box 1553, Madison Square Station, New York, NY 10159, (212) 979-6057
- National Vulvodynia Association, PO Box 9309, Silver Spring, MD 20916-9309, (301) 460-6407

Handouts

- Commercially available products
  - Progressive Therapeutics (1333 W. 120th Avenue, Suite 304, Westminister, CO 80234)
    - *Urinary Incontinence Handout Manual Step by Step*
  - Krames Communications (1100 Grundy Lane, San Bruno, CA 94066)
    - *Understanding Pelvic Organ Prolapse*

- Specific home program
  - Bladder diary
  - Bladder retraining
  - Techniques to defer urgency
  - Pelvic floor strengthening—tonic and phasic contractions
- Functional considerations
  - Use of pelvic brace with movements, transfers, lifting, and before activities of increased abdominal pressure—coughing, sneezing, and laughing
  - Proper voiding habits
  - Diaphragmatic breathing—avoiding valsalva

Direct Interventions

Treatment Phase: 5–12 Visits
- Therapeutic exercise
  - Aerobic endurance
  - Body mechanics and ergonomics avoiding valsalva
  - Breathing exercises: Diaphragmatic
  - Gait, locomotion, and balance training
  - Neuromuscular education or reeducation of pelvic floor—with or without biofeedback
  - Postural awareness training to decrease lordosis
  - Strengthening of pelvic floor
    - Active: With or without biofeedback
    - Assistive: Manual facilitation, overflow from associated muscles, electrical stimulation
    - Resistive: Vaginal weights
  - Stretching and strengthening of specific pelvic, hip, and trunk muscles
- Manual therapy techniques
  - Connective tissue massage: Internal vaginal or rectal myofascial release, external myofascial release, craniosacral, visceral mobilization
  - Joint mobilization and manipulation
  - Manual traction
  - Soft-tissue mobilization and manipulation: Muscle energy
  - Therapeutic massage
- Electrotherapeutic modalities
  - Biofeedback: EMG and pressure
  - Electrical muscle stimulation: Internal probe or surface electrodes
  - Neuromuscular electrical stimulation: Internal or surface
  - Transcutaneous electrical nerve stimulation

- Physical agents and mechanical modalities
  - Athermal modalities: Pulsed ultrasound
  - Cryotherapy
  - Deep thermal modalities
  - Hydrotherapy: Sitz bath
  - Superficial thermal modalities
  - Traction
  - Vaginal and rectal dilators
- Community training

Functional Carryover
- Instruction in progression for return to maximum vocational, recreational, and sports activities
- ADLs training while maintaining pelvic brace (pelvic floor contraction with abdominal contraction)
- Transitional movements without leakage

DISCHARGE PLANNING AND PATIENT RESPONSIBILITY

Criteria for Discharge
- Patient has reached all goals with exception of voiding schedule of every 3–4 hours but has understanding of progressing schedule independently
- Ability to use home unit for biofeedback or electrical stimulation

Circumstances Requiring Additional Visits
- Decreased pelvic floor contraction and incoordination of pelvic floor contraction/relaxation
- History of previous injury or surgery to related area

Home Program
- Aerobic conditioning
- Strengthening/relaxation of pelvic floor muscles
- Biofeedback or electrical stimulation as appropriate
- Strengthening and stretching of appropriate hip and abdominal muscles

Monitoring
- Instruct patient to call for advice should progression halt or a negative trend occur
- Patient to recheck/call at 2–4 weeks post-discharge to ensure progression toward achieving all rehab goals
- Schedule clinic visit as needed if symptoms return

REFERENCES

1. American Physical Therapy Association. *Guide to Physical Therapist Practice*. Alexandria, VA: APTA; 1997.

2. Baker PK. Musculoskeletal origins of chronic pelvic pain: diagnosis and treatment. *Obstet Gyn Clin North Am*. 1993;20:719-741.

3. Everett T, McIntosh J, Grant A. Ultrasound therapy for persistent post-natal perineal pain and dyspareunia. *Physiotherapy*. 1992;78(4):163-167.

4. Gourley Stevenson R, Shelly ER. Women's health. In: Wilder E, ed. *The Gynecological Manual*. American Physical Therapy Association: Alexandria, VA; 1997.

5. Gray H; Williams PL, ed. *Gray's Anatomy*. 38th ed. New York, NY: Churchill Livingstone; 1995.

6. Hart A, Hopkins C, Ford B. *ICD-9-CM Expert For Physicians, Volume 1&2*. 7th ed. USA: Ingenix; 2005.

7. Hartmann D. Vulvodynia: when making love hurts and physical therapy helps. *Adv Phys Therapists*. 1998;9(14):11-13.

8. Schussler B, Laycock J, Norton P. *Pelvic Floor Re-education: Principles and Practice*. New York, NY: Springer-Verlag; 1994.

POSTOP. REHAB. OF THE LUMBAR SPINE
SUMMARY OVERVIEW

ICD-9

722.80   722.83   737.12   737.22   V45.4

APTA Preferred Practice Pattern: **4B, 4G, 4H, 4J**

EXAMINATION

- History and Systems Review
- Tests and Measures
  Systems review per APTA's *Guide to Physical Therapy Practice*
  - Anthropometric characteristics
  - Gait, locomotion, and balance
  - Integumentary integrity
  - Joint integrity and mobility
  - Muscle performance
  - Pain
  - Posture
  - ROM
  - Reflex integrity
  - Sensory integrity
  - Special tests
- Establish Plan of Care

GOALS/OUTCOMES

- Patient displays understanding of proper posture and body mechanics
- Pain: 2/10 or less
- ROM
- Strength: 4/5 on manual muscle test for back extensors, gluteals, abdominals
- Functional lower-extremity ROM
- Avoidance of movements causing a reoccurence of symptoms
- Return to previous functional status for ADLs and vocational, recreational, and sports activities as identified by patient
- Independence in a progressive home exercise program emphasizing function

INTERVENTION
Number of Visits: 7–12

- Patient Instruction
  - Basic Anatomy and Biomechanics
  - Handouts
  - Functional Considerations
- Direct Interventions
  - Acute Phase: 3–6 Visits
  - Subacute Phase: 4–6 Visits
- Functional Carryover

DISCHARGE PLANNING AND PATIENT RESPONSIBILITY

- Criteria for Discharge
  - Patient is able to perform exercises in mechanically correct fashion and is compliant with exercise program as instructed
  - All goals/outcomes have been achieved with the possible exception of return to sport/recreational activities
  - Patient demonstrates proper body mechanics and understands their relation to daily activity
- Circumstances Requiring Additional Visits
  - Pain and/or muscle weakness that prohibits the patient from performing exercises and functional activities safely
  - Persistent functional motor performance deficit or 3/5 on manual muscle test
  - History of previous injury/surgery to related area
  - Persistent radicular symptoms or neurological deficit
  - Severe deconditioning
  - Special occupational needs requiring extensive fitness/strengthening
  - Instability at fracture/surgical site
  - Postoperative infection/complication
  - Severe postoperative scarring
  - Multiple fracture/injury sites
  - Arthritic conditions
  - Severe traumatic injury with persistent functional/occupational deficits
- Home Program
  - Flexibility exercises
  - Strengthening/stabilization exercises
  - Cardiovascular conditioning
  - Use of modalities for occasional flare-ups
- Monitoring

Summary Overview | Lumbar Spine | Postop. Rehab. Of The Lumbar Spine   255

POSTOP. REHAB. OF THE LUMBAR SPINE

ICD-9

722.80	Postlaminectomy syndrome, unspecified region
722.83	Postlaminectomy syndrome, lumbar region
737.12	Kyphosis, postlaminectomy
737.22	Other postsurgical lordosis
V45.4	Postprocedural arthrodesis status

APTA Preferred Practice Pattern: 4B, 4G, 4H, 4J

EXAMINATION

History and Systems Review

- History of current condition
  - Date of surgery
  - Mechanism of injury/onset
  - Date of injury/onset
  - Location, nature, and behavior of symptoms
    - Pre and post surgical
    - Radiating symptoms
    - Aggravating/relieving factors
    - a.m./p.m. changes
  - Obtain operative report if available
  - Presence of cauda equina symptoms
  - Postoperative rehabilitation and restrictions as outlined by physician
- Past history of current condition
  - History of injury prior to surgery
  - Hospitalization
  - Surgical intervention
  - Lower-extremity problems
  - Bracing injections, etc.
- Past medical/surgical history
  - Systemic pathology
    - Appendix
    - Abdominal
    - Pancreas
    - Large intestine
    - Kidney
    - Genital/urinary
      a. Bladder
      b. Ureter
      c. Prostate gland
      d. Cervix
      e. Uterus

- Functional status and activity level: current/prior
- Patient's functional goals

Tests and Measures

Systems review per APTA's *Guide to Physical Therapy Practice*

Testing will be dependent upon the acuteness of symptoms or precautions as identified by physician

- Anthropometric characteristics
  - Leg length discrepancy
    - Supine
    - Weight-bearing
- Gait, locomotion, and balance
  - Asymmetrical gait pattern
    - Arm swing
    - Hip transverse plane motion
    - Knee extension in stance phase
    - Knee flexion in swing phase
    - Early heel off
    - Excessive pronation
    - Lumbar-sacroiliac weight bearing: Mobility
    - Balance
  - Drop foot
    - Repeated calf raise unilaterally
    - Ability to raise up on tip toes
- Integumentary integrity
  - Observation/palpation of incision
  - Edema/tenderness
  - Integrity of scar tissue, fluid drainage
  - Skin/scar mobility
- Joint integrity and mobility
  - Stress tests (if appropriate given surgical procedure) It is recommended that stress tests be performed at those segments that are hypomobile or that the therapist intends to mobilize to end range (Grades III–V)
  - Palpation, including key landmarks

256   POSTOP REHAB OF THE LUMBAR SPINE | LUMBAR SPINE

- Central posterior to anterior glides (appropriate per symptoms/procedure)
  In prone position, with posterior to anterior pressure on spinous or transverse process
  - Flexion/extension
  - Side bend
  - Rotation
- Muscle performance
  - Resisted testing
  - Key muscle tests
  To determine possible palsy, utilize a combination of resistance and repetition
    - Hip flexion (L2)
    - Quadriceps (L3)
    - Tibialis anterior (L4)
    - Extensor hallicus longus (L5)
    - Peroneals (S1)
    - Gastrocnemius and hip extensors, S1–S2
    - Abdominals
    - Spinal extensors
    - Hip extensor
    - Inner unit
- Pain
  - Measured on visual analog scale
- Posture
  - Anterior, posterior, side
  - Bony landmarks
  - Scoliosis, sway back, flat back
  - Pelvic asymmetry
- ROM
  - Active
    - Flexion
    - Extension
    - Side bend
    - Rotation
  - Overpressure (passive)
- Reflex integrity
  - Reflex testing
    - Patellar tendon (L3)
    - Hamstring tendon (L5)
    - Achilles tendon (S1)
  - Rule out upper motor neuron lesion
    - Babinski
    - Clonus
- Sensory integrity
  - Sensation, L2–S2

- Special tests
  - Dural tension tests
  - Traction
  - Patrick/FABRE
    - Patient is supine in FABRE position
    - Inguinal pain implicates hip joint pathology or muscular restrictions
    - To stress the sacroiliac joint, place one hand on the flexed knee and the other on the opposite ASIS and press down

Establish Plan of Care
- Based on history, tests, and measures

GOALS/OUTCOMES
- Patient displays understanding of proper posture and body mechanics as evidenced by pain-free performance of ADLs and vocational activities
- Pain: 2/10 or less
- ROM
  - Hip ROM: Within normal limits when possible
  - Lumber ROM: restore maximum symptom-free motion, given surgical procedure, or achieve a minimum of 80% of AMA guides

	Normal	*80%*
Flexion	60°	50°
Extension	25°	20°
Side bend	25°	20°

- Strength: 4/5 on manual muscle test for back extensors, gluteals, abdominals
  - Abdominals
  - Spinal extensor
  - Gluteals
  - Inner unit (able to hold for 10 seconds for 10 repetitions)
  Or specific functional motor performance, such as
  - Squat to 90°
  - Retrieve object from floor
  - Perform work task (weight- and repetition-specific)

- Functional lower-extremity ROM:
  - Hip
    - Flexion: 125°
    - Extension: 0°
    - Internal rotation in neutral: 20°
    - External rotation in neutral: 30°
  - Knee
    - Flexion: 120°
    - Extension: 5°
  - Ankle
    - Dorsiflexion: 8° in subtalar neutral with knee extended
- Avoidance of movements causing a reoccurence of symptoms
- Return to previous functional status for ADLs and vocational, recreational, and sports activities as identified by patient
- Independence in a progressive home exercise program emphasizing function

INTERVENTION
NUMBER OF VISITS: 7–12

Coordination, Communication, and Documentation
- Provision of services between admission and discharge that facilitate cost-effective and efficient integration or reintegration to home, community, or work
- Documentation of therapeutic intervention is required for each episode of care and serves as the basic foundation for communication
- Coordination and additional communication will depend on the patient's impairment and home/work/ community/leisure situation and requirements. Such services may include:
  - Case management
  - Coordination of care and collaboration with those integral to the patient's rehabilitation program
  - Coordination and monitoring of the delivery of available resources
  - Referrals to other health-care professionals
  - Identification of resources, support groups, or advocacy services
  - Provision of educational or training information
  - Technical assistance

Patient Instruction

Basic Anatomy and Biomechanics
- Spinal musculature, ligaments, and disc anatomy
- Pertinent Gray's Anatomy (Gray. 1995. 510–516, 526–528, 534–537, 809–813, 819–827)
- Healing process post surgery

Handouts
- Postoperative restrictions
- Commercially available products, such as:
  - Krames Communications (1100 Grundy Lane, San Bruno, CA 94066)
    - *Lumbar Disc Surgery*
    - *Spine Surgery for Your Lower Back*
    - *The Post-Op Back Book*
- Specific home program

Functional Considerations
- Review of body mechanics and posture to minimize spinal stress
- Avoidance of activities or positions that cause pain
- Maintain normal and pain-free spinal curves during
  - Sitting/driving
  - Sleeping
  - Walking
  - Recreational activities

Direct Interventions
Therapist should consult referring physician regarding precautions/progression given the specific procedure performed.

Acute Phase: 3–6 Visits
- Therapeutic exercise and home program
  - Stretching within pain-free range
    - Knee to chest
    - Piriformis
    - Straight-leg raise to stretch hamstring
      a. Maintain sciatic nerve mobility
    - External rotators of the hip
    - Pelvic movement (cat/camel)
    - Press-up if appropriate
    - Quadriceps
    - Iliopsoas
    - Iliotibial band

258   PostOp Rehab of the Lumbar Spine | Lumbar Spine

- Posture
  - Pelvic stabilization
  - Proper pelvic positions
- Strength
  - Abdominal/extensor stabilization
    a. Supine
    b. Hooklying/bridging
    c. Modified plantigrade
    d. Quadruped
  - Lower-extremity strengthening with bracing
- Cardiovascular conditioning
  - Upper body ergometer
  - Progressive walking
- Transversus abdominis and multifidus training
- Manual therapy techniques
  - Soft-tissue techniques—use patient tolerance as guide over surgical site
  - Joint mobilization
    - Grades I–II distraction for pain relief at surgical site
      a. Exception: spinal fusion
    - Grades I–V as appropriate for specific spinal hypomobilities above and below surgical site
    - Hip mobilization as indicated
  - Positional isometric exercises for pain reduction and initiation of stabilization
  - Graded neural tension maneuvers as tolerated
- Electrotherapeutic modalities
- Physical agents and mechanical modalities
  - Cryotherapy/superficial thermal modalities
  - Ultrasound
- Goals/outcomes
  - Lumbar AROM: 60% of AMA guides
    - Flexion: 35°
    - Extension: 15°
    - Side bend: 15°
  - Pain: 2/10 at rest; 4/10 with activity
  - Pain-free ambulation for 10 minutes on a level surface
  - Voluntary abdominal control (neutral spine) in supine, sitting, and standing
  - Alleviate radicular symptoms

Subacute Phase: 4–6 Visits
- Therapeutic exercise and home program
  - Flexibility
    - Straight-leg raises to restore hamstring and sciatic nerve mobility

- Restore extension range
  a. Press-up
  b. Static press-up
  c. Mobilization press-up
- Rotation
- Lower trunk rotation
- Rising sun
  Begin right side-lying with both shoulders flexed to 90°, left hip and knee flexed to 90°, right hip and knee extended, horizontally abduct the left arm, rotating the trunk to the left. Do not allow the left knee to leave the surface. Maintain the stretch for 10 breaths. Repeat to the opposite side
- Flexion
- Strength
  - Lumbar stabilization exercises
    a. Curl-up progression to leg lifts
    b. Continued progression of transversus abdominus and multifidus training
  - Beginning rotation
  - Beginning side bend
  - Lower extremities
  - Lumbar extensors (prone back extension)
  - Progressive strengthening
    a. Manually resisted intensive back program (Brown, 1970)
    b. Weight machines
  - Closed-kinetic chain
    a. Squats
    b. Multidirectional lunges
    c. Balance/reach
  - Therapeutic ball
- Neuromuscular/balance/proprioceptive reeducation
  - Quadruped opposite arm/leg lift
  - Modified plantigrade opposite arm/leg lift
  - Unilateral stance balancing, reaching one or both arms in various directions to maximum distance, avoiding use of other leg for counterbalance
    a. Anterior reach: Stimulates hamstrings, soleus, gastrocnemius, and hip/back extensors (depending on height of reach)
    b. Posterior overhead reach: Stimulates abdominals
    c. Lateral rotational reach: Stimulates hip abductors and lateral trunk stabilizers

- Unilateral stance balancing, reaching opposite leg in various directions to maximum distance
    a. Anterior reach: Stimulates quadriceps, soleus
    b. Posterior reach: Stimulates gluteals, quadriceps, hip/back extensors
    c. Rotational reach to side: Stimulates gluteals, quadriceps, trunk stabilizers, hip abductors, abdominals
  - Cardiovascular conditioning
    - Treadmill/walking program
    - Upper or lower-extremity cycling
    - Stair machine
    - Ski machine
    - Swimming/aquatic therapy
  - Work simulation/conditioning
  - Exercise oriented toward specific postural dysfunction/limitations
    - Lordotic back
      a. Strengthen abdominals to control pelvic positioning
      b. Stretch lumbar extensors and hip flexors
      c. Mobilize hip into extension
    - Flat back
      a. Strengthen lumbar and hip extensors
      b. Stretch abdominal and hip musculature as necessary
      c. Mobilize lumbar spine into extension
    - Hypermobile back or segment
      a. Strengthen trunk musculature within controlled ROM to promote spinal stabilization
      b. Stretch musculature as necessary
      c. Mobilize hypomobilities above and below
    - Deconditioned back
      a. Cardiovascular conditioning
      b. Motor performance/stabilization
      c. Flexibility
- Manual therapy techniques
  - Soft-tissue techniques
    - Soft-tissue mobilization
    - Contract/hold relax
    - Trigger-point techniques
    - Strain/counterstrain
    - Myofascial release
    - Friction massage

- Joint mobilization
    - Progress grade of mobilization to specific hypomobilities as indicated
      a. Lumbar spine
      b. Thoracic spine
      c. Hip
  - Neural tension stretches
- Physical agents and mechanical modalities
  - Continue effective modalities as in Acute Phase, with increased emphasis on use as needed at home
- Goals/outcomes
  - Lumbar AROM: restore maximum symptom-free motion given surgical procedure or achieve a minimum of 80% of AMA guides
  - Attain functional lower-extremity ROM
  - Pain: 2/10 or less with activity, 0/10 during rest in all positions
  - Strength: 4/5 on manual muscle test for abdominals, spinal extensors, and rotators, or achieve a predetermined functional motor performance parameter
  - Achieve pain-free activity when using proper body mechanics

Functional Carryover

- Incorporation of bracing/stabilization into ADLs and vocational activities
- Importance of utilizing proper body mechanics to avoid aggravation of condition
- Ergonomic modification of work site including chair, desk height, or computer placement

DISCHARGE PLANNING AND PATIENT RESPONSIBILITY

Criteria for Discharge

- Patient is able to perform exercises in mechanically correct fashion and is compliant with exercise program as instructed
- All goals/outcomes have been achieved with the possible exception of return to sport/recreational activities
- Patient demonstrates proper body mechanics and understands their relation to daily activity

Circumstances Requiring Additional Visits

- Pain and/or muscle weakness that prohibits the patient from performing exercises and functional activities safely
- Persistent functional motor performance deficit or 3/5 on manual muscle test
- History of previous injury/surgery to related area
- Persistent radicular symptoms or neurological deficit
- Severe deconditioning
- Special occupational needs requiring extensive fitness/strengthening
- Instability at fracture/surgical site
- Postoperative infection/complication
- Severe postoperative scarring
- Multiple fracture/injury sites
- Arthritic conditions
- Severe traumatic injury with persistent functional/occupational deficits

Home Program

- Flexibility exercises
  - Hip flexors/extensors
  - Spinal extensors
  - Knee flexors/extensors
  - Gastrocnemius/soleus
- Strengthening/stabilization exercises
  - Therapeutic ball progression
  - Closed-kinetic chain
  - Health club
- Cardiovascular conditioning
- Use of modalities for occasional flare-ups

Monitoring

- Instruct patient to call for advice should progression halt or a negative trend occur
- Patient is to recheck/call at 2–4 weeks post-discharge to ensure progression toward return to previous functional status
- Schedule follow-up visit as needed if symptoms persist or patient is unable to resume previous activity level

REFERENCES

1. American Physical Therapy Association. *Guide to Physical Therapist Practice.* Alexandria, VA: APTA; 1997.
2. Atlas SJ, Deyo RA, Keller RB, et al. The Maine lumbar spine study, part III: 1-year outcomes of surgical and nonsurgical management of lumbar spinal stenosis. *Spine.* 1996;21:1787-1795.
3. Brown I. Intensive exercise for the low back. *J Am Phys Ther Assoc.* 1970;50(4):487-498.
4. Connolly PJ, Grob D. Bracing of patients after fusion for degenerative problems of the lumbar spine—yes or no? *Spine.* 1998;23:1426-1428.
5. Deen HG, Zimmerman RS, Lyons MK, et al. Use of the exercise treadmill to measure baseline functional status and surgical outcome in patients with severe lumbar spinal stenosis. *Spine.* 1998;23:244-248.
6. Ferreira PH, Ferreira ML, Hodges PW. Changes in recruitment of the abdominal muscles in people with low back pain: ultrasound measurement of muscle activity. *Spine;* 2004;29:2560-6.
7. Gluck NI. Passive care and active rehabilitation in a patient with failed back surgery syndrome. *J Manipulative Physiol Ther.* 1996;19:41-47.
8. Gray H; Williams PL, ed. *Gray's Anatomy.* 38th ed. New York, NY: Churchill Livingstone; 1995.
9. Hart A, Hopkins C, Ford B. *ICD-9-CM Expert For Physicians, Volume 1&2.* 7th ed. USA: Ingenix; 2005.
10. Herno A, Airaksinen O, Sarri T. Long-term results of surgical treatment of lumbar spinal stenosis. *Spine.* 1993;18:1471-1474.
11. Hides J, Wilson S, Stanton W, et al. An MRI investigation into the function of the transversus abdominis muscle during "drawing-in" of the abdominal wall. *Spine* 2006; 31:175-8.
12. Hodges PW, Richardson CA. Altered trunk recruitment in people with low back pain with upper limb movement at different speeds. *Arch Phys Med Rehabil.* 1999;80:1005-12.
13. Hu RW, Jaglal S, Axcell T, Anderson G. A population based study of reoperations after back surgery. *Spine.* 1997;22:2265-2270.
14. Katz JN, Lipson SJ, Chang LC, et al. Seven-to-10-year outcome of decompressive surgery for degenerative lumbar spinal stenosis. *Spine.* 1996;21:92-98.
15. Kuslich SD, Ulstrom CL, Griffith SL, Ahern JW, Dowdle JD. The Bagby and Kuslich method of lumbar interbody fusion: history, techniques, and 2-year

follow-up results of a united states prospective, multicenter trial. *Spine.* 1998;23:1267-1278.

16. Manniche C. Assessment and exercise in low back pain: with special reference to the management of pain and disability following first time lumbar disc surgery. *Dan Med Bull.* 1995;42:301-313.

17. Manniche C, Skall HF, Braendholt L, et al. Clinical trial of postoperative dynamic back exercises after first lumbar discectomy. *Spine.* 1993;18:92-97.

18. Manniche C, Asmussen K, Lauritsen B, et al. Intensive dynamic back exercises with or without hyperextension in chronic back pain after surgery for lumbar disc protrusion: a clinical trial. *Spine.* 1993;18:560-567.

19. Moseley GL, Hodges PW, Gandevia SC. Deep and superficial fibers of the lumbar multifidus muscle are differentially active during voluntary arm movements. *Spine.* 2002; 27: 29-36.

20. Richardson CA, Snijders CJ, Hides JA, et al. The relation between the transversus abdominis muscles, sacroiliac joint mechanics, and low back pain. *Spine.* 2002;27:399-405.

21. Slotman GJ, Stein SC. Laminectomy compared with laparoscopic discectomy and outpatient laparoscopic discectomy for herniated L5-S1 intervertebral disks. *J Laparoendosc Adv Surg Technol A.* 1998;8:261-267.

22. Timm KE. A randomized-control study of active and passive treatments for chronic low back pain following L5 laminectomy. *J Orthop Sports Med.* 1994;20:276-286.

23. Urquhart DM, Hodges PW. Differential activity of regions of the transversus abdominis during trunk rotation. *Eur Spine J.* 2005;14:393-400.

24. Waddell G, Reilly S, Torsney B, et al. Assessment of the outcome of low back surgery. *J Bone Joint Surg.* 1988;70:723-727.

25. Weiner BK, Fraser RD. Spine update: lumbar interbody cages. *Spine.* 1998;23:634-640.

26. Zdelblick TA. A prospective, randomized study of lumbar fusion: preliminary results. *Spine.* 1993;18:983-991.

27. Zindrick MR. The role of transpedicular fixation systems for stabilization of the lumbar spine. *Orthop Clin North Am.* 1991;22:333-344.

POSTURAL DYSFUNCTION
SUMMARY OVERVIEW

ICD-9

524.9   723.1   724.1   724.2   729.1   840.8

APTA Preferred Practice Pattern: 4B, 4C, 4D, 4E, 4F, 4G, 4J

EXAMINATION

- History and Systems Review
- Tests and Measures
  Systems review per APTA's *Guide to Physical Therapy Practice*
  - Anthropometric characteristics
  - Gait, locomotion, and balance
  - Joint integrity and mobility
  - Muscle performance
  - Pain
  - Postural assessment
  - ROM
  - Reflex integrity
  - Sensory integrity
  - Special tests
- Establish Plan of Care

GOALS/OUTCOMES

- Patient displays understanding of proper posture and body mechanics
- Pain: 2/10 or less
- Pain-free spinal ROM: A minimum of 80% of AMA guides
- Strength: 4/5 on manual muscle test for back extensors, gluteals, abdominals, inner unit, or specific functional strength
- Functional upper- and lower-extremity ROM
- Avoidance of movements causing a reoccurrence of symptoms
- Return to previous functional status for ADLs and vocational, recreational, and sports activities as identified by patient
- Independence in a progressive home exercise program emphasizing function

INTERVENTION
NUMBER OF VISITS: 5–11

- Patient Instruction
  - Basic Anatomy and Biomechanics
  - Handouts
  - Functional Considerations
- Direct Interventions
  - Acute Phase: 2–6 Visits
  - Subacute Phase: 3–5 Visits
- Functional Carryover

DISCHARGE PLANNING AND PATIENT RESPONSIBILITY

- Criteria for Discharge
  - Patient understands the importance of and implements stress management and relaxation techniques
  - Patient understands the need for regular stretching/strengthening exercises to combat negative effects of specific daily postures
  - Cardiovascular conditioning: Preferably 3 times per week for a minimum of 20 minutes
  - All goals/outcomes have been achieved
- Circumstances Requiring Additional Visits
  - Persistent functional strength deficit or 3/5 on manual muscle test
  - History of previous injury/surgery to related area
  - Severe deconditioning
  - Special occupational needs requiring extensive fitness/strengthening
  - Spinal instability
- Home Program
  - Aware of proper postures and 30 minute reminders to change habits
  - Stretching/strengthening exercises for maintenance of postural balance
  - Cardiovascular conditioning
  - Proper body mechanics and posturing specific activities
- Monitoring

SUMMARY OVERVIEW | LUMBAR SPINE | POSTURAL DYSFUNCTION   263

POSTURAL DYSFUNCTION

ICD-9

524.9	Unspecified dentofacial anomalies
723.1	Cervicalgia
724.1	Pain in thoracic spine
724.2	Lumbago
729.1	Myalgia and myositis, unspecified
840.8	Sprain of other specified sites of shoulder and upper arm

APTA Preferred Practice Pattern: 4B, 4C, 4D, 4E, 4F, 4G, 4J

EXAMINATION

History and Systems Review

- History of current conditions
  - Mechanics of injury/onset
  - Date of injury/onset
  - Other postural problems
  - Location, nature, and behavior of symptoms
    - Radiating symptoms
    - Aggravating/relieving factors
    - a.m./p.m.
  - Presence of cauda equina symptoms
- Past history of current condition
  - Hospitalization
  - Surgical intervention
  - Lower-extremity problems
  - Bracing, injections, etc.
  - Cervical
  - Thoracic
  - Lumbar
  - Lower extremity
  - Pregnancy/childbirth
    - C-section
- Past medical/surgical history
  - Systemic pathology
    - Appendix
    - Abdominal
    - Pancreas
    - Large intestine
    - Kidney
    - Genital/urinary
      a. Bladder
      b. Ureter
      c. Prostate gland
      d. Cervix
      e. Uterus

- Health status
  - Change in work position/posture
  - Recent weight gain
- Functional status and activity level: current/prior
  - Exercise habits
  - Hobbies
- Patient's functional goals

Tests and Measures

Systems review per APTA's *Guide to Physical Therapy Practice*

- Anthropometric characteristics
  - Leg length discrepancy
    - Supine
    - Weight-bearing
- Gait, locomotion, and balance
- Joint integrity and mobility
  - Central posterior to anterior glides
    In prone position, with posterior to anterior pressure on spinous or transverse processes
  - Flexion/extension
  - Side bend
  - Rotation
  - Stress tests
    It is recommended that stress tests be performed at those segments that are hypomobile or that the therapist intends to mobilize to end range (Grades III–V)
  - Passive intervertebral motion T10–S1
  - Palpation, including key landmarks
- Muscle performance
  - Key muscle tests
    To determine possible palsy, utilize a combination of resistance and repetition
    - Hip flexion (L2)
    - Quadriceps (L3)

264 POSTURAL DYSFUNCTION | LUMBAR SPINE

- Tibialis Anterior (L4)
- Extensor Hallicus Longus (L5)
- Peroneals (S1)
- Gastrocnemius (S1)
  - Abdominals
  - Spinal extensors
  - Hip extensor
  - Inner unit
  - Soft-tissue observation
    - Atrophy
    - Hypertrophy
    - Spasm
- Pain
  - Measured on visual analog scale
- Postural assessment
  - Anterior, posterior, side
  - Bony landmarks
  - Scoliosis, sway back, flat back
  - Thoracic curvature
  - Pelvic asymmetry
  - Relaxed calcaneal posture
  - Sitting
  - Lying
- ROM
  - Active lumbar
    - Flexion
    - Extension
    - Side bend
  - Hip flexion
  - Hip internal/external rotation
- Reflex integrity
  - Reflex testing
    - Patellar tendon (L3)
    - Achilles tendon (S1)
  - Rule out upper motor neuron lesion
    - Clonus
    - Babinski
- Sensory integrity
  - Sensory assessment (T12–S2)
- Special tests
  - Compression overload
    - In supine position with hips and knees flexed to end range
    - Apply overpressure to lower extremities in superior direction

- Patrick/FABRE
  - Patient is supine in FABRE position
  - Inguinal pain implicates hip joint pathology or muscular restrictions
  - To stress the sacroiliac joint, place one hand on the flexed knee and the other on the opposite ASIS and press down
  - Dural tension tests (see description under "Special Tests" in *Low Back General Pain* guideline)
  - Grind test
  - Standing sacroiliac test
  - Thomas test

Establish Plan of Care
- Based on history, tests, and measures

GOALS/OUTCOMES
- Patient displays understanding of proper posture and body mechanics as evidenced by pain-free performance of ADLs and vocational activities
- Pain: 2/10 or less
- Pain-free spinal ROM: A minimum of 80% of AMA guides

Cervical	Normal	80%
Flexion	60°	50°
Extension	75°	60°
Rotation	80°	65°
Side bend	45°	35°

Lumbar	Normal	80%
Flexion	60°	50°
Extension	25°	20°
Side bend	45°	35°

Thoracic	Normal	80%
Flexion	40°	30°
Extension	No AMA guides established	
Rotation	30°	25°
Side bend	10°	8°

- Strength: 4/5 on manual muscle test for back extensors, gluteals, abdominals, inner unit, or specific functional strength
  - Squat to 90°
  - Retrieve object from floor
  - Perform work task (weight and repetition-specific)

- Functional upper and lower-extremity ROM:
  - Hip
    - Flexion: 125°
    - Extension: 0°
  - Shoulder
    - Flexion: 160°
    - External Rotation: 60°
  - Foot/Ankle
    - Dorsiflexion: 8° in subtalar neutral with knee extended
- Avoidance of movements causing a reoccurrence of symptoms
- Return to previous functional status for ADLs and vocational, recreational, and sports activities as identified by patient
- Independence in a progressive home exercise program emphasizing function

INTERVENTION
NUMBER OF VISITS: 5–11

Coordination, Communication, and Documentation

- Provision of services between admission and discharge that facilitate cost-effective and efficient integration or reintegration to home, community, or work
- Documentation of therapeutic intervention is required for each episode of care and serves as the basic foundation for communication
- Coordination and additional communication will depend on the patient's impairment and home/work/community/leisure situation and requirements. Such services may include:
  - Case management
  - Coordination of care and collaboration with those integral to the patient's rehabilitation program
  - Coordination and monitoring of the delivery of available resources
  - Referrals to other health-care professionals
  - Identification of resources, support groups, or advocacy services
  - Provision of educational or training information
  - Technical assistance

Patient Instruction

Basic Anatomy and Biomechanics
- Anatomical review for appropriate body regions
- Importance of proper posture and biomechanics in the reduction of spinal pain
- Integration of proper upper and lower quarter alignment in the promotion of proper posture throughout the kinetic chain

Handouts
- Commercially available products, such as:
  - Iglarsh et al, 111 N. Fairfax, Alexandria, VA 22314-1488, *The Secret of Good Posture*
  - Krames Communications (1100 Grundy Lane, San Bruno, CA 94066)
    - *Poor Posture Hurts*
    - *Back Tips for People Who Sit*
- Specific home program

Functional Considerations
- Review movement patterns and postures contributing to malalignment, such as chronic forward head with repetitive trunk flexion
- Instruct in proper body mechanics and movement patterns

Direct Interventions

Acute Phase: 2–6 Visits
- Therapeutic exercise and home program
  - Self-mobilization
  - Cervical and shoulder retraction maintaining normal cervical curvature
    - Emphasis on C6–T2
    - Craniovertebral flexion
  - Upper back strengthening
    - Latissimus dorsi
    - Rhomboids
    - Mid and lower trapezius
  - Stretching to appropriate muscle groups indicated above
  - Cardiovascular conditioning
    - Emphasis on pain-free, upright posture
  - Diaphragmatic breathing
    - Relaxation of upper rib cage and cervical musculature

266   POSTURAL DYSFUNCTION | LUMBAR SPINE

- Lumbar stabilization exercises as appropriate
  - Down train global muscles
  - Up train the inner unit
- Pelvic clock exercises to establish position of comfort
  - Pelvic tilt
- Manual therapy techniques
  - Soft-tissue techniques
    - Soft-tissue mobilization
    - Trigger-point techniques
    - Strain/counterstrain
    - Myofascial release
    - Manual traction
    - Muscle energy techniques
  - Joint mobilization
    - Grades I–V manipulations for hypomobilities
  - Assisted passive stretching as appropriate
    - Pectoralis
    - Latissimus dorsi
    - Spinal extensors
    - Suboccipitals
    - Hamstrings
    - Hip flexors
    - Quadriceps
    - Gastrocnemius
    - Soleus
- Electrotherapeutic modalities
- Physical agents and mechanical modalities
  - Cryotherapy/thermal modalities
  - Ultrasound
- Goals/outcomes
  - Pain: 5/10 or less
  - Exercises performed with proper body alignment and in pain-free range
  - Patient understands and can follow through with altering poor postures and body mechanics contributing to pain
  - Strength: 3+/5 for abdominals and spinal extensors
  - Initiate cardiovascular conditioning without exacerbation of symptoms

Subacute Phase: 3–5 Visits
- Therapeutic exercise and home program
  - Cardiovascular conditioning
    - Treadmill/walking program
    - Upper or lower-extremity cycling

- Ski machine
- Stair machine
- Swimming/aquatic therapy
  - Neuromuscular/balance/proprioceptive reeducation
    - Quadriped opposite arm/leg lift
    - Unilateral stance balancing, reaching one or both arms in various directions to maximum distance, avoiding use of other leg for counterbalance
      a. Anterior reach: Stimulates hamstrings, soleus, gastrocnemius, and hip/back extensors (depending on height of reach)
      b. Posterior overhead reach: Stimulates abdominals
      c. Lateral rotational reach: Stimulates hip abductors and lateral trunk stabilizers
    - Unilateral stance balancing, reaching opposite leg in various directions to maximum distance
      a. Anterior reach: Stimulates quadriceps, soleus
      b. Posterior reach: Stimulates gluteals, quadriceps, hip/back extensors
      c. Rotational reach to side: Stimulates gluteals, quadriceps, trunk stabilizers, hip abductors, abdominals
  - Progress strengthening with increased repetitions and weight
    - Squats
    - Multidirectional lunges
    - Pulley, resistive band, or free-weight resisted scapular retraction
    - Therapeutic ball activities
      a. Abdominals
      b. Spinal extensors
      c. Hip musculature
      d. Scapular retractors/depressors
    - Abdominals
      a. Supine
      b. Standing
    - Spinal extensors
  - Progress stretching techniques to areas of continued tightness
  - Relaxation techniques (for further information, see *Stress Management* guideline)
    - Diaphragmatic breathing
    - Contract/relax
    - Visualization/guided imagery
    - Relaxation tapes

LUMBAR SPINE | POSTURAL DYSFUNCTION   267

- Manual therapy techniques
  - Continue effective soft-tissue techniques
  - Progress assisted stretching
  - Joint mobilization
    - Continue Grades III–V to specific hypomobilities
    - Specifically address atlanto/occipital joint, C6–T4 and T10–L1
  - Proprioceptive neuromuscular facilitation techniques
- Physical agents and mechanical modalities
  Continue effective modalities as in Acute Phase with increased emphasis on use as needed at home
- Goals/outcomes
  - Pain: 2/10 or less
  - Establish a cardiovascular conditioning program 3 times weekly for a minimum of 20 minutes per session
  - Patient able to recognize and avoid postures that have been determined to aggravate/promote symptoms
  - Functional ROM to perform ADLs and recreational activities safely
  - Strength: 4/5 on manual muscle test for abdominals, hip/spinal extensors, and scapular retractors, or achieve a predetermined functional motor performance measure

Functional Carryover

- Patient is aware of the importance of:
  - A firm mattress
  - Support to the cervical and lumbar lordosis
  - Good shoes for providing support and improving general biomechanical alignment
  - Utilization of a supportive chair
  - Ergonomic relationship in the work environment
  - Proper lifting techniques
- Refer patient to physician or nutritionist for consultation for weight management if appropriate
- Ergonomic modification of home and work site as indicated

DISCHARGE PLANNING AND PATIENT RESPONSIBILITY

Criteria for Discharge

- Patient understands the importance of and implements stress management and relaxation techniques
- Patient understands the need for regular stretching/strengthening exercises to combat negative effects of specific daily postures
- Cardiovascular conditioning: Preferably 3 times per week for a minimum of 20 minutes
- All goals/outcomes have been achieved

Circumstances Requiring Additional Visits

- Persistent functional strength deficit or 3/5 on manual muscle test
- History of previous injury/surgery to related area
- Severe deconditioning
- Special occupational needs requiring extensive fitness/strengthening
- Spinal instability

Home Program

- Aware of proper postures and 30-minute reminders to change habits
- Stretching/strengthening exercises for maintenance of postural balance
- Cardiovascular conditioning
- Proper body mechanics and posturing specific activities, such as:
  - Sitting at a computer
  - Lifting
  - Reading

Monitoring

- Instruct patient to call for advice should progression halt or a negative trend occur
- Patient is to phone at 2–4 weeks post-discharge to report progress and address any residual symptoms or difficulty with the home program, with clinic follow-up visit if needed
- Schedule clinic follow-up at 3 months to ensure maintenance of postural balance and progress home program

REFERENCES

1. Alexander KM, LaPier TL. Differences in static balance and weight distribution between normal subjects and subjects with chronic unilateral low back pain. *J Orthop Sports Phys Ther.* 1998;28(6):378-383.

2. American Physical Therapy Association. *Guide to Physical Therapist Practice.* Alexandria, VA: APTA; 1997.

3. Beling J, Wolfe GA, Allen KA, Boyle JM. Lower extremity preference during gross and fine motor skills performed in sitting and standing postures. *J Orthop Sports Phys Ther.* 1998;28(6):400-404.

4. Dettori JR, Bullock SH, Sutlive TG, Franklin RJ, Patience T. The effects of spinal flexion and extension exercises and their associated postures in patients with acute low back pain. *Spine.* 1995;20:2303-2312.

5. Dolan KJ, Green A. Lumbar spine reposition sense: the effect of a "slouched" posture. *Man Ther.* 2006; 11(3):202-7.

6. Gray, H; Williams PL, ed. *Gray's Anatomy.* 38th ed. New York, NY: Churchill Livingstone; 1995.

7. Grieve G. *Modern Manual Therapy of The Vertebral Column.* New York, NY: Churchill Livingstone; 1986:504, 555, 592, 641, 701, 706.

8. Hart A, Hopkins C, Ford B. *ICD-9-CM Expert For Physicians, Volume 1&2.* 7th ed. USA: Ingenix; 2005.

9. Heino JG, Godges JJ, Carter CL. Relationship between hip extension ROM and postural alignment. *J Orthop Sports Phys Ther.* 1990;12(6):243-247.

10. Iglarsh A, Kendall F, Lewis C, Sahrmann S. *The Secret of Good Posture.* Alexandria, VA: American Physical Therapy Association; 1985.

11. Itoi E, Sinaki M. Effect of back strengthening exercise on posture in healthy women 49 to 65 years of age. *Mayo Clin Proc.* 1994;69:1054-1059.

12. Lee D. *The Pelvic Girdle.* New York, NY: Churchill Livingstone; 1999:81-143.

13. Levine D, Whittle MW. The effects of pelvic movement on lumbar lordosis in the standing position. *J Orthop Sports Phys Ther.* 1996;24(3):130-135.

14. Popa T, Bonfifazi M, Della Volpe R, Rossi A, Mazzocchio R. Adaptive changes in postural strategy selection in chronic low back pain. *Exp Brain Res.* September 15, 2006.

15. Richardson C, Jull G, Hodges P, Hide S. *Therapeutic Exercises For Spinal Segmental Stabilization In Low Back Pain.* New York, NY: Churchill Livingstone; 1999.

16. Riegger-Krugh C, Keysor JJ. Skeletal malalignments of the lower quarter: correlated and compensatory motions and postures. *J Orthop Sports Phys Ther.* 1996;23(2):164-170.

17. Sparto PJ, Parnianpour M, Reinsel TE, Simon S. The effect of fatigue on multijoint kinematics, coordination, and postural stability during a repetitive lifting test. *J Orthop Sports Phys Ther.* 1997;25(1):3-12.

18. Vleeming A, Mooney V, Dorman T, Snyders C, Stoeckart R. *Movement, Stability and Low Back Pain.* New York, NY: Churchill Livingstone; 1997.

SACROILIAC DYSFUNCTION
SUMMARY OVERVIEW

ICD-9

719.45   724.6   739.4   846.1   846.8   846.9   847.3   847.9

APTA Preferred Practice Pattern: 4B, 4C, 4E, 4F, 4G, 4J, 7A

EXAMINATION

- History and Systems Review
- Tests and Measures
  Systems review per APTA's *Guide to Physical Therapy Practice*
  - Anthropometric characteristics
  - Gait, locomotion, and balance
  - Joint integrity and mobility
  - Muscle performance
  - Pain
  - Posture
  - ROM
  - Reflex integrity
  - Sensory integrity
  - Special tests
- Establish Plan of Care

GOALS/OUTCOMES

- Patient displays understanding of proper posture and body mechanics
- Pain-free lumbar ROM: A minimum of 80% of AMA guides
- Pain: 2/10 or less
- Strength: 4/5 on manual muscle test for back extensors, gluteals, abdominals
- Functional AROM
- Restore pelvic and leg length symmetry if mechanical
- Avoidance of movements causing a reoccurence of symptoms
- Return to previous functional status for ADLs and vocational, recreational, and sports activities as identified by patient
- Independence in a progressive home exercise program emphasizing function

INTERVENTION
NUMBER OF VISITS: 5–12

- Patient Instruction
  - Basic Anatomy and Biomechanics
  - Handouts
  - Functional Considerations

- Direct Interventions
  - Acute Phase: 3–6 Visits
  - Subacute Phase: 2–6 Visits
- Functional Carryover

DISCHARGE PLANNING AND PATIENT RESPONSIBILITY

- Criteria for Discharge
  - All goals/outcomes have been met with the exception of return to previous status for recreational and sports activities
  - Patient has initiated return to recreation and sports activities
  - Patient demonstrates competency in use of proper posture and body mechanics and in display of home exercise program
- Circumstances Requiring Additional Visits
  - Persistent functional strength deficit or 3/5 on manual muscle test
  - History of previous injury/surgery to related area
  - Severe deconditioning
  - Special occupational needs requiring extensive fitness/strengthening
  - Multiple injury sites including lower extremity
  - Severe traumatic injury with persistent functional/occupational deficits
  - Spinal instability
  - Biomechanical lower-extremity dysfunction
- Home Program
  - Closed-kinetic chain strengthening for lower extremity
  - Abdominal strengthening
  - Flexibility
  - Self-mobilization/muscle energy techniques for maintenance of pelvic symmetry
  - Utilization of immobilization belt as needed
- Monitoring

SUMMARY OVERVIEW | LUMBAR SPINE | SACROILIAC DYSFUNCTION   271

SACROILIAC DYSFUNCTION

ICD-9

719.45	Pain in joint, pelvic region and thigh
724.6	Disorders of sacrum
739.4	Nonallopathic lesions, not elsewhere classified, sacral region
846.1	Sacroiliac ligament sprain
846.8	Sprain of other specified sites of sacroiliac region
846.9	Sprain of unspecified site of sacroiliac region
847.3	Sprain of sacrum
847.9	Sprain of unspecified site of back

APTA Preferred Practice Pattern: 4B, 4C, 4E, 4F, 4G, 4J, 7A

EXAMINATION

History and Systems Review

- History of current condition
  - Mechanism of injury/onset
  - Date of injury/onset
  - Location, nature, and behavior of symptoms
    - Radiating symptoms
    - Aggravating/relieving factors
  - Presence of cauda equina symptoms
- Past history of current condition
  - Hospitalization
  - Surgical intervention
  - Lower-extremity problems
  - Bracing, injections, etc.
  - History of lower-extremity dysfunction
  - Pregnancy/childbirth
    - C-section
- Medications
- Past medical/surgical history
  - Systemic pathology
    - Appendix
    - Abdominal
    - Pancreas
    - Large intestine
    - Kidney
    - Genital/urinary
      a. Bladder
      b. Ureter
      c. Prostate gland
      d. Cervix
      e. Uterus
    - Iritis
    - Cardiac

- Respiratory
- Central nervous system disorders
- Psoriasis
- Irritable bowel symptoms
- Functional status and activity level (current/prior)
- Patient's functional goals

Tests and Measures

Systems review per APTA's *Guide to Physical Therapy Practice*

- Anthropometric characteristics
  - Leg length discrepancy
    - Supine
    - Weight-bearing: There should be consistency between weight-bearing and non-weight-bearing sacroiliac ROM tests if a hypomobility is present. Inconsistency suggests a hypermobility/instability
- Gait, locomotion, and balance
  - Asymmetrical gait pattern
    - Arm swing
    - Hip transverse plane motion
    - Knee extension in stance phase
    - Knee flexion in swing phase
    - Early heel off
    - Excessive pronation
    - Lumbar/sacroiliac weight-bearing mobility
  - Balance
  - Stereotypic postural movements
- Joint integrity and mobility
  - Palpation, including key landmarks
    - Iliac crests
    - ASIS
    - PSIS
      a. Point tenderness

272 SACROILIAC DYSFUNCTION | LUMBAR SPINE

- Ischial tuberosity
- Sacral sulcus
- Inferior lateral angle of sacrum
- Pubic symphysis
- L5 spinous process and transverse processes
- Sacrotuberous ligament
  - AROM—supine
    - Supine to long-sit
  - AROM—prone
    - Knee flexion test (iliosacral)
    - Press-up (sacroilial) extension
    - Kneeling, buttocks on heels (sacroilial) flexion
  - Passive intervertebral motion, T10–S1
  - Stress test hypermobile segments
  - Passive sacroiliac stress tests
    - Anterior gapping
    - Posterior gapping
    - Rotary
    - Distraction
  - Supine—knee flex and palpate L5 Sacrum
  - Standing muscle test (Gillet)
- Muscle performance
  - Resisted testing
  - Key muscle tests
  To determine possible palsy, utilize a combination of resistance and repetition
    - Hip flexion (L2)
    - Quadriceps (L3)
    - Tibialis Anterior (L4)
    - Extensor Hallicus Longus (L5)
    - Peroneals (S1)
    - Gastrocnemius (S1)
  - Abdominals
  - Spinal extensors
  - Hip extensor
  - Inner unit
- Pain
  - Measured on visual analog scale
- Posture
  - Anterior, posterior, side
  - Bony landmarks
  - Scoliosis, sway back, flat back
  - Pelvic asymmetry
- ROM
  - Flexion/extension
  - Side bend
  - Overpressure

- Reflex integrity
  - Reflex testing
    - Patellar tendon (L3)
    - Achilles tendon (S1)
  - Rule out upper motor neuron lesion
    - Clonus
    - Babinski
- Sensory integrity
  - Sensation, T12–S1
- Special tests
  - Dural tension tests
  - Patrick/FABRE
    - Patient is supine in FABRE position
    - Inguinal pain implicates hip joint pathology or muscular restrictions
    - To stress the sacroiliac joint, place one hand on the flexed knee and the other on the opposite ASIS and press down
  - Squatting
  - Sacroiliac tests
    - Marching tests
    - Straight leg raise test
    - Standing sacroiliac test
    - Standing rotation test
    - Sitting test

Establish Plan of Care
- Based on history, tests, and measures

GOALS/OUTCOMES
- Patient displays understanding of proper posture and body mechanics as evidenced by pain-free performance of ADLs and vocational activities
- Pain-free lumbar ROM: A minimum of 80% of AMA guides

	Normal	80%
Flexion	60°	50°
Extension	25°	20°
Side bend	25°	20°
Rotation	30°	25°

- Pain: 2/10 or less
- Strength: 4/5 on manual muscle test for back extensors, gluteals, abdominals
  - Abdominal
  - Spinal extensor
  - Gluteals
  - Inner unit (able to hold for 10 seconds for 10 repetitions)

Or specific functional motor performance, such as
- Squat to 90°
- Retrieve object from floor
- Perform work task (weight- and repetition-specific)
- Functional AROM
  - Hip
    - Flexion: 125°
    - Extension: 0°
    - Internal rotation: 20°
    - External rotation: 30°
  - Knee
    - Flexion: 120°
    - Extension: 5°
- Restore pelvic and leg length symmetry if mechanical
- Avoidance of movements causing a reoccurence of symptoms
- Return to previous functional status for ADLs and vocational, recreational, and sports activities as identified by patient
- Independence in a progressive home exercise program emphasizing function

INTERVENTION
NUMBER OF VISITS: 5–12

Coordination, Communication, and Documentation
- Provision of services between admission and discharge that facilitate cost-effective and efficient integration or reintegration to home, community, or work
- Documentation of therapeutic intervention is required for each episode of care and serves as the basic foundation for communication
- Coordination and additional communication will depend on the patient's impairment and home/work/community/leisure situation and requirements. Such services may include:
  - Case management
  - Coordination of care and collaboration with those integral to the patient's rehabilitation program
  - Coordination and monitoring of the delivery of available resources
  - Referrals to other health-care professionals
  - Identification of resources, support groups, or advocacy services
  - Provision of educational or training information
  - Technical assistance

Patient Instruction

Basic Anatomy and Biomechanics
- Relationship of sacrum, ilium, pelvis, hip, and lumbar vertebrae
- Ligamentous structures and the concept of hypermobility if applicable
- Pertinent Gray's Anatomy (Gray. 1995. 510–516, 526–531, 534–537, 809–813, 819–827)
- Importance of adequate ROM of all joints in the kinetic chain (spine, pelvis, hip, lower-extremity) to reduce the stress on the involved sacroiliac joint

Handouts
- Patient education
- Specific home program
- Commercially available products, such as:
  - Krames Communications (1100 Grundy Lane, San Bruno, CA 94066)
    - *Back to Basics*
    - *Your Back Is Always Working*
    - *Safety Zone: Using Natural Limits to Protect Your Back*

Functional Considerations
- Avoidance of activities and positions causing pain, e.g., extended periods of deep squats, bending, or crossing legs
- Relationship of proper body mechanics to daily activities
- Utilization of abdominal contraction to stabilize lumbar spine/sacroiliac region for lift tasks

Direct Interventions

Acute Phase: 3–6 Visits
- Therapeutic exercise and home program
  - Sacroiliac belt for immobilization during activity
    - Walking
    - Especially during flexion/extension activities
  - Home self-mobilization techniques
  - Flexibility exercises/stabilizing exercises
    - Lumbar
    - Hip
    - Lower extremity
  - Instruction in postures to be avoided

- Manual therapy techniques
  - Soft-tissue techniques
    - Soft-tissue mobilization
    - Trigger-point techniques
    - Strain/counterstrain
    - Myofascial release
    - Muscle energy technique
    - Contract or hold/relax
  - Assisted stretching techniques
    - Hip
    - Lower extremity
  - Joint mobilization
    - Grades I–V mobilization to the spine, sacrum, ilium, and hip as indicated in mobility examination
- Electrotherapeutic modalities
  - Iontophoresis
- Physical agents and mechanical modalities
  - Cryotherapy/superficial thermal modalities
  - Ultrasound
- Goals/outcomes
  - Pain: 5/10 or less
  - Awareness of proper posture and of postural influences on exacerbation of symptoms
  - Proper lifting mechanics utilizing abdominal stabilization
  - Lumbar AROM: 60% of AMA guides
    - Flexion: 35°
    - Extension: 15°
    - Side bend: 15°
    - Rotation: 20°
  - Hip AROM
    - Flexion: 90°
    - Extension: 5° (short of neutral)
    - Internal rotation: 10°
    - External rotation: 15°
  - Able to do pelvic tilt

Subacute Phase: 2–6 Visits

- Therapeutic exercise and home program
  - Trunk stabilization with a therapeutic ball/pelvic neutral
  - Stretching for tight muscle groups or joint tightness
  - Motor performance/stabilization
    - Squats
    - Multidirectional lunges

- Spinal extensors
- Abdominals
  a. Three-position partial sit-ups
  b. Stabilization progression
  c. Standing pelvic neutral overhead reach
- Aquatic therapy
- Initiate spinal stabilization
  - Inner unit
  - Bracing: co-contraction of trunk musculature
  - Pelvic tilt for abdominal strengthening/pelvic neutral
  - Functional activities
    a. Bed mobility
    b. Sit to stand
    c. Supine to sit
- Cardiovascular conditioning with use of immobilization belt as necessary
- Neuromuscular/balance/proprioceptive reeducation
  - Quadruped opposite arm/leg lift
  - Unilateral stance balancing, reaching one or both arms in various directions to maximum distance, avoiding use of other leg for counterbalance
    a. Anterior reach: Stimulates hamstrings, soleus, gastrocnemius, and hip/back extensors (depending on height of reach)
    b. Posterior overhead reach: Stimulates abdominals
    c. Lateral rotational reach: Stimulates hip abductors and lateral trunk stabilizers
  - Unilateral stance balancing, reaching opposite leg in various directions to maximum distance
    a. Anterior reach: Stimulates quadriceps, soleus
    b. Posterior reach: Stimulates gluteals, quadriceps, hip/back extensors
    c. Rotational reach to side: Stimulates gluteals, quadriceps, trunk stabilizers, hip abductors, abdominals
- Task-oriented exercises specifically related to work, home, and recreation

LUMBAR SPINE | SACROILIAC DYSFUNCTION   275

- Manual therapy techniques
  - Continue effective soft-tissue techniques
    - Emphasis on hip rotators, quadratus lumborum, tensor fasciæ latæ, gluteals, hip flexors, and piriformis
    - Muscle energy techniques to areas of hypomobility
  - Joint mobilization to areas of hypomobility
    - Lumbar
    - Sacroiliac
    - Hip
  - Continue assisted stretching techniques
- Therapeutic devices and equipment
  - For immobilization as needed
- Physical agents and mechanical modalities
  Continue effective modalities as in Acute Phase with increased emphasis on use as needed at home
- Goals/outcomes
  - Pain: 2/10 or less with ADLs 0/10 at rest
  - Return to previous functional status for ADLs and vocational activity
  - Strength: Minimum of 4/5 on manual muscle test for spinal/hip extensors and abdominals, or achieve a specific functional motor performance measure
  - Pain-free lumbar ROM: At 80% of AMA guides
  - Pain-free functional hip ROM
  - Normal sacroiliac joint ROM/negative special tests for sacroiliac

Functional Carryover

- Ergonomic evaluation as indicated for ADLs and vocational postures
- Patient understands the function of pelvic stabilization exercises and use of belt as well as the importance of continuation/progression during indicated activities
- Modification of cardiovascular and recreational activities as necessary until healing/stabilization occurs

DISCHARGE PLANNING AND PATIENT RESPONSIBILITY

Criteria for Discharge

- All goals/outcomes have been met with the exception of return to previous status for recreational and sports activities
- Patient has initiated return to recreation and sports activities
- Patient demonstrates competency in use of proper posture and body mechanics and in display of home exercise program

Circumstances Requiring Additional Visits

- Persistent functional strength deficit or 3/5 on manual muscle test
- History of previous injury/surgery to related area
- Severe deconditioning
- Special occupational needs requiring extensive fitness/strengthening
- Multiple injury sites including lower extremity
- Severe traumatic injury with persistent functional/occupational deficits
- Spinal instability
- Biomechanical lower-extremity dysfunction

Home Program

- Closed-kinetic chain strengthening for lower extremity
- Abdominal strengthening
- Flexibility
- Self-mobilization/muscle energy techniques for maintenance of pelvic symmetry
- Utilization of immobilization belt as needed

Monitoring

- Patient is to recheck/call at 2–4 weeks post-discharge to ensure progression toward achieving all goals/outcomes
- Schedule clinic visit as needed if symptoms return or patient is unable to resume recreational and sports activities
- Physician visit

276 SACROILIAC DYSFUNCTION | LUMBAR SPINE

REFERENCES

1. Alderink GJ. The sacroiliac joint: review of anatomy, mechanics and function. *J Orthop Sports Phys Ther.* 1991;13(2):71-84.

2. American Physical Therapy Association. *Guide to Physical Therapist Practice.* Alexandria, VA: APTA; 1997.

3. Cummings G, Scholz JP, Barnes K. The effect of imposed leg length difference on pelvic bone symmetry. *Spine.* 1993;18:368-373.

4. Daum WJ. The sacroiliac joint: an underappreciated pain generator. *Am J Orthop.* 1995;24:475-478.

5. Douglas S. Sciatic pain and piriformis syndrome. *Nurse Pract.* 1997;22(5):166-168, 170.

6. Fortin JD, Falco FJ. The Fortin finger test: an indicator of sacroiliac pain. *Am J Orthop.* 1997;26:477-480.

7. Gray H; Williams PL, ed. *Gray's Anatomy.* 38th ed. New York, NY: Churchill Livingstone; 1995.

8. Hart A, Hopkins C, Ford B. *ICD-9-CM Expert For Physicians, Volume 1&2.* 7th ed. USA: Ingenix; 2005.

9. Lee D. *The Pelvic Girdle.* New York, NY: Churchill Livingstone; 1999:81-143.

10. Maigne JY, Aivaliklis A, Pfefer F. Results of sacroiliac joint double block and value of sacroiliac pain provocation tests in 54 patients with low back pain. *Spine.* 1996;21:1889-1992.

11. Parziale JR, Hudgins TH, Fishman LM. The piriformis syndrome. *Am J Orthop.* 1996;25:819-823.

12. Richardson C, Jull G, Hodges P, Hide S. *Therapeutic Exercises For Spinal Segmental Stabilization In Low Back Pain.* New York, NY: Churchill Livingstone; 1999.

13. Tullberg T, Blomberg S, Branth B, Johnson R. Manipulation does not alter the position of the sacroiliac joint: a Roentgen stereophotogrammetric analysis. *Spine.* 1998;23:1124-1129.

14. Vleeming A, Mooney V, Dorman T, Snyders C, Stoeckart R. *Movement, Stability and Low Back Pain.* New York, NY: Churchill Livingstone; 1997.

SPINAL STENOSIS
SUMMARY OVERVIEW

ICD-9

724.00   724.01   724.02

APTA Preferred Practice Pattern: **4F, 4G, 4J**

EXAMINATION
- History and Systems Review
- Tests and Measures
  Systems review per APTA's *Guide to Physical Therapy Practice*
  - Anthropometric characteristics
  - Gait, locomotion, and balance
  - Joint integrity and mobility
  - Muscle performance
  - Pain
  - Posture
  - ROM
  - Reflex integrity
  - Sensory integrity
  - Special tests
  - Special consideration for geriatric population
- Establish Plan of Care

GOALS/OUTCOMES
- Patient displays understanding of proper posture and body mechanics
- Pain: 2/10 or less
- ROM
- Functional spinal stability and endurance as evidenced by symptom-free tolerance of postural requirements during normal ADLs and vocational activities
- Trunk strength: 4/5 on manual muscle
- Functional lower-extremity ROM
- Avoidance of movements causing a reoccurence of symptoms
- Return to previous functional status for ADLs and vocational, recreational, and sports activities as identified by patient
- Independence in a progressive home exercise program emphasizing function

INTERVENTION
NUMBER OF VISITS: 8–12

- Patient Instruction
  - Basic Anatomy and Biomechanics
  - Handouts
  - Functional Considerations
- Direct Interventions
  - Acute Phase: 4–6 Visits
  - Subacute Phase: 4–6 Visits
- Functional Carryover

DISCHARGE PLANNING AND PATIENT RESPONSIBILITY
- Criteria for Discharge
  - Patient demonstrates compliance with home exercise program. Ability to perform exercises in mechanically correct fashion.
  - All goals/outcomes have been achieved with the exception of return to previous functional level for recreational activities or sports activities
- Circumstances Requiring Additional Visits
  - Persistent functional motor performance deficit or 3/5 on manual muscle test
  - History of previous injury/surgery to related area
  - Severe deconditioning
  - Special occupational needs requiring extensive fitness/strengthening
  - Unable to maintain erect posture
  - Arthritic conditions
  - Hip dysfunction
  - Special consideration for geriatric population
  - Patient likely has long history of low back pain and consideration for additional recovery time will be extended
- Home Program
  - Modalities as needed
  - Cardiovascular conditioning
  - Flexibility exercises to prevent increased lordosis
  - Motor performance/stabilization
  - Home traction
- Monitoring

SUMMARY OVERVIEW | LUMBAR SPINE | SPINAL STENOSIS   279

SPINAL STENOSIS

ICD-9

724.00	Spinal stenosis, unspecified region
724.01	Spinal stenosis, thoracic region
724.02	Spinal stenosis, lumbar region

APTA Preferred Practice Pattern: 4F, 4G, 4J

EXAMINATION

History and Systems Review

- History of current condition
  - Mechanism of injury/onset
  - Date of injury/onset
  - Location, nature, and behavior of symptoms
    - Radiating symptoms into the buttock or leg
    - Increased pain with walking and standing aggravating or relieving factors
    - Pain relieved with sitting or squatting
  - Presence of cauda equina symptoms
- Past history of current condition
  - Hospitalization
  - Surgical intervention
  - Lower-extremity problems
  - Bracing, injections, etc.
  - Corset use
  - Involvement of other spinal or lower-extremity joint problems
  - Previous therapeutic intervention
- Other tests and measures
  - Diagnostic procedures
- Past medical/surgical history
  - Systemic pathology
    - Appendix
    - Abdominal
    - Pancreas
    - Large intestine
    - Kidney
    - Genital/urinary
      a. Bladder
      b. Ureter
      c. Prostate gland
      d. Cervix
      e. Uterus
- Functional status and activity level (current/prior)
- Patient's functional goals

Tests and Measures

Systems review per APTA's *Guide to Physical Therapy Practice*

- Anthropometric characteristics
  - Leg length discrepancy
    - Supine
    - Weight-bearing
- Gait, locomotion, and balance
  - Asymmetrical gait pattern
    - Arm swing
    - Hip transverse plane motion
    - Knee extension in stance phase
    - Knee flexion in swing phase
    - Early heel off
    - Excessive pronation
  - Lumbar-sacroiliac weight bearing: Mobility
  - Balance
- Joint integrity and mobility
  - Central posterior to anterior glides
    In prone position, with posterior to anterior pressure on spinous or transverse processes
  - Passive intervertebral motion
    - Flexion/extension
    - Side bend
    - Rotation
  - Stress tests
    It is recommended that stress tests be performed at those segments that are hypomobile or that the therapist intends to mobilize to end range (Grades III–V)
- Muscle performance
  - Resisted testing
  - Key muscle test
    To determine possible palsy, utilize a combination of resistance and repetition
    - Hip flexion (L2)
    - Quadriceps (L3)
    - Tibialis anterior (L4)
    - Extensor hallicus longus (L5)

280   SPINAL STENOSIS | LUMBAR SPINE

- Peroneals (S1)
- Gastrocnemius (S1)
  - Abdominals
  - Spinal extensors
  - Hip extensors
  - Inner unit
  - Squat
  - Lunge knee to floor and recover
- Pain
  - Measured on visual analog scale
- Posture
  - Anterior, posterior, side
  - Bony landmarks
  - Scoliosis, sway back, flat back, lordosis
  - Pelvic asymmetry
  - Palpation, including key landmarks
- ROM
  - Active
    - Flexion
    - Extension
    - Side bend
    - Rotation
  - Overpressure (passive)
- Reflex integrity
  - Reflex testing
    - Patellar tendon (L3)
    - Hamstring tendon (L5)
    - Achilles tendon (S1)
  - Rule out upper motor neuron lesion
    - Clonus
    - Babinski
- Sensory integrity
  - Sensory assessment
- Special tests
  - Dural tension tests
  - Compression overload
    - In supine position with hips and knees flexed to end range
    - Apply overpressure to lower extremities in superior direction
  - Traction
  - Lower-extremity special tests
  - Sacroiliac tests
  - Patrick/FABRE
    - Patient is supine in FABRE position
    - Inguinal pain implicates hip joint pathology or muscular restrictions

- To stress the sacroiliac joint, place one hand on the flexed knee and the other on the opposite ASIS and press down
- Special consideration for geriatric population

Establish Plan of Care
- Based on history, tests, and measures

GOALS/OUTCOMES
- Patient displays understanding of proper posture and body mechanics as evidenced by pain-free performance of ADLs and vocational activities
- Pain: 2/10 or less
- Pain-free lumbar/thoracic ROM: A minimum of 80% of AMA guides

Lumbar	Normal	80%
Flexion	60°	50°
Extension	25°	20°
Side bend	25°	20°

Thoracic	Normal	80%
Flexion	40°	30°
Extension	no AMA guides established	
Side bend	10°	8°
Rotation	30°	25°

- Functional spinal stability and endurance as evidenced by symptom-free tolerance of postural requirements during normal ADLs and vocational activities
- Trunk strength: 4/5 on manual muscle
  - Abdominals
  - Spinal extensors
  - Gluteals
  - Inner unit (able to hold for 10 seconds for 10 repetitions)

Or specific functional motor performance, such as
  - Squat to 90°
  - Retrieve object from floor
  - Perform work task (weight- and repetition-specific)
- Functional lower-extremity ROM
  - Hip
    - Flexion: 125°
    - Extension: 0°
    - Internal rotation: 20°
    - External rotation: 30°
  - Knee
    - Flexion: 120°
    - Extension: 5°

LUMBAR SPINE | SPINAL STENOSIS

- Avoidance of movements causing a reoccurence of symptoms
- Return to previous functional status for ADLs and vocational, recreational, and sports activities as identified by patient
- Independence in a progressive home exercise program emphasizing function

INTERVENTION
NUMBER OF VISITS: 8–12

Coordination, Communication, and Documentation
- Provision of services between admission and discharge that facilitate cost-effective and efficient integration or reintegration to home, community, or work
- Documentation of therapeutic intervention is required for each episode of care and serves as the basic foundation for communication
- Coordination and additional communication will depend on the patient's impairment and home/work/ community/leisure situation and requirements. Such services may include:
  - Case management
  - Coordination of care and collaboration with those integral to the patient's rehabilitation program
  - Coordination and monitoring of the delivery of available resources
  - Referrals to other health-care professionals
  - Identification of resources, support groups, or advocacy services
  - Provision of educational or training information
  - Technical assistance

Patient Instruction

Basic Anatomy and Biomechanics
- Back anatomy (Back Views video or personal instruction)
- Anatomy of the spine
- Biomechanics of lumbar spine and relationship of symptoms to mechanisms of injury
- Segmental mobility dysfunction
- Muscle weakness or imbalance
- Postural or lower-extremity biomechanical effects
- Pertinent Gray's Anatomy (Gray. 1995. 510–516, 526–531, 534–537, 809–813, 819–827)

Handouts
- Patient education
- Specific help
- Commercially available products, such as:
  - Krames Communications (1100 Grundy Lane, San Bruno, CA 94066)
    - *Back Basics*
    - *Back Owner's Manual*
- Special considerations for geriatric population
  - Handouts on all exercises, body mechanics, and other instructions will help eliminate problems with short-term memory loss

Functional Considerations
- Review of aggravating positions and activities
- Instruction on positioning for relief of symptoms
- Avoidance of positions and postures that reproduce symptoms, such as prolonged standing, walking, or extension activities
- Modification of body mechanics to encourage pelvic tilt and flexion bracing
- Instruction on posture and body mechanics for ADLs

Direct Interventions

Acute Phase: 4–6 Visits
- Therapeutic exercise and home program
  Special consideration for geriatric population (See *Geriatric Rehabilitation* guidelines)
  Targeting use of *neutral spine*
  - Patient may have multiple joint and systemic involvement, which may limit use of treatment positions, exercise tolerance, and use of proper body mechanics
  - Home use of superficial thermal modalities and cryotherapy
  - Flexion exercise
    - Knee-to-chest
    - Pelvic tilt
  - ADLs training
    - Sleeping position
    - Frequent sitting
    - Transfer technique
  - Abdominal strengthening
    - Initiate lumbar stabilization
    - Inner unit
    - Bracing co-contraction of trunk musculature
    - Pelvic neutral

282   SPINAL STENOSIS | LUMBAR SPINE

- ○ Extensor strengthening
  - ▪ Bridging
  - ▪ Modified plantigrade opposite arm/leg lift
  - ▪ Quadruped opposite arm/leg lift
- ○ Functional activities
- ○ Manual therapy techniques
  - ▪ Soft-tissue mobilization
  - ▪ Assisted ROM and stretching to hip and lower extremity
  - ▪ Joint mobilization
    - a. Grade I or II
    - b. Specific traction
- • Electrotherapeutic modalities
- • Physical agents and mechanical modalities
  - ○ Thermal modalities/cryotherapy
  - ○ Mechanical traction
  - ○ Ultrasound
- • Goals/outcomes
  - ○ Pain: 5/10 or less
  - ○ Exercises performed in pain-free range
  - ○ Patient understands the importance of ADLs techniques and of modifying his/her environment
    - ▪ Sit frequently, correct sitting posture
    - ▪ Pace activities
    - ▪ Sleep in a fetal position—pillow placement
    - ▪ Transfer techniques
    - ▪ Voluntary trunk co-contraction with neutral spine

Subacute Phase: 4–6 Visits

- • Therapeutic exercise and home program
  - ○ Cardiovascular conditioning
    - ▪ Treadmill
    - ▪ Forward
    - ▪ Backward
    - ▪ Walking progression
    - ▪ Swimming or aquatic exercise
    - ▪ Stationary cycling
    - ▪ Upper body ergometer
  - ○ Abdominal strengthening
    - ▪ Three-position partial sit ups
    - ▪ Stabilization progression
    - ▪ Pelvic neutral overhead reach
      - a. Standing
      - b. Single leg standing
  - ○ Flexion stretches to lumbar region

- ○ Functional closed-kinetic chain progression with abdominal stabilization
  - ▪ Squats
  - ▪ Multidirectional lunges
- • Manual therapy techniques
  - ○ Joint mobilization
    - ▪ Progress grade to maximize mobility
    - ▪ Clear thoracic/lumbar junction
    - ▪ Maximize hip ROM
  - ○ Soft-tissue mobilization
  - ○ Assisted stretching
    - ▪ Torso rotation
    - ▪ Hip rotators
    - ▪ Psoas
    - ▪ Quadriceps
  - ○ Proprioceptive neuromuscular facilitation
- • Physical agents and mechanical modalities
  Continue effective modalities as in Acute Phase with increased emphasis on use as needed at home
- • Goals/outcomes
  - ○ Lumbar/thoracic AROM: 80% of AMA guides
  - ○ Trunk strength: 4/5 on manual muscle test or achieve predetermined motor performance parameter
  - ○ Return to normal work, recreation, and ADLs
  - ○ Improve awareness of proper body mechanics
  - ○ Pain: 2/10 or less and absence of radiating symptoms with ADLs

Functional Carryover

- • Task-oriented exercise dependent on home, work, and recreational activities
- • Patient understands the role of posterior pelvic tilt and lumbar flexion in decreasing radiating symptoms

DISCHARGE PLANNING AND PATIENT RESPONSIBILITY

Criteria for Discharge

- • Patient demonstrates compliance with home exercise program. Ability to perform exercises in mechanically correct fashion.
- • All goals/outcomes have been achieved with the exception of return to previous functional level for recreational activities or sports activities

LUMBAR SPINE | SPINAL STENOSIS   283

Circumstances Requiring Additional Visits

- Persistent functional motor performance deficit or 3/5 on manual muscle test
- History of previous injury/surgery to related area
- Severe deconditioning
- Special occupational needs requiring extensive fitness/strengthening
- Unable to maintain erect posture
- Arthritic conditions
- Hip dysfunction
- Special consideration for geriatric population
- Patient likely has long history of low back pain and consideration for additional recovery time will be extended

Home Program

- Modalities as needed
- Cardiovascular conditioning
- Flexibility exercises to prevent increased lordosis
- Motor performance/stabilization
- Home traction

Monitoring

- Patient is to phone for follow-up at 2–4 weeks post-discharge to ensure progression toward achieving all goals/outcomes
- Schedule clinic follow-up as needed if symptoms return or patient is unable to achieve return to recreational activities

REFERENCES

1. American Physical Therapy Association. *Guide to Physical Therapist Practice.* Alexandria, VA: APTA; 1997.
2. Ferreira PH, Ferreira ML, Hodges PW. Changes in recruitment of the abdominal muscles in people with low back pain: ultrasound measurement of muscle activity. *Spine.* 2004;29:2560-6.
3. Fritz JM, Erhard RE, Vignovic M. A nonsurgical treatment approach for patients with lumbar spinal stenosis. *Phys Ther.* 1997;77:962-973.
4. Fritz JM, Delitto A, Welch WC, Erhard RE. Lumbar spinal stenosis: a review of current concepts in evaluation, management, and outcome measurements. *Arch Phys Med Rehab.* 1998;79:700-708.
5. Gray H; Williams PL, ed. *Gray's Anatomy.* 38th ed. New York, NY: Churchill Livingstone; 1995.
6. Hart A, Hopkins C, Ford B. *ICD-9-CM Expert For Physicians, Volume 1&2.* 7th ed. USA: Ingenix; 2005.
7. Herno A, Airaksinen O, Saari T. Long-term results of surgical treatment of lumbar spinal stenosis. *Spine.* 1993;18:1471-1474.
8. Hides J, Wilson S, Stanton W, et al. An MRI investigation into the function of the transversus abdominis muscle during "drawing-in" of the abdominal wall. *Spine.* 2006;31:175-8.
9. Hodges PW, Richardson CA. Altered trunk muscle recruitment in people with low back pain with upper limb movement at different speeds. *Arch Phys Med Rehabil.* 1999;80:1005-12.
10. Moseley GL, Hodges PW, Gandevia SC. Deep and superficial fibers of the lumbar multifidus muscle are differentially active during voluntary arm movements. *Spine.* 2002;27:29-36.
11. Nagler W, Hausen HS. Conservative management of lumbar spinal stenosis: identifying patients likely to do well without surgery. *Postgrad Med.* 1998;103:69-71, 76, 81-83.
12. Nowakowski P, Delitto A, Erhard RE. Lumbar spinal stenosis. *Phys Ther.* 1996;76:187-190.
13. Onel D, Sari H, Donmez C. Lumbar spinal stenosis: clinical/radiologic therapeutic evaluation in 145 patients; conservative treatment or surgical intervention? *Spine.* 1993;18:291-298.
14. Porter RW, Ward D. Cauda equina dysfunction: the significance of two-Level pathology. *Spine.* 1992;17:9-15.
15. Radu AS, Menkes CJ. Update on lumbar spinal stenosis: retrospective study of 62 patients and review of the literature. *Rev Rheum Engl Ed.* 1998;65:337-345.
16. Richardson CA, Snijders CJ, Hides JA, et al. The relation between the transversus abdominis muscles, sacroiliac joint mechanics, and low back pain. *Spine.* 2002;27:399-405.
17. Urquhart DM, Hodges PW. *Eur Spine J.* 2005;14:393-400.

SPONDYLOLISTHESIS
SUMMARY OVERVIEW

ICD-9

738.4   756.12

APTA Preferred Practice Pattern: **4B, 4G, 4J**

EXAMINATION

- History and Systems Review
- Tests and Measures
  Systems review per APTA's *Guide to Physical Therapy Practice*
  - ○ Anthropometric characteristics
  - ○ Gait, locomotion, and balance
  - ○ Joint integrity and mobility
  - ○ Motor function
  - ○ Muscle performance
  - ○ Pain
  - ○ Posture
  - ○ Palpation
  - ○ ROM
  - ○ Reflex integrity
  - ○ Sensory integrity for neurological examination
  - ○ Special tests
- Establish Plan of Care

GOALS/OUTCOMES

- Patient displays understanding of proper posture and body mechanics
- Pain: 2/10 or less
- Pain-free lumbar ROM: A minimum of 80% of AMA guides with the ability to stabilize involved segment sufficiently to avoid pain
- Strength: 4/5 on manual muscle test for back extensors, gluteals, abdominals
- Functional lower-extremity ROM
- Avoidance of movements causing a reoccurence of symptoms
- Return to previous functional status for ADLs and vocational, recreational, and sports activities as identified by patient
- Independence in a progressive home exercise program emphasizing function

INTERVENTION
NUMBER OF VISITS: 5–11

- Patient Instruction
  - ○ Basic Anatomy and Biomechanics
  - ○ Handouts
  - ○ Functional Considerations
- Direct Interventions
  - ○ Acute Phase: 2–5 Visits
  - ○ Subacute Phase: 3–6 Visits
- Functional Carryover

DISCHARGE PLANNING AND PATIENT RESPONSIBILITY

- Criteria for Discharge
  - ○ Patient displays full understanding of positions of preference for ADLs
  - ○ Patient demonstrates proper body mechanics during simulated ADLs and vocational postures
  - ○ All goals/outcomes have been achieved except as described in the guideline
  - ○ Patient recognizes symptoms and appropriately modifies home program and activities
- Circumstances Requiring Additional Visits
  - ○ Persistent functional motor performance deficit or 3/5 on manual muscle test
  - ○ History of previous injury/surgery to related area
  - ○ Persistent radicular symptoms or neurological deficit
  - ○ Severe deconditioning
  - ○ Special occupational needs requiring extensive fitness/strengthening
  - ○ Instability
  - ○ Arthritic conditions
  - ○ Severe traumatic injury with persistent functional/occupational deficits
- Home Program
  - ○ Stabilization and strengthening exercise
  - ○ Cardiovascular conditioning program
  - ○ Flexibility exercises
- Monitoring

SUMMARY OVERVIEW | LUMBAR SPINE | SPONDYLOLISTHESIS   285

SPONDYLOLISTHESIS

ICD-9

738.4	Acquired spondylolisthesis
756.12	Congenital spondylolisthesis

APTA Preferred Practice Pattern: **4B, 4G, 4J**

EXAMINATION

History and Systems Review

- History of current condition
  - Mechanism of injury/onset
  - Date of injury/onset
  - Location, nature, and behavior of symptoms
    - Radiating symptoms
    - Aggravating/relieving factors
      a. Postures
    - Presence of cauda equina symptoms
- Past history of current condition
  - Hospitalization
  - Surgical intervention
  - Lower-extremity problems
  - Bracing, injections, etc.
- Other tests and measures
  - X-rays, stress x-rays, MRI, bone scan
- Past medical/surgical history
  - Systemic pathology
    - Appendix
    - Abdominal
    - Pancreas
    - Large intestine
    - Kidney
    - Genital/urinary
      a. Bladder
      b. Ureter
      c. Prostate gland
      d. Cervix
      e. Uterus
- Functional status and activity level: current/prior
- Patient's functional goals

Tests and Measures

Systems review per APTA's *Guide to Physical Therapy Practice*

- Anthropometric characteristics
  - Leg length discrepancy
    - Supine
    - Weight-bearing
    - Prone

- Gait, locomotion, and balance
  - Asymmetrical gait pattern
    - Arm swing
    - Hip transverse plane motion
    - Knee extension in stance phase
    - Knee flexion in swing phase
    - Early heel off
    - Excessive pronation
    - Lumbar-sacroiliac weight bearing: Mobility
  - Balance
- Joint integrity and mobility (as appropriate given diagnosis grade of spondylolisthesis)
  - Central posterior to anterior glides (may be questionable test if gross instability is present): In prone position, with posterior to anterior pressure on spinous or transverse processes
  - Sidelying shear test
  - Flexion/extension
  - Side bend
  - Rotation
  - Stress tests
    It is recommended that stress tests be performed at those segments that are hypomobile or that the therapist intends to mobilize to end range (Grades III–V)
- Motor function
  - Dynamic lordosis
- Muscle performance
  - Resisted testing
  - Key muscle tests : To determine possible palsy, utilize a combination of resistance and repetition
    - Hip flexion (L2)
    - Quadriceps (L3)
    - Tibialis anterior (L4)
    - Extensor hallicus longus (L5)
    - Peroneals (S1)
    - Gastrocnemius and hip extensors, S1–S2
  - Abdominals
  - Spinal extensors
  - Hip extensor
  - Inner unit

286 SPONDYLOLISTHESIS | LUMBAR SPINE

- Pain
  - Measured on visual analog scale
- Posture
  - Anterior, posterior, side
  - Bony landmarks
  - Scoliosis, sway back, flat back
  - Pelvic asymmetry
  - Static lordosis
- Palpation, including key landmarks
- ROM
  - Active
    - Flexion
    - Extension
    - Side bend
    - Rotation
    - Possible visual or palpable anterior shear at one lumbosacral segment while patient is in position of forward bending
  - Overpressure (passive)
- Reflex integrity
  - Reflex testing
    - Patellar tendon (L3)
    - Achilles tendon (S1)
  - Rule out upper motor neuron lesion
    - Babinski
    - Clonus
- Sensory integrity for neurological examination
  - Sensory assessment (T12–S2)
- Special tests
  - Sacroiliac tests
    - Standing
    - Marching
    - Sitting
  - Compression overload
    - In supine position with hips and knees flexed to end range
    - Apply overpressure to lower extremities in superior direction
  - Traction—manual supine
    - Hooklying vs. straight leg
  - Patrick/FABRE
    - Patient is supine in FABRE position
    - Inguinal pain implicates hip joint pathology or muscular restrictions
    - To stress the sacroiliac joint, place one hand on the flexed knee and the other on the opposite ASIS and press down

- Thomas test
  - Quad tightness
  - Psoas tightness
- Dural tension tests

Establish Plan of Care
- Based on history, tests, and measures

GOALS/OUTCOMES
- Patient displays understanding of proper posture and body mechanics as evidenced by pain-free performance of ADLs and vocational activities
- Pain: 2/10 or less
- Pain-free lumbar ROM: A minimum of 80% of AMA guides with the ability to stabilize involved segment sufficiently to avoid pain

	Normal	*80%*
Flexion	60°	50°
Extension	25°	20°
Lateral flexion	25°	20°

- Strength: 4/5 on manual muscle test for back extensors, gluteals, abdominals
  - Abdominals
  - Spinal extensor
  - Gluteals
  - Inner unit (able to hold for 10 seconds for 10 repetitions)

  Or specific functional motor performance, such as:
  - Squat to 90°
  - Retrieve object from floor demonstrating proper body mechanics
  - Perform work task (weight and repetition specific)
- Functional lower-extremity ROM
  - Hip
    - Flexion: 125°
    - Extension: 0°
    - Internal rotation: 20°
    - External rotation: 30°
  - Knee
    - Flexion: 120°
    - Extension: 5°
  - Ankle
    - Dorsiflexion: 8° in subtalar neutral with knee extended

- Avoidance of movements causing a reoccurence of symptoms
- Return to previous functional status for ADLs and vocational, recreational, and sports activities as identified by patient
- Independence in a progressive home exercise program emphasizing function

INTERVENTION
NUMBER OF VISITS: 5–11

Coordination, Communication, and Documentation
- Provision of services between admission and discharge that facilitate cost-effective and efficient integration or reintegration to home, community, or work
- Documentation of therapeutic intervention is required for each episode of care and serves as the basic foundation for communication
- Coordination and additional communication will depend on the patient's impairment and home/work/community/leisure situation and requirements. Such services may include:
  - Case management
  - Coordination of care and collaboration with those integral to the patient's rehabilitation program
  - Coordination and monitoring of the delivery of available resources
  - Referrals to other health-care professionals
  - Identification of resources, support groups, or advocacy services
  - Provision of educational or training information
  - Technical assistance

Patient Instruction

Basic Anatomy and Biomechanics
- Pertinent Gray's Anatomy (Gray. 1995. 510–516, 526–528, 534–537, 809–813, 819–827)
- Description of spondylolisthesis, for example,
  - *Physical Examination of the Spine and Extremities* (Hoppenfield. 1976. 241)
  - *Textbook of Disorders and Injuries of the Musculoskeletal System* (Salter. 1999. 317)
  - Illustrations of postures to be avoided

Handouts
- Specific home program
- Commercially available products, such as:
  - Krames Communications (1100 Grundy Lane, San Bruno, CA 94066)
    - *Poor Posture Hurts*
    - *Back Owner's Manual*

Functional Considerations
- Restriction of vigorous activity until pain/spasm decreases
- Bracing/stabilization during gait, transfers, and ADLs

Direct Interventions
Note: If anterior shear is positive in neutral and flexion, patient will exercise and perform body mechanics in neutral. If anterior shear is positive in neutral and negative in flexion, patient will exercise and perform body mechanics with a posterior pelvic tilt.

Acute Phase: 2–5 Visits
- Therapeutic exercise and home program
  - Flexibility exercises
    - Upper-extremity and lower-extremity stretching, especially:
      a. Hip joints
      b. Hamstrings
      c. Hip flexors
  - Initiate lumbar stabilization as appropriate
  - Posture awareness training
    - Bracing with sit-to-stand
    - Instruction on bed mobility
    - Bracing with ADLs
  - Progressive walking with bracing as tolerated
- Manual therapy techniques
  - Soft-tissue techniques
    - Soft-tissue mobilization
    - Trigger-point techniques
    - Myofascial release
    - Strain/counterstrain
    - Muscle energy techniques
  - Joint mobilization
    - Grades III–V as necessary above and below site of instability
    - Grades I–II at level of instability for pain relief
    - Thoracic spine and hips as necessary
    - Supine 90°/90° manual traction for pain relief
  - Assisted lower-extremity flexibility exercises

288 SPONDYLOLISTHESIS | LUMBAR SPINE

- Electrotherapeutic modalities
- Physical agents and mechanical modalities
  - Cryotherapy/superficial thermal modalities
  - Ultrasound
- Goals/outcomes
  - Voluntary abdominal control in supine, sitting, and standing
  - Ambulation for 10 minutes on level surface
  - Strength: 4/5 on manual muscle test for abdominals and extensors
  - Pain: 5/10 or less with activities
  - Pain: 5/10 or less with performance of functional activities
    - Proper bed mobility
    - Proper posture and body mechanics with ADLs

Subacute Phase: 3–6 Visits

- Therapeutic exercise and home program
  - Progressive abdominal strengthening/stabilization
    - Curl-ups
    - Manually resisted proprioceptive neuromuscular facilitation patterns
    - Pulley
    - Therapeutic ball
      a. Supine
      b. Quadruped
  - Aggressive extensor strengthening/stabilization
    - Prone extension over pillows to neutral
    - Quadruped activities
    - Pulley
    - Therapeutic ball
  - Closed-kinetic chain strengthening with stabilization
    - Squatting
    - Multidirectional lunges
    - Kneeling
    - Step up/step down
  - Isotonic strengthening for:
    - Latissimus dorsi
    - Quadriceps
    - Hamstrings
    - Gluteals
    - Erector spinæ
  - Upper extremity/lower-extremity stretching program
    - Emphasize gastrocnemius and hip flexors

- Neuromuscular/balance/proprioceptive reeducation
  - Quadruped opposite arm/leg lift
  - Unilateral stance balancing, reaching one or both arms in various directions to maximum distance, avoiding use of other leg for counterbalance
    a. Anterior reach: Stimulates hamstrings, soleus, gastrocnemius, and hip/back extensors (depending on height of reach)
    b. Posterior overhead reach: Stimulates abdominals
    c. Lateral rotational reach: Stimulates hip abductors and lateral trunk stabilizers
  - Unilateral stance balancing, reaching opposite leg in various directions to maximum distance
    a. Anterior reach: Stimulates quadriceps, soleus
    b. Posterior reach: Stimulates gluteals, quadriceps, hip/back extensors
    c. Rotational reach to side: Stimulates gluteals, quadriceps, trunk stabilizers, hip abductors, abdominals
  - Cardiovascular conditioning
    - Treadmill/walking program
    - Swimming/aquatic therapy
    - Cycling
- Manual therapy techniques
  - Continue effective soft-tissue techniques
  - Joint mobilization as appropriate given diagnosis
    - Grades I–II at level of instability
    - Grades III–V to hypomobile levels of thoracic and lumbar spines, pelvis
    - Hip mobilization as indicated
  - Hip and lower-extremity assisted passive stretching
- Physical agents and mechanical modalities
  Continue effective modalities as in Acute Phase with increased emphasis on use as needed at home
- Goals/outcomes
  - Lower-extremity ROM: Within normal limits except for hip extension, flexion with knee straight
  - Strength: 4/5 abdominals, spinal extensors, and lower extremities or achieve predetermined functional motor performance parameter
  - Pain: 2/10 or less
  - Functional activity
    - Patient demonstrates avoidance of excesses of range during gait, transfers, ADLs, and vocational activities
  - Patient achieves pain-free activity when using proper body mechanics

LUMBAR SPINE | SPONDYLOLISTHESIS   **289**

Functional Carryover

- Avoidance of activities involving extreme lumbar ROM
- Depending on residual segmental stability, patient is instructed in appropriate pelvic position for daily activities
- Instructions in proper progression for return to ADLs and vocational, recreational, and sports activities

DISCHARGE PLANNING AND PATIENT RESPONSIBILITY

Criteria for Discharge

- Patient displays full understanding of positions of preference for ADLs
- Patient demonstrates proper body mechanics during simulated ADLs and vocational postures
- All goals/outcomes have been achieved except:
  - Return to previous vocational activity may be delayed depending upon physical demands
  - Limited return to previous status for recreational and sports activities
- Patient recognizes symptoms and appropriately modifies home program and activities

Circumstances Requiring Additional Visits

- Persistent functional motor performance deficit or 3/5 on manual muscle test
- History of previous injury/surgery to related area
- Persistent radicular symptoms or neurological deficit
- Severe deconditioning
- Special occupational needs requiring extensive fitness/strengthening
- Instability
- Arthritic conditions
- Severe traumatic injury with persistent functional/occupational deficits

Home Program

- Stabilization and strengthening exercise
  - Therapeutic ball
  - Resistive tubing/cords
  - Free-weights or health club equipment
- Cardiovascular conditioning program
- Flexibility exercises
  - Gastrocnemius/soleus
  - Hip flexors/rotators
  - Spinal and hip extensors

Monitoring

- Patient is instructed in the progressive condition and its symptomatology requiring physician consultation
- Instruct patient to call at 4 weeks post-discharge to ensure progression toward attaining all goals/outcomes
- Schedule clinic follow-up at 2–3 months if there are recurring symptoms

REFERENCES

1. Aihara T, Takahashi K, Yamagata M, Moriya H. Fracture-dislocation of the fifth lumbar vertebra: a new classification. *J Bone Joint Surg Br.* 1998;80:840-845.
2. American Physical Therapy Association. *Guide to Physical Therapist Practice.* Alexandria, VA: APTA; 1997.
3. Cinotti G, Postacchini F, Fassari F, Urso S. Predisposing factors in degenerative spondylolisthesis. A radiographic and CT study. *Ind Orthop.* 1997;21:337-342.
4. Cyriax J. *Textbook of Orthopedic Medicine. Vol I: Diagnosis of Soft Tissue Lesions.* 8th ed. London, England: Balliere Tindall; 1982.
5. Fennered K. Isthmic spondylolisthesis among patients receiving disability pension under the diagnosis of chronic low back pain syndromes. *Spine.* 1994;19:2766-2769.
6. Gray H; Williams PL, ed. *Gray's Anatomy.* 38th ed. New York, NY: Churchill Livingstone; 1995.
7. Hart A, Hopkins C, Ford B. *ICD-9-CM Expert For Physicians, Volume 1&2.* 7th ed. USA: Ingenix; 2005.
8. Hoppenfeld S. *Physical Examination of the Spine and Extremities.* Norwalk, CT: Appleton & Lange; 1976.
9. Hu SS, Bradford DS, Transfeldt EE, Cohen M. Reduction of high-grade spondylolisthesis using Edwards instrumentation. *Spine.* 1996;21:367-371.
10. Ishikawa S, Kumar SJ, Torres BC. Surgical treatment of dysplastic spondylolisthesis: results after in situ fusion. *Spine.* 1994;19:1691-1696.
11. Nagaosa Y, Kikuchi S, Hasue M, Sato S. Pathoanatomic mechanisms of degenerative spondylolisthesis: a radiographic study. *Spine.* 1998;23:1447-1451.
12. O'Sullivan PB, Phyty GD, Twomey LT, Allison GT. Evaluation of specific stabilizing exercise in the treatment of chronic low back pain with radiologic diagnosis of spondylolysis of spondylolisthesis. *Spine.* 1997;22:2959-2967.
13. Pettine KA, Salib RM, Walker SG. External electrical stimulation and bracing for treatment of spondylolysis: a case report. *Spine.* 1993;18:436-439.

14. Salter RB. *Textbook of Disorders And Injuries Of The Musculoskeletal System: An Introduction To Orthopaedics, Fractures, and Joint Injuries, Rheumatology, and Metabolic Bone Disease and Rehabilitation*. 3rd Ed. Philadelphia, PA: Lippincott Williams & Wilkins; 1999.

15. Schwab FJ, Farcy JP, Roye DP Jr. The sagittal pelvic tilt as a criterion in the evaluation of spondylolisthesis: preliminary observations. *Spine* 1997;22:1661-1667.

16. Shipley JA, Beukes CA. The nature of the spondylolytic defect: demonstration of a communication synovial pseudarthrosis in the pars interarticularis. *J Bone Joint Surg Br.* 1998;80:662-664.

17. Sinaki M, Lutness MP, Ilstrup DM, Chu CP, Gramse RR. Lumbar spondylolisthesis: retrospective comparison and three year follow-up of two conservative treatment programs. *Arch Phys Med Rehabil.* 1989;70;594-598.

18. Spratt KF, Weinstein JN, Lehmann TR, Woody J, Sayre H. Efficacy of flexion and extension treatments incorporating braces for low back pain patients with retrodisplacement, spondylolisthesis, or normal sagittal translation. *Spine.* 1993;18:1839-1849.

19. Weber MD, Woodall WR. Spondylogenic disorders in gymnasts. *J Orthop Sports Phys Ther.* 1991;14(1):6-13.

292   SPONDYLOLISTHESIS | LUMBAR SPINE

Cervical/Thoracic

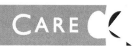

CERVICAL/THORACIC SPINE

Cervical/Thoracic General Pain	295
Cervical Disc Pathology	301
Cervical Spondylolysis with Myelopathy	308
Cervical Stenosis	313
Compression Fracture	319
Craniovertebral Stability Tests	325
Objective Measurement of Forward Head Posture	327
Osteoporosis	329
Postoperative/Postfracture Rehabilitation of the Cervical/Thoracic Spine	335
Rib Dysfunction	341
Scoliosis	347
Thoracic Outlet Syndrome	353
Whiplash Syndrome	359

294   CERVICAL/THORACIC SPINE

CERVICAL/THORACIC GENERAL PAIN
SUMMARY OVERVIEW

ICD-9

715.90 715.98 721.0 723.1 724.1 729.1 739.1 739.2 840.8
847.0 847.1

APTA Preferred Practice Pattern: 4B, 4C, 4D, 4E, 4F, 4G, 4H, 4I, 4J, 5F, 6B

EXAMINATION

- History and Systems Review
- Tests and Measures
  Systems review per APTA's *Guide to Physical Therapy Practice*
  - Aerobic capacity and endurance
  - Joint integrity and mobility
  - Muscle performance
  - Pain
  - Posture
  - ROM
  - Reflex integrity
  - Sensory integrity
  - Special tests
- Establish Plan of Care

GOALS/OUTCOMES

- Pain: 2/10 or less
- ROM: At least 80% of AMA guides and equal bilaterally
- Adequate spinal strength and stability to prevent reinjury: 4+/5 on manual muscle test of cervical and scapular muscles
- Return to previous functional status for ADLs and vocational, recreational, and sports activities as identified by patient
- Independence in a progressive home exercise program emphasizing function
- Minimize/resolve any neurological deficits

INTERVENTION
NUMBER OF VISITS: 6–12

- Patient Instruction
  - Basic Anatomy and Biomechanics
  - Handouts
  - Functional Considerations

- Direct Interventions
  - Acute Phase: 3–6 Visits
  - Subacute Phase: 3–6 Visits
- Functional Carryover

DISCHARGE PLANNING AND PATIENT RESPONSIBILITY

- Criteria for Discharge
  - Patient demonstrates independence in home exercise program
  - All goals/outcomes have been achieved with the exception of return to previous status for recreational and sports activities
  - Patient displays understanding of the role of proper posture and body mechanics in prevention of reinjury
- Circumstances Requiring Additional Visits
  - Persistent functional strength deficit or 3/5 on manual muscle test
  - History of previous injury/surgery to related area
  - Persistent radicular symptoms or neurological deficit
  - Severe deconditioning
  - Special occupational needs requiring extensive fitness/strengthening
  - Ligamentous injury (whiplash)
  - Head/facial impact in motor vehicle accident
  - Multiple injury sites
  - Craniovertebral instability
  - Referral to PT > 6 weeks post-onset
- Home Program
  - Flexibility exercises for maintenance of postural balance
  - Increase repetitions/intensity and provide strengthening progression to challenge patient's current level and achieve all goals/outcomes
  - Self-mobilization techniques
  - Use of modalities at home as needed for occasional flare-ups
  - Progression/maintenance aerobic endurance
- Monitoring

SUMMARY OVERVIEW | CERVICAL/THORACIC SPINE | CERVICAL/THORACIC GENERAL PAIN   295

CERVICAL/THORACIC GENERAL PAIN

ICD-9

715.90	Osteoarthrosis, unspecified whether generalized or localized, site unspecified
715.98	Osteoarthrosis, unspecified whether generalized or localized, other specified sites
721.0	Cervical spondylosis without myelopathy
723.1	Cervicalgia
724.1	Pain in thoracic spine
729.1	Myalgia and myositis, unspecified
739.1	Nonallopathic lesions, not elsewhere classified, cervical region
739.2	Nonallopathic lesions, not elsewhere classified, thoracic region
840.8	Sprain of other specified sites of shoulder and upper arm
847.0	Neck sprain
847.1	Thoracic sprain

APTA Preferred Practice Pattern: 4B, 4C, 4D, 4E, 4F, 4G, 4H, 4I, 4J, 5F, 6B

EXAMINATION

History and Systems Review

- History of current condition
  - Location, nature, and behavior of symptoms
    - Radiating symptoms
    - Aggravating/relieving factors
  - Presence of cardinal signs
- Past history of current condition
- Other tests and measures
  - X-ray
  - MRI
- Medications
- Past medical/surgical history
  - Inquire regarding areas of possible systemic pathology such as:
    - Heart
    - Lung
    - Liver
    - Gall bladder
    - Kidney
    - Gastrointestinal
- Functional status and activity level (current/prior)
  - Postural tolerance
  - Sleep disruption
  - Vocational activities
  - ADLs
- Patient's functional goals

Tests and Measures

Systems review per APTA's *Guide to Physical Therapy Practice*

- Aerobic capacity and endurance
- Joint integrity and mobility
  - Craniovertebral stability tests
  - C0–T12
- Muscle performance
  - Grip motor performance
  - Key muscle tests C3–T1
  - Resisted
    - Cervical
    - Thoracic
    - Scapular
- Pain
  - Measured on visual analog scale
  - With palpation
- Posture
  - Sitting
  - Standing
  - Vocational/recreational postures
- ROM
  - Cervical/thoracic
    - Active ROM
    - PROM
    - Overpressure
  - Functional ROM
    - Patient demonstrates ability to touch mid-back with the shoulder flexed/externally rotated and extended/internally rotated

296 CERVICAL/THORACIC GENERAL PAIN | CERVICAL/THORACIC SPINE

- Inspiration/expiration in flexion and extension
  These tests are used to assess spinal contribution to symptoms. For example:
  a. If full inspiration (which extends the spine) is painful in extension but not in flexion, the spine is implicated
  b. If it is painful in both full flexion and extension, a costal problem is implied
  c. Applies to forced expiration in full flexion vs. both flexion and extension
- Reflex integrity
  ○ Biceps (C6)
  ○ Triceps (C7)
  ○ Brachioradialis (C5–6)
- Sensory integrity
  ○ Sensation, C3–T1
- Special tests
  ○ Upper limb tension test

Establish Plan of Care
- Based on history, tests, and measures

GOALS/OUTCOMES
- Pain: 2/10 or less
- ROM: At least 80% of AMA guides and equal bilaterally

Cervical	Normal	80%
Flexion	60°	50°
Extension	75°	60°
Rotation	80°	65°
Side bend	45°	35°

Thoracic	Normal	80%
Flexion	40°	30°
Extension	No AMA guides established	
Rotation	30°	25°
Side bend	10°	8°

- Adequate spinal strength and stability to prevent reinjury: 4+/5 on manual muscle test of cervical and scapular muscles
- Return to previous functional status for ADLs and vocational, recreational, and sports activities as identified by patient
- Independence in a progressive home exercise program emphasizing function
- Minimize/resolve any neurological deficits

INTERVENTION
NUMBER OF VISITS: 6–12

Coordination, Communication, and Documentation
- Provision of services between admission and discharge that facilitate cost-effective and efficient integration or reintegration to home, community, or work
- Documentation of therapeutic intervention is required for each episode of care and serves as the basic foundation for communication
- Coordination and additional communication will depend on the patient's impairment and home/work/community/leisure situation and requirements. Such services may include:
  ○ Case management
  ○ Coordination of care and collaboration with those integral to the patient's rehabilitation program
  ○ Coordination and monitoring of the delivery of available resources
  ○ Referrals to other health-care professionals
  ○ Identification of resources, support groups, or advocacy services
  ○ Provision of educational or training information
  ○ Technical assistance

Patient Instruction

Basic Anatomy and Biomechanics
- Anatomy of cervical and thoracic spine
- Mechanism of injury and importance of protection and rehabilitation of the stabilizing structures
- Importance of adequate motor performance, postural alignment, and ROM of the kinetic chain in the alleviation of symptoms
- Distinction between stretching and strengthening exercises
- Pertinent Gray's Anatomy (Gray. 1995. 510-522, 537, 803–805, 807–813, 835–838)

Handouts
- Commercially available products, such as:
  ○ Krames Communications (1100 Grundy Lane, San Bruno, CA 94066):
    - *Neck Basics*
    - *Fit Neck Workout*
    - *Neck Owners Manual*

- McKenzie (PO Box 93, Waikanae, New Zealand)
  - *Treat Your Own Neck*
- Saunders (4250 Norex Drive, Chaska, MN 55318)
  - *For Your Own Neck*
- Home program
  - ROM
  - Stretching
  - Strength/stabilization exercises

Functional Considerations

- Importance of maintaining normal and pain-free cervical and thoracic curves with support during:
  - Sitting
  - Sleeping
  - Driving
  - Speaking
  - Breathing
- Importance of proper body mechanics and limitation/ avoidance of aggravating upper-extremity activity and prolonged head postures
- Stabilization/prevention of reinjury
  - Alteration of ADLs

Direct Interventions

Acute Phase: 3–6 Visits

- Therapeutic exercise and home program
  - Stretching exercises
  - Strengthening exercises as appropriate. Active assistive progressing to active, progressing to resistive
  - Postural awareness and body mechanics training
  - Aerobic exercise for tissue healing
  - Home program
    - Gentle axial extension maintaining
    - Scapular ROM/shoulder rolls
    - Self-positional distraction
    - Home traction
    - Home use of cryotherapy
  - Diaphragmatic breathing and relaxation techniques
  - Supported active exercise in pain-free ROM, supine or standing
    - Scapular
    - Upper extremity
    - Cervical
    - Thoracic
  - Walking or other aerobic exercise as tolerated

- Manual therapy
  - Soft-tissue mobilization
  - Joint mobilization
    - Grades I–II to relieve pain
    - Specific traction at involved segment performed in a position of comfort
    - Grades III–V if needed to hypomobile segments above and below involved segment
    - Positional isometric techniques for ROM and pain reduction
- Electrotherapeutic modalities
- Physical agents and mechanical modalities
  - Superficial thermal/cryotherapy
  - Deep thermal: Ultrasound
  - Mechanical traction
- Goals/outcomes
  - Pain: Reduced 50% from initial rating
  - ROM: 50% of AMA guides and equal bilaterally
    - Cervical
      a. Flexion: 30°
      b. Extension: 40°
      c. Rotation: 40°
      d. Side bend: 25°
    - Thoracic
      a. Flexion: 20°
      b. Extension: No AMA guides established
      c. Rotation: 15°
      d. Side bend: 5°
  - Pain-free postural alignment during rest and basic ADLs
  - Improve cervical stabilization to prevent reinjury

Subacute Phase: 3–6 Visits

- Physical agents and mechanical modalities
  - Continue effective modalities as in acute phase with increased emphasis on use as needed at home
- Manual therapy
  - Soft-tissue techniques
    - Soft-tissue mobilization
    - Trigger-point techniques
    - Strain/counterstrain
    - Myofascial release
    - Friction massage
  - Joint mobilization
    - Progressive Grades III–V to hypomobile joints as indicated
    - Progress graded specific traction to irritable joints

- Manually resisted exercises including proprioceptive neuromuscular facilitation patterns
- Assisted passive techniques
  - Muscle stretching
  - Neural tension
- Therapeutic exercise
  - Continue ROM exercises using increased range
  - Instruct in self-mobilization exercises as appropriate for lower cervical and thoracic regions
  - Initiate self-resisted strengthening exercises or gravity-resisted strengthening exercises as appropriate
    - Cervical isometrics
    - Therapeutic ball exercises
    - Pulley exercises
    - Resistive band
  - Emphasize cardiovascular conditioning with postural balance
    - Upper- and lower-extremity cycling
    - Treadmill/walking program
    - Ski machine
    - Aquatic therapy
- Goals/outcomes
  - Pain: 2/10 or less
  - ROM: At least 80% of AMA guides and equal bilaterally
    - Cervical
      a. Flexion: 50°
      b. Extension: 60°
      c. Rotation: 65°
      d. Side bend: 35°
    - Thoracic
      a. Flexion: 30°
      b. Extension: No AMA guides established
      c. Rotation: 25°
      d. Side bend: 8°
  - Adequate spinal strength and stability to prevent reinjury: 4+/5 on manual muscle test of cervical and scapular muscles
  - Return to previous functional status for ADLs and vocational, recreational, and sports activities as identified by patient

Functional Carryover

- Instruction regarding use of cervical or lumbar support for proper postural alignment during work, driving, and ADLs
- Ergonomic evaluation of the work site if necessary, such as chair, desk height, and computer placement

DISCHARGE PLANNING AND PATIENT RESPONSIBILITY

Criteria for Discharge

- Patient demonstrates independence in home exercise program
- All goals/outcomes have been achieved with the exception of return to previous status for recreational and sports activities
- Patient displays understanding of the role of proper posture and body mechanics in prevention of reinjury

Circumstances Requiring Additional Visits

- Persistent functional strength deficit or 3/5 on manual muscle test
- History of previous injury/surgery to related area
- Persistent radicular symptoms or neurological deficit
- Severe deconditioning
- Special occupational needs requiring extensive fitness/strengthening
- Ligamentous injury (whiplash)
- Head/facial impact in motor vehicle accident
- Multiple injury sites
- Craniovertebral instability
- Referral to PT > 6 weeks post onset

Home Program

- Flexibility exercises for maintenance of postural balance
- Increase repetitions/intensity and provide strengthening progression to challenge patient's current level and achieve all goals/outcomes
- Self-mobilization techniques
- Use of modalities at home as needed for occasional flare-ups
- Progression/maintenance of aerobic endurance

Monitoring

- Instruct patient to call for advice should progression halt or a negative trend occur
- Follow up at 4–8 weeks post-discharge to ensure expected return to function and progression toward attaining all goals/outcomes

CERVICAL/THORACIC SPINE | CERVICAL/THORACIC GENERAL PAIN

REFERENCES

1. American Physical Therapy Association. *Guide to Physical Therapist Practice*. Alexandria, VA: APTA; 1997.

2. Aprill C, Bogduk N. The prevalence of cervical zygapophyseal joint pain: a first approximation. *Spine*. 1992;17:744-747.

3. Assendelft WJ, Bouter LM, Knipschild PG. Complications of spinal manipulation: a comprehensive review of the literature. *J Fam Pract*. 1996;42:475-480.

4. Edmondson S, Allison G, Althorpe B, McConnell D, Samuel K. Comparison of ribcage and posteroanterior thoracic spine stiffness: an investigation of the normal response. *Manual Therapy*. August 1999;4(3):157-62.

5. Gray H; Williams PL, ed. *Gray's Anatomy*, 38th ed. New York, NY: Churchill Livingstone; 1995.

6. Gross AR, Aker PD, Quartly C. Manual therapy in the treatment of neck pain. *Rheum Dis Clin North Am*. 1996;22:579-598.

7. Hart A, Hopkins C, Ford B. *ICD-9-CM Expert For Physicians, Volume 1&2*. 7th ed. USA: Ingenix; 2005.

8. Honet JC, Puri K. Cervical radiculitis: treatment and results in 82 patients. *Arch Phys Med Rehabil*. 1976;57:12-16.

9. Iai H, Moriya H, Goto S, et al. Three-dimensional motion analysis of the upper cervical spine during axial rotation. *Spine*. 1993;18:2388-2392.

10. Jordan A, Bendix T, Nielsen H, Hansen FR, Host D, Winkel A. Intensive training, physiotherapy, or manipulation for patients with chronic neck pain. A prospective, single-blinded, randomized clinical trial. *Spine*. 1998;23:311-318; discussion, 319.

11. Koes BW, Bouter LM, van Mameren H, et al. A randomized clinical trial of manual therapy and physiotherapy for persistent band and neck complaints: subgroup analysis and relationship between outcome measures. *J Manipulative Physiol Ther*. 1993;16:211-219.

12. Lee D. *The Pelvic Girdle*. New York, NY: Churchill Livingstone; 1999:81-143.

13. Lord SM, Barnsley L, Wallis BJ, Bogduk N. Chronic cervical zygapopysial joint pain after whiplash: a placebo controlled prevalence study. *Spine*. 1996;21:1737-1744.

14. McKenzie R. *Treat Your Own Neck*. 2nd ed. Waikanae, New Zealand: Spinal Publications; 1983.

15. Nakajima M, Hirayama K. Midcervical central cord syndrome: numb and clumsy hands due to midline cervical disk protrusion at the C3-4 intervertebral level. *J Neurol Neurosurg Psychiatry*. 1995;58:607-613.

16. Pearson ND, Walmsley RP. Trial into the effects of repeated neck retractions in normal subjects. *Spine*. 1995;20:1245-1251.

17. Rheault W, Albright B, Byers C, et al. Intertester reliability of the cervical ROM device. *J Orthop Sports Phys Ther*. 1992;13(3):147-150.

18. Richardson C, Jull G, Hodges P, Hide S. *Therapeutic Exercises For Spinal Segmental Stabilization In Low Back Pain*. New York, NY: Churchill Livingstone; 1999.

19. Riddle DL, Stratford PW. Use of generic versus region-specific functional status measures on patients with cervical spine disorders. *Phys Ther*. 1998;78:951-963.

20. Sandmark H, Nisell R. Validity of five neck pain provoking tests. *Scand J Rehabil Med*. 1995;27(3):131-136.

21. Saunders HD. *Self-help Manual For Your Neck*. Chaska, MN: The Saunders Group, Inc; 1992.

22. Saunders HD. Use of spinal traction in the treatment of neck and back conditions. *Clin Orthop* 1983:31-38.

23. Senter BS. Cervical discogenic syndrome: a cause of chronic head and neck pain. *J Miss State Med Assoc*. 1995;36:231-234.

24. Sran M, Khan K, Zhu Q, McKay H, Oxlan T. Failure characteristics of the thoracic spine with a posterioranterior load: investigating the safety of spinal mobilization. *Spine*. November 2004;29(21):2382-8.

25. Swezey RL. Chronic neck pain. *Rheum Dis Clin North Am*. 1996;22:411-437.

26. Taylor JR, Twomey LT. Acute injuries to cervical joints: an autopsy study of neck sprain. *Spine*. 1993;18:1115-1122.

27. Vleeming A, Mooney V, Dorman T, Snyders C, Stoeckart R. *Movement, Stability and Low Back Pain*. New York, NY: Churchill Livingstone; 1997.

28. Yoo JU, Zou D, Edwards WT, Bayley J, Yuan HA. Effect of cervical spine motion on the neuroforaminal dimensions of human cervical spine. *Spine*. 1992;17:1131-1136.

29. Youdas JW, Carey JR, Garrett TR. Reliability of measurements of cervical spine ROM—comparison of three methods. *Phys Ther*. 1991;71:98-104; discussion, 105-106.

30. Youdas JW, Garrett TR, Suman VJ, et al. Normal ROM of the cervical spine: an initial goniometric study. *Phys Ther*. 1992;72:770-780.

CERVICAL DISC PATHOLOGY
SUMMARY OVERVIEW

ICD-9

722.0   722.4   722.71   723.4

APTA Preferred Practice Pattern: **4A, 4B, 4F, 4G, 4H, 4J, 5F**

EXAMINATION

- History and Systems Review
  Systems review per APTA's *Guide to Physical Therapy Practice*
- Tests and Measures
  - Joint integrity and mobility
  - Muscle performance
  - Pain
  - Posture
  - ROM
  - Reflex integrity
  - Sensory integrity
- Establish Plan of Care

GOALS/OUTCOMES

- Centralized pain: 2/10 or less with alleviation of radicular signs and symptoms
- ROM: at least 80% of AMA guides and equal bilaterally
- Balanced posture (head position, shoulder position, and spinal curvatures) and understanding of in-postural effects on condition
- Spinal strength and stability to prevent reinjury: 4+/5 on manual muscle test of the cervical and scapular muscles
- Return to previous functional status for ADLs and vocational, recreational, and sports activities as identified by patient
- Independence in a progressive home exercise program emphasizing function
- Minimize neurological deficits
- Symmetrical cervical rotation and side flexion

INTERVENTION
NUMBER OF VISITS: 6–12

- Patient Instruction
  - Basic Anatomy and Biomechanics
  - Handouts
  - Functional Considerations

- Direct Interventions
  - Acute Phase: 3–6 Visits
  - Subacute Phase: 3–6 Visits
- Functional Carryover

DISCHARGE PLANNING AND PATIENT RESPONSIBILITY

- Criteria for Discharge
  - Patient displays understanding of the role of proper posture and body mechanics in the prevention of reinjury
  - All goals/outcomes have been achieved with the exception of a return to previous functional status for recreational and sports activities
- Circumstances Requiring Additional Visits
  - Persistent functional strength deficit or 3/5 on manual muscle test
  - History of previous injury/surgery to related area
  - Persistent radicular symptoms or neurological deficit
  - Severe deconditioning
  - Special occupational needs requiring extensive fitness/ strengthening
  - Restriction in segmental joint mobility
  - Surgery is indicated, however the patient is not a surgical candidate due to risk factors
  - Bilateral upper-extremity radiculopathy
  - Presence of fracture
  - Deferred referral to PT > 6 weeks since onset
  - Inability to maintain normal posture
  - Inhibition of soft tissue that does not allow normal mobility
- Home Program
  - Flexibility exercises for maintenance of postural balance
  - Increase repetitions/intensity and provide strengthening progression
  - Self-mobilization techniques
  - Use of modalities at home
  - Use of home traction on as-needed basis
  - Progression/maintenance of aerobic endurance
  - Sleeping postures/positions
  - Correct breathing pattern instruction
- Monitoring

SUMMARY OVERVIEW | CERVICAL/THORACIC SPINE | CERVICAL DISC PATHOLOGY   301

CERVICAL DISC PATHOLOGY

ICD-9

722.0	Displacement of cervical intervertebral disc without myelopathy
722.4	Degeneration of cervical intervertebral disc
722.71	Intervertebral disc disorder with myelopathy, cervical region
723.4	Brachial neuritis or radiculitis NOS

APTA Preferred Practice Pattern: 4A, 4B, 4F, 4G, 4H, 4J, 5F

EXAMINATION

History and Systems Review

- History of current condition
  - Presence of cardinal signs
  - Location, nature, and behavior of symptoms
    - Aggravating/relieving factors (postural, motions, ADLs)
    - Radiating symptoms
- Past history of current condition
  - Involvement of other spinal or upper-extremity joints
  - Therapeutic intervention
- Other tests and measures
  - X-ray
  - MRI
- Medications
- Past medical/surgical history
  - Systemic pathology
    - Heart
    - Lung
    - Liver
    - Gall bladder
    - Kidney
    - Gastrointestinal
- Functional status and activity level (current/prior)
  - Effect on sleep
  - Independent mobility, such as driving
  - Work and ADL postural tolerance
- Patient's functional goals

Tests and Measures

Systems review per APTA's *Guide to Physical Therapy Practice*

- Joint integrity and mobility
  - C0–T6
  - Craniovertebral stability tests

- Muscle performance
  - Key muscle tests, C3–T1
  - Resisted
    - Cervical
    - Thoracic
    - Scapular
  - Grip strength
- Pain
  - Measured on visual analog scale
  - With palpation
- Posture
  - Static
  - Dynamic
- ROM
  - Cervical/thoracic
  - Active ROM
  - PROM
  - Overpressure
  - Functional ROM
  - Patient demonstrates ability to touch mid-back with the shoulder flexed/externally rotated and extended/internally rotated
- Reflex integrity
  - Biceps (C6)
  - Triceps (C7)
  - Brachioradialis (C5–6)
  - Hoffman's
  - Babinski
  - Clonus
- Sensory integrity
  - Sensation, C5–T1

Establish Plan of Care

- Based on history, tests, and measures

GOALS/OUTCOMES

- Centralized pain: 2/10 or less with alleviation of radicular signs and symptoms
- ROM to at least 80% of AMA guides and equal bilaterally

Cervical	Normal	80%
Flexion	60°	50°
Extension	75°	60°
Rotation	80°	65°
Side bend	45°	35°

Thoracic	Normal	80%
Flexion	40°	30°
Extension	No AMA guides established	
Rotation	30°	25°
Side bend	10°	8°

- Balanced posture (head position, shoulder position, and spinal curvatures) and understanding of in-postural effects on condition
- Spinal strength and stability to prevent reinjury: 4+/5 on manual muscle test of the cervical and scapular muscles
- Return to previous functional status for ADLs and vocational, recreational, and sports activities as identified by patient
- Independence in a progressive home exercise program emphasizing function
- Minimize neurological deficits
- Symmetrical cervical rotation and side flexion

INTERVENTION
NUMBER OF VISITS: 6–12

Coordination, Communication, and Documentation

- Provision of services between admission and discharge that facilitate cost-effective and efficient integration or reintegration to home, community, or work
- Documentation of therapeutic intervention is required for each episode of care and serves as the basic foundation for communication
- Coordination and additional communication will depend on the patient's impairment and home/work/community/leisure situation and requirements. Such services may include:
  - Case management
  - Coordination of care and collaboration with those integral to the patient's rehabilitation program
  - Coordination and monitoring of the delivery of available resources
  - Referrals to other health-care professionals
  - Identification of resources, support groups, or advocacy services
  - Provision of educational or training information
  - Technical assistance

Patient Instruction

Idea of "centralization" of symptoms vs. aggravation of radiating signs and symptoms: A sudden change or progression of neurological signs necessitates consultation with physician.

Basic Anatomy and Biomechanics

- Anatomy of cervical and thoracic spine: vertebrae, discs, nerve roots, and soft tissues
  - Pertinent Gray's Anatomy (Gray. 1995. 510-518, 537, 803–804, 807–813, 835–888)
- Mechanism of injury/dysfunction and importance of protection and rehabilitation of the stabilizing structures

Handouts

- Commercially available products, such as:
  - Krames Communications (1100 Grundy Lane, San Bruno, CA 94066):
    - *Neck Basics*
    - *Neck Exercises for a Healthy Neck*
    - *Neck Owner's Manual*
    - *Fit Neck Workout*
    - *Cervical Disc Surgery*
  - McKenzie (PO Box 93, Waikanae, New Zealand)
    - *Treat Your Own Neck*
  - Saunders (4250 Norex Drive, Chaska, MN 55318)
    - *For Your Neck*
- Home program
  - ROM
  - Flexibility
  - Self mobilization
  - Stabilization
  - Exercises as appropriate
  - Future self-care program

Functional Considerations

- Importance of maintaining normal and pain-free cervical and thoracic curves with support during:
  - Sitting/driving

- Sleeping
- Walking
- Importance of utilizing proper body mechanics; limitation/avoidance of aggravating upper-extremity or cervical activities and prolonged head postures, such as:
  - Lifting
  - Overhead activity
  - Reading, television, phone, movies
  - Workstation postures

Direct Interventions

Acute Phase: 3–6 Visits
- Therapeutic exercise
  - ROM
  - Stretching exercises
  - Strengthening exercises as appropriate: Active assistive, progressing to active, progressing to resistive
  - Postural awareness and body mechanics training
  - Neuromuscular re-education of longus coli, serratus anterior, scalenes, etc.
  - Aerobic exercises for tissue healing
  - Home program
    - Gentle axial extension maintaining normal cervical curvature
    - Scapular ROM/shoulder rolls
    - Self-positional distraction
    - Home traction
    - Home use of cryotherapy
- Manual therapy techniques
  - Soft-tissue mobilization
  - Joint mobilization
    - Grade I or II with intent of pain relief
    - Specific traction at involved segment performed in a position of comfort
    - Grades III–V if necessary to hypomobile segments above and below involved segment. Must be able to maintain comfort/stability at involved segment.
- Electrotherapeutic modalities
- Physical agents and mechanical modalities
  - Superficial thermal/cryotherapy
  - Deep thermal: Ultrasound
  - Traction
    - Static mechanical
- Goals/outcomes
  - Pain: ⅔–½ of initial rating
  - Centralize radicular signs and symptoms

- Cervical ROM to 60% of AMA guides:
  - Flexion: 35°
  - Extension: 45°
  - Rotation: 50°
  - Side bend: 30°
- Improve postural awareness and body mechanics as evidenced by avoidance of symptom aggravation with daily activity
- Prevent reinjury
- Independent in home program for symptom management, flexibility, and strengthening. Exercise as appropriate.

Subacute Phase: 3–6 Visits
- Therapeutic exercise
  - Stretching program for cervical, thoracic, and upper extremities
  - Aerobic endurance
    - Upper body ergometer
    - Walking
    - Treadmill
    - Stationary bike
    - Stair machine
    - Ski machine
  - Neuromuscular reeducation/proprioceptive/balance training
  - Stabilization activities
  - Strengthening exercises, resisted
    - Cervical isometrics
    - Concentric and eccentric strengthening
    - Cervical/thoracic/scapular therapeutic ball exercises
    - Upper-extremity diagonal patterns
  - Home traction
  - Home program
- Manual therapy techniques
  - Soft-tissue techniques
    - Soft-tissue mobilization
    - Trigger-point techniques
    - Myofascial release
    - Strain/counterstrain

304   CERVICAL DISC PATHOLOGY | CERVICAL/THORACIC SPINE

- Joint mobilization
  - Grades III–V to appropriate cervical and thoracic segments
  - Specific traction at involved segment, progressing from position of comfort to restoration of normal segmental mobility
  - Dural-neural mobilization techniques
- Physical agents and mechanical modalities
  - Continue effective modalities as in acute phase, with increased emphasis on use as needed at home
- Goals/outcomes
  - To include exercises as above as appropriate
  - Centralize pain: 2/10 or less with alleviation of radicular signs and symptoms
  - ROM at least 80% of AMA guides and equal bilaterally
    - Cervical
      a. Flexion: 50°
      b. Extension: 60°
      c. Rotation: 65°
      d. Side bend: 35°
    - Thoracic
      a. Flexion: 30°
      b. Rotation: 25°
      c. Side bend: 8°
  - Grip strength: Within 10% of uninvolved extremity
  - Balanced posture (head position, shoulder position, and spinal curvatures)
  - Spinal strength and stability to prevent reinjury: 4/5 on manual muscle test of the cervical and scapular muscles
  - Return to previous functional status for ADLs and vocational activities

Functional Carryover

- Integration of home exercise program into vocational environment
- Completion of ergonomic adjustments to home, automobile, and vocational areas
- Incorporation of proper posture and body mechanics to avoid exacerbation of symptoms
- Recognition/avoidance of activities that increase or exacerbate radiating symptoms

DISCHARGE PLANNING AND PATIENT RESPONSIBILITY

Criteria for Discharge

- Patient displays understanding of the role of proper posture and body mechanics in the prevention of reinjury
- All goals/outcomes have been achieved with the exception of a return to previous functional status for recreational and sports activities

Circumstances Requiring Additional Visits

- Persistent functional strength deficit or 3/5 on manual muscle test
- History of previous injury/surgery to related area
- Persistent radicular symptoms or neurological deficit
- Severe deconditioning
- Special occupational needs requiring extensive fitness/strengthening
- Restriction in segmental joint mobility
- Surgery is indicated, however the patient is not a surgical candidate due to risk factors
- Bilateral upper-extremity radiculopathy
- Presence of fracture
- Deferred referral to PT > 6 weeks since onset
- Inability to maintain normal posture
- Inhibition of soft tissue that does not allow normal mobility

Home Program

- Flexibility exercises for maintenance of postural balance
- Increase repetitions/intensity and provide strengthening progression to challenge patient's current level and achieve all goals/outcomes
- Self-mobilization techniques
- Use of modalities at home as needed for occasional flare-ups
- Use of home traction on as-needed basis
- Progression/maintenance of aerobic endurance
- Sleeping postures/positions
- Correct breathing pattern instruction

Monitoring

- Instruct patient to call for advice should progression halt or a negative trend occur
- Follow up at 4–8 weeks post-discharge to ensure expected return to function and progression toward attaining all goals/outcomes

REFERENCES

1. American Physical Therapy Association. *Guide to Physical Therapist Practice*. Alexandria, VA: APTA; 1997.

2. Assendelft WJ, Bouter LM, Knipschild PG. Complications of spinal manipulation: a comprehensive review of the literature. *J Fam Pract*. 1996;42:475-480.

3. Basmajian JV, Nyberg R, eds. Rational manual therapies. Baltimore, MD: Williams & Wilkins; 1993.

4. Bland JH, Boushey DR. Anatomy and physiology of the cervical spine. *Arthritis Rheum*. 1990;20(1):1-20.

5. Cipriano JJ. *Photographic Manual of Regional Orthopedic and Neurological Tests*. 2nd ed. Baltimore, MD: Williams & Wilkins; 1991.

6. Cyriax JH, Cyriax PJ. *Cyriax's Illustrated Manual of Orthopedic Medicine*. 2nd ed. Boston, MA: Butterworth-Heinemann; 1993.

7. Dalton PA, Tull GA. The distribution and characteristics of neck-arm pain in patients with and without a neurological deficit. *Aust J Physiother*. 1989;35:3-8.

8. Gilman S, Newman SW. *Manter and Gatz's Essentials of Clinical Neuroanatomy and Neurophysiology*. 7th ed. Philadelphia, PA: FA Davis; 1987.

9. Gray H; Williams PL, ed. *Gray's Anatomy*, 38th ed. New York, NY: Churchill Livingstone; 1995.

10. Gross AR, Aker PD, Quartly C. Manual therapy in the treatment of neck pain. *Rheum Dis Clin of North Am*. 1996;22:579-598.

11. Guyton AC. Basic neuroscience: anatomy and physiology. Philadelphia, PA: WB Saunders; 1987.

12. Hart A, Hopkins C, Ford B. *ICD-9-CM Expert For Physicians, Volume 1&2*. 7th ed. USA: Ingenix; 2005.

13. Honet JC, Puri K. Cervical radiculitis: treatment and results in 82 patients. *Arch Phys Med Rehabil*.1976;57:12-16.

14. Hoppenfeld S. Physical examination of the spine and extremities. Norwalk, CT: Appleton-Century-Crofts; 1976.

15. Jordan A, Bendix T, Nielsen H, et al. Intensive training, physiotherapy, or manipulation for patients with chronic neck pain. A prospective, single-blinded, randomized clinical trial. *Spine*. 1998;23:311-318; discussion 319.

16. Kendall FP, McCreary EK. *Muscles: Testing and Function*. 3rd ed. Baltimore, MD: Williams & Wilkins; 1983.

17. Kessler RM, Hertling D. *Management of Common Musculoskeletal Disorders: Physical Therapy Principles and Methods*. Philadelphia, PA: Harper & Row; 1983.

18. McKenzie R. *Treat Your Own Neck*. 2nd ed. Waikanae, New Zealand: Spinal Publications; 1983.

19. Morishita Y, Hide S, Naito M, Matsushima U. Evaluation of cervical spondylotic myelopathy using somatosensory-evoked potentials. *Int Orthop*. December 2005;29(6):343-6.

20. Maitland GD. *Vertebral manipulation*. 5th ed. Boston, MA: Butterworths; 1986.

21. Nakajima M, Hirayama K. Midcervical central cord syndrome: numb and clumsy hands due to midline cervical disk protrusion at the C3-4 intervertebral level. *J Neurol Neurosurg Psychiatry*. 1995;58:607-613.

22. Panjabi MM, Ito S, Pearson A, Ivancic P. Injury mechanisms of the cervical intervertebral disc during simulated whiplash. *Spine*. June 2004;29(11):1217-25.

23. Riddle DL, Stratford PW. Use of generic versus region-specific functional status measures on patients with cervical spine disorders. *Phys Ther*. 1998;78:951-963.

24. Sandmark H, Nisell R. Validity of five common manual neck pain provoking tests. *Scand J Rehabil Med*. 1995;27(3):131-136.

25. Saunders HD. *Evaluation, Treatment, and Prevention of Musculoskeletal Disorders*. Minneapolis, MN: Viking Press; 1988.

26. Saunders HD. Use of spinal traction in the treatment of neck and back conditions. *Clin Orthop Rel Res*. 1983:31-38.

27. Senter BS. Cervical discogenic syndrome: a cause of chronic head and neck pain. *J Miss State Med Assoc*. 1995;36:231-234.

28. Swezey RL. Chronic neck pain. *Rheum Dis Clin North Am*. 1996;22:411-437.

29. Youdas JW, Carey JR, Garrett TR. Reliability of measurements of cervical spine ROM: comparison of three methods. *Phys Ther*. 1991;71:98-104; discussion 105-106.

30. Youdas JW, Garrett TR, Suman VJ, et al. Normal ROM of the cervical spine: an initial goniometric study. *Phys Ther*. 1992;72:770-780.

CERVICAL SPONDYLOLYSIS WITH MYELOPATHY
SUMMARY OVERVIEW

ICD-9

721.1   721.91

APTA Preferred Practice Pattern: 4F, 5H, 4I

EXAMINATION

- History and Systems Review
- Tests and Measures
  Systems review per APTA's *Guide to Physical Therapy Practice*
  - Circulation
  - Cranial and peripheral nerve integrity
  - Environmental, home, and work barriers
  - Ergonomics and body mechanics
  - Gait, locomotion, and balance
  - Joint integrity and mobility
  - Motor function
  - Muscle performance
  - Pain
  - Posture
  - ROM
  - Reflex integrity
  - Self-care and home management
  - Sensory integrity
  - Work (job/school/play), community, and leisure integration or reintegration
- Establish Plan of Care

GOALS/OUTCOMES

- Pain: 2/10 or less and absence of radiating symptoms
- Cervical and thoracic ROM: 80% of AMA guidelines
- Functional spinal stability and endurance: Able to tolerate postural requirements of work, recreation, and household duties
- Spine, scapular, and upper-extremity strength 4+/5 manual muscle test
- Return to previous functional status for all ADLs including sports, recreation, and vocational activities
- Independence with home exercise program
- Negative upper-limb tension tests
- Grip strength to be restored to 90% of the uninvolved side
- Restore normal breathing patterns
- Lumbopelvic stability

INTERVENTION
NUMBER OF VISITS: 5–10

- Patient Instruction
  - Basic Anatomy and Biomechanics
  - Handouts
  - Functional Considerations
- Direct Interventions
  - Acute Phase: 1–4 Visits
  - Subacute Phase: 4–6 Visits
- Functional Carryover

DISCHARGE PLANNING AND PATIENT RESPONSIBILITY

- Criteria for Discharge
  - All goals have been met in the subacute phase
  - Patient has returned to work, daily ADLs without aggravation of symptoms
  - Patient demonstrates a level of independence with ADLs and return to work
  - Patient returns to sports activities
  - Patient has no radicular symptoms or radiating symptoms into upper extremities
  - Patient demonstrates independence with home exercise program
  - Patient understands biomechanics and is aware of what activities to avoid secondary to symptoms/limitations/weakness
- Circumstances Requiring Additional Visits
  - Severe degenerative changes
  - History of other upper-quadrant pathology
  - Presence of other medical conditions influencing cell healing, muscle tone, or upper-quadrant posture
  - Contractures of the musculoskeletal system
  - Cognitive limitations or impairments
  - Postoperative complications
  - Excessive environmental barriers to discharge
- Home Program
  - Provide an individually developed written home exercise instruction, complete with pictures and text explanations
  - Home program should be based on functional goals
- Monitoring

SUMMARY OVERVIEW | CERVICAL/THORACIC SPINE | CERVICAL SPONDYLOLYSIS WITH MYELOPATHY   307

CERVICAL SPONDYLOLYSIS WITH MYELOPATHY

ICD-9:

    721.1   Cervical spondylosis with myelopathy

    721.91   Spondylosis of unspecified site, with myelopathy

APTA Preferred Practice Pattern: 4F, 5H, 4I

EXAMINATION

History and Systems Review

- History of current condition
- Past history of current and related conditions
- Other tests and measures
- Medications
- Past medical/surgical history
- Functional status and activity level (current/prior), including any upper-extremity functional limitations
- Patient's functional goals

Tests and Measures

Systems review per APTA's *Guide to Physical Therapy Practice*

- Circulation (arterial, venous, lymphatic) of the upper quadrant
- Cranial and peripheral nerve integrity
- Environmental, home, and work (job/school/play) barriers
- Ergonomics and body mechanics, especially as they relate to sitting and upper-extremity function
- Gait, locomotion, and balance
- Joint integrity and mobility of the cervical and thoracic spine, as well as the rib cage and, in some cases, the lumbopelvic ring
- Motor function (motor control and motor learning) of the deep neck flexors, cervical movers, thoracic and rib control system, and the scalar stabilization system
- Muscle performance (including strength, power, and endurance) of all upper-extremity functions
- Pain
- Posture in sitting, standing, walking, and over head activities
- ROM (including muscle length) of the cervical, thoracic, and lumbar spine, as well as all motions of the upper extremity
- Reflex integrity
  - Levator scapula (C4)
  - Deltoid (C5)
  - Biceps (C6)
  - Triceps (C7)
- Self-care and home management (including ADLs and instrumental ADLs)
- Sensory integrity biased to the upper extremities, cervical spine, and upper thoracic spine
- Work (job/school/play), community, and leisure integration or reintegration (including instrumental ADLs)

Establish Plan of Care

- Based on history, tests, and measures

GOALS/OUTCOMES

- Pain: 2/10 or less and absence of radiating symptoms
- Cervical and thoracic ROM: 80% of AMA guidelines
- Functional spinal stability and endurance: Able to tolerate postural requirements of work, recreation, and household duties
- Spine, scapular, and upper-extremity strength: 4+/5 on manual muscle test
- Return to previous functional status for all ADLs, including sports, recreation, and vocational activities
- Independence with home exercise program
- Negative upper limb tension tests
- Grip strength to be restored to 90% of the uninvolved side
- Restore normal breathing patterns
- Lumbopelvic stability

INTERVENTION

NUMBER OF VISITS: 5–10

Coordination, Communication, and Documentation

- Provision of services between admission and discharge that facilitate cost-effective and efficient integration or reintegration to home, community, or work

308   CERVICAL SPONDYLOLYSIS WITH MYELOPATHY | CERVICAL/THORACIC SPINE

- Documentation of therapeutic intervention is required for each episode of care and serves as the basic foundation for communication
- Coordination and additional communication will depend on the patient's impairment and home/work/community/leisure situation and requirements. Such services may include:
  - Case management
  - Coordination of care and collaboration with those integral to the patient's rehabilitation program
  - Coordination and monitoring of the delivery of available resources
  - Referrals to other health-care professionals
  - Identification of resources, support groups, or advocacy services
  - Provision of educational or training information
  - Technical Assistance

Patient Instruction

Basic Anatomy and Biomechanics
- Cervical spine
  - Vertebrae
  - Disc
  - Nerve root compression signs and symptoms
  - Soft tissue
  - Spinal cord
- Pertinent Gray's Anatomy (Gray, 1995. 510-518, 537, 803–805, 807–813, 835–838)
- Importance of segmental stabilization and protection (vertebrae, ligamentous structures, peripheral nerves, disc material, soft tissue)
- Etiologies of spondylolysis with myelopathy

Handouts
- Commercially available products, such as:
  - Krames Communications (1100 Grundy Lane, San Bruno CA 94066
    - *Neck Basics*
    - *Neck Exercises For The Healthy Neck*
    - *Neck Owner's Manual*
    - *Fit Neck Workout*
    - *Cervical Disc Surgery*
  - McKenzie (PO Box 93, Waikanae, New Zealand)
    - *Treat Your Own Neck*

- Home program
  - Home exercise program should begin with initial treatment, should be developed individually, and should be specifically based on treatment and condition progression
  - Final routine to be set up with guidelines/timelines for independent exercise and return to gym when appropriate
  - Functional considerations to include:
    - Maintaining proper posture
    - Maintaining full cervical and thoracic ROM
    - Improving lumbopelvic stability and function
    - Correct postures during sleep, walking, sitting, etc.
    - Specific instruction on how to minimize or avoid lifting, overhead work, reading, and workstation posture that may aggravate existing condition

Functional Considerations
- Posture (sitting, standing, sleeping, driving): Consider an ergonomic assessment of work station
- Assistive devices: Temporary use of a soft collar may assist in early symptom reduction (collars)
- Precautions: Closely monitor for progressing neurological signs and symptoms
- Alteration of ADLs to unload cervical and thoracic spine
- Avoidance of prolonged postures, especially sitting
- Positioning for relief of symptoms
- Body mechanic instruction for lifting, pushing, pulling, etc.
- Training recommendations to maintain or improve cardiovascular activity to promote systemic cell health

Direct Interventions

Acute Phase: 1–4 Visits
- Therapeutic exercise and activities
  - Cervical and thoracic PROM and AROM activities in a pain-free ROM
  - Shoulder AROM activities in a pain-free ROM
  - Postural awareness and body mechanics instruction
  - Home exercise program: Diaphragmatic breathing and relaxation work, cervical AROM in a pain-free ROM, shoulder rolls (posterior to prevent shrugging), home traction (instruction to family member or friend), postural correction

- Manual therapy
  - Soft-tissue mobilization—to affected soft tissue in neck, upper back, and shoulders, myofascial release
  - Joint mobilization—Grade I–II for pain relief. Direction of mobilization to open foramina, reducing pressure on nerve root, Grade II–V mobilization to uninvolved segments. Contraindications of joint mobilization to include radicular symptoms or upper cervical dysfunction.
  - Assisted stretching to cervical and thoracic soft tissue
  - Neural tension techniques in a pain-free ROM (when decreasing radicular signs are present)
- Modalities
  - Ultrasound, interferential current, TENS unit, cryotherapy, mechanical traction (when no instability is present)
- Goals/outcomes
  - Pain: Reduced by 50% from initial rating by patient
  - Cervical and thoracic ROM
    - To be 50% of AMA guidelines for both regions

Subacute Phase: 4–6 Visits

- Therapeutic exercise and activities
  - Cervical and thoracic, scapular and shoulder AROM
  - Upper quadrant exercise with emphasis to thoracic and scapula movement corrective patterning
  - Lower quadrant exercise to create a stable lumbopelvic region
  - Mutli-plane stretching to facilitate proper function and alignment
  - Cardiovascular exercises that do not produce compromised postural changes
  - Therapeutic activities to improve tolerance to prolonged postures, sleep, work, and recreational activities
  - Neuromuscular training with proper cervical rotation, side bending, flexion, and extension
  - Breathing, corrective exercise training (e.g. capnography)
- Manual therapy work
  - Soft-tissue mobilization through myofascial and neural fascial techniques
  - Articular mobilizations Grade II–V to the lumbopelvic region, thoracic and cervical spine to facilitate proper alignment and function (avoiding manipulations to unstable or hypermobile segments)

- Neuromuscular training with an emphasis to up-training the longus coli and down-training the global musculature
- Modalities
  - Ultrasound, interferential current, TENS, cryotherapy, and mechanical traction (dependent on patient tolerance and absence of cervical instability)
- Goals/outcomes
  - Pain: 2/10 or less and absence of radicular symptoms into upper extremity
  - AROM to be 80% of AMA guidelines for the cervical and thoracic spine
  - Strength to be 4+/5 or better in all upper-extremity manual muscle tests
  - Negative upper limb tension testing

Functional Carryover

- Integration of home exercise program into vocational environment
- Completion of ergonomic adjustments to home, automobile, and vocational areas
- Incorporation of proper posture and body mechanics to avoid exacerbation of symptoms
- Recognition/avoidance of activities that increase or exacerbate radiating symptoms, especially with overhead activities

DISCHARGE PLANNING AND PATIENT RESPONSIBILITY

Criteria for Discharge

- All goals have been met in the sub-acute phase
- Patient has returned to work, daily ADLs without aggravation of symptoms
- Patient demonstrates a level of independence with ADLs and return to work
- Patient returns to sports activities
- Patient has no radicular symptoms or radiating symptoms into upper extremities
- Patient demonstrates an independence with home exercise program
- Patient understands biomechanics and has an awareness of what activities to avoid secondary to symptoms/limitations/weakness

Circumstances Requiring Additional Visits

- Severe degenerative changes
- History of other upper-quadrant pathology
- Presence of other medical conditions influencing cell healing, muscle tone, or upper-quadrant posture
- Contractures of the musculoskeletal system
- Cognitive limitations or impairments
- Postoperative complications
- Excessive environmental barriers to discharge

Home Program

- Provide an individually developed written home exercise instruction, complete with pictures and text explanations
- A home program should be based on functional goals

Monitoring

- Instruct the patient to call or email for advice if the condition persists or is aggravated
- The clinician may elect to schedule a follow-up visit at the expected time of readiness for exercise progression

REFERENCES

1. American Physical Therapy Association. *Guide to Physical Therapist Practice.* Alexandria, VA: APTA; revised 2003.
2. Gray H; Williams PL, ed. *Gray's Anatomy.* 38th ed. New York, NY: Churchill Livingstone; 1995.
3. Gross AR, Aker PD, Quartly C. Manual therapy in the treatment of neck pain. *Rheum Dis Clin North Am.* 1996;22:579-598.
4. Hart A, Hopkins C, Ford B. *ICD-9-CM Expert For Physicians, Volume 1&2.* 7th ed. USA: Ingenix; 2005.
5. Levine DN. Pathogenesis of cervical spondylotic myelopathy. *J Neurol Neurosurg Psychiatry.* April 1997;62(4):334-340.
6. McKenzie R. *Treat Your Own Neck.* 2nd ed. Waikanae, New Zealand: Spinal Publications; 1983.
7. Nordin M, Frankel VH. *Basic Biomechanics of The Musculoskeletal System.* Malvern, PA: Lea & Febiger; 1989.
8. Meadows J. *Orthopedic Differential Diagnosis In Physical Therapy: A Case Study Approach.* New York, NY: McGraw-Hill; 1999.
9. Orr RD, Zdeblick TA. Cervical spondylotic myelopathy. Approaches to surgical treatment. *Clin Orthop Related Res.* February 1999; (359):58-66.
10. Riddle DL, Stratford PW. Use of generic versus region—specific functional status measures on patients with cervical spine disorders. *Phys Ther.* 1998;78:951-963.
11. Youdas JW, Carey JR, Garrett TR. Reliability of measurements of cervical spine ROM: comparison of three methods. *Phys Ther.* 1991;71:98-104; discussions 105-106.
12. Youdas JW, Garrett TR, Suman VJ, et al. Normal ROM of the cervical spine: an initial goniometric study. *Phys. Ther.* 1992;72:770-780.

312   CERVICAL SPONDYLOLYSIS WITH MYELOPATHY | CERVICAL/THORACIC SPINE

CERVICAL STENOSIS
SUMMARY OVERVIEW

ICD 9:

723.0

APTA Preferred Practice Pattern: **4G**

EXAMINATION

- History and Systems Review
- Tests and Measures
  Systems review per APTA's *Guide to Physical Therapy Practice*
  - Joint integrity and mobility
  - Muscle performance
  - Pain
  - Posture
  - ROM
  - Reflex integrity
  - Sensory integrity
  - Special tests
- Establish Plan of Care

GOALS/OUTCOMES

- Pain: 2/10 or less and absence of radiating symptoms with ADLs
- Cervical and thoracic ROM: At least 80% of AMA guides
- Functional spinal stability and endurance as evidenced by symptom-free tolerance of postural requirements during normal ADLs and vocational activities
- Spinal and scapular strength: 4+/5 on manual muscle test
- Return to previous functional status for ADLs and vocational, recreational, and sports activities as identified by patient
- Independence in a progressive home exercise program emphasizing function
- Negative upper-limb tension signs

INTERVENTION
NUMBER OF VISITS: 7–12

- Patient Instruction
  - Basic Anatomy and Biomechanics
  - Handouts
  - Functional Considerations
- Direct Interventions
  - Acute Phase: 4–6 Visits
  - Subacute Phase: 3–6 Visits
- Functional Carryover

DISCHARGE PLANNING AND PATIENT RESPONSIBILITY

- Criteria for Discharge
  - All goals/outcomes have been achieved with the exception of return to previous recreational and sports activities
  - Demonstrates independence in home program and exercise program
  - Displays understanding of role of posture and body mechanics in avoidance of re-aggravation
- Circumstances Requiring Additional Visits
  - Persistent functional strength deficit or 3/5 on manual muscle test
  - History of previous injury/surgery to related area
  - Persistent radicular symptoms or neurological deficit
  - Severe deconditioning
  - Special occupational needs requiring extensive fitness/strengthening
  - Unable to maintain normal head/neck posture
  - Presence of lower-extremity signs and symptoms
  - Arthritic conditions
  - Significant loss of cervical-thoracic junction mobility
- Home Program
  - Modalities as needed
  - Flexibility exercises and strengthening progression incorporating posture correction techniques
  - Cardiovascular conditioning
  - Home traction
- Monitoring

SUMMARY OVERVIEW | CERVICAL/THORACIC SPINE | CERVICAL STENOSIS   313

CERVICAL STENOSIS

ICD 9:

    723.0   Spinal stenosis in cervical region

APTA Preferred Practice Pattern: 4G

EXAMINATION

History and Systems Review

- History of current condition
  - Location, nature, and behavior of symptoms
    - Aggravating/relieving factors
    - Radiating symptoms
  - Presence of cardinal signs
- Past history of current condition
  - Involvement of other spinal or upper-extremity joints
  - Therapeutic intervention
- Other tests and measures
  - X-ray
  - MRI
  - Scans
- Past medical/surgical history
- Functional status and activity level (current/prior)
  - Work and ADL postural tolerance
  - Independent mobility
- Patient's functional goals

Tests and Measures

Systems review per APTA's *Guide to Physical Therapy Practice*

- Joint integrity and mobility
  - Craniovertebral stability tests
  - C0–T6
- Muscle performance
  - Key muscle tests, C3–T1
  - Grip strength
  - Resisted tests
    - Cervical
    - Scapular
- Pain
  - Measured on visual analog scale
  - With palpation
- Posture
  - Static
  - Dynamic

- ROM
  - Cervical and thoracic
    - Active
    - Passive
    - Overpressure
- Reflex integrity
  - Upper and lower extremity
  - Abnormal reflexes
    - Babinski
    - Hoffman's
    - Clonus
- Sensory integrity
  - C3–T1
- Special tests
  - Upper limb tension test

Establish Plan of Care

- Based on history, tests, and measures

GOALS/OUTCOMES

- Pain: 2/10 or less and absence of radiating symptoms with ADLs
- Cervical and thoracic ROM: at least 80% of AMA guides

Cervical	Normal	80%
Flexion	60°	50°
Extension	75°	60°
Rotation	80°	65°
Side bend	45°	35°

Thoracic	Normal	80%
Flexion	40°	30°
Rotation	30°	25°
Side bend	10°	8°
Extension	No AMA guides established	

314   CERVICAL STENOSIS | CERVICAL/THORACIC SPINE

- Functional spinal stability and endurance as evidenced by symptom-free tolerance of postural requirements during normal ADLs and vocational activities
- Spinal and scapular strength: 4+/5 on manual muscle test
- Return to previous functional status for ADLs and vocational, recreational, and sports activities as identified by patient
- Independence in a progressive home exercise program emphasizing function
- Negative upper-limb tension signs

INTERVENTION
NUMBER OF VISITS: 7–12

Coordination, Communication, and Documentation
- Provision of services between admission and discharge that facilitate cost-effective and efficient integration or reintegration to home, community, or work
- Documentation of therapeutic intervention is required for each episode of care and serves as the basic foundation for communication
- Coordination and additional communication will depend on the patient's impairment and home/work/community/leisure situation and requirements. Such services may include:
  - Case management
  - Coordination of care and collaboration with those integral to the patient's rehabilitation program
  - Coordination and monitoring of the delivery of available resources
  - Referrals to other health-care professionals
  - Identification of resources, support groups, or advocacy services
  - Provision of educational or training information
  - Technical assistance

Patient Instruction

Basic Anatomy and Biomechanics
- Cervical spine
  - Vertebræ
  - Disc
  - Nerve root
  - Soft tissue

- Pertinent Gray's Anatomy (Gray. 1995. 510-518, 537, 803–805, 807–813, 835–838)
- Dysfunction and the importance of protection and rehabilitation of the stabilizing structures
- Etiologies of central canal vs. lateral stenosis and importance of restoring the balance of spinal joint mobility to decrease stress on individual segments
  - Educate patient with central canal stenosis regarding warning signs of cord compression, such as bilateral or quadrilateral paresthesia

Handouts
- Commercially available products, such as:
  - Krames Communications (1100 Grundy Lane, San Bruno, CA 94066):
    - *Neck Basics*
    - *Neck Exercises for a Healthy Neck*
    - *Neck Owner's Manual*
  - McKenzie (PO Box 93, Waikanae, New Zealand)
    - *Treat Your Own Neck*
- Specific home program

Functional Considerations
- Posture
  - Maintenance of normal and pain-free posture with use of cervical collar as indicated for symptom relief
  - Alteration of ADLs to avoid aggravating postures
- Body mechanics
  - Avoidance of aggravating upper-extremity activities and prolonged head postures

Direct Interventions

Acute Phase: 4–6 Visits
- Therapeutic exercise
  - Stretching exercises
  - Cervical, thoracic, and shoulder ROM exercises as appropriate: Active assistive progressing to active
  - Postural awareness and body mechanics training
  - Aerobic exercises for tissue healing
  - Home program
    - Diaphragmatic breathing and relaxation techniques
    - Cervical AROM
    - Shoulder rolls or scapular retraction/depression
    - Home traction
    - Postural correction program

CERVICAL/THORACIC SPINE | CERVICAL STENOSIS   315

- Manual therapy techniques
  - Soft-tissue techniques
    - Soft-tissue mobilization
    - Trigger-point techniques
    - Myofascial release
  - Joint mobilization (lateral stenosis)
    - Grade I or II to involved segments (lateral stenosis), emphasis on traction/flexion range with stabilization of involved segments
    - Grades II–V to uninvolved segments Contraindicated in the presence of bilateral upper-extremity symptoms unless central stenosis has been ruled out
  - Assisted upper-extremity and cervical stretching
  - Neural tension maneuvers
- Electrotherapeutic modalities
- Physical agents and mechanical modalities
  - Superficial thermal: Cryotherapy/thermal modalities
  - Deep thermal: Ultrasound
  - Static mechanical traction
    - Position, duration, and intensity dependent upon patient tolerance
- Goals/outcomes
  - Pain: 50% reduction from initial rating with a centralizing trend
  - Cervical ROM: 50% of AMA guides
    - Flexion: 30°
    - Extension: 40°
    - Rotation: 40°
    - Side bend: 25°

Subacute Phase: 3–6 Visits
- Therapeutic exercise and home program
  - Active flexibility exercises in pain-free ROM
    - Cervical rotation, side bend, and forward diagonals
    - Upper-extremity elevation/external rotation
    - Thoracic rotation, extension
    - Scapular retraction/depression
    - Pectoral stretching
  - Cardiovascular conditioning
    - Walking program/treadmill
    - Upper or lower-extremity cycling
    - Aquatic therapy
    - Ski machine
  - Postural training
  - Strengthening exercises
    - Cervical isometrics

- Cervical/thoracic/scapular therapeutic ball exercises
- Overhead activities
- Upper-extremity diagonal patterns
  - Neuromuscular/balance/proprioceptive reeducation
  - Home traction
- Manual therapy techniques
  - Continued soft-tissue techniques
  - Grades II–V joint mobilizations to cervical and thoracic spine
    - Contraindicated in the presence of bilateral upper-extremity symptoms unless central stenosis has been ruled out
- Physical agents and mechanical modalities
  - Continue effective modalities as in acute phase, with increased emphasis on use as needed at home
- Goals/outcomes
  - Pain: 2/10 or less and absence of radiating symptoms with ADLs
  - AROM: 80% of AMA guides for the cervical/thoracic spine
  - Strength: 4+/5 for cervical and scapular musculature
  - Negative upper limb tension signs

Functional Carryover
- Integration of home exercise program into vocational environment
- Completion of ergonomic adjustments to home and vocational areas
- Incorporation of proper posture and body mechanics for functional activities to avoid exacerbation of symptoms

DISCHARGE PLANNING AND PATIENT RESPONSIBILITY

Criteria for Discharge
- All goals/outcomes have been achieved with the exception of return to previous recreational and sports activities
- Patient demonstrates independence in home program and exercise program
- Patient displays understanding of role of posture and body mechanics in avoidance of re-aggravation

Circumstances Requiring Additional Visits

- Persistent functional strength deficit or 3/5 on manual muscle test
- History of previous injury/surgery to related area
- Persistent radicular symptoms or neurological deficit
- Severe deconditioning
- Special occupational needs requiring extensive fitness/strengthening
- Unable to maintain normal head/neck posture
- Presence of lower-extremity signs and symptoms
- Arthritic conditions
- Significant loss of cervical-thoracic junction mobility

Home Program

- Modalities as needed
- Flexibility exercises and strengthening progression incorporating posture correction techniques
- Cardiovascular conditioning
- Home traction

Monitoring

- Instruct patient to call for advice should progression halt or a negative trend occur
- Follow up at 4–8 weeks post-discharge to ensure expected return to function and progression toward attaining all goals/outcomes
- Patient educated on when to seek intervention (avoid exacerbations on a long-term basis)

REFERENCES

1. American Physical Therapy Association. *Guide to Physical Therapist Practice.* Alexandria, VA: APTA; 1997.
2. Cantu RC. Stingers, transient quadriplegia, and cervical spinal stenosis: return to play criteria. *Med Sci Sports Exerc.* 1997;29(suppl):S233-S235.
3. Gray H; Williams PL, ed. *Gray's Anatomy,* 38th ed. New York, NY: Churchill Livingstone; 1995.
4. Gross AR, Aker PD, Quartly C. Manual therapy in the treatment of neck pain. *Rheum Dis Clin North Am.* 1996;22:579-598.
5. Hart A, Hopkins C, Ford B. *ICD-9-CM Expert For Physicians, Volume 1&2.* 7th ed. USA: Ingenix; 2005.
6. Heller JG. The syndromes of degenerative cervical disease. *Orthop Clin North Am.* 1992;23:381-394.
7. McKenzie R. *Treat Your Own Neck.* 2nd ed. Waikanae, New Zealand: Spinal Publications; 1983.
8. Meyer SA, Schulte KR, Callaghan JJ, et al. Cervical spinal stenosis and stingers in collegiate football players. *Am J Sports Med.* 1994;22:158-166.
9. Riddle DL, Stratford PW. Use of generic versus region-specific functional status measures on patients with cervical spine disorders. *Phys Ther.* 1998;78:951-963.
10. Sandmark H, Nisell R. Validity of five common manual neck pain provoking tests. *Scand J Rehabil Med.* 1995;27(3):131-136.
11. Saunders HD. Use of spinal traction in the treatment of neck and back conditions. *Clin Orthop Rel Res.* October 1983:31-38.
12. Sekhon LH. Posterior cervical decompression and fusion for circumferential spondylotic cervical stenosis: review of 50 consecutive cases. *J of Clinical Neuroscienc.* January 2006;13(1):23-30.
13. Swezey RL. Chronic neck pain. *Rheum Dis Clin North Am.* 1996;22:411-437.
14. Youdas JW, Carey JR, Garrett TR. Reliability of measurements of cervical spine ROM—comparison of three methods. *Phys Ther.* 1991;71:98-104;discussion 105-106.
15. Youdas JW, Garrett TR, Suman VJ, et al. Normal ROM of the cervical spine: an initial goniometric study. *Phys Ther.* 1992;72:770-780.

318   CERVICAL STENOSIS | CERVICAL/THORACIC SPINE

COMPRESSION FRACTURE
SUMMARY OVERVIEW

ICD-9
> 733.13　　805.0　　805.2

APTA Preferred Practice Pattern: **4D, 4H, 4J**

EXAMINATION

- History and Systems Review
- Tests and Measures
  Systems review per APTA's *Guide to Physical Therapy Practice*
  - Muscle performance
  - Pain
  - Posture
  - ROM
  - Reflex integrity
  - Sensory integrity
  - Ventilation, respiration, and circulation (if thoracic spine involved)
- Establish Plan of Care

GOALS/OUTCOMES

- ROM: At least 80% of AMA guides
- Improve postural balance and awareness as evidenced by avoidance of symptomatic flexed positioning
- Independence in a progressive home exercise program emphasizing function
- Return to previous functional status for ADLs and vocational, recreational, and sports activities as identified by patient
- Pain: 2/10 or less with normal ADLs and vocational activities
- Strength: A minimum of 4+/5 on manual muscle test for cervical and trunk musculature

INTERVENTION
NUMBER OF VISITS: 6–10

- Patient Instruction
  - Basic Anatomy and Biomechanics
  - Handouts
  - Functional Considerations
- Direct Interventions
  - Acute Phase: 3–5 Visits
  - Subacute Phase: 3–5 Visits
- Functional Carryover

DISCHARGE PLANNING AND PATIENT RESPONSIBILITY

- Criteria for Discharge
  - Patient demonstrates compliance with home program
  - Patient tolerates ADLs and home exercise program, as evidenced by avoidance of aggravating activities and avoidance of symptoms with progression of home program
  - Patient demonstrates understanding of condition, including prognosis and necessary lifestyle adjustments
  - All goals/outcomes have been achieved, with the possible exception of return to previous recreational/ sports activities
- Circumstances Requiring Additional Visits
  - Persistent functional strength deficit or 3/5 on manual muscle test
  - History of previous injury/surgery to related area
  - Persistent radicular symptoms or neurological deficit
  - Severe deconditioning
  - Special occupational needs requiring extensive fitness/ strengthening
  - Severe traumatic injury with persistent functional/ occupational deficits
  - Multiple injury/fracture sites
  - Arthritic conditions
  - Extreme kyphotic posture
  - Unable to maintain erect weight-bearing postures
  - Instability
- Home Program
  - Physical agents and mechanical modalities at home as needed for flare-ups
  - Self-mobilization, flexibility exercises
  - Progression of strengthening exercises, balance, and proprioceptive exercises
  - Cardiovascular conditioning
- Monitoring

SUMMARY OVERVIEW | CERVICAL/THORACIC SPINE | COMPRESSION FRACTURE

COMPRESSION FRACTURE

ICD-9

733.13	Pathologic fracture of vertebrae
805.0	Closed fracture of cervical vertebra without mention of spinal cord injury
805.2	Closed fracture of dorsal [thoracic] vertebra without mention of spinal cord injury

APTA Preferred Practice Pattern: **4D, 4H, 4J**

EXAMINATION

History and Systems Review

- History of current condition
  - Traumatic vs. insidious
    - If insidious, assume loss of bone density and follow precautions in *Osteoporosis* guideline
    - If surgical; type, immobilization, protocol for mobilization (active, passive)
  - Location, nature, and behavior of symptoms
    - Radicular signs/symptoms
    - Aggravating/relieving factors
    - Postures
    - Activities
- Past history of current condition
  - Spinal injury/surgery
  - Therapeutic interventions
- Other tests and measures
  - X-ray
  - Scans
- Medications
- Past medical/surgical history
- Functional status and activity level (current/prior)
  - Postural tolerance: vocational and ADLs
  - Independent mobility
  - Personal care
- Patient's functional goals

Tests and Measures

Systems review per APTA's *Guide to Physical Therapy Practice*

- Muscle performance
  - Key muscle tests
    - Upper extremity: C3–T1
    - Lower extremity: L2–S1
  - Isometric strength spinal musculature
- Pain
  - Measured on visual analog scale
  - With palpation

- Posture
  Flexion will be painful and should be avoided in treatment positioning
  - Static
  - Dynamic
  - Standing
  - Sitting
  - Preferred sleeping position
  - Inclinometer readings for standing and sitting thoracic kyphosis/cervical lordosis
- ROM
  - Active
  - Passive
    - Spinal
      a. Cervical
      b. Thoracic
      c. Lumbar
    - Shoulder
    - Scapular
- Reflex integrity
  - Upper and lower extremity
- Sensory integrity
  - Upper and lower extremity
- Ventilation, respiration, and circulation (if thoracic spine involved)
  - Chest wall mobility and expansion
    - Adult male: At least 2"
    - Adult female: At least 1½"

Establish Plan of Care

- Based on history, tests, and measures

GOALS/OUTCOMES

- ROM: At least 80% of AMA guides

Cervical	Normal	80%
Flexion	60°	45°
Extension	75°	60°
Rotation	80°	65°
Side bend	45°	35°

320   COMPRESSION FRACTURE | CERVICAL/THORACIC SPINE

Thoracic	*Normal*	*80%*
Extension	No AMA guides established	
Rotation	30°	25°
Side bend	10°	8°

- Improve postural balance and awareness, as evidenced by avoidance of symptomatic flexed positioning
- Independence in a progressive home exercise program emphasizing function
- Return to previous functional status for ADLs and vocational, recreational, and sports activities as identified by patient
- Pain: 2/10 or less with normal ADLs and vocational activities
- Strength: a minimum of 4+/5 on manual muscle test for cervical and trunk musculature

INTERVENTION
NUMBER OF VISITS: 6–10
Note: Type of fracture, method of fixation/immobilization, healing state, x-ray findings will be paramount in determining the appropriateness of treatment. Consult with the referring physician.

Coordination, Communication, and Documentation

- Provision of services between admission and discharge that facilitate cost-effective and efficient integration or reintegration to home, community, or work
- Documentation of therapeutic intervention is required for each episode of care and serves as the basic foundation for communication
- Coordination and additional communication will depend on the patient's impairment and home/work/community/leisure situation and requirements. Such services may include:
  - Case management
  - Coordination of care and collaboration with those integral to the patient's rehabilitation program
  - Coordination and monitoring of the delivery of available resources
  - Referrals to other health-care professionals
  - Identification of resources, support groups, or advocacy services
  - Provision of educational or training information
  - Technical assistance

Patient Instruction

Basic Anatomy and Biomechanics
- Cervical and thoracic spine: Vertebral bodies, disc and nerve roots, soft tissues
- Pertinent Gray's Anatomy (Gray. 1995. 510-518, 537, 803–805, 807–813, 835–838)
- Patient education in prognosis: The compression fracture is usually stable, but the vertebral body deformity is permanent, and care must be taken to avoid aggravating postures and activities

Handouts
- Commercially available products, such as:
  - Krames Communications (1100 Grundy Lane, San Bruno, CA 94066)
    - *Back Basics*
    - *Poor Posture Hurts*
    - *Back Tips for People Who Sit*
    - *Neck Owner's Manual*
    - *Arranging Your Work Station to Fit You*
- Specific home program

Functional Considerations
- Posture
  - Standing, sitting, and sleeping postures
  - Maintain normal and pain-free posture with use of cervical collar or brace to decrease symptoms
  - Alteration of ADLs
  - Avoidance of prolonged flexed postures
- Body mechanics
  - Proper lifting techniques to minimize spinal stress
  - Restriction of activities which may exacerbate symptoms, such as vigorous rotational or impact activities

Direct Interventions

Acute Phase: 3–5 Visits
- Therapeutic exercise
  - Active flexibility exercises within pain-free ROM
  - Graded spinal extensor strengthening as tolerated
  - Home program
    - Instruction in modalities as needed at home
    - Instruction positions of relief, postural modifications

CERVICAL/THORACIC SPINE | COMPRESSION FRACTURE

- Manual therapy techniques
  - Soft-tissue mobilization with care near fracture site
  - Joint mobilization as appropriate given any stabilization procedures performed, follow-up x-rays to determine stage of healing, clearance by surgeon.
    - Specific traction at involved segment performed in a position of comfort: Grades I–II with intent of pain relief
    - Grades III–V to hypomobile segments above and below involved segment
- Electrotherapeutic modalities
- Physical agents and mechanical modalities
  - Superficial thermal: Cryotherapy/thermal modalities
  - Deep thermal: Ultrasound
- Goals/outcomes
  - Pain: 50% reduction from initial rating
  - Avoidance of aggravating activities
  - Patient exhibits ability to remain pain-free in postures encountered in ADLs at home (with supportive equipment as necessary)
    - Standing
    - Sitting
    - Side-lying
    - Supine
    - Prone
  - Patient demonstrates knowledge of isometric/active spinal strengthening exercise progression

Subacute Phase: 3–5 Visits
- Therapeutic exercise
  - Continue active exercise in pain-free ROM
  - Progress self-resisted and stabilization exercises as appropriate
  - Instruct in self-mobilization exercises as appropriate for regions above and below injury site
  - Neuromuscular/balance/proprioceptive reeducation
    - Quadruped opposite arm/leg lift
    - Unilateral stance balancing, reaching one or both arms in various directions to maximum distance, avoiding use of other leg for counterbalance
      a. Anterior reach: Stimulates hamstrings, soleus, gastrocnemius, and hip/back extensors (depending on height of reach)
      b. Posterior overhead reach: Stimulates abdominals
      c. Lateral rotational reach: Stimulates hip abductors and lateral trunk stabilizers

- Unilateral stance balancing, reaching opposite leg in various directions to maximum distance
  a. Anterior reach: Stimulates quadriceps, soleus
  b. Posterior reach: Stimulates gluteals, quadriceps, hip/back extensors
  c. Rotational reach to side: Stimulates gluteals, quadriceps, trunk stabilizers, hip abductors, abdominals
- Cardiovascular conditioning
- Manual therapy techniques
  - Soft-tissue techniques
    - Soft-tissue mobilization
    - Trigger-point techniques
    - Strain/counterstrain
    - Myofascial release
  - Joint mobilization: See precautions listed above in acute phase
    - Progressive Grades III–V joint mobilization to any persistent specific hypomobilities above and below injury site
    - Progress graded specific traction to irritable joints
- Physical agents and mechanical modalities
  - Continue effective modalities as in acute phase, with increased emphasis on as needed use at home
- Goals/outcomes
  - Pain: 2/10 or less
  - Cervical and thoracic spine ROM: 80% of AMA guides
  - Strength: A minimum of 4+/5 on manual muscle test for cervical and scapular musculature
  - Maintain pain-free postures during vocational activities

Functional Carryover
- Clinical or on-site ergonomic evaluation of the workstation
- Modification of ADLs and recreational and exercise activities to avoid exacerbation of symptoms

DISCHARGE PLANNING AND PATIENT RESPONSIBILITY

Criteria for Discharge
- Patient demonstrates compliance with home program
- Patient tolerates ADLs and home exercise program, as evidenced by avoidance of aggravating activities and

322   COMPRESSION FRACTURE | CERVICAL/THORACIC SPINE

avoidance of symptoms with progression of home program

- Patient demonstrates understanding of condition, including prognosis and necessary lifestyle adjustments
- All goals/outcomes have been achieved, with the possible exception of return to previous recreational/sports activities

Circumstances Requiring Additional Visits

- Persistent functional strength deficit or 3/5 on manual muscle test
- History of previous injury/surgery to related area
- Persistent radicular symptoms or neurological deficit
- Severe deconditioning
- Special occupational needs requiring extensive fitness/strengthening
- Severe traumatic injury with persistent functional/occupational deficits
- Multiple injury/fracture sites
- Arthritic conditions
- Extreme kyphotic posture
- Unable to maintain erect weight-bearing postures
- Instability

Home Program

- Physical agents and mechanical modalities at home as needed for flare-ups
- Self-mobilization, flexibility exercises
- Progression of strengthening exercises, balance, and proprioceptive exercises
- Cardiovascular conditioning

Monitoring

- Instruct patient to call for advice should progression halt or negative trend occur
- Recheck by phone within 3 months post-discharge to review home program and assess any further modifications to daily activities or work site

REFERENCES

1. American Physical Therapy Association. *Guide to Physical Therapist Practice*. Alexandria, VA: APTA; 1997.
2. Cooper C, O'Neill T, Silman A. The epidemiology of vertebral fractures. *Bone*. 1993;14(1):S89-S97.
3. Garfin S, Buckley R, Ledlie J. Balloon kyphoplasty for symptomatic vertebral body compression fractures results in rapid, significant, and sustained improvements in back pain, function, and quality of life for elderly patients. *Spine*. September 2006.
4. Gray H; Williams PL, ed. *Gray's Anatomy*. 38th ed. New York, NY: Churchill Livingstone; 1995.
5. Gross AR, Aker PD, Quartly C. Manual therapy in the treatment of neck pain. *Rheum Dis Clin North Am*. 1996;22:579-598.
6. Harrop J, Prpa B, Reinhardt M. Primary and secondary osteoporosis' incidence of subsequent vertebral compression fractures after kyphoplasty. *Spine*. October 2004.
7. Hart A, Hopkins C, Ford B. *ICD-9-CM Expert For Physicians, Volume 1&2*. 7th ed. USA: Ingenix; 2005.
8. Lukert BP. Vertebral compression fractures: how to manage pain, avoid disability. *Geriatrics*. 1994;49(2):22-26.
9. Phillips F. Minimally invasive treatments of osteoporotic vertebral compression fractures. *Spine*. August 2003;28(15 Suppl):S45-53.
10. Prather H, Dillen L, Metzler J, et. al. Prospective measurement of function and pain in patients with non-neoplastic compression fractures treated with vertebroplasty. *J Bone Joint Surg Am*. February 2006.
11. Riddle DL, Stratford PW. Use of generic versus region-specific functional status measures on patients with cervical spine disorders. *Phys Ther*. 1998;78:951-963.
12. Sandmark H, Nisell R. Validity of five common manual neck pain provoking tests. *Scand J Rehabil Med*. 1995;27(3):131-136.
13. Saunders HD. *Evaluation, Treatment, and Prevention of Musculoskeletal Disorders*. Minneapolis, MN: Viking Press; 1988.
14. Shih-Tseng Lee. Closed reduction vertebroplasty for the treatment of osteoporotic vertebral compression fractures. Technical note. *J Neurosurg*. April 2004.
15. Youdas JW, Carey JR, Garrett TR. Reliability of measurements of cervical spine ROM—comparison of three methods. *Phys Ther*. 1991;71:98-104; discussion, 105-106.
16. Youdas JW, Garrett TR, Suman VJ, et al. Normal ROM of the cervical spine: an initial goniometric study. *Phys Ther*. 1992;72:770-780.

324   COMPRESSION FRACTURE | CERVICAL/THORACIC SPINE

CRANIOVERTEBRAL STABILITY TESTS

It is recommended that these tests be performed on appropriate patients with a cervical diagnosis in the presence of trauma, subjective reports of cardinal signs or symptoms, or when treatment will include manual therapy techniques that approach end range of motion. Note that this test has inherent risks and the decision to perform should be based on post-graduate orthopedic manual physical therapy training.

CARDINAL SIGNS

Craniovertebral instability manifests itself with the presence of cardinal signs that suggest either arterial insufficiency or cervical spinal cord compression.

- Loss of balance without loss of consciousness/drop attacks
- Lip paresthesia
- Bilateral or quadrilateral limb paresthesia
- Nystagmus

Cardinal signs or symptoms reproduced during the craniovertebral stability tests indicate serious pathology, and the patient should be referred immediately to the physician.

NONCARDINAL SIGNS

Other noncardinal signs and symptoms that may be associated with craniovertebral instability:

- Lump in throat
- Inconsistent swallowing
- Nausea/vomiting
- Severe headache
- Marked spasm
- Empty endfeel
- Dizziness
- Vertigo
- Lightheadedness
- Blurred vision
- Tinnitus
- Fainting
- Hoarseness
- Drowsiness

The reproduction of noncardinal signs warrants caution but does not contraindicate continued treatment.

CRANIOVERTEBRAL STABILITY TESTS

These tests check the ability of the bony and ligamentous structures of the craniovertebral joints to prevent excessive accessory motion.

- General compression
  - Tests for fracture/joint integrity
- General traction
  - Tests the longitudinal ligamentous stability
- General traction in flexion
- Specific traction
  - Fix axis (C2) and apply traction in neutral
  - Fix axis (C2) and apply traction in flexion
- Occiput anterior on atlas
  - Tests the anterior capsule and membranes of C0–1
  - Fix atlas anterior with thumbs and squeeze occiput upward with fingertips
- Occiput posterior on atlas
  - Tests the posterior capsule and membranes of C0–1
  - Fix posterior arch of atlas and squeeze down on the occiput with thenar eminence
- Atlas anterior on axis
  - Tests the transverse ligament
  - Nonspecific: Lift atlas and occiput anteriorly; if positive symptoms, then retest in flexion
  - Specific: Fix axis (C2) anteriorly with thumbs and squeeze atlas anteriorly
- Dens integrity test
  - Fix axis (C2) and laterally shear atlas. Do both sides.
- Alar ligament test
  - Firm stabilization of axis (C2) and then side bend the occiput. Do both sides.
    - Neutral
    - Flexion
    - Extension

CERVICAL/THORACIC SPINE | CRANIOVERTEBRAL STABILITY TESTS   325

VERTEBRAL ARTERY TEST

Note: Vertebral basilar insufficiency testing may place the artery under greater stress with testing than is necessary or safe. Each clinician should develop a strategy for when to test and when not to test. This information may be obtained by post-graduate orthopedic manual physical therapy training.

When testing, it is recommended that the vertebral artery be progressively stressed:
- The patient keeps his or her eyes open during the entire test
- Each position is held until the patient complains of arterial occlusion symptoms or for 30 seconds, whichever comes first
- Rotate the head as far as possible to one side, hold 10–30 seconds, and repeat to the other side
- Maintaining lower cervical flexion, rotate and extend the upper cervical spine (this takes the stress off of the lower part of the vertebral artery while testing the upper portion). Repeat to the opposite side.
- Maintaining upper cervical flexion, test the lower portion of the artery by rotating and extending the lower cervical spine
- Maintaining extension of the entire cervical spine, rotate the head to one side, hold, and repeat to the opposite side
- If the above positions do not reproduce symptoms, the vertebral artery is maximally stressed by the addition of traction to the fully extended and rotated cervical spine
- Remember that in the presence of considerable loss of cervical ROM, the vertebral artery cannot be fully stressed. Therefore, as gains are made in the available ROM, the vertebral artery must be retested until full range is achieved.

OBJECTIVE MEASUREMENT OF FORWARD HEAD POSTURE

The patient stands in his/her normal postural position, and the following measurements are recorded:

X: The distance from a vertical line from the mentonian symphysis (chin) to the sternal notch.
Y: The distance from a vertical line from the most prominent aspect of the thoracic spine to the apex of the cervical spine (usually C3).

These measurements can be taken with a standard metric ruler and recorded in centimeters. There is also a measuring instrument available through the Rocabodo Institute that is adjustable and has a level incorporated.

Mentonian Symphysis Vertical from Thoracic	*to Sternal Notch*	*to the Apex of Cervical*
Normal	1.5–3 cm	5–7 cm
Mild	4–5 cm	8–9 cm
Moderate	6–7 cm	10–11 cm
Marked	>7 cm	>11 cm

You can then correct the patient's posture and remeasure. This allows you to record his/her potential for posture correction and set appropriate, objective goals.

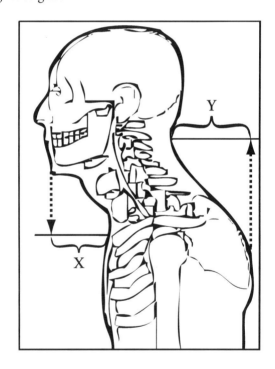

328 OBJECTIVE MEASUREMENT OF FORWARD HEAD POSTURE | CERVICAL/THORACIC SPINE

OSTEOPOROSIS
SUMMARY OVERVIEW

ICD-9

733.0   733.10   733.13   733.19   733.2   733.40   733.49   733.7   733.90

733.91   733.95   733.99

APTA Preferred Practice Pattern: **4A, 4B, 4C, 4G, 4H**

EXAMINATION

- History and Systems Review
- Tests and Measures
  Systems review per APTA's *Guide to Physical Therapy Practice*
  - Anthropometric characteristics
  - Gait, locomotion, and balance
  - Motor performance
  - Pain
  - Posture
  - ROM
  - Ventilation, respiration, and circulation
- Establish Plan of Care

GOALS/OUTCOMES

- Improve body mechanics and postural awareness as evidenced by symptom-free tolerance of postural requirements during normal ADLs and vocational activities
- Maintain or increase aerobic capacity and endurance
- Pain: 2/10 or less
- Restore ROM to a minimum of 80% of AMA guides Normal age-related decrease in ROM should be considered.
- Achieve 30-second stance time on balance tests
- Strength: 4+/5 on manual muscle test for trunk musculature or the ability to demonstrate specific motor performance as listed in guidelines
- Return to previous functional status for ADLs and vocational and recreational activities as identified by patient
- Independence in a progressive home exercise program emphasizing function

INTERVENTION
NUMBER OF VISITS: 4–8

- Patient Instruction
  - Basic Anatomy and Biomechanics
  - Handouts
  - Functional Considerations
- Direct Interventions
  - Active Treatment Phase: 4–8 Visits
- Functional Carryover

DISCHARGE PLANNING AND PATIENT RESPONSIBILITY

- Criteria for Discharge
  - All goals/outcomes have been met, with possible exceptions as listed in guideline
  - Patient demonstrates appropriate body mechanics for daily activities
  - Patient is able to distinguish appropriate/ inappropriate activities for the osteoporotic condition
- Circumstances Requiring Additional Visits
  - Persistent functional strength deficit or 3/5 on manual muscle test
  - History of previous injury/surgery to related area
  - Persistent radicular symptoms or neurological deficit
  - Severe deconditioning
  - Special occupational needs requiring extensive fitness/ strengthening
  - Presence of compression fracture
  - Balance deficits
  - Extreme kyphotic posture
  - Presence of osteoarthritis
  - Unable to maintain erect weight-bearing posture
  - Severe chronic obstructive pulmonary disease
- Home Program
  - Regular weight-bearing exercise activities, such as a walking program, monitoring exertion levels
  - Strengthening exercises targeting the back extensors and abdominals
  - Stretching to appropriate muscles
- Monitoring

OSTEOPOROSIS

ICD-9

733.0	Osteoporosis
733.10	Pathologic fracture, unspecified site
733.13	Pathologic fracture of vertebrae
733.19	Pathologic fracture of other specified site
733.2	Cyst of bone
733.40	Aseptic necrosis of bone, site unspecified
733.49	Aseptic necrosis of bone, other
733.7	Algoneurodystrophy
733.90	Disorder of bone and cartilage, unspecified
733.91	Arrest of bone development or growth
733.95	Stress fracture of other bone
733.99	Other disorder of bone and cartilage

APTA Preferred Practice Pattern: 4A, 4B, 4C, 4G, 4H

EXAMINATION

History and Systems Review

- History of current condition
  - Date of diagnosis or mechanism of exacerbation
  - Location, nature, and behavior of symptoms
    - Aggravating/relieving factors
  - Presence of cardinal signs
- Past history of current condition
  - History of fractures or stooped postures
  - Onset of menopause before the age of 45
- Other tests and measures
  - Radiologic exam: 40% loss of bone density occurs before evident on x-rays
- Medications
- Past medical/surgical history
  - Systemic pathology
- Functional status and activity level (current/prior)
  - Work and ADL postural tolerance
  - Personal care
- Social habits
  - Diet low in calcium
  - Inactive lifestyles
  - Smoker
  - Excessive use of alcohol
  - Excessive use of certain medications, including thyroid hormone, glucocorticosteroids, anti-seizure, anti-coagulants, and laxatives
- Family history
  - History of early estrogen deficiency

- General demographics
  - Advanced age
  - Caucasian and Asian women
- Patient's functional goals

Tests and Measures

Systems review per APTA's *Guide to Physical Therapy Practice*

In addition to a general cervical/thoracic spine evaluation (see *Cervical/Thoracic General Pain* guideline), the following are performed:

- Anthropometric characteristics
  - Body type: Thin, small boned
- Gait, locomotion, and balance
  - Single-leg stance time with eyes open
    - Goal of 30 seconds independently
  - Tandem-leg stance time with eyes open
    - Goal of 30 seconds independently
  - 2 x 20 ft walking with change of direction and no loss of balance
- Motor performance
  - Specific functional motor performance, such as:
    - Squat to 90°
    - Transfer in/out of car
    - Retrieve object from floor
- Pain
  - Measured on visual analog scale
  - With palpation
- Posture
  - Static

330   OSTEOPOROSIS | CERVICAL/THORACIC SPINE

- ROM
  - Inclinometer ROM for thoracic kyphosis
- Ventilation, respiration, and circulation
  - Chest expansion
    - Adult male: Normal 2"
    - Adult female: Normal 1½"
  - Assessment of diaphragmatic breathing in supine and sitting positions

Establish Plan of Care

- Based on history, tests, and measures

GOALS/OUTCOMES

- Improve body mechanics and postural awareness as evidenced by symptom-free tolerance of postural requirements during normal ADLs and vocational activities
- Maintain or increase aerobic capacity and endurance
  - Perform cardiovascular conditioning 3 times per week for a minimum of 20 minutes per session
- Pain: 2/10 or less
- Restore ROM to a minimum of 80% of AMA guides Normal age-related decrease in ROM should be considered.

Lumbar	Normal	80%
Flexion	60°	50°
Extension	25°	20°
Side bend	20°	15°

Thoracic	Normal	80%
Flexion	40°	30°
Extension	No AMA guides established	
Side bend	10°	8°
Rotation	30°	25°

Cervical	Normal	80%
Flexion	60°	50°
Extension	75°	60°
Side bend	45°	35°
Rotation	80°	65°

- Achieve 30-second stance time on balance tests
- Strength: 4+/5 on manual muscle test for trunk musculature or the ability to demonstrate the following motor performance:
  - Independent stair negotiation
  - Independent transfer to/from sitting (squat 90°)
  - Retrieve object from floor
  - Perform work/ADL tasks (weight and repetition-specific)
- Return to previous functional status for ADLs and vocational and recreational activities as identified by patient
- Independence in a progressive home exercise program emphasizing function

INTERVENTION
NUMBER OF VISITS: 4–8

Coordination, Communication, and Documentation

- Provision of services between admission and discharge that facilitate cost-effective and efficient integration or reintegration to home, community, or work
- Documentation of therapeutic intervention is required for each episode of care and serves as the basic foundation for communication
- Coordination and additional communication will depend on the patient's impairment and home/work/community/leisure situation and requirements. Such services may include:
  - Case management
  - Coordination of care and collaboration with those integral to the patient's rehabilitation program
  - Coordination and monitoring of the delivery of available resources
  - Referrals to other health-care professionals
  - Identification of resources, support groups, or advocacy services
  - Provision of educational or training information
  - Technical assistance

Patient Instruction

Basic Anatomy and Biomechanics

- Anatomy of cervical and thoracic spine, rib cage, and shoulder girdle
- Disease progression, possible sequalæ and the importance of avoiding/eliminating behavioral risk factors
- Additional resource/support group information on diagnosis and treatment
  - National Arthritis Foundation, 1314 Spring Street NW, Atlanta, GA 30309, 1-800-933-7023
  - National Osteoporosis Foundation, M. Street NW, Suite 602, Washington, DC 20037 (202)-223-2226

Handouts

- Commercially available products, such as:
  - *Self Balance Hints for Older Persons*
  - *The Secret of Good Posture*
  - National Osteoporosis Foundation (1232 22nd Street NW, Washington, DC 20037)
    - *Avoiding Falls and Other Injuries*
  - Krames Communications (1100 Grundy Lane, San Bruno, CA 94066)
    - *Woman's Guide to Osteoporosis*
    - *Back Basics*

Functional Considerations

- Implementation of positive behavioral habits to reduce risk
  - Supplement calcium in diet per medical advice
  - Initiate regular exercise program
  - Smoking cessation
  - Reduce alcohol consumption
- Utilization of erect posture during ADLs

Direct Interventions

Active Treatment Phase: 4–8 Visits

- Therapeutic exercise and home program
  - Breathing techniques to increase aerobic capacity and endurance
  - Flexibility exercises—Encourage spinal extension
    - Pectoralis major and minor
    - Hip flexors
    - Latissimus dorsi
    - Trunk rotators
  - Strengthening exercises—Progress from static to dynamic activities
    - Abdominals
    - Spinal extensors
    - Scapular retractors/depressors
    - Gluteals
  - Cardiovascular conditioning
    - Treadmill/walking program
    - Aquatic therapy
    - Upper or lower-extremity cycling
    - Structured exercise class
  - Neuromuscular/balance/proprioceptive reeducation
    - Quadruped opposite arm/leg lift
    - Unilateral stance balancing, reaching one or both arms in various directions to maximum distance, avoiding use of other leg for counterbalance
      a. Anterior reach stimulates hamstrings, soleus, gastrocnemius, and hip/back extensors (depending on height of reach)
      b. Posterior overhead reach stimulates abdominals
      c. Lateral rotational reach stimulates hip abductors and lateral trunk stabilizers
    - Unilateral stance balancing, reaching opposite leg in various directions to maximum distance
      a. Anterior reach stimulates quadriceps, soleus
      b. Posterior reach stimulates gluteals, quadriceps, hip/back extensors
      c. Rotational reach to side stimulates gluteals, quadriceps, trunk stabilizers, hip abductors, abdominals
- Manual therapy techniques
  - Soft-tissue techniques
    - Soft-tissue mobilization
    - Myofascial release
    - Acupressure
  - Progressive joint mobilization (must use care with direct pressure, especially over ribs)
    - Cervicothoracic junction
    - Thoracolumbar junction
  - Manual traction
  - Assisted passive stretching
  - Proprioceptive neuromuscular facilitation
- Electrotherapeutic modalities

332   OSTEOPOROSIS | CERVICAL/THORACIC SPINE

- Physical agents and mechanical modalities
  - If acute flare-up of symptoms
  - Superficial cryotherapy/thermal modalities
    - Avoiding osteoporotic sites
  - Deep thermal: Ultrasound

Functional Carryover

- Ergonomic modifications with emphasis on proper sitting and standing posture
- Implementation of measures to promote safety at home and in community activities
- Task-oriented exercise dependent on home, work, recreation, and athletic activities
- Replacement of clothing that may cause constriction, such as:
  - Narrow bra straps
  - Girdles

DISCHARGE PLANNING AND PATIENT RESPONSIBILITY

Criteria for Discharge

- All goals/outcomes have been met with the following possible exceptions:
  - May discharge at 4-/5 on manual muscle test
  - May discharge prior to achievement of cardiovascular goal as long as program has been initiated
  - May discharge with less than 80% ROM if all other goals/outcomes have been achieved
- Patient demonstrates appropriate body mechanics for daily activities
- Patient is able to distinguish appropriate/inappropriate activities for the osteoporotic condition

Circumstances Requiring Additional Visits

- Persistent functional strength deficit or 3/5 on manual muscle test
- History of previous injury/surgery to related area
- Persistent radicular symptoms or neurological deficit
- Severe deconditioning
- Special occupational needs requiring extensive fitness/strengthening
- Presence of compression fracture
- Balance deficits
- Extreme kyphotic posture
- Presence of osteoarthritis
- Unable to maintain erect weight-bearing posture
- Severe chronic obstructive pulmonary disease

Home Program

- Regular weight-bearing exercise activities, such as a walking program, monitoring exertion levels
- Strengthening exercises targeting the back extensors and abdominals
- Stretching to appropriate muscles

Monitoring

- Instruct patient to call for advice should progression halt or a negative trend occur
- Follow up with a clinic visit at 3–6 months post-discharge to assess functional status and compliance with regular exercise program

REFERENCES

1. American Physical Therapy Association. *Guide to Physical Therapist Practice.* Alexandria, VA: APTA; 1997.

2. Cooper C, O'Neill T, Silman A. The epidemiology of vertebral fractures. *Bone.* 1993;14(1):S89-S97.

3. Gray H; Williams PL, ed. *Gray's Anatomy.* 38th ed. New York, NY: Churchill Livingstone; 1995.

4. Hart A, Hopkins C, Ford B. *ICD-9-CM Expert For Physicians, Volume 1&2.* 7th ed. USA: Ingenix; 2005.

5. Iglarsh A, Kendall F, Lewis C, Sahrmann S. *The Secret of Good Posture.* Alexandria, VA: American Physical Therapy Association; 1985.

6. Lewis CB. *Self Balance Hints For Older Persons.* Gaithersburg, MD: Aspen Publishers.

7. Lewis CB, Knortz KA. *Orthopedic Assessment and Treatment of the Geriatric Patient.* St. Louis, MO: Mosby-Yearbook; 1993.

8. Lind B, Sihlbom H. Normal ROM of the cervical spine. *Arch Phys Ther Rehabil.* 1989;70:692-695.

9. Mac Kinnon JL. Osteoporosis: a review. *Phys Ther.* 1988;68:1533-1541.

10. Millard PS, Rosen CJ, Johnson KH. Osteoporotic vertebral fractures in postmenopausal women. *Am Fam Physician.* 1997;55:1315-1322.

11. Riddle DL, Stratford PW. Use of generic versus region-specific functional status measures on patients with cervical spine disorders. *Phys Ther.* 1998;78:951-963.

12. Sandmark H, Nisell R. Validity of five common manual neck pain provoking tests. *Scand J Rehabil Med.* 1995;27(3):131-136.

13. Smidt GL, O'Dwyer KD, Lin S, Blanpied PR. The effect of trunk resistive exercise on muscle strength in postmenopausal women. *J Orthop Sports Phys Ther.* 1991;13(6):300-309.

14. Swezey RL. Chronic neck pain. *Rheum Dis Clin North Am.* 1996;22:411-437.

15. Von Feldt JM. Managing osteoporotic fractures: minimizing pain and disability. *Rev Rhum Eng Ed.* 1997;64(6 suppl):78s-80s.

16. Wyke B. Cervical articular contributions to posture and gait: their relation to senile disequilibrium. *Age Aging.* 1979;8:251-258.

17. Youdas JW, Carey JR, Garrett TR. Reliability of measurements of cervical spine ROM—comparison of three methods. *Phys Ther.* 1991;71:98-104; discussion, 105-106.

18. Youdas JW, Garrett TR, Suman VJ, et al. Normal ROM of the cervical spine: an initial goniometric study. *Phys Ther.* 1992;72:770-780.

POSTOPERATIVE / POSTFRACTURE REHABILITATION OF THE CERVICAL / THORACIC SPINE

SUMMARY OVERVIEW

ICD-9

722.81   722.82   805.0   805.1   805.2   805.3   807   V45.4

APTA Preferred Practice Pattern: 4D, 4G, 4H, 4J

EXAMINATION

- History and Systems Review
- Tests and Measures

  Systems review per APTA's *Guide to Physical Therapy Practice*
  - ROM
  - Integumentary integrity
  - Joint integrity and mobility
  - Sensory integrity
  - Pain
  - Posture
  - Reflex integrity
  - Motor performance
  - Special tests
  - Ventilation/respiration
- Establish Plan of Care

GOALS/OUTCOMES

- Pain: 2/10 or less
- ROM: Restore maximum symptom-free motion given surgical procedure, or achieve a minimum of 80% of AMA guides
- Spinal and scapular muscle strength: 4+/5 on manual muscle test
- Achieve functional spinal stability and endurance as evidenced by symptom-free tolerance of postural requirements during normal ADLs and vocational activities
- Return to previous functional status for ADLs and vocational, recreational, and sports activities as identified by patient
- Independence in a progressive home exercise program emphasizing function

INTERVENTION
NUMBER OF VISITS: 6–14

- Patient Instruction
  - Basic Anatomy and Biomechanics
  - Handouts
  - Functional Considerations
  - Description of Surgical Procedure
- Direct Interventions
  - Acute Phase: 4–6 Visits
  - Subacute Phase: 2–8 Visits
- Functional Carryover

DISCHARGE PLANNING AND PATIENT RESPONSIBILITY

- Criteria for Discharge
  - All goals/outcomes have been achieved with the exception of return to previous status for recreational and sports activities
- Circumstances Requiring Additional Visits
  - Persistent functional strength deficit or 2+/5 on manual muscle test
  - History of previous injury/surgery to related area
  - Persistent radicular symptoms or neurological deficit
  - Severe deconditioning
  - Special occupational needs requiring extensive fitness/strengthening
  - Instability at fracture/surgical site
  - Postoperative infection/complication
  - Severe postoperative scarring
  - Presence of surgical hardware
  - Multiple fracture/injury sites
  - Head injury
  - Arthritic conditions
  - Multilevel fracture, surgical involvement
  - Residual signs and symptoms
  - Necessary to return to normal work status (no modified duty available)
- Home Program
  - Flexibility exercises for maintenance of postural balance
  - Progressive strengthening exercises to challenge patient's current level
  - Self-mobilization techniques
  - Use of modalities at home as needed for occasional flare-ups
  - Progression of aerobic endurance exercise
- Monitoring

SUMMARY OVERVIEW | CERVICAL/THORACIC SPINE | POSTOPERATIVE/POSTFRACTURE REHAB OF THE CERVICAL/THORACIC SPINE   335

POSTOPERATIVE / POSTFRACTURE REHABILITATION OF THE CERVICAL / THORACIC SPINE

ICD-9

722.81	Postlaminectomy syndrome, cervical region
722.82	Postlaminectomy syndrome, thoracic region
805.0	Closed fracture of cervical vertebra without mention of spinal cord injury
805.1	Open fracture of cervical vertebra without mention of spinal cord injury
805.2	Closed fracture of dorsal [thoracic] vertebra without mention of spinal cord injury
805.3	Open fracture of dorsal [thoracic] vertebra without mention of spinal cord injury
807	Fracture of rib(s), sternum, larynx, and trachea
V45.4	Postprocedural arthrodesis status

APTA Preferred Practice Pattern: **4D, 4G, 4H, 4J**

EXAMINATION

History and Systems Review

- History of current condition
  - Date and type of surgical procedure if applicable
  - Location, nature, and behavior of symptoms
    - Radiating symptoms
    - Aggravating/relieving factors
  - Presence of cardinal signs
- Other tests and measures
- Medications
- Past history of cervical/thoracic problems
- Functional status and activity level (current/prior)
  - Postoperative restrictions
- Patient's functional goals

Tests and Measures

Systems review per APTA's *Guide to Physical Therapy Practice*

- ROM
  - Cervical/thoracic
    - AROM
    - PROM
  - Functional upper-extremity ROM
    - Patient demonstrates ability to touch mid-back with the shoulder flexed/externally rotated and extended/internally rotated
- Integumentary integrity
  - Edema/tenderness
  - Integrity of scar tissue
  - Skin/scar mobility
  - Drainage, inflammation

- Joint integrity and mobility
  - Levels above and below fracture or surgery site
  - Craniovertebral stability tests
- Sensory integrity
  - Sensory integrity, C3–T1
- Pain
  - Measured on visual analog scale
  - Palpation
- Posture
  - Head, shoulder positioning
  - Cervical, thoracic, and lumbar curves
- Reflex integrity
  - Biceps (C6)
  - Triceps (C7)
  - Brachioradialis (C5–6)
  - Hoffman's
  - Babinski
  - Clonus
- Motor performance
  - Key muscle tests, C3–T1
  - Grip strength
- Special tests
  - Upper limb tension tests (ULTTs):
    - ULTT 1 (median nerve dominant)
      a. With patient supine, depress shoulder, abduct to approximately 110°, supinate forearm, extend wrist, fingers, and elbow
      b. Side bend head both toward and away
      c. Assess normal vs. abnormal responses (see Butler. 1991)

336   POSTOPERATIVE/POSTFRACTURE REHAB OF THE CERVICAL/THORACIC SPINE | CERVICAL/THORACIC SPINE

- ULTT 2 (radial nerve dominant)
  a. Patient supine, depress shoulder, shoulder abducted and internally rotated, pronate forearm, extend elbow, and flex the wrist
  b. Side bend head both toward and away
  c. Assess normal vs. abnormal responses (see Butler. 1991)
  - ULTT 3 (ulnar nerve dominant)
    a. Patient is supine; extend wrist, supinate forearm, fully flex elbow, depress shoulder, abduct shoulder
    b. Side bend head both toward and away
    c. Assess normal vs. abnormal responses (see Butler. 1991)
- Ventilation/respiration
  ○ Chest expansion
    - Adult male: Normal 2"
    - Adult female: Normal 1½"

Establish Plan of Care
- Based on history, tests, and measures

GOALS/OUTCOMES
- Pain: 2/10 or less
- ROM: Restore maximum symptom-free motion given surgical procedure or achieve a minimum of 80% of AMA guides:

Cervical	Normal	80%
Flexion	60°	50°
Extension	75°	60°
Rotation	80°	65°
Side bend	45°	35°

Thoracic	Normal	80%
Flexion	40°	30°
Extension	No AMA guides established	
Rotation	30°	25°
Side bend	10°	8°

- Spinal and scapular muscle strength: 4+/5 on manual muscle test
- Achieve functional spinal stability and endurance as evidenced by symptom-free tolerance of postural requirements during normal ADLs and vocational activities
- Return to previous functional status for ADLs and vocational, recreational, and sports activities as identified by patient
- Independence in a progressive home exercise program emphasizing function

INTERVENTION
NUMBER OF VISITS: 6–14

Coordination, Communication, and Documentation
- Provision of services between admission and discharge that facilitate cost-effective and efficient integration or reintegration to home, community, or work
- Documentation of therapeutic intervention is required for each episode of care and serves as the basic foundation for communication
- Coordination and additional communication will depend on the patient's impairment and home/work/community/leisure situation and requirements. Such services may include:
  ○ Case management
  ○ Coordination of care and collaboration with those integral to the patient's rehabilitation program
  ○ Coordination and monitoring of the delivery of available resources
  ○ Referrals to other health-care professionals
  ○ Identification of resources, support groups, or advocacy services
  ○ Provision of educational or training information
  ○ Technical assistance

Patient Instruction

Basic Anatomy and Biomechanics
- Cervical and thoracic spine, rib cage, and shoulder girdle
- Pertinent Gray's Anatomy (Gray. 1995. 510-522, 537, 803–805, 807–813, 835–838)
- Importance of:
  ○ Initiation of pain-free motion for joint and muscle nutrition
  ○ Restoration of functional motion for tolerance of ADLs

Handouts
- Commercially available products, such as:
  ○ Krames Communications (1100 Grundy Lane, San Bruno, CA 94066)
    - *Cervical Disc Surgery*
    - *Spinal Surgery*
    - *Neck Basics*
    - *Fit Neck Workout*

- Specific home program for appropriate ROM, stabilization, aerobic exercises
- Postoperative restrictions

Functional Considerations
- Maintain normal and pain-free cervical and thoracic curves during:
  - Sitting
  - Sleeping
  - Driving
- Body mechanics: Limitation/avoidance of aggravating upper-extremity activity and prolonged head postures
- Stabilization/prevention of reinjury
  - Cervical soft collar/hard collar as indicated, per MD orders
  - Alteration of ADLs

Description of Surgical Procedure
- Review of operative procedure and relation to joint biomechanics, rehabilitation, and function

Direct Interventions

Acute Phase: 4–6 Visits
- Therapeutic exercise and home program
  - ROM exercises as appropriate: Active assistive progressing to active
  - Postural awareness and body mechanics training
  - Aerobic exercises for tissue healing
  - Home program
    - Active exercise in pain-free ROM
      a. Cervical/thoracic (supported as needed)
      b. Scapular/glenohumeral
    - Cervical isometrics
    - Postural reeducation exercises
    - Home use of thermal modalities/cryotherapy, supported postures, and avoidance of prolonged activities/postures
- Manual therapy techniques
  - Soft-tissue mobilization
    - Use patient tolerance as guide over fracture/surgical site
  - Joint mobilization
    - Grades I–II for pain relief at surgical site
      a. Exception: cervical fusion
    - Grades III–IV for hypomobilities above and below injury site

- Positional isometric exercises for pain reduction and initiation of stabilization
- Graded neural tension maneuvers as tolerated
- Electrotherapeutic modalities
- Physical agents and mechanical modalities
  - Superficial thermal/cryotherapy
  - Deep thermal: Ultrasound
- Goals/outcomes
  - Pain: 50% reduction from initial rating
  - Decrease muscle guarding as evidenced by improved pain-free AROM
  - Improve spinal awareness and stabilization to prevent reinjury

Subacute Phase: 2–8 Visits
- Therapeutic exercise and home program
  - Continue active exercise in pain-free ROM
  - Self-mobilization exercises as appropriate for regions above and below injury site
  - Strengthening exercises
    - Isometrics
    - Resistive band
      a. Proprioceptive neuromuscular facilitation, upper-extremity diagonals
      b. Scapular retraction/depression
    - Therapeutic ball
    - Plyometrics, such as ball toss in various positions
  - Neuromuscular/balance/proprioceptive reeducation
  - Cardiovascular conditioning with emphasis on postural balance
    - Walking program/treadmill
    - Upper or lower-extremity cycling
    - Aquatic therapy/swimming
    - Ski machine
- Manual therapy techniques
  - Soft-tissue techniques
    - Soft-tissue mobilization
    - Trigger-point techniques
    - Myofascial release
    - Strain/counterstrain
    - Friction massage for incision as tolerated
  - Joint mobilization
    - Progress grade to specific hypomobilities as indicated

- Manually resisted stabilization exercises, emphasizing:
  - 6–10-second hold
  - Repetitions to fatigue
  - Performance in pain-free range
- Progress neural tension maneuvers
- Physical agents and mechanical modalities
  - Continue effective modalities as in acute phase, with increased emphasis on use as needed at home
- Goals/outcomes
  - Pain: 2/10 or less
  - ROM: Restore maximum symptom-free motion, given surgical procedure or achieve a minimum of 80% of AMA guides
    - Cervical
      a. Flexion: 50°
      b. Extension: 60°
      c. Rotation: 65°
      d. Side bend: 35°
    - Thoracic
      a. Flexion: 30°
      b. Extension: No AMA guides established
      c. Rotation: 25°
      d. Side bend: 8°
  - Spinal stabilization, strength, and endurance: 4+/5 on manual muscle test
  - Return to previous functional status for ADLs and vocational, recreational, and sports activities as tolerated

Functional Carryover

- Instruction regarding use of cervical or lumbar support for proper postural alignment during work, driving, and ADLs
- Ergonomic evaluation of the work site if necessary: For example, chair, desk height, computer placement, etc.
- Modification of vocational, recreational, and sports activities as necessary due to residual limitations

DISCHARGE PLANNING AND PATIENT RESPONSIBILITY

Criteria for Discharge

- All goals/outcomes have been achieved with the exception of return to previous status for recreational and sports activities

Circumstances Requiring Additional Visits

- Persistent functional strength deficit or 2+/5 on manual muscle test
- History of previous injury/surgery to related area
- Persistent radicular symptoms or neurological deficit
- Severe deconditioning
- Special occupational needs requiring extensive fitness/strengthening
- Instability at fracture/surgical site
- Postoperative infection/complication
- Severe postoperative scarring
- Presence of surgical hardware
- Multiple fracture/injury sites
- Head injury
- Arthritic conditions
- Multilevel fracture, surgical involvement
- Residual signs and symptoms
- Necessary to return to normal work status (no modified duty available)

Home Program

- Flexibility exercises for maintenance of postural balance
- Progressive strengthening exercises to challenge patient's current level, including increasing:
  - Repetitions
  - Duration
  - Resistance
- Self-mobilization techniques
- Use of modalities at home as needed for occasional flare-ups
- Progression of aerobic endurance exercise

Monitoring

- Instruct patient to call for advice should progression halt or a negative trend occur
- Patient is to recheck/call at 2–4 weeks post-discharge to ensure expected return to function

CERVICAL/THORACIC SPINE | POSTOPERATIVE/POSTFRACTURE REHAB OF THE CERVICAL/THORACIC SPINE

REFERENCES

1. American Physical Therapy Association. *Guide to Physical Therapist Practice*. Alexandria, VA: APTA; 1997.

2. Butler DS. *Mobilization of The Nervous System*. Melbourne, Australia: Churchill Livingstone; 1991.

3. Chesnut RM, Abitol JJ, Garfin SR. Surgical management of cervical radiculopathy: indication, techniques, and results. *Orthop Clin North Am*. 1992;23:461-473.

4. Ching RP, Watson NA, Carter JW, Tencer AF. The effect of post-injury spinal position on canal occlusion in a cervical spine burst fracture model. *Spine*. 1997;22:1710-1715.

5. Corrigan B, Maitland GD. *Practical Orthopedic Medicine*. London, England: Butterworths; 1983.

6. Gray H; Williams PL, ed. *Gray's Anatomy*. 38th ed. New York, NY: Churchill Livingstone; 1995.

7. Gross AR, Aker PD, Quartly C. Manual therapy in the treatment of neck pain. *Rheum Dis Clin North Am*. 1996;22:579-598.

8. Hart A, Hopkins C, Ford B. *ICD-9-CM Expert For Physicians, Volume 1&2*. 7th ed. USA: Ingenix; 2005.

9. Jordan A, Bendix T, Nielsen H, Hansen FR, Host D, Winkel A. Intensive training, physiotherapy, or manipulation for patients with chronic neck pain. a prospective, single-blinded, randomized clinical trial. *Spine*. 1998;23:311-318; discussion, 319.

10. Kurz LT, Herkowitz HN. Surgical management of myelopathy. *Orthop Clin of North Am*. 1992;23:495-504.

11. Nowinski GP, Visarius H, Nolte LP, Herkowitz HN. A biomechanical comparison of cervical laminaplasty and cervical laminectomy with progressive facetectomy. *Spine*. 1993;18:1995-2004.

12. Prall JA, Winston KR, Brennan R. Spine and spinal cord injuries in downhill skiers. *J Trauma*. 1995;39:1115-1118.

13. Riddle DL, Stratford PW. Use of generic versus region-specific functional status measures on patients with cervical spine disorders. *Phys Ther*. 1998;78:951-963.

14. Sandmark H, Nisell R. Validity of five common manual neck pain provoking tests. *Scand J Rehabil Med*. 1995 Sep;27(3):131-136.

15. Snow RB, Weiner H. Cervical laminectomy and foraminectomy as surgical treatment of cervical spondylosis. *J Spin Disord*. 1993;6:245-250.

16. Youdas JW, Carey JR, Garrett TR. Reliability of measurements of cervical spine ROM—comparison of three methods. *Phys Ther*. 1991;71:98-104; discussion, 105-106.

17. Youdas JW, Garrett TR, Suman VJ, et al. Normal ROM of the cervical spine: an initial goniometric study. *Phys Ther*. 1992;72:770-780.

RIB DYSFUNCTION
SUMMARY OVERVIEW

ICD-9

353.8   807   848.3

APTA Preferred Practice Pattern: 4D, 4E, 4F, 4H, 5D

EXAMINATION

- History and Systems Review
- Tests and Measures
  Systems review per APTA's *Guide to Physical Therapy Practice*
  - Joint integrity and mobility
  - Muscle performance
  - Pain
  - Posture
  - ROM
  - Special tests
  - Ventilation, respiration, and circulation
- Establish Plan of Care

GOALS/OUTCOMES

- Pain: 2/10 or less
- Thoracic ROM: At least 80% of AMA guides
- Normal aerobic capacity and endurance
- Full, pain-free inspiration and expiration
- Trunk strength: 4+/5 on manual muscle test for spinal extensors and abdominals
- Return to previous functional status for ADLs and vocational, recreational, and sports activities as identified by patient
- Independence in a progressive home exercise program emphasizing function

INTERVENTION
NUMBER OF VISITS: 4–8

- Patient Instruction
  - Basic Anatomy and Biomechanics
  - Handouts
  - Functional Considerations
- Direct Interventions
  - Acute Phase: 2–4 Visits
  - Subacute Phase: 2–4 Visits
- Functional Carryover

DISCHARGE PLANNING AND PATIENT RESPONSIBILITY

- Criteria for Discharge
  - All goals/outcomes have been met
  - Patient demonstrates understanding of importance of proper breathing mechanics
- Circumstances Requiring Additional Visits
  - Persistent functional strength deficit or 3/5 on manual muscle test
  - History of previous injury/surgery to related area
  - Severe deconditioning
  - Special occupational needs requiring extensive fitness/strengthening
  - Persistent pain with normal respiration
  - Instability
  - Rib fracture
  - Cartilagenous separation
  - Multiple injury sites
- Home Program
  - Use of home modalities for flare-ups
  - Thoracic and scapular stabilization/strengthening exercises
  - Cardiovascular conditioning
  - Self-mobilization exercise techniques
  - Flexibility exercises
- Monitoring

SUMMARY OVERVIEW | CERVICAL/THORACIC SPINE | RIB DYSFUNCTION   341

RIB DYSFUNCTION

ICD-9
353.8	Other nerve root and plexus disorders
807	Fracture of rib(s), sternum, larynx, and trachea
848.3	Sprain of ribs

APTA Preferred Practice Pattern: 4D, 4E, 4F, 4H, 5D

EXAMINATION

History and Systems Review
- History of current condition
  - Location, nature, and behavior of symptoms
    - Radiating symptoms
      a. Anterior radiation often implicates spine
    - Aggravating/relieving factors
      a. Spinal motion
      b. Respiration
      c. Postures, activities
- Past history of current condition
- Other tests and measures
- Medications
- Past medical/surgical history
  - Inquire regarding systemic pathology
    - Tuberculosis
    - Ankylosing spondylitis
    - Rheumatoid arthritis
    - Shingles
    - Pleurisy
    - Bronchitis
    - Cardiac
    - Gall bladder
- Functional status and activity level (current/prior)
  - Effect on sleep
  - Work/ADL postural tolerance
  - Personal care
- Patient's functional goals

Tests and Measures
Systems review per APTA's *Guide to Physical Therapy Practice*

Unless a rib fracture is proven or suspected, the thoracic spine must be assessed concurrently with specific ribs. Rib problems commonly occur secondary to thoracic spine dysfunction.

- Joint integrity and mobility
  - Passive thoracic segmental motion
    - Central and unilateral posterior to anterior
  - Costovertebral posterior to anterior glide
- Muscle performance
  - Isometric motor performance testing of trunk motions
  - Resisted testing
- Pain
  - Measured on visual analog scale
  - Palpation
    - Static
      a. Intercostal musculature
      b. Ribs
      c. Inferior margins
      d. Superior margins
      e. Rib angles
    - Dynamic with full inspiration and expiration
      a. Costovertebral junction
      b. Sternocostal junction
- Posture
  - Head position
  - Scoliosis
  - Thoracic kyphosis inclinometer reading
- ROM
  - Cervical, thoracic rib, and shoulder
  - AROM
  - PROM
  - Overpressure
- Special tests
  - Dural mobility tests
    - Slump test
    - Straight leg raise test
- Ventilation, respiration, and circulation
  - Chest expansion
    - Adult male: Normal 2"
    - Adult female: Normal 1½"

342   RIB DYSFUNCTION | CERVICAL/THORACIC SPINE

○ Inspiration/expiration in flexion/extension
  ▪ These tests are used to assess spinal contribution to symptoms. For example:
    a. If full inspiration (which extends the spine) is painful in extension but not in flexion, the spine is implicated
    b. If it is painful in both full flexion and extension, a costal problem is implied

Establish Plan of Care
- Based on history, tests, and measures

GOALS/OUTCOMES
- Pain: 2/10 or less
- Thoracic ROM: At least 80% of AMA guides

	Normal	*80%*
Flexion	40°	30°
Extension	No AMA guides established	
Rotation	30°	25°
Side bend	10°	8°

- Normal aerobic capacity and endurance
- Full, pain-free inspiration and expiration
- Trunk strength: 4+/5 on manual muscle test for spinal extensors and abdominals
- Return to previous functional status for ADLs and vocational, recreational, and sports activities as identified by patient
- Independence in a progressive home exercise program emphasizing function

INTERVENTION
NUMBER OF VISITS: 4–8

Coordination, Communication, and Documentation
- Provision of services between admission and discharge that facilitate cost-effective and efficient integration or reintegration to home, community, or work
- Documentation of therapeutic intervention is required for each episode of care and serves as the basic foundation for communication
- Coordination and additional communication will depend on the patient's impairment and home/work/community/leisure situation and requirements. Such services may include:
  ○ Case management
  ○ Coordination of care and collaboration with those integral to the patient's rehabilitation program

○ Coordination and monitoring of the delivery of available resources
○ Referrals to other health-care professionals
○ Identification of resources, support groups, or advocacy services
○ Provision of educational or training information
○ Technical assistance

Patient Instruction

Basic Anatomy and Biomechanics
- Anatomy of the thoracic spine, ribs, intercostal muscles, and diaphragm
- Pertinent Gray's Anatomy (Gray. 1995. 540-545, 811–815)
- Biomechanical relationship of ribs and spine
- Normal breathing mechanics vs. chest breathing

Handouts
- Specific home program

Functional Considerations
- Protection of injury site during healing time
- Proper breathing mechanics
- Techniques for symptom management during cough, sneeze, or valsalva maneuver as indicated

Direct Interventions

Acute Phase: 2–4 Visits
- Therapeutic exercise and home program
  ○ Abdominal breathing exercises, initially in supine
  ○ Thoracic spine flexibility exercises
  ○ Home program
    ▪ Minimize painful chest motions
    ▪ Self-mobilization exercises for specific thoracic hypomobilities
    ▪ Continued abdominal breathing exercises
  ○ Teach stretching exercises in neural tension test positions for upper and lower extremities
- Manual therapy techniques
  ○ Soft-tissue mobilization
    ▪ Positional isometric techniques
    ▪ Muscle energy techniques
    ▪ Trigger-point acupressure

CERVICAL/THORACIC SPINE | RIB DYSFUNCTION 343

○ Joint mobilization
  ▪ Spinal joint mobilization Grades I–III
    a. Specific traction
    b. Posterior to ankle glide
    c. Side bend/rotation
  ▪ Costovertebral joint mobilization, Grades I–II as tolerated
○ Rib mobility techniques using passive upper-extremity elevation and respiration
○ Neural mobilization
• Electrotherapeutic modalities
○ TENS may be beneficial for intercostal neuralgia
• Physical agents
○ Superficial thermal/cryotherapy
○ Deep thermal: Ultrasound
• Goals
○ Pain: 50% reduction from initial rating
○ Consistent utilization of diaphragmatic breathing mechanics
○ Thoracic ROM: a minimum of 50% of AMA guides
  ▪ Flexion: 20°
  ▪ Extension: No AMA guides established
  ▪ Side bend: 5°
  ▪ Rotation: 15°
○ Patient demonstrates adequate protective and stabilization measures for prevention of reinjury or aggravation with daily activities

Subacute Phase: 2–4 Visits
• Therapeutic exercise and home program
○ Cardiovascular conditioning
  ▪ Level of exertion not to exceed pain-free respiration
○ Active thoracic flexibility exercises
  ▪ Rising sun
    a. Begin right side-lying with both shoulders flexed to 90°; left hip and knee flexed to 90°, right hip and knee extended
    b. Horizontally abduct the left arm, rotating the trunk to the left. Do not allow the left knee to leave the surface.
    c. Maintain the stretch for 10 breaths
    d. Repeat to the opposite side
○ Thoracic self-mobilization as needed
○ Active thoracic strengthening in pain-free extension, flexion, rotation, and side bending using resistive tubing

○ Shoulder girdle strengthening exercises
○ Progress abdominal breathing exercises to functional/exercise postures
• Manual therapy techniques
○ Continue effective soft-tissue mobilization
○ Joint mobilization
  ▪ Progressive Grades III–V to hypomobile joints
  ▪ Progress graded specific traction to irritable joints
  ▪ Continue rib mobilization if indicated
○ Progress use of neural tension stretching as effective
• Physical agents to thoracic spine as needed
○ Continue effective modalities as in acute phase, with increased emphasis on use as needed at home
• Goals
○ Pain: 2/10 or less
○ Thoracic ROM: a minimum of 80% of AMA guides
  ▪ Flexion: 30°
  ▪ Extension: No AMA guides established
  ▪ Rotation: 25°
  ▪ Side bend: 8°
○ Return to pain-free ADLs and vocational activities
○ Demonstrates knowledge of progression of conditioning exercises: For example, exertion is limited by pain-free breathing
○ Scapular and spinal motor performance equal and painless bilaterally: Primary concern is restoration of painful motions tested isometrically in the initial examination

Functional Carryover
• Instruction regarding use of cervical or lumbar support for proper postural alignment during work, driving, and ADLs
• Integration of proper body mechanics into ADL/vocational activities
• Ergonomic modification of work site, including chair, desk height, and computer placement

DISCHARGE PLANNING AND PATIENT RESPONSIBILITY

Criteria for Discharge
• All goals/outcomes have been met
• Patient demonstrates understanding of importance of proper breathing mechanics

Circumstances Requiring Additional Visits

- Persistent functional strength deficit or 3/5 on manual muscle test
- History of previous injury/surgery to related area
- Severe deconditioning
- Special occupational needs requiring extensive fitness/strengthening
- Persistent pain with normal respiration
- Instability
- Rib fracture
- Cartilagenous separation
- Multiple injury sites

Home Program

- Use of home modalities for flare-ups
- Thoracic and scapular stabilization/strengthening exercises
- Cardiovascular conditioning
- Self-mobilization exercise techniques
- Flexibility exercises

Monitoring

- Instruct patient to call for advice should progression halt or a negative trend occur
- Patient is to recheck/call at 4–6 weeks post-discharge to assess progress toward previous functional status

REFERENCES

1. American Physical Therapy Association. *Guide to Physical Therapist Practice.* Alexandria, VA: APTA; 1997.
2. Gray H; Williams PL, ed. *Gray's Anatomy.* 38th ed. New York, NY: Churchill Livingstone; 1995.
3. Hart A, Hopkins C, Ford B. *ICD-9-CM Expert For Physicians, Volume 1&2.* 7th ed. USA: Ingenix; 2005.
4. Lee D. *Manual Therapy For The Thorax: A Biomechanical Approach.* Delta, British Columbia, Canada: DOPC; 1994.
5. Riddle DL, Stratford PW. Use of generic versus region-specific functional status measures on patients with cervical spine disorders. *Phys Ther.* 1998;78:951-963.
6. Sandmark H, Nisell R. Validity of five neck pain provoking tests. *Scand J Rehabil Med.* 1995;27(3):131-136.
7. Youdas JW, Carey JR, Garrett TR. Reliability of measurements of cervical spine ROM—comparison of three methods. *Phys Ther.* 1991;71:98-104; discussion, 105-106.
8. Youdas JW, Garrett TR, Suman VJ, et al. Normal ROM of the cervical spine: an initial goniometric study. *Phys Ther.* 1992;72:770-780.

SCOLIOSIS
SUMMARY OVERVIEW

ICD-9

356.1   732.0   732.1   732.8   732.9   737.3   737.4   754.2

APTA Preferred Practice Pattern: 4A, 4B, 4F, 4G, 4H, 4J, 5E, 6F

EXAMINATION

- History and Systems Review
- Tests and Measures
  Systems review per APTA's *Guide to Physical Therapy Practice*
  - Gait, locomotion, and balance
  - Muscle performance
  - Pain
  - Posture
  - ROM
  - Reflex integrity
  - Sensory integrity
  - Special tests
- Establish Plan of Care

GOALS/OUTCOMES

- Pain: 1/10 or less
- Maximize stable spinal ROM
- Stop progression of structural curve
- Independence in a progressive home exercise program emphasizing function
- Strength: 4+/5 on manual muscle test for abdominal, scapular, and hip/spinal extensor muscle groups
- Return to previous functional status for ADLs and vocational, recreational, and sports activities as identified by patient

INTERVENTION
NUMBER OF VISITS: 4–9

- Patient Instruction
  - Basic Anatomy and Biomechanics
  - Handouts
  - Functional Considerations
  - Description of Surgical Procedure
- Direct Interventions
  - Phase I: 2–6 Visits
  - Phase II: 2–3 Visits
- Functional Carryover

DISCHARGE PLANNING AND PATIENT RESPONSIBILITY

- Criteria for Discharge
  - Patient demonstrates understanding of proper postural alignment
  - Patient demonstrates knowledge and understanding of brace use if appropriate
  - All goals/outcomes have been achieved
- Circumstances Requiring Additional Visits
  - Persistent functional strength deficit or 3/5 on manual muscle test
  - History of previous injury/surgery to related area
  - Severe deconditioning
  - Special occupational needs requiring extensive fitness/ strengthening
  - Arthritic conditions
  - Instability
  - Traumatic injury with persistent functional/ occupational deficits
- Home Program
  - Postural instruction
  - Strengthening
  - Flexibility
  - Diaphragmatic breathing
- Monitoring

SCOLIOSIS

ICD-9

356.1	Peroneal muscular atrophy
732.0	Juvenile osteochondrosis of spine
732.1	Juvenile osteochondrosis of hip and pelvis
732.8	Other specified forms of osteochondropathy
732.9	Unspecified osteochondropathy
737.3	Kyphoscoliosis and scoliosis
737.4	Curvature of spine associated with other conditions
754.2	Certain congenital musculoskeletal deformities of spine

APTA Preferred Practice Pattern: 4A, 4B, 4F, 4G, 4H, 4J, 5E, 6F

EXAMINATION

History and Systems Review

- History of current condition
  - Congenital
  - Progressive
  - Posttraumatic
  - Location, nature, and behavior of symptoms
    - Aggravating/relieving factors
- Past history of current condition
  - Curve behavior or progression
  - Use of brace
  - Date and type of surgical procedure if applicable
- Other tests and measures
  - X-ray findings
  - Degree and direction of curvature
- Medications
- Past medical/surgical history
  - Presence of congenital or acquired neuropathic or myopathic disorders
  - Possible systemic pathology
- Functional status and activity level (current/prior)
  - Independent mobility
  - Work and ADL postural tolerance
- Patient's functional goals
- Reported cardiopulmonary status
  - Rib cage ROM
  - Vital/total lung capacity
  - Right ventricle/atrium hypertrophy from pulmonary hypertension

Tests and Measures

Systems review per APTA's *Guide to Physical Therapy Practice*

- Gait, locomotion, and balance
  - Asymmetrical gait pattern
    - Arm swing
    - Hip transverse plane motion
    - Knee extension in stance phase
    - Knee flexion in swing phase
    - Early heel off
    - Excessive pronation
- Muscle performance
  - Key muscle tests
  - Abdominal
    - Obliques
    - Rectus abdominis
    - Pelvic tilt isolation
  - Erector spinae and thoracolumbar musculature
  - Scapular musculature
  - Quadratus lumborum
  - Iliopsoas
- Pain
  - Measured on visual analog scale
  - With palpation
- Posture
  - Shoulder, scapulothoracic, and pelvis symmetry
    - Direction, degree of curvature within spine (use inclinometer for kyphosis measurements)
    - Spinal level of curve apex
    - Compensatory changes
      a. Arm length
      b. Asymmetries in stance
      c. Distance between arms and body
      d. Head and neck alignment
      e. Multiple curvature
  - Leg length discrepancy
    - Supine
    - Weight-bearing

348   SCOLIOSIS | CERVICAL/THORACIC SPINE

- ROM
  - Spine, hip, shoulder
  - Active ROM rib hump measurement
    - Structural vs. functional scoliosis
      a. *Structural scoliosis* is a lateral and rotational curvature that cannot be corrected by positioning or voluntary effort. Forward bending produces posterior rib hump (greater than or equal to 1 cm) at the convexity of the thoracic curve, anterior rib cage prominence on concave side and associated spine. Structural changes may also occur, such as vertebral body wedging.
      b. *Functional scoliosis* is reversible with forward or side bending or with changes in spine or pelvic alignment with muscle contraction. It may also reverse in supine. No rib hump is evident.
  - PROM
  - Overpressure
    - Ribs
    - Spine
- Reflex integrity
- Sensory integrity
- Special tests
  - Dural tension tests

Establish Plan of Care

- Based on history, tests, and measures

GOALS/OUTCOMES

- Pain: 1/10 or less
- Maximize stable spinal ROM
- Stop progression of structural curve
- Independence in a progressive home exercise program emphasizing function
- Strength: 4+/5 on manual muscle test for abdominal, scapular, and hip/spinal extensor muscle groups
- Return to previous functional status for ADLs and vocational, recreational, and sports activities as identified by patient

INTERVENTION

NUMBER OF VISITS: 4–9

Coordination, Communication, and Documentation

- Provision of services between admission and discharge that facilitate cost-effective and efficient integration or reintegration to home, community, or work
- Documentation of therapeutic intervention is required for each episode of care and serves as the basic foundation for communication
- Coordination and additional communication will depend on the patient's impairment and home/work/community/leisure situation and requirements. Such services may include:
  - Case management
  - Coordination of care and collaboration with those integral to the patient's rehabilitation program
  - Coordination and monitoring of the delivery of available resources
  - Referrals to other health-care professionals
  - Identification of resources, support groups, or advocacy services
  - Provision of educational or training information
  - Technical assistance

Patient Instruction

Basic Anatomy and Biomechanics
- Spinal anatomy, normal movement patterns, and scoliotic limitations
- Diagnosis and prognosis
- National Scoliosis Foundation (72 Mt. Auburn St, Watertown, MA 97172, 617-926-0397)
- Scoliosis Association (PO Box 51353, Raleigh, NC 27609, 919–846-2639)
- Scoliosis Program, Children's Hospital at Stanford University Orthopedic Rehabilitation Service (20 Willow Road, Palo Alto, CA 94304)
- Scoliosis Research Society (222 South Prospect, Suite 127, Park Ridge, IL 60068, 708-698-1627)
- Standards for Scoliosis Screening in California Public Schools, Publication Sales Department of Education (PO Box 271, Sacramento, CA 95802-0271)

CERVICAL/THORACIC SPINE | SCOLIOSIS

Handouts

- American Physical Therapy Association (1111 N. Fairfax Street, Alexandria VA 22314)
  - *Scoliosis*
  - *The Secret of Good Posture*
- Specific home exercises, postural instruction

Functional Considerations

- If curve greater than or equal to 40°, may consider bracing depending on curve behavior and age of patient
  - Milwaukie brace
  - Body jacket
- Postural awareness for ADLs and recreational activities
- Preoperative education, flexibility, and motor performance training as appropriate

Description of Surgical Procedure

- Review of operative procedure and relation to joint biomechanics, rehabilitation, and function

Direct Interventions

Phase I: 2–6 Visits

- Therapeutic exercise and home program
  - Strengthening exercises as appropriate: Progress active/assisted, to active, to resistive
  - Postural awareness and body mechanics training
  - Aerobic exercises for tissue healing
  - Home program
    - Home pain management procedures
      a. Thermal modalities/cryotherapy
      b. TENS
    - Postural awareness
  - Abdominal and trunk strengthening
    - Pelvic tilt
      a. Supine
      b. Hook lying
      c. Standing
    - Trunk or pelvis shift: Stand with arms at side and shift trunk or pelvis to correct concavity
    - Side-lying trunk elevation (lateral trunk flexors on convexity strengthened)
    - Abdominal crunches forward and diagonally to each side
    - Quadruped or prone trunk extensor strengthening
    - Therapeutic ball program

- Hip extensor strengthening
    a. Squats
    b. Multidirectional lunges
  - Flexibility
    - Heel sit with arms reaching forward, laterally bend trunk and arms away from concavity
    - Stand facing a wall, elongate spine with arms overhead, emphasizing stretch on concave side of curvature
    - Rising sun
      a. Begin right side-lying with both shoulders flexed to 90°, left hip and knee flexed to 90°, right hip and knee extended
      b. Horizontally abduct the left arm, rotating the trunk to the left. Do not allow the left knee to leave the surface.
      c. Maintain the stretch for 10 breaths
      d. Repeat to the opposite side
      e. Perform 2:1 ratio lying on side of convexity
  - Side-lying on convex side over a pillow
  - Hip flexors
  - Erector spinae
    - Hamstrings
    - Pectorals
    - Sternocleidomastoid
    - Scalenes
  - Diaphragmatic breathing
    - Supine
    - Sitting
    - Combine with concave side segmental breathing during unilateral stretch or with bilateral pectoral stretch
- Manual therapy techniques
  - Soft-tissue mobilization
    - Trigger-point techniques
    - Strain/counterstrain
    - Myofascial release
    - Friction massage
  - Joint mobilization
    - Progressive Grades III–V joint mobilization to hypomobile joints
    - Graded specific traction to irritable joints
  - Assisted stretching for tight muscles
- Electrotherapeutic modalities
  - TENS

- Physical agents and mechanical modalities
  - Superficial thermal/cryotherapy
  - Deep thermal: Ultrasound
- Goals/outcomes
  - Pain: 1/10 or less
  - Strength: 4-/5 on manual muscle test for abdominal, scapular, and hip/spinal extensor muscle groups
  - Maximize stable spinal ROM

Phase II: 2–3 Visits
- Review ADLs and recreational postural awareness
- Reassess rib hump, ROM, and motor performance tests for comparison to initial screenings
- Progress home exercise program for maximal challenge with maintenance postural alignment
- Reinforce need for consistent daily performance of home exercise program

Functional Carryover
- Modification of cardiovascular or recreational activities as necessary to diminish compressive forces
- Instruction regarding proper body mechanics for ADLs and recreational activities, including lifting and sitting
- Instruction in applying trunk stabilization or diaphragmatic breathing during sports or dynamic activities
- Referral of patient to appropriate support groups

DISCHARGE PLANNING AND PATIENT RESPONSIBILITY

Criteria for Discharge
- Patient demonstrates understanding of proper postural alignment
- Patient demonstrates knowledge and understanding of brace use if appropriate
- All goals/outcomes have been achieved

Circumstances Requiring Additional Visits
- Persistent functional strength deficit or 3/5 on manual muscle test
- History of previous injury/surgery to related area
- Severe deconditioning
- Special occupational needs requiring extensive fitness/strengthening
- Arthritic conditions
- Instability
- Traumatic injury with persistent functional/occupational deficits

Home Program
- Postural instruction
- Strengthening
- Flexibility
- Diaphragmatic breathing

Monitoring
- Patient is to recheck or call at 3- and 6-month intervals to ensure continued consistency with home exercise program and progression toward full functional status
- Patient is to come in for 1–2 visits to:
  - Review ADLs and recreational postural awareness
  - Reassess rib hump, ROM, and motor performance tests for comparison to initial screenings
  - Progress home exercise program for maximal challenge with maintenance postural alignment
  - Reinforce need for consistent daily performance of home exercise program

REFERENCES

1. Connolly BH, Lezberg SF, Weiler DR. *Scoliosis.* American Physical Therapy Association; Alexandria, VA; 1985.

2. Focarile FA, Bondaldi A, Giarolo MA, et al. Effectiveness of non-surgical treatment for idiopathic scoliosis: overview of available evidence. *Spine.* 1991;16:395-401.

3. Gray H; Williams PL, ed. *Gray's Anatomy.* 38th ed. New York, NY: Churchill Livingstone; 1995.

4. Hart A, Hopkins C, Ford B. *ICD-9-CM Expert For Physicians, Volume 1&2.* 7th ed. USA: Ingenix; 2005.

5. Iglarsh A, Kendall F, Lewis C, Sahrmann S. *The Secret of Good Posture.* American Physical Therapy Association; Alexandria, VA; 1985.

6. King HA. Analysis and treatment of type II idiopathic scoliosis. *Orthop Clin North Am.* 1994;25:225-238.

7. Perdiolle R, Becchetti S, Vidal J, Lopez P. Mechanical process and growth cartilages: essential factors in the progression of scoliosis. *Spine.* 1993;18:343-349.

8. Poussa M, Mellin G. Spinal mobility and posture in adolescent idiopathic scoliosis at three stages of curve magnitude. *Spine.* 1992;17:757-760.

9. Salter RB. *Textbook of Disorders And Injuries of The Musculoskeletal System.* 2nd ed. 315-316.

10. Simons ED, Kowalski JM, Simmons EH. The results of surgical treatment for adult scoliosis. *Spine.* 1993;18:718-724.

11. Willers U, Normelli H, Aaro S, Svensson O, Hedlund R. Long-term results of Boston brace treatment on vertebral rotation in idiopathic scoliosis. *Spine.* 1993;18:432-435.

12. Winter RB. The pendulum has swung too far: bracing for adolescent idiopathic scoliosis in the 1990s. *Orthop Clin North Am.* 1994;25:195-204.

THORACIC OUTLET SYNDROME
SUMMARY OVERVIEW

ICD-9

  353.0   353.2   353.3   353.5   353.8   353.9

APTA Preferred Practice Pattern: **4F, 5D**

EXAMINATION

- History and Systems Review
- Tests and Measures
  Systems review per APTA's *Guide to Physical Therapy Practice*
  - Anthropometric characteristics
  - Integumentary integrity
  - Joint integrity and mobility
  - Muscle performance
  - Pain
  - Posture
  - ROM
  - Reflex integrity
  - Sensory integrity
  - Special tests
- Establish Plan of Care

GOALS/OUTCOMES

- Pain: 2/10 or less
- Functional joint mobility as well as connective tissue and muscle flexibility of the rib cage, thoracic, and cervical spines
- Cervical and thoracic ROM: A minimum of 80% of AMA guides
- Shoulder ROM: A minimum of 90% of AMA guides
- Negative response with special circulation and neural mobility tests
- Restore postural symmetry as evidenced by observation of proper sitting and standing postures
- Improve body mechanics as evidenced by patient recognition and avoidance of aggravating postures
- Strength: 4+/5 on manual muscle test for abdominals, hip/back extensors, and scapular retractors/elevators
- Return to previous functional status for ADLs and vocational, recreational, and sports activities as identified by patient
- Independence in a progressive home exercise program emphasizing function

INTERVENTION
NUMBER OF VISITS: 6–12

- Patient Intervention
  - Basic Anatomy and Biomechanics
  - Handouts
  - Functional Considerations
- Direct Interventions
  - Acute Phase: 3–6 Visits
  - Subacute Phase: 3–6 Visits
- Functional Carryover

DISCHARGE PLANNING AND PATIENT RESPONSIBILITY

- Criteria for Discharge
  - Patient demonstrates ability to perform exercises correctly and reports intent to continue performance until strength, pain-free ROM, and functional level have returned to normal
  - Patient understands that in most cases there is no "cure," but rather, that this is a management issue and that symptoms occur due to inflammation near pain-sensitive structures (such as Brachial Plexus)
  - All goals/outcomes have been achieved with the exception of return to previous level for recreational and sports activities
- Circumstances Requiring Additional Visits
  - Persistent functional strength deficit or 3/5 on manual muscle test
  - History of previous injury or surgery to related area
  - Persistent radicular symptoms
  - Severe deconditioning
  - Special occupational needs requiring extensive fitness/ strengthening
- Home Program
  - Diaphragmatic breathing
  - Self-mobilization
  - Flexibility/strengthening exercises for maintenance of postural balance
- Monitoring

SUMMARY OVERVIEW | CERVICAL/THORACIC SPINE | THORACIC OUTLET SYNDROME   353

THORACIC OUTLET SYNDROME

ICD-9

353.0	Brachial plexus lesions
353.2	Cervical root lesions, not elsewhere classified
353.3	Thoracic root lesions, not elsewhere classified
353.5	Neuralgic amyotrophy
353.8	Other nerve root and plexus disorders
353.9	Unspecified nerve root and plexus disorder

APTA Preferred Practice Pattern: 4F, 5D

EXAMINATION

History and Systems Review
- History of current condition
  - Location, nature, and behavior of symptoms
    - Neurogenic symptoms, predominately C8/T1 distribution
      a. Paresthesia
      b. Numbness and tingling
      c. Pain (aching or sharp)
      d. Sensory or motor loss
    - Presence of release phenomena
      a. Pain at night
    - Pain usually unilateral but can be bilateral
    - Supraclavicular area
    - Shoulder
    - Arm
    - Hypothenar area
    - Hand
    - 5th digit
    - Chest wall
    - Aggravating/relieving factors
  - Fine motor coordination
  - Signs of arterial obstruction
    - Possible coolness or cold sensitivity in hands
  - Signs of venous obstruction
    - Cyanotic discoloration
    - Edema
    - Stiffness
    - Feeling of heaviness
  - Exertional fatigue
- Past history of current condition
  - Including interventions for Thoracic Outlet Syndrome

- Other tests and measures
- Medications
- Functional status and activity level (current/prior)
  - Combing hair
  - Reaching
  - Holding a book, telephone, or steering wheel
  - Carrying a purse/briefcase/bag
- Patient's functional goals

Tests and Measures
Systems review per APTA's *Guide to Physical Therapy Practice*
- Anthropometric characteristics
  - Atrophy/hypertrophy
  - Edema
- Integumentary integrity
  - Skin
    - Color changes
    - Scars
- Joint integrity and mobility
  - Cervical/thoracic spine:
    - Particularly C3 and C4 levels both ipsilateral and contralateral to upper-extremity symptoms
    - Craniovertebral stability
  - Shoulder, acromioclavicular joint, sternoclavicular joint
- Muscle performance
  - Key muscle tests, C3–T1
    - Specifically thenar, hypothenar, and interosseous muscles
- Pain
  - Measured on visual analog scale
  - Palpation of muscles, tendons, and ligaments
    - Trigger-points with or without referral
  - Positional changes

354 THORACIC OUTLET SYNDROME | CERVICAL/THORACIC SPINE

- Posture
  - Head, neck, and shoulder symmetry
  - Asymmetry of extremities, e.g., protraction of the shoulder girdle
  - Rotoscoliosis of thoracolumbar spine
- ROM
  - Active
  - Passive
  - Thoracic and cervical motion
  - Rib ROM
    - With shoulder elevation
    - With breathing
- Reflex integrity
  - Biceps (C6)
  - Triceps (C7)
  - Brachioradialis (C5–6)
  - Hoffman's
  - Babinski
  - Clonus
- Sensory integrity
  - Hypesthesia may occur in C8–T1 dermatomes
- Special tests
  - Circulation (radial pulse)
    - Hyperabduction/Wright's test
      a. Compare radial pulse with arm resting at side to pulse with shoulder abducted to end range
    - Costoclavicular test
      a. Find radial pulse while sitting, then have patient retract shoulders maximally and flex chin to chest. Reassess radial pulse.
    - Adson test
      a. Lateral flexion of the head to the contralateral side; reassess pulse
    - Exaggerated military position test
      a. Depression of shoulder girdle; reassess pulse
    - Hands-up/abduction external rotation test
      a. Abduct shoulder and externally rotate to 90°; reassess pulse
  - Neural mobility
    - Upper limb tension tests (ULTTs)
      a. ULTT 1 (median nerve dominant)
        - With patient supine, depress shoulder, abduct to approximately 110°, supinate forearm, extend wrist, fingers, and elbow
        - Side bend head both toward and away
        - Assess normal vs. abnormal responses (see Butler. 1991)

  b. ULTT 2 (radial nerve dominant)
    - Patient supine, depress shoulder, shoulder abducted and internally rotated, pronate forearm, extend elbow, and flex the wrist
    - Side bend head both toward and away
    - Assess normal vs. abnormal responses (see Butler. 1991)
  c. ULTT 3 (ulnar nerve dominant)
    - Patient is supine; extend wrist, supinate forearm, fully flex elbow, depress shoulder, abduct shoulder
    - Side bend head both toward and away
    - Assess normal vs. abnormal responses (see Butler. 1991)
  - Ventilation
    - Diaphragmatic function, breathing patterns

Establish Plan of Care
- Based on history, tests, and measures

GOALS/OUTCOMES
- Pain: 2/10 or less
- Functional joint mobility as well as connective tissue and muscle flexibility of the rib cage, thoracic, and cervical spines
- Cervical and thoracic ROM: A minimum of 80% of AMA guides

Cervical	Normal	80%
Flexion	60°	50°
Extension	75°	60°
Rotation	80°	65°
Side bend	45°	35°

Thoracic	Normal	80%
Flexion	40°	30°
Extension	No AMA guides established	
Rotation	30°	25°
Side bend	10°	8°

- Shoulder ROM: A minimum of 90% of AMA guides

	Normal	90%
Flexion	180°	160°
Extension	50°	45°
Abduction	170+°	155°
Internal rotation	80+°	70°
External rotation	80+°	70°

- Negative response with special circulation and neural mobility tests

- Restore postural symmetry as evidenced by observation of proper sitting and standing postures
- Improve body mechanics as evidenced by patient recognition and avoidance of aggravating postures
- Strength: 4+/5 on manual muscle test for abdominals, hip/back extensors, and scapular retractors/elevators
- Return to previous functional status for ADLs and vocational, recreational, and sports activities as identified by patient
- Independence in a progressive home exercise program emphasizing function

INTERVENTION

NUMBER OF VISITS: 6–12

Coordination, Communication, and Documentation

- Provision of services between admission and discharge that facilitate cost-effective and efficient integration or reintegration to home, community, or work
- Documentation of therapeutic intervention is required for each episode of care and serves as the basic foundation for communication
- Coordination and additional communication will depend on the patient's impairment and home/work/community/leisure situation and requirements. Such services may include:
  - Case management
  - Coordination of care and collaboration with those integral to the patient's rehabilitation program
  - Coordination and monitoring of the delivery of available resources
  - Referrals to other health-care professionals
  - Identification of resources, support groups, or advocacy services
  - Provision of educational or training information
  - Technical assistance

Patient Intervention

Basic Anatomy and Biomechanics

- Contents of the thoracic outlet and mechanism of compression
- Pertinent Gray's Anatomy (Gray. 1995. 808–809, 1266–1270, 1530)

Handouts

- Specific home exercise instruction
- Commercially available products, such as:
  - Krames Communications (1100 Grundy Lane, San Bruno, CA 94066):
    - *Arranging Your Work Station to Fit You*
    - *Poor Posture Hurts*
    - *Back Tips for People Who Sit*

Functional Considerations

- Effects of poor posture on thoracic outlet syndrome symptoms
- Avoidance of activities, such as pushing, pulling, or carrying with shoulder strap and lifting overhead
- Effects of poor stress management on exacerbation of symptoms
- Avoidance of bra straps and seat belts that are too tight
- Caution regarding repetitive activities

Direct Interventions

Acute Phase: 3–6 Visits

- Therapeutic exercise with home program carryover
  - Self-mobilization of 1st rib with use of a tennis ball or mobilization strap
  - Shoulder elevation activities
  - Cervical ROM exercises
  - Stretching for sternocleidomastoid and scalene muscles
  - Diaphragmatic breathing
  - Relaxation techniques and tapes
- Manual therapy techniques
  - Soft-tissue techniques
    - Direct and indirect trigger-point techniques
    - Soft-tissue mobilization
    - Muscle energy techniques
    - Myofascial release
  - Proprioceptive neuromuscular facilitation
  - Joint mobilization (Grades I–IV)
    - 1st rib
    - Clavicle
    - Cervical/thoracic spine
- Electrotherapeutic modalities
  - Biofeedback
  - Muscle stimulation
- Physical agents and mechanical modalities
  - Superficial thermal/cryotherapy
  - Deep thermal: Ultrasound

356   THORACIC OUTLET SYNDROME | CERVICAL/THORACIC SPINE

- Goals/outcomes
  - Pain: 50% decrease from initial rating, including night symptoms
  - Cervical/thoracic AROM: 50% of AMA guides, increased to 60% or 70%
    - Cervical
      a. Flexion: 30°
      b. Extension: 40°
      c. Side bend: 25°
      d. Rotation: 40°
    - Thoracic
      a. Flexion: 20°
      b. Extension: No AMA guides established
      c. Side bend: 5°
      d. Rotation: 15°
  - Shoulder ROM: 80% of AMA guides
    - Flexion: 145°
    - Extension: 40°
    - Abduction: 135°
    - Internally rotated: 65°
    - Externally rotated: 65°
  - Posture normalization

Subacute Phase: 3–6 Visits

- Therapeutic exercise, home program
  - Self-mobilization with tennis ball
  - Diaphragmatic breathing and relaxation exercises
  - Cervical strengthening and ROM activities
  - Postural exercises
    - Craniovertebral flexion
    - C7/T1 extension
    - Pectoral stretching
    - Scapular retraction/depression strengthening
- Manual therapy techniques
  - Soft-tissue techniques
    - Soft-tissue mobilization
    - Myofacial release
    - Direct or indirect trigger-point techniques
  - Proprioceptive neuromuscular facilitation
  - Assisted passive stretching to the cervical and pectoral musculature
  - Joint mobilization
    - Progress grade of mobilization to patient's tolerance
- Physical agents and mechanical modalities
  - Continue effective modalities as in acute phase, with increased emphasis on use as-needed at home

- Goals/outcomes
  - Pain: 2/10 or less
  - Increase tissue extensibility and circulation to the extremities as evidenced by negative response on special tests
  - Increase exercise tolerance and upper quarter strength to minimum of 4+/5 on manual muscle test
  - Independent function in household, occupational, and recreational activities
  - ROM: 80% of AMA guides
  - Shoulder ROM: 90% of AMA guides

Functional Carryover

- Ergonomic evaluation for proper sitting and standing posture
- Utilization of stress management techniques in the home and work environment
- Instruction in sleep postures to avoid exacerbation of symptoms
- Task-oriented exercise, specifically related to work, home, and recreation

DISCHARGE PLANNING AND PATIENT RESPONSIBILITY

Criteria for Discharge

- Patient demonstrates ability to perform exercises correctly and reports intent to continue performance until strength, pain-free ROM, and functional level has returned to normal
- Patient understands that in most cases there is no "cure," but rather that this is a management issue and that symptoms occur due to inflammation near pain-sensitive structures (such as Brachial Plexus)
- All goals/outcomes have been achieved with the exception of return to previous level for recreational and sports activities

Circumstances Requiring Additional Visits

- Persistent functional strength deficit or 3/5 on manual muscle test
- History of previous injury or surgery to related area
- Persistent radicular symptoms
- Severe deconditioning
- Special occupational needs requiring extensive fitness/strengthening

CERVICAL/THORACIC SPINE | THORACIC OUTLET SYNDROME   357

Home Program

- Diaphragmatic breathing
- Self-mobilization
- Flexibility/strengthening exercises for maintenance of postural balance

Monitoring

- Instruct patient to call for advice should progression halt or a negative trend occur
- Patient is to recheck/call at 2 weeks post-discharge to report progression with home program
- Schedule clinic follow-up as needed if patient is unable to return to recreational/sports activities

REFERENCES

1. Aligne C, Barral X. Rehabilitation of patients with thoracic outlet syndrome. *Ann Vasc Surg.* 1992;6:381-389.

2. American Physical Therapy Association. *Guide to Physical Therapist Practice.* Alexandria, VA: APTA; 1997.

3. Atasoy E. Thoracic outlet compression syndrome. *Orthop Clin North Am.* 1996;27:265-303.

4. Butler D, Gifford L. The concept of adverse mechanical tension in the nervous system, part 2: examination and treatment. *Physiotherapy.* 1989;75:629-636.

5. Butler DS. Adverse mechanical tension in the nervous system: a model for assessment and treatment. *Aust J Physiother.* 1989;35:227-238.

6. Dawson DM. Entrapment neuropathies: clinical overview. *Hosp Pract (Office Ed).* 1995;30(8):37-40, 43-44.

7. Fechter JD, Kuschner SH. The thoracic outlet syndrome. *Orthopedics.* 1993;16:1243-1251.

8. Gray H; Williams PL, ed. *Gray's Anatomy.* 38th ed. New York, NY: Churchill Livingstone; 1995.

9. Hart A, Hopkins C, Ford B. *ICD-9-CM Expert For Physicians, Volume 1&2.* 7th ed. USA: Ingenix; 2005.

10. Hoppenfeld S. *Physical Examination of The Spine And Extremities.* Norwalk, CT: Appleton-Century-Crofts; 1976.

11. Howell JW. Evaluation and management of thoracic outlet syndrome. In: Donatelli R, ed. *Physical Therapy of the Shoulder. Vol II. Clinics in Physical Therapy.* New York, NY: Churchill Livingstone; 1986.

12. Jamieson WG, Chinnick G. Thoracic outlet syndrome: fact or fancy? A review of 409 consecutive patients who underwent operation. *Can J Surg.* 1996;39:321-326.

13. Kendall FP, McCreary EK. *Muscles: Testing and Function.* 3rd ed. Baltimore, MD: Williams & Wilkins; 1983.

14. Kenny RA, Traynor GB, Withington D, Keegan DJ. Thoracic outlet syndrome: a useful exercise treatment option. *Am J Surg.* 1993;165:282-284.

15. Lindgren KA. Conservative treatment of thoracic outlet syndrome: a two-year follow-up. *Arch Phys Med Rehabil.* 1997;78:373-378.

16. Nathan PA. Outcome following conservative management of thoracic outlet syndrome. *J Hand Surg.* 1995;20:542-548.

17. Nichols AW. The thoracic outlet syndrome in athletes. *J Am Board Fam Pract.* 1996;9:346-355.

18. Novak CB, Mackinnon SE. Thoracic outlet syndrome. *Orthop Clin North Am.* 1996;27:747-762.

19. Pratt NE. Neurovascular entrapment in the regions of the shoulder and posterior triangle of the neck. *Phys Ther.* 1986;66:1894-1900.

20. Rayan BM, Jensen C. Thoracic outlet syndrome: provocative examination maneuvers in a typical population. *J Shoulder Elbow Surg.* 1995;4:113-117.

21. Riddle DL, Stratford PW. Use of generic versus region-specific functional status measures on patients with cervical spine disorders. *Phys Ther.* 1998;78:951-963.

22. Sandmark H, Nisell R. Validity of five common manual neck pain provoking tests. *Scand J Rehabil Med.* 1995;27(3):131-136.

23. Walsh MT. Therapist management of thoracic outlet syndrome. *J Hand Ther.* 1994;7:131-144.

24. Youdas JW, Carey JR, Garrett TR. Reliability of measurements of cervical spine ROM—comparison of three methods. *Phys Ther.* 1991;71:98-104; discussion, 105-106.

25. Youdas JW, Garrett TR, Suman VJ, et al. Normal ROM of the cervical spine: an initial goniometric study. *Phys Ther.* 1992;72:770-780.

WHIPLASH SYNDROME
SUMMARY OVERVIEW

ICD-9

847.0

APTA Preferred Practice Pattern: 4G

EXAMINATION

- History and Systems Review
- Tests and Measures
  Systems review per APTA's *Guide to Physical Therapy Practice*
  - Joint integrity
  - Muscle performance
  - Pain
  - Posture
  - ROM
  - Reflex integrity
  - Sensory integrity
- Establish Plan of Care

GOALS/OUTCOMES

- Pain: 2/10 or less
- ROM: at least 80% of AMA guides and equal bilaterally
- Spinal muscle strength and stability to prevent re-injury: 4+/5 on manual muscle test for cervical and scapular muscles
- Return to previous functional status for ADLs and vocational, recreational, and sports activities as identified by patient
- Independence in a progressive home exercise program emphasizing function

INTERVENTION
NUMBER OF VISITS: 12–24

- Patient Instruction
  - Basic Anatomy and Biomechanics
  - Handouts
  - Functional Considerations
- Direct Interventions
  - Acute Phase: 4–8 Visits
  - Subacute Phase: 8–16 Visits
- Functional Carryover

DISCHARGE PLANNING AND PATIENT RESPONSIBILITY

- Criteria for Discharge
  - All goals/outcomes have been achieved with the possible exception of return to previous sports/recreational activities
  - Patient displays understanding of the role of proper posture and body mechanics in prevention of reinjury
- Circumstances Requiring Additional Visits
  - Persistent functional motor performance deficit or 3/5 on manual muscle test
  - History of previous injury/surgery to related area
  - Persistent radicular symptoms or neurological deficit
  - Bilateral upper-extremity radiculopathy
  - Severe deconditioning
  - Special occupational needs requiring extensive fitness/strengthening
  - Head/facial impact in motor vehicle accident
  - Craniovertebral instability
  - Multiple injury sites
  - Restriction in segmental joint mobility
  - Arthritic conditions
  - Necessary to return to normal work status (no modified duty available)
- Home Program
  - Flexibility exercises
  - Increase repetitions/intensity and provide strengthening progression to challenge patient's current level and achieve all goals/outcomes
  - Self-mobilization techniques
  - Use of modalities at home as needed for occasional flare-ups
- Monitoring

SUMMARY OVERVIEW | CERVICAL/THORACIC SPINE | WHIPLASH SYNDROME

WHIPLASH SYNDROME

ICD-9

847.0   Neck sprain

APTA Preferred Practice Pattern: 4G

EXAMINATION

History and Systems Review

- History of current condition
  - Body position at impact
  - Direction of impact
  - Seat belt
  - Airbag
  - Loss of consciousness
  - Location, nature, and behavior of symptoms
    - Radiating symptoms
    - Aggravating/relieving factors
  - Presence of cardinal and non-cardinal signs
- Past history of current condition
  - Previous injury/surgery
- Other tests and measures
  - Inquire about open mouth films for C1 and C2 integrity
- Medications
- Past medical/surgical history
- Functional status and activity level (current/prior)
  - Positional tolerance
  - Sleep disruption
  - ADLs
- Patient's functional goals

Tests and Measures

Systems review per APTA's *Guide to Physical Therapy Practice*

- Joint integrity
  - Craniovertebral scan

    Purpose: To identify the acute patient who may have a serious life-threatening injury and should receive immediate emergency medical attention. This will be important for patients who present with recent injury, collar, x-rays that were negative. Patient is reluctant to move head and has great difficulty lying down or lifting head from pillow.
    - Scan is actively performed with patient sitting and with minimal "hands on" by the therapist
      a. Neck rotation and flexion
      b. Upper cervical side bending

      c. Extension
      d. Compression/distraction
         If these tests do not produce cardinal signs and the patient can lie down, progress to passive craniovertebral stability tests.
  - C0–T12—anterior/posterior stability test
  - Craniovertebral stability tests
  - Dizziness screen
  - Palpation
    - Suboccipital region
    - Anterior neck musculature
    - Joint capsules
    - Supraspinous ligament
- Muscle performance
  - Key muscle tests, C5–T1
    - Grip strength
  - Resisted testing
    - Cervical
    - Thoracic
    - Scapular
- Pain
  - Measured on visual analog scale
  - With palpation
- Posture
  - Sitting
  - Standing
  - Vocational/recreational postures
- ROM

  Performed per clinician's judgment
  - Active ROM of the cervical and thoracic spine
  - PROM
  - Overpressure (to assess soft-tissue involvement)
  - Functional upper-extremity ROM
    - Patient demonstrates ability to touch mid-back with the shoulder flexed/externally rotated and extended/internally rotated
- Reflex integrity
  - Biceps (C5–6)
  - Brachioradialis (C5–6)
  - Triceps (C7)
- Sensory integrity
  - Sensation, C3–T1

360   WHIPLASH SYNDROME | CERVICAL/THORACIC SPINE

Establish Plan of Care

- Based on history, tests, and measures

GOALS/OUTCOMES

- Pain: 2/10 or less
- ROM: at least 80% of AMA guides and equal bilaterally

Cervical	Normal	80%
Flexion	60°	50°
Extension	75°	60°
Rotation	80°	65°
Side bend	45°	35°

Thoracic	Normal	80%
Flexion	40°	30°
Extension	No AMA guides established	
Rotation	30°	25°
Side bend	10°	10°

- Spinal muscle strength and stability to prevent re-injury: 4+/5 on manual muscle test for cervical and scapular muscles
- Return to previous functional status for ADLs and vocational, recreational, and sports activities as identified by patient
- Independence in a progressive home exercise program emphasizing function

INTERVENTION

NUMBER OF VISITS: 12–24

Coordination, Communication, and Documentation

- Provision of services between admission and discharge that facilitate cost-effective and efficient integration or reintegration to home, community, or work
- Documentation of therapeutic intervention is required for each episode of care and serves as the basic foundation for communication
- Coordination and additional communication will depend on the patient's impairment and home/work/community/leisure situation and requirements. Such services may include:
  - Case management
  - Coordination of care and collaboration with those integral to the patient's rehabilitation program
  - Coordination and monitoring of the delivery of available resources
  - Referrals to other health-care professionals

  - Identification of resources, support groups, or advocacy services
  - Provision of educational or training information
  - Technical assistance

Patient Instruction

Basic Anatomy and Biomechanics

- Anatomy of cervical and thoracic spine
- Pertinent Gray's Anatomy (Gray. 1995. 510-522, 537, 803–805, 807–813, 835–838)
- Importance of adequate strength, postural alignment, and ROM of the kinetic chain in the alleviation of symptoms
- Mechanism of injury and importance of protection and rehabilitation of the stabilizing structures
- Distinction between stretching and strengthening exercises

Handouts

- Commercially available products, such as:
  - Krames Communications (1100 Grundy Lane, San Bruno, CA 94066)
    - *Neck Basics*
    - *Neck Owner's Manual*
    - *Fit Neck Workout*
  - McKenzie (PO Box 93, Waikane, New Zealand)
    - *Treat Your Own Neck*
  - Saunders (4250 Norex Drive, Chaska, MN 55318)
    - *For Your Neck*
- Specific home program for appropriate ROM, stretching, and stabilization exercises

Functional Considerations

- Importance of maintaining normal and pain-free cervical and thoracic curves. Support during:
  - Sitting
  - Sleeping
  - Driving
  - Speaking
  - Breathing
- Importance of proper body mechanics and limitation/avoidance of aggravating upper-extremity activity and prolonged head postures
- Stabilization/prevention of reinjury
  - Cervical soft collar if indicated
  - Alteration of ADLs

CERVICAL/THORACIC SPINE | WHIPLASH SYNDROME   361

Direct Interventions

- Depending on the nature and severity of ligamentous injury, in the presence of constant high-level pain, the patient may benefit from an initial instructional visit in:
  - Home cryotherapy
  - Supported rest positions/postures
  - Avoidance of aggravating factors
- The patient would then return home for 3–5 days prior to initiation of the acute phase of clinical treatment

Acute Phase: 4–8 Visits

- Therapeutic exercise and home program
  - Strengthening exercises as appropriate: active assistive progressing to active progressing to resistive
  - Postural awareness and body mechanics training
  - Aerobic exercises for tissue healing
  - Home program
    - Home use of cryotherapy and supported postures
    - Diaphragmatic breathing and relaxation techniques
    - Supported active exercise in pain-free ROM, supine or standing
      a. Scapular
      b. Upper extremity
      c. Cervical
      d. Thoracic
    - Walking or other aerobic exercises as tolerated
- Manual therapy techniques
  - Soft-tissue techniques
    - Soft-tissue mobilization
    - Trigger-point techniques
    - Myofascial release
    - Strain/counterstrain
  - Joint mobilization
    - Grades I–II, including specific traction compression with the intent of pain relief
  - Positional isometric techniques for ROM and pain reduction
  - ROM in pain-free range
- Electrotherapeutic modalities
- Physical agents and mechanical modalities
  - Superficial thermal: Cryotherapy, thermal modalities
  - Deep thermal: Ultrasound
- Goals/outcomes
  - Pain: Reduced 40% from initial rating
  - Cervical ROM: 50% of AMA guides and equal bilaterally
    - Flexion: 30°
    - Extension: 40°
    - Rotation: 40°
    - Side bend: 25°
  - Achieve supported pain-free postural alignment during rest and basic ADLs
  - Cervical stabilization to prevent reinjury

Subacute Phase: 8–16 Visits

- Therapeutic exercise and home program
  - Progress active, isometric, and resisted exercises to tolerance
  - Emphasize cardiovascular conditioning
    - Upper or lower-extremity cycling
    - Treadmill/walking program
    - Ski machine
    - Aquatic therapy
  - Neuromuscular/balance/proprioceptive reeducation
  - Home program
    - Continue ROM exercises using increased range
    - Specific postural correction exercises
      a. Axial extension maintaining normal cervical curvature
      b. Scapular retraction/depression
      c. Pectoral stretching
    - Instruct in self-mobilization exercises to appropriate levels, including craniovertebral and cervicothoracic junction
    - Initiate self-resisted strengthening exercises or gravity-resisted strengthening exercises as appropriate
      a. Cervical isometrics
      b. Therapeutic ball exercises
      c. Resisted exercises utilizing pulleys, resistive band, or free-weights
      d. Plyometric activities with cervical stabilization, such as throwing activities
- Manual therapy techniques
  - Soft-tissue techniques
    - Soft-tissue mobilization
    - Myofascial release
    - Trigger-point techniques
    - Strain/counterstrain
    - Muscle energy techniques
    - Friction massage
  - Joint mobilization
    - Grades I–V as appropriate for stage of ligamentous healing

- Manually resisted exercises, including proprioceptive neuromuscular facilitation patterns
- Assisted passive techniques
  - Muscle stretching
  - Neural tension maneuvers
- Physical agents and mechanical modalities
  - Continue effective modalities as in acute phase, with increased emphasis on use as needed at home
- Goals/outcomes
  - Pain: 2/10 or less
  - ROM: at least 80% of AMA guides and equal bilaterally:
    - Cervical
      a. Flexion: 50°
      b. Extension: 60°
      c. Rotation: 65°
      d. Side bend: 35°
    - Thoracic
      a. Flexion: 30°
      b. Extension: No AMA guides established
      c. Rotation: 25°
      d. Side bend: 8°
  - Spinal strength and stability to prevent reinjury: 4/5 on manual muscle test of cervical and scapular muscles
  - Return to previous functional status for ADLs and vocational and recreational activities as identified by patient

Functional Carryover

- Use of cervical or lumbar support for proper postural alignment during work, driving, and ADLs
- Ergonomic evaluation of the work site as needed, including chair, desk height, and computer placement
- Implementation of stress management techniques during ADLs and vocational activities
- Awareness of activity level/pacing and its influence on exacerbation of symptoms

DISCHARGE PLANNING AND PATIENT RESPONSIBILITY

Criteria for Discharge

- All goals/outcomes have been achieved with the possible exception of return to previous sport/recreational activities
- Patient displays understanding of the role of proper posture and body mechanics in prevention of reinjury

Circumstances Requiring Additional Visits

- Persistent functional motor performance deficit or 3/5 on manual muscle test
- History of previous injury/surgery to related area
- Persistent radicular symptoms or neurological deficit
- Bilateral upper-extremity radiculopathy
- Severe deconditioning
- Special occupational needs requiring extensive fitness/strengthening
- Head/facial impact in motor vehicle accident
- Craniovertebral instability
- Multiple injury sites
- Restriction in segmental joint mobility
- Arthritic conditions
- Necessary to return to normal work status (no modified duty available)

Home Program

- Flexibility exercises
- Increase repetitions/intensity and provide strengthening progression to challenge patient's current level and achieve all goals/outcomes
- Self-mobilization techniques
- Use of modalities at home as needed for occasional flare-ups

Monitoring

- Instruct patient to call for advice should progression halt or a negative trend occur
- Follow up at 4–8 weeks post-discharge to ensure expected return to function and progression toward attaining all goals/outcomes

CERVICAL/THORACIC SPINE | WHIPLASH SYNDROME

REFERENCES

1. American Physical Therapy Association. *Guide to Physical Therapist Practice.* Alexandria, VA: APTA; 1997.

2. Assendelft WJ, Bouter LM, Knipschild PG. Complications of spinal manipulation: a comprehensive review of the literature. *J Fam Pract.* 1996;42:475-480.

3. Borchgrevink GE, Kaasa A, McDonagh D, et al. Acute treatment of whiplash neck sprain injuries. a randomized trial of treatment during the first fourteen days after a car accident. *Spine.* 1998:23:25-31.

4. Bogduk N. Epidemiology of Whiplash. *Ann Rheum Dis.* May 2000;59(5):394-395.

5. Brault JR, Wheeler JB, Siegmund GP, Brault EJ. Clinical response of human subjects to rear-end automobile collisions. *Arch Phys Med Rehab.* 1998:79:72-80.

6. Brison RJ, Hartling L, Dostaler S. A randomized controlled trial of an educational intervention to prevent the chronic pain of whiplash associated disorders following rear-end motor vehicle collisions. *Spine.* August 15, 2005;30(16):1799-807.

7. Derrick LJ, Chesworth BM. Post-motor vehicle accident alar ligament laxity. *J Orthop Sports Phys Ther.* 1992;16(1):6-11.

8. Evans RW. Some observations on whiplash injuries. *Neurologic Clin.* 1992:10:975-997.

9. Gennis P, Miller L, Gallagher EJ, et al. The effect of soft cervical collars on persistent neck pain in patients with whiplash injury. *Acad Emerg Med.* 1996:3:568-573.

10. Gray H; Williams PL, ed. *Gray's Anatomy.* 38th ed. New York, NY: Churchill Livingstone; 1995.

11. Hart A, Hopkins C, Ford B. *ICD-9-CM Expert For Physicians, Volume 1&2.* 7th ed. USA: Ingenix; 2005.

12. Holm LW, Carroll LJ, Cassidy JD. Factors influencing neck pain intensity in whiplash-associated disorders. *Spine.* February 2006.

13. Jonsson H, Cesarini K, Sahlstedt B, Rauschining W. Findings and outcome in whiplash-type neck distortions. *Spine.* 1994;19:2733-2743.

14. Lord SM, Barnsley L, Wallis BJ, Bogduk N. Chronic cervical zygapopysial joint pain after whiplash. a placebo controlled prevalence study. *Spine.* 1996;21:1737-1744.

15. McKenzie R. *Treat Your Own Neck,* 2nd ed. Waikanae, New Zealand: Spinal Publications; 1983.

16. Pettersson K, Karrholm J, Toolanen G, Hildingsson C. Decreased width of the spinal canal in patients with chronic symptoms after whiplash injury. *Spine.* 1995;20:1664-1667.

17. Pho C, Godges JJ. Management of WAD addressing thoracic and cervical spine impairments: a case report. *J Ortho Sports Phys Ther.* 2004;34(9):511-523.

18. Riddle DL, Stratford PW. Use of generic versus region-specific functional status measures on patients with cervical spine disorders. *Phys Ther.* 1998;78:951-963.

19. Sandmark H, Nisell R. Validity of five neck pain provoking tests. *Scand J Rehabil Med* 1995;27(3):131-136.

20. Saunders HD. *Self Help Manual For Your Back.* Chasta, MN: The Saunders Group, Inc; 1992.

21. Sterling M, Jull G, Vicenzino B, Kenardy J. Characterization of acute whiplash-associated disorders. *Spine.* January 15, 2004;29(2):182-8.

22. Taylor JR, Twomey LT. Acute injuries to cervical joints: an autopsy study of neck sprain. *Spine.* 1993;18:1115-1122.

23. Treleaven J, Jull G, LowChoy N. The relationship of cervical joint position error to balance and eye movement disturbances in persistent whiplash. *Man Ther.* May 2006;11(2):99-106.

24. Youdas JW, Carey JR, Garrett TR. Reliability of measurements of cervical spine ROM—comparison of three methods. *Phys Ther.* 1991;71:98-104; discussion, 105-106.

25. Youdas JW, Garrett TR, Suman VJ, et al. Normal ROM of the cervical spine: an initial goniometric study. *Phys Ther.* 1992;72:770-780.

TMJ/Headache/Stress

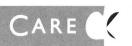

TMJ/Headache/Stress

Headache	367
Postoperative Rehabilitation of the Temporomandibular Joint (Orthognathic, Arthroplasty, or Arthroscopic)	373
Relaxation and Stress Management	381
Stress Management	384
Temporomandibular Dysfunction	389

366   TMJ/Headache/Stress

HEADACHE
SUMMARY OVERVIEW

ICD-9

307.81   346   350.2   784.0

APTA Preferred Practice Pattern: 4B, 4C, 4D, 4E, 4F, 4G, 4I, 5D

EXAMINATION

- History and Systems Review
- Tests and Measures
  Systems review per APTA's *Guide to Physical Therapy Practice*
  - Muscle performance
  - Pain
  - ROM
  - Reflex integrity
  - Sensory integrity
  - Special tests
- Establish Plan of Care

GOALS/OUTCOMES

- Pain: 2/10 or less
- Reduce frequency of headaches to 2/7 days or less
- Normal orthostatic posture
- ROM: A minimum of 80% of AMA guides
- Shoulder ROM: A minimum of 90% of AMA guides
- Cervical and scapular strength: 4/5 on manual muscle test
- Cardiovascular conditioning: A minimum of 20 minute duration 3 times per week
- Independence in a progressive home exercise program emphasizing function
- Return to previous functional status for ADLs and vocational, recreational, and sports activities as identified by patient

INTERVENTION
NUMBER OF VISITS: 4–12

- Patient Instruction
  - Basic Anatomy and Biomechanics
  - Handouts
  - Functional Considerations
- Direct Interventions
  - Acute Phase: 2–6 Visits
  - Subacute Phase: 2–6 Visits
- Functional Carryover

DISCHARGE PLANNING AND PATIENT RESPONSIBILITY

- Criteria for Discharge
  - Patient displays understanding of the role of proper posture and body mechanics in prevention of symptoms
  - All goals/outcomes have been achieved with possible exceptions listed in the guidelines
- Circumstances Requiring Additional Visits
  - Persistent functional motor performance deficit or 3/5 on manual muscle test
  - History of previous injury/surgery to related area
  - Severe deconditioning
  - Special occupational needs requiring extensive fitness/strengthening
  - Arthritic conditions
  - Craniovertebral instability
  - Ligamentous injury
  - Head/facial impact in motor vehicle accident
  - Multiple injury sites
  - Psychosocial and socioeconomic complicating factors
  - Level of patient/client adherence to the intervention program
  - Pre-existing systemic conditions of diseases
- Home Program
  - Fitness program at local health club
  - Flexibility/strengthening exercises for maintenance of postural balance
  - Self-mobilization techniques
  - Use of modalities as needed for flare-ups
  - Cardiovascular conditioning 20 minutes, 3 times per week
- Monitoring

SUMMARY OVERVIEW | TMJ/HEADACHE/STRESS | HEADACHE   367

HEADACHE

ICD-9

307.81	Tension headache
346	Migraine
350.2	Atypical face pain
784.0	Headache

APTA Preferred Practice Pattern: 4B, 4C, 4D, 4E, 4F, 4G, 4I, 5D

EXAMINATION

History and Systems Review

- History of current condition
  - Location, nature, and behavior of symptoms
    - Location of head/neck pain
      a. Vertex
      b. Frontal
      c. Temporal
      d. Occipital
      e. Parietal
      f. Base of cranium
      g. Zygomatic arch
      h. Thorax
      i. Upper maxilla
      j. Palate
      k. Angle of mandible
      l. Throat
      m. Anterior/lateral/posterior neck
    - Presence of aura
    - Pattern over a 24 hour period
      a. Constant
      b. Intermittent
      c. Increasing
      d. Decreasing
    - Presence over 7 days
    - Aggravating/relieving factors
    - TMJ pain symptoms
      a. Crepitation, clicking, or popping
      b. Pain with opening, closing, mastication, or speech
- Presence of cardinal signs
- Other tests and measures
- Medications
- Functional status and activity level (current/prior)
  - Occupational/employment
    - Ergonomic environment
  - ADLs
  - Recreational/sport
- Social history
- Patient's functional goals

Tests and Measures

Systems review per APTA's *Guide to Physical Therapy Practice*

- Muscle performance
  - Palpation
    - Temporalis
    - Medial pterygoid
    - Masseter
    - Tongue muscles
    - Scalenes
    - Sternocleidomastoid
    - Trapezius
    - Digastric
    - Longus colli
    - Levator scapulae
    - Posterior cervical
    - Suboccipitals (lateral to medial)
      a. Longissimus capitis
      b. Semispinalis capitis
      c. Obliquus capitis superior
      d. Obliquus capitis inferior
         - Very common cause of headaches
      e. Rectus capitis posterior major
      f. Rectus capitis posterior minor
         - Posture
  - Resisted
    - Cervical
    - Thoracic
    - Scapular
- Pain

368   HEADACHE | TMJ/HEADACHE/STRESS

- ROM performed per clinician's judgment
  - Cervical AROM
  - Cervical PROM
  - TMJ scan
    - Mandibular AROM (lateral exclusion, protrusion, opening)
    - Presence of joint sounds (crepitation, opening click, closing click)
  - Overpressure (cervical and mandibular)
  - Upper-extremity functional ROM
    - Patient demonstrates ability to touch mid-back with the shoulder flexed/externally rotated and extended/internally rotated
- Reflex integrity
  - Reflexes
  - Upper motor neuron
    - Hoffman's test: Flick the patient's middle finger into extension, and if the thumb and index finger come together, this is considered a positive test
    - Clonus
      a. Supination of forearm
      b. Dorsiflexion
    - Babinski
- Sensory integrity
  - Sensation
- Special tests
  - Craniovertebral stability tests
    Purpose: To identify the acute patient who may have a serious life-threatening injury and should receive immediate emergency medical attention. Patient presents with recent injury, collar, and x-rays that were negative. Patient is reluctant to move head and has great difficulty lying down or lifting head from pillow.
    - Scan is actively performed with patient sitting and with minimal "hands on" by the therapist
      a. Neck rotation
      b. Upper cervical side bending
      c. Extension
    - If these tests do not produce cardinal signs and the patient can lie down, progress to passive craniovertebral stability tests
  - Vascular tests
    - Hautard's test
      a. A modification of Rhomberg's test for cerebellar dysfunction

b. Used to differentiate the vertebral artery from other causes
c. The patient is sitting with the arms elevated to 90° anteriorly
d. The patient then closes his or her eyes, and the therapist observes for a drop in position of one or both arms. This phase, if positive, indicates a nonvascular cerebellar dysfunction.
e. If negative, the patient is then asked to maintain the elevated arm position while rotating (or a combination of rotating and extending) the head and neck, while the therapist observes for a drop in position of the arm(s). A positive test implicates a vasculogenic cerebellar dysfunction.
    - Vertebral artery test
    - Pulses
    - Adson's test
  - Neural mobility/sensitivity
    - Dural stretch, T1: Full scapular retraction with arms at side
    - Neural tension scan: Compare shoulder abduction performed with head in midline with shoulder abduction performed with head side bent contralaterally. Suspect neural tension component if first test is pain-free and second test reproduces symptoms.
    - Slump test

Establish Plan of Care
- Based on history, tests, and measures

GOALS/OUTCOMES
- Pain: 2/10 or less
- Reduce frequency of headaches to 2/7 days or less
- Normal orthostatic posture
- ROM: A minimum of 80% of AMA guides

Cervical	Normal	80%
Flexion	60°	50°
Extension	75°	60°
Rotation	80°	65°
Side bend	45°	35°

Thoracic	Normal	80%
Flexion	40°	30°
Extension	No AMA guides established	
Rotation	30°	25°
Side bend	10°	8°

TMJ/Headache/Stress | Headache   369

- Shoulder ROM: A minimum of 90% of AMA guides

	Normal	90%
Flexion	180°	160°
Extension	50°	45°
Abduction	170+°	155°
Internal rotation	80+°	70°
External rotation	80+°	70°

- Cervical and scapular strength: 4/5 on manual muscle test
- Cardiovascular conditioning: A minimum of 20 minute, 3 times per week
- Independence in a progressive home exercise program emphasizing function
- Return to previous functional status for ADLs and vocational, recreational, and sports activities as identified by patient

INTERVENTION
NUMBER OF VISITS: 4–12

Coordination, Communication, and Documentation

- Provision of services between admission and discharge that facilitate cost-effective and efficient integration or reintegration to home, community, or work
- Documentation of therapeutic intervention is required for each episode of care and serves as the basic foundation for communication
- Coordination and additional communication will depend on the patient's impairment and home/work/ community/leisure situation and requirements. Such services may include:
  - Case management
  - Coordination of care and collaboration with those integral to the patient's rehabilitation program
  - Coordination and monitoring of the delivery of available resources
  - Referrals to other health-care professionals
  - Identification of resources, support groups, or advocacy services
  - Provision of educational or training information
  - Technical assistance

Patient Instruction

Basic Anatomy and Biomechanics
- Anatomy of cervical and thoracic spine as well as the craniomandibular complex

Handouts
- Commercially available products, such as:
  - Krames Communications (1100 Grundy Lane, San Bruno, CA 94066):
    - *Poor Posture Hurts*
    - *Neck Exercises for a Healthy Neck*
    - *Migraine and Tension Headaches: Strategies for Coping with the Pain*
  - McKenzie (PO Box 93, Waikanae, New Zealand)
    - *Treat Your Own Neck*
  - Saunders (4250 Norex Drive, Chaska, MN 55318)
    - *For Your Neck*

Functional Considerations
- Rationale for pharmacologic management
- Role of dietary factors in onset or exacerbation of symptoms
- Proper posture/body mechanics
  - Sitting
  - Lifting
  - Standing
- Ergonomic workstation adjustment
- Importance of frequent positional changes, preferably every hour
- Recognition of stressors in everyday life
- Identification of precipitating factors

Direct Interventions

Acute Phase: 2–6 Visits
- Therapeutic exercise and home program
  - Diaphragmatic breathing and relaxation techniques
  - Initiate walking program as tolerated
  - Posture training
  - Upper quarter AROM/flexibility exercises
- Manual therapy techniques
  - Joint mobilization
    - Grades III–IV to hypomobile segments of the cervical and thoracic spines as well as to the shoulder joint
    - Especially C3 and up

- Soft-tissue techniques
  - Soft-tissue mobilization
  - Trigger-point work
  - Acupressure
  - Myofascial release
  - Assisted passive techniques
    - Muscle stretching
    - Neural tension maneuvers
  - Positional isometric techniques for increasing ROM and pain reduction
    - Inhibitive distraction
- Therapeutic devices and equipment
  - Intraoral appliance as needed
  - Soft cervical collar as needed
- Electrotherapeutic modalities
  - Biofeedback
  - Mechanical traction
- Physical agents and mechanical modalities
  - Cryotherapy/thermal modalities
  - Ultrasound
- Goals/outcomes
  - Pain: 5/10 or less
  - Reduction in frequency of headaches (specific goals to be determined based on current frequency)
  - ROM: 60% of AMA guides for cervical/thoracic spine

Cervical	Normal	60%
Flexion	60°	35°
Extension	75°	45°
Rotation	80°	50°
Side bend	45°	30°

Thoracic	Normal	60%
Flexion	40°	25°
Extension	No AMA guides established	
Rotation	30°	20°
Side bend	10°	5°

  - Strength: 3+/5 on manual muscle test for cervical/scapular musculature
  - Develop awareness of proper postural position
  - Safe work site ergonomics
  - Initiate cardiovascular conditioning program

Subacute Phase: 2–6 Visits

- Therapeutic exercise and home program
  - Cervical/scapular stabilization exercises
  - Posture exercises
  - Stretching/strengthening for lower quarter
  - Cardiovascular conditioning
- Manual therapy techniques
  - Continue effective soft-tissue techniques
  - Progressive Grades III–V joint mobilization to hypomobile joints
- Physical agents and mechanical modalities
  - Continue effective modalities as in acute phase, only if necessary with increased emphasis on use as needed at home
- Goals/outcomes
  - Pain: 2/10 or less
  - Reduce frequency of headaches to 2/7 days or less
  - Normal orthostatic posture
  - Cervical and scapular strength/stability: 4/5 on manual muscle test
  - Cardiovascular conditioning: A minimum of 20 minutes, 3 times per week

Functional Carryover

- Instruction regarding use of cervical or lumbar support for proper postural alignment during work, driving, and ADLs
- Ergonomic modification of the work site if necessary, including chair, desk height, and computer placement
- Stress management skills incorporated into ADLs/vocational activities
- Address sleep disturbances/postures that may interfere with management of chronic condition

DISCHARGE PLANNING AND PATIENT RESPONSIBILITY

Criteria for Discharge

- Patient displays understanding of the role of proper posture and body mechanics in prevention of symptoms
- All goals/outcomes have been achieved with the following exceptions:
  - Patient may be discharged prior to attaining cardiovascular goal as long as program has been initiated
  - Patient may not have returned to previous status for recreational/sports activities

Circumstances Requiring Additional Visits
- Persistent functional motor performance deficit or 3/5 on manual muscle test
- History of previous injury/surgery to related area
- Severe deconditioning
- Special occupational needs requiring extensive fitness/strengthening
- Arthritic conditions
- Craniovertebral instability
- Ligamentous injury
- Head/facial impact in motor vehicle accident
- Multiple injury sites
- Psychosocial and socioeconomic complicating factors
- Level of patient/client adherence to the intervention program
- Pre-existing systemic conditions of diseases

Home Program
- Fitness program at local health club
- Flexibility/strengthening exercises for maintenance of postural balance
- Self-mobilization techniques
- Use of modalities as needed for flare-ups
- Cardiovascular conditioning a minimum of 20 minutes, 3 times per week

Monitoring
- Instruct patient to call for advice should progression halt or a negative trend occur
- Follow up at 4–8 weeks post-discharge to ensure expected return to function and progression toward attaining all goals/outcomes

REFERENCE
1. American Physical Therapy Association. *Guide to Physical Therapist Practice.* Alexandria, VA: APTA; 1997.
2. Arena JE, Bruno GM, Hannah SL, Meador KJ. A comparison of frontal electromyographic biofeedback training, trapezius electromyographic biofeedback training and progressive relaxation therapy in the treatment of tension headache. *Headache.* 1995;35:411-419.
3. Aspinall W. Clinical testing for cervical mechanical disorders which produce ischemic vertigo. *J Orthop Sports Phys Ther.* 1989;11(5):176-182.
4. Boline PD, Kassak K, Bronfort G, Nelson C, Anderson AV. Spinal manipulation versus amitriptyline for the treatment of chronic tension-type headaches: a randomized clinical trial. *J Manipulative Physiol Ther.* 1995;18(3):148-154.
5. Eggleton T, Langton D. *Advanced Physical Therapy Management of Craniomandibular and Vertebral Dysfunction.* October 1-3, 1993. Coursework, Edmonds, WA; Ursa Foundation.
6. Engel JM. Relaxation training: a self-help approach for children with headaches. *Am J Occup Ther.* 1992;46:591-596.
7. Gary WJ, Brunsen J, Branson SJ. The effectiveness of physical therapy in the treatment of chronic daily headaches. *Headache.* 1989;29:156-162.
8. Gray H; Williams PL, ed. *Gray's Anatomy.* 38th ed. New York, NY: Churchill Livingstone; 1995.
9. Hamill JM, Cook TM, Rosecrance JC. Effectiveness of a physical therapy regime in the treatment of tension-type headache. *Headache.* 1996;36:149-153.
10. Hart A, Hopkins C, Ford B. *ICD-9-CM Expert for Physicians, Volume 1&2.* 7th ed. USA: Ingenix; 2005.
11. Iai H, Moriya H, Goto S, et al. Three-dimensional motion analysis of the upper cervical spine during axial rotation. *Spine.* 1993;18:2388-2392.
12. Lehrer PM, Carr R, Sargunaraj D, Woolfolk RL. Stress management techniques: are they all equivalent, or do they have specific effects? *Biofeedback Self Regul.* 1994;19:353-401.
13. McKenzie R. *Treat Your Own Neck.* 2nd ed. Waikanae, New Zealand: Spinal Publications; 1983.
14. Nilsson N. The prevalence of cervicogenic headache in a random population sample of 20-59 year olds. *Spine.* 1995;20:1884-1888.
15. Schonensee SK, Jensen G, Nicholson G, Gossman M, Katholi C. The effect of mobilization on cervical headaches. *J Orthop Sports Phys Ther.* 1995;21(4):184-196.

POSTOPERATIVE REHABILITATION OF THE TEMPOROMANDIBULAR JOINT (ORTHOGNATHIC, ARTHROPLASTY, OR ARTHROSCOPIC)

SUMMARY OVERVIEW

ICD-9

524.6   802.2   830.0

APTA Preferred Practice Pattern: 4I, 4J

EXAMINATION

- History and Systems Review
- Tests and Measures
  Systems review per APTA's *Guide to Physical Therapy Practice*
  - Aerobic capacity and endurance
  - Anthropometric characteristics
  - Integumentary integrity
  - Joint integrity and mobility
  - Motor function
  - Muscle performance
  - Pain
  - Posture
  - ROM
  - Reflex integrity
  - Sensory integrity for neurological examination
  - Special tests
- Establish Plan of Care

GOALS/OUTCOMES

- Pain: 2/10 or less
- Decrease frequency of headaches to 2/7 days or less
- Normalization of muscle balance (cervical, upper quadrant, and masticatory) to achieve normal postural alignment
- Effective implementation of stress management practices
- Functional strength and endurance of jaw musculature to allow normal mastication
- Normalization of mandibular dynamics emphasizing normal joint ROM and symmetry of motion to achieve 40 mm of pain-free, symmetrical mandibular opening
- Resolution of inflammatory process
- Achieve functional cervical/thoracic AROM or 80% of AMA guides
- Return to previous functional status for ADLs and vocational, recreational, and sports activities as identified by patient
- Independence in a progressive home exercise program emphasizing function

- Cardiovascular conditioning a minimum of 20 minutes, 3 times per week

INTERVENTION
NUMBER OF VISITS: 12–20

- Patient Instruction
  - Basic Anatomy and Biomechanics
  - Handouts/Home Exercise Program
  - Functional Considerations
  - Description of Surgical Procedure
- Direct Interventions
  - Acute Phase: 4–8 Visits, Weeks 1–4
  - Subacute Phase: 8–12 Visits, Weeks 5–8
- Functional Carryover

DISCHARGE PLANNING AND PATIENT RESPONSIBILITY

- Criteria for Discharge
  - All goals/outcomes have been achieved with possible exceptions listed in the guidelines
  - Patient demonstrates understanding of orthotics utilization, proper posture, and continuation of home program
- Circumstances Requiring Additional Visits
  - Persistent functional motor performance deficit or 3/5 on manual muscle test
  - History of previous injury/surgery to related area
  - Severe deconditioning
  - Special occupational needs requiring extensive fitness/ strengthening
  - Craniovertebral instability
  - Head/facial impact in motor vehicle accident
  - Multiple injury sites
  - Severe postoperative scarring
  - Postoperative infection/complication
  - Persistent radicular symptoms
  - Level of patient/client adherence to intervention program
  - Psychosocial and socioeconomic complicating factors

- Home Program
  - Flexibility
  - Strength
  - Cardiovascular conditioning 3 times per week
  - Self-therapies
  - Daily practice of relaxation techniques
- Monitoring

POSTOPERATIVE REHABILITATION OF THE TEMPOROMANDIBULAR JOINT (ORTHOGNATHIC, ARTHROPLASTY, OR ARTHROSCOPIC)

ICD-9

524.6	Temporomandibular joint disorders
802.2	Fracture of mandible, closed
830.0	Closed dislocation of jaw

APTA Preferred Practice Pattern: 4I, 4J

EXAMINATION

History and Systems Review

- History of current condition
  - Date and type of surgical procedure
  - Location, nature, and behavior of symptoms
    - Headaches, ear, or oral symptoms
    - Dizziness
    - Other radiating symptoms
    - Aggravating/relieving factors
- Past history of current condition
  - Previous therapeutic intervention
- Other tests and measures
- Medications
- Past medical/surgical history
- Functional status and activity level (current/prior)
  - Occupation/employment
    - Ergonomic environment
  - ADLs
  - Recreational/sport
- Social history
- Patient's functional goals

Tests and Measures

Systems review per APTA's *Guide to Physical Therapy Practice*

- Aerobic capacity and endurance
  - Respiration and alteration in nasal diaphragmatic breathing
- Anthropometric characteristics
  - Edema
- Integumentary integrity
  - Discoloration
  - Scars
- Joint integrity and mobility
  - Cervical segmental testing, C0–T3
  - Temporomandibular joint (TMJ)

- Loading for the reproduction of pain: Place palms of hands under the mandible and gently apply pressure superiorly up and through the TMJ
  - Joint end feel
    a. Distraction
    b. Anteriomedial glides
    c. Lateral glides
- Motor function
  - Tongue rest position
  - Swallowing pattern
  - Lip closure position
  - Mandibular and condylar rest position
  - Presence of tongue thrust
- Muscle performance
  - Key muscle tests, C3–T1
  - Palpation of the facial, head, and cervical regions
    - Muscles
      a. Trigger-points, with or without referral, hyperactivity, hypertrophy, and atrophy
    - Ligaments
    - Fascia
    - Via the ear canals
- Pain
- Posture
  - General
    - Swayback
    - Lordosis
    - Flatback
  - Forward head posture (see "Objective Measurement of Forward Head Posture" in *Cervical/Thoracic General Pain* guideline)
- ROM
  - Cervical
    - Flexion
    - Extension
    - Side bending
    - Rotation

○ Mandibular
Note any deflections, the moment of translation, and available rotation
  ▪ Opening
  ▪ Protrusion
  ▪ Overjet
  ▪ Overbite
  ▪ Laterotrusion
    a. Normal Mandibular ROM
    b. Opening: 40–50 mm
    c. Laterotrusion: 7–12 mm
    d. Protrusion: 2–6 mm
  ▪ Auscultation for popping, clicking, and crepitation (should be minimal postoperatively)
○ Seated thoracic rotation
○ Upper-extremity functional ROM
  ▪ Patient demonstrates ability to touch mid-back with the shoulder flexed/externally rotated and extended/internally rotated
• Reflex integrity
  ○ Reflexes
• Sensory integrity for neurological examination
  ○ Sensation, C1–T1
• Special tests
  ○ Clear cervical spine and upper extremities
  ○ Craniovertebral stress tests
  ○ Vertebral artery test

Establish Plan of Care
• Based on history, tests, and measures

GOALS/OUTCOMES
• Pain: 2/10 or less
• Decrease frequency of headaches to 2/7 days or less
• Normalization of muscle balance (cervical, upper quadrant, and masticatory) to achieve normal postural alignment
• Effective implementation of stress management practices
• Functional strength and endurance of jaw musculature to allow normal mastication
• Normalization of mandibular dynamics emphasizing normal joint ROM and symmetry of motion to achieve 40 mm of pain-free, symmetrical mandibular opening
• Resolution of inflammatory process

• Achieve functional cervical/thoracic AROM or 80% of AMA guides

Cervical	Normal	80%
Flexion	60°	50°
Extension	75°	60°
Side bend	45°	35°
Rotation	80°	65°

Thoracic	Normal	80%
Flexion	40°	30°
Extension	No AMA guides established	
Side bend	10°	8°
Rotation	30°	25°

• Return to previous functional status for ADLs and vocational, recreational, and sports activities as identified by patient
• Independence in a progressive home exercise program emphasizing function
• Cardiovascular conditioning a minimum of 20 minutes, 3 times per week

INTERVENTION

NUMBER OF VISITS: 12–20

Coordination, Communication, and Documentation
• Provision of services between admission and discharge that facilitate cost-effective and efficient integration or reintegration to home, community, or work
• Documentation of therapeutic intervention is required for each episode of care and serves as the basic foundation for communication
• Coordination and additional communication will depend on the patient's impairment and home/work/community/leisure situation and requirements. Such services may include:
  ○ Case management
  ○ Coordination of care and collaboration with those integral to the patient's rehabilitation program
  ○ Coordination and monitoring of the delivery of available resources
  ○ Referrals to other health-care professionals
  ○ Identification of resources, support groups, or advocacy services
  ○ Provision of educational or training information
  ○ Technical assistance

- Specific coordination and communication provisions:
  - Dentist/oral surgeon regarding intraoral appliance
  - Biofeedback specialist
  - Counseling

Patient Instruction

Basic Anatomy and Biomechanics
- Biomechanics of the craniomandibular complex; fibrocartilagenous disc, ligaments, capsule, and surrounding musculature
- Pertinent Gray's Anatomy (Gray. 1995. 578–582, 799–805)
- *Myofascial Pain Dysfunction: The Trigger Point Manual* (Travell, Simons. 1983)

Handouts/Home Exercise Program
- Specific home program
- Commercially available products, such as:
  - Krames Communications (1100 Grundy Lane, San Bruno, CA 94066):
    - *TM Disorders*
    - *Poor Posture Hurts*
  - Dinner Through a Straw: A Handbook for Maxillary Trauma
  - Let's Do Lunch: A Handbook of Instructions and Recipes for Patients of Oral Surgery and Others Requiring Soft Foods or Liquid Diets
- List of postoperative precautions

Functional Considerations
- Effects of bruxing on the TMJ and surrounding soft tissue
- Purpose of intraoral appliance and importance of compliance with use
- Effects of poor posture resulting in increased temporomandibular joint compression
- Dietary influences on temporomandibular joint compression
- Adherence to postoperative precautions
  - Sleeping supine and elevated until edema dissipates
  - Mastication restrictions
  - Lifting restrictions

Description of Surgical Procedure
- Review operative procedure and relation to joint biomechanics, rehabilitation, and function

Direct Interventions

Acute Phase: 4–8 Visits, Weeks 1–4
The initiation of postoperative treatment is physician dependent. The optimal time of treatment initiation is 1–48 hours for arthroscopic procedures, 1–2 weeks post arthroplasty, and 2–3 weeks post-orthognathic surgery.
- Therapeutic exercise and home program
  - Self-intraoral massage
  - Self-trigger-point acupressure
  - Tongue rest position
  - Controlled opening
  - Scapular retraction/depression
  - Axial extension
  - Cervical exercises as appropriate
  - Begin regular opening if patient is able to perform within a pain-free ROM
- Manual therapy techniques
  - Soft-tissue techniques
    - Soft-tissue mobilization to the cervical and facial musculature
    - Direct and indirect trigger-point techniques
    - Intraoral massage
  - Joint mobilization
    - TMJ
      a. Arthroscopic: Graded to patient tolerance
      b. Arthroplastia: Grade I for pain relief
      c. Orthognathic: None
    - Cervical
      a. Grades I–IV to segmental hypomobilities
      b. Especially C0-3
- Electrotherapeutic modalities
  - Iontophoresis
  - Biofeedback
- Physical agents and mechanical modalities
  - Cryotherapy/superficial thermal
  - Ultrasound
- Goals/outcomes
  - Pain: 5/10 or less
  - Decrease spasm and inflammation
  - Restore functional jaw AROM: Achieve a minimum of 30 mm mandibular opening

TMJ/HEADACHE/STRESS | POSTOP REHAB OF THE TMJ (ORTHOGNATHIC, ARTHROPLASTY, OR ARTHROSCOPIC)

○ Achieve a minimum of 50% of AMA guides for cervical/thoracic AROM:

	Cervical	*Thoracic*
Flexion	30°	20°
Extension	40°	*
Rotation	40°	15°
Side bend	23°	5°

* No AMA guides established

○ Restore proper mandibular dynamics (rotation/translation)
○ Implement proper posture for sitting, sleeping, and ADLs
○ Prevent adhesion formation
○ Decrease frequency of headaches to 4/7 days or less

Subacute Phase: 8–12 Visits, Weeks 5–8

Treatment frequency is now 1–2 times a week, dependent on rate of progression toward achieving the goals.

- Therapeutic exercise and home program
  ○ Self-intraoral massage
  ○ Rest position of tongue
  ○ Cervical ROM
  ○ Cervical isometrics
  ○ Mandibular ROM
  ○ Mandibular isometrics, progressing to resistance throughout the ROM
  ○ Self-mobilization of the TMJ using tongue depressors
  ○ Pectoral stretching
  ○ Scapular and spinal extensor strengthening
    ▪ Therapeutic ball stabilization exercises
    ▪ Resistive band diagonals
    ▪ Overhead press
  ○ Cardiovascular conditioning
    ▪ Walking
    ▪ Upper body cycle ergometry
- Manual therapy techniques
  ○ Soft-tissue techniques
    ▪ Soft-tissue mobilization to the cervical and masticatory regions
    ▪ Trigger-point work
    ▪ Myofascial release
    ▪ Intraoral massage
  ○ Proprioceptive neuromuscular facilitation
  ○ Joint mobilization
    ▪ TMJ
      a. Arthroscopic procedure
         As needed

b. Arthroplastic procedure
   Progress grade and add anteriomedial and lateral glides
c. Orthognathic procedure
   Initiate and progress to Grade IV as quickly as tolerated
  ▪ Cervical
  ▪ Thoracic
  ▪ Glenohumeral
- Physical agents and mechanical modalities
  ○ Continue effective modalities as in acute phase with increased emphasis on use as needed at home.
- Goals/outcomes
  ▪ Mandibular AROM: 40 mm of pain-free, symmetrical opening
  ○ Pain: 2/10 or less
  ○ Decrease frequency of headaches to 2/7 days or less
  ○ Achieve a minimum of 80% of AMA guides for cervical/thoracic AROM
  ○ Functional status: Patient is able to chew soft foods without exacerbation of symptoms (dependent upon surgeon's postoperative standards for mastication)
  ○ Patient displays independence in maintaining proper posture
  ○ Initiate cardiovascular conditioning program

Functional Carryover

- Instruction regarding progression to mastication with normal foods and continued avoidance of extremely hard or textured foods
- Integration of home program into ADLs and vocational and recreational activities to ensure continuation for a minimum of 1 month post-discharge
- Specific instruction regarding progressive posturing for sleep, ADLs, and vocational activities
- Continued utilization of relaxation and stress management tools on a daily basis (see Patient Information Sheet *Relaxation and Stress Management*)

DISCHARGE PLANNING AND PATIENT RESPONSIBILITY

Criteria for Discharge
- All goals/outcomes have been achieved with the exception of:
  - Patient may continue a soft-chew diet
  - Patient may be discharged at 35 mm of symmetrical opening
  - Patient may be discharged prior to attaining cardiovascular conditioning goal, but program must be initiated
  - Patient may not have returned to previous functional status for recreational and sports activities
- Patient demonstrates understanding of orthotics utilization, proper posture, and continuation of home program

Circumstances Requiring Additional Visits
- Persistent functional motor performance deficit or 3/5 on manual muscle test
- History of previous injury/surgery to related area
- Severe deconditioning
- Special occupational needs requiring extensive fitness/strengthening
- Cranioidvertebral instability
- Head/facial impact in motor vehicle accident
- Multiple injury sites
- Severe postoperative scarring
- Postoperative infection/complication
- Persistent radicular symptoms
- Level of patient/client adherence to the intervention program
- Psychosocial and socioeconomic complicating factors

Home Program
- Flexibility
  - Mandibular
  - Cervical/thoracic
  - Pectoral
- Strength
  - Mandibular
    - Progression to chewing as a mode of strengthening
  - Cervical
  - Scapular stabilizers and spinal extensors
- Cardiovascular conditioning 3 times per week
- Self-therapies
  - Thermal/cryotherapy
  - Mobilization
  - Intraoral massage
- Daily practice of relaxation techniques

Monitoring
- Patient is counseled that a continued curve of progression should prevail, and should exacerbation occur that is not alleviated with the home program within 2–3 days, he/she should call for advice
- Patient is to recheck/call at 2 weeks post-discharge to report progression toward functional status and activity level
- Patient is to recheck with physician on a regularly scheduled basis for orthotic adjustments and reevaluation

REFERENCES

1. American Physical Therapy Association. *Guide to Physical Therapist Practice*. Alexandria, VA: APTA; 1997.
2. Austin BD, Shupe SM. The role of physical therapy in recovery after temporomandibular joint surgery. *J Oral Maxillofac Surg*. 1993;51:495-498.
3. Bertolucci LE. Postoperative physical therapy post-arthroscopic TMJ management (update). *J Craniomandib Pract*. 1992;10;130-137.
4. Bertolucci LE. Postoperative physical therapy in temporomandibular joint arthroplasty. *J Craniomandib Pract*. 1992;10:211-220.
5. Eggleton T, Langton D. *Introduction to Craniomandibular Disorders and Dysfunction of the Temporomandibular Joint*. March 22-24, 1991. Edmonds, WA; Ursa Foundation.
6. Eggleton T, Langton D. *Advanced Physical Therapy Management of Craniomandibular and Vertebral Dysfunction*. October 1-3, 1993. Edmonds, WA; Ursa Foundation.
7. Friedman MH, Weisberg J, Weber FL. Postsurgical temporomandibular joint hypomobility. *Oral Surg Oral Med Oral Path*. 1993;75:24-28.
8. Gray H; Williams PL, ed. *Gray's Anatomy*. 38th ed. New York, NY: Churchill Livingstone; 1995.
9. Hart A, Hopkins C, Ford B. *ICD-9-CM Expert for Physicians, Volume 1&2*. 7th ed. USA: Ingenix; 2005.
10. Helland M. Anatomy and function of the temporomandibular joint. In: Grieve G, ed. *Modern*

Manual Therapy of the Vertebral Column. New York, NY: Churchill Livingstone; 1986:64-76.

11. Kuwahara T, Bessette R, Maruyama T. The influence of postoperative treatment on the results of TMJ menisectomy. Part II: comparison of chewing movement. *J Craniomandib Pract.* 1996;14:121-131.

12. Rocabado M. *Musculoskeletal Approach to Maxillofacial Pain*. Philadelphia, PA: JB Lippincott; 1991.

13. Travell JG, Simons DG. *Myofascial Pain Dysfunction: The Trigger Point Manual*. Philadelphia, PA: Lippincott, Williams & Wilkins; 1983:203-281.

14. Trott P. Examination of the temporomandibular joint. In: Grieve G, ed. *Modern Manual Therapy of the Vertebral Column*. New York, NY: Churchill Livingstone; 1986:521-529.

15. Waide FL, Bade DM, Lovasko J, Montana J. Clinical management of a patient following temporomandibular joint arthroscopy. *Phys Ther.* 1992;72:355-364.

16. Wilk BR, McCain JP. Rehabilitation of the temporomandibular joint after arthroscopic surgery. *Oral Surg Oral Med Oral Path.* 1992;73:531-536.

RELAXATION AND STRESS MANAGEMENT

INTRODUCTION

Stress, physical and emotional, is an inherent part of everyday life. Our reaction to stress is usually unconscious and controlled by the autonomic nervous system, which regulates heart rate, respiration, perspiration, and digestion. The response most commonly associated with stress is "fight or flight" and literally is designed to prepare the body to physically attack or run from the perceived threat. Muscles become tense, heart rate and respiration become more rapid, and digestion slows in preparation for the anticipated threat. When this response becomes chronic, muscles remain tense for a prolonged period, and this can lead to physical discomfort. Some of the more common areas of chronic tension are facial, neck, shoulder, and upper back muscles. In addition, muscle tension can reveal itself through trigger points, referred pain, and bruxism (grinding and clenching the teeth). Understanding how stress affects your body both psychologically and physiologically can enhance your ability to adjust your body's reaction to stress.

There are many sources for assistance in learning how to reduce and manage stress; the following list is not all-inclusive but is meant to be a starting point.

- Counseling
- Support groups
- Hypnosis
- Biofeedback
- Self-guided relaxation techniques

STRESS REDUCTION

Recognizing Stress

Identify the sources of stress in your life. These may include schedules, individuals, projects, or physical labor, to name a few. Once you have identified a source, consider how frequently you encounter it. If it is a frequent source of stress, then make a note of it. Not all sources of stress are under our control; however, in many cases we can make minor adjustments to a situation and change our perception and response to it. The next time you encounter one of the things that you have identified as a frequent source of stress, note how you respond to it. Do you sense your shoulders going up? Are you clenching your teeth? Does your stomach feel tight or upset? Do you crave or shun food? Once you become aware of your response to stress, you can begin to make some adjustments. Setting realistic limitations on your schedule, organizing projects, delegating responsibility, adjusting your workstation to fit you, and opening the channels of communication are all techniques used to minimize the incidence of stress in our lives. Another is to set aside some time for relaxation and release.

RELEASE • RELAX • REGROUP

Physical exercise is one form of release that allows the energy of the fight-or-flight response to be dissipated naturally. The exercise does not need to be strenuous to accomplish this. For most of us, walking is the most natural and accessible form of exercise and can be incorporated into our routine with minimal effort. However, any activity that keeps your body in rhythmic motion for 20 minutes or more will suffice. Dancing, swimming, skating, running, cross-country skiing, and bicycling are a few of the more popular forms of aerobic exercise. Weight lifting, gardening, and tennis will also accomplish the goal of dissipating excess stress, though they may not be aerobic in nature. Discuss with your physical therapist or exercise specialist which form is best for you, and make the commitment to work it into your routine. One of the many benefits of regular exercise is that by releasing muscle tension, it enhances your body's ability to relax.

SELF-GUIDED RELAXATION

The first step is to set aside a time and place to practice your relaxation. Don't be fooled; it will require practice! A warm and quiet environment with a comfortable, supportive chair or bed will help you let go. The next step

TMJ/HEADACHE/STRESS | RELAXATION AND STRESS MANAGEMENT 381

is to make yourself comfortable and begin diaphragmatic (belly) breathing. As you inhale through your nose and mouth, your diaphragm pulls down into the belly, pushing your abdomen out. When you exhale, your diaphragm retracts to its resting position under the lungs, and your abdomen flattens again.

As you practice the belly breathing, check to see that you are letting go physically and mentally. Let your mind rest, and focus only on breathing. Start with your toes and work toward the top of your head, checking each body part for hidden tension. It may take as little as 10 minutes or as much as an hour to work from head to toe. If you're not sure a part is relaxed, try tightening your muscles and feeling the difference between a muscle that is contracted and one that is relaxed. For example, clench your fist tightly and notice how you feel a tension in your hand that travels up your arm into your shoulder. Relax your fist and make note of how different that feels. Areas that need particular attention will differ from person to person, so ask your physical therapist to help you identify your areas of chronic tension. Identifying muscle tension sometimes takes practice, but you will soon be able to relax your muscles without needing to tense them first. Once you have become adept at this form of relaxation, you can incorporate it into your routine throughout the day, learning to release excess muscle tension whenever it becomes apparent. Breaking the cycle of chronic muscle tension is vital to relieving your pain.

STRESS MANAGEMENT
SUMMARY OVERVIEW

ICD-9

    307.81   346   350.2   524.6   524.9   728.9   729.1   784   847

APTA Preferred Practice Pattern: 4B, 4C, 4D, 4E, 4F, 4G, 4I, 5D, 7A

EXAMINATION

- History and Systems Review
- Tests and Measures
  Systems review per APTA's *Guide to Physical Therapy Practice*
  - Gait, locomotion, and balance
  - Muscle performance
  - Pain
  - Posture
  - ROM
  - Visible signs of tension
- Establish Plan of Care

GOALS/OUTCOMES

- Pain: 2/10 or less with activity, 0/10 with ADLs
- Ability to identify sources of stress
- Self-awareness of patient's reactions to stress and ability to implement a plan for changing these responses
- Demonstrates proper body mechanics and postures for ADLs
- Strength: 4/5 for all lower extremity, upper extremity, abdominal, and spinal extensor musculature
- Returns to previous functional status for ADLs and vocational, recreational, and sports activities as identified by patient
- Independence in a progressive home exercise program emphasizing function
- Functional levels of spinal ROM: A minimum of 80% of AMA guides
- Functional upper and lower extremity ROM

INTERVENTION
NUMBER OF VISITS: 6–12

- Patient Instruction
  - Basic Anatomy and Biomechanics
  - Handouts
  - Functional Considerations
- Direct Intervention
  - Treatment Phase: 6–12 Visits
  - Functional Carryover

DISCHARGE PLANNING AND PATIENT RESPONSIBILITY

- Criteria for Discharge
  - Understanding that changing stress reaction habits takes time and that the home program must continue for a minimum of 60 days
  - All goals/outcomes have been achieved
- Circumstances Requiring Additional Visits
  - Severe deconditioning
  - Special occupational needs requiring extensive fitness/strengthening
  - Psychosocial and socioeconomic complicating factors
  - Level of patient/client adherence to the intervention program
  - Preexisting systemic conditions of diseases
- Home Program
  - Flexibility
  - Strengthening
  - Cardiovascular conditioning
  - Self-guided relaxation techniques
- Monitoring

SUMMARY OVERVIEW | TMJ/HEADACHE/STRESS | STRESS MANAGEMENT   383

STRESS MANAGEMENT

ICD-9

307.81	Tension headache
346	Migraine
350.2	Atypical face pain
524.6	Temporomandibular joint disorders
524.9	Unspecified dentofacial anomalies
728.9	Unspecified disorder of muscle, ligament, and fascia
729.1	Myalgia and myositis, unspecified
784	Symptoms involving head and neck
847	Sprains and strains of other and unspecified parts of back

APTA Preferred Practice Pattern: **4B, 4C, 4D, 4E, 4F, 4G, 4I, 5D, 7A**

EXAMINATION

History and Systems Review

- History of current condition
  - Location, nature, and behavior of symptoms
    - Pain
    - Fatigue
    - Headaches
    - Sleeplessness
    - Abdominal distress
    - Sudden loss or gain of weight
- Past history of current condition
- Past medical/surgical history
- Other tests and measures
- Medication
  - History of substance abuse
  - Current use of antidepressant medication
- Functional status and activity level (current/prior)
  - Vocational requirements
  - Recreational pursuits
  - ADLs limitations
- Social history
  - Significant life changes
  - Divorce
  - Death of a loved one
  - Relocation
  - Vocational
    - New job
    - Workstation change
    - Promotion
    - Transfer
    - Termination
- Patient's functional goals

Tests and Measures

Systems review per APTA's *Guide to Physical Therapy Practice*

- Gait, locomotion, and balance
  - Gait analysis
- Muscle performance
  - Abdominals
  - Spinal extensors
  - Scapular retractors/depressors
  - Gluteals
  - Lower extremity
  - Upper extremity
- Pain
- Posture
  - Forward head/rounded shoulders
  - Thoracic kyphosis
  - Lumbar lordosis
  - Genu recurvatum
  - Calcaneal varus/valgus
- ROM (active and passive)
  - Cervical/thoracic
  - Lumbar
  - Upper extremity
  - Lower extremity
- Visible signs of tension
  - Inability to sit still during initial evaluation
  - Clenching of teeth
  - Rapid speech
  - Frequent blinking
  - Distractibility

384   STRESS MANAGEMENT | TMJ/HEADACHE/STRESS

Establish Plan Of Care

- Based on history, tests, and measures

GOALS/OUTCOMES

- Pain: 2/10 or less with activity, 0/10 with ADLs
- Ability to identify sources of stress
- Self-awareness of patient's reactions to stress and ability to implement a plan for changing these responses
- Demonstrates proper body mechanics and postures for ADLs
- Strength: 4/5 for all lower extremity, upper extremity, abdominal, and spinal extensor musculature
- Returns to previous functional status for ADLs and vocational, recreational, and sports activities as identified by patient
- Independence in a progressive home exercise program emphasizing function
- Functional levels of spinal ROM: A minimum of 80% of AMA guides

Cervical	Normal	80%
Flexion	60°	50°
Extension	75°	60°
Rotation	80°	65°
Side bend	45°	35°

Thoracic	Normal	80%
Flexion	40°	30°
Extension	no AMA guides established	
Rotation	30°	25°
Side bend	10°	8°

Lumbar	Normal	80%
Flexion	60°	50°
Extension	25°	20°
Side bend	25°	20°

- Functional upper and lower extremity ROM
  - Hip
    - Flexion: 125°
    - Extension: 0°
  - Shoulder
    - Flexion: 160°
    - External rotation: 60°
    - Internal rotation: 60°
  - Foot/ankle
    - Dorsiflexion: 8° in subtalar neutral with knee extended

INTERVENTION

NUMBER OF VISITS: 6–12

Coordination, Communication, and Documentation

- Provision of services between admission and discharge that facilitate cost-effective and efficient integration or reintegration to home, community, or work
- Documentation of therapeutic intervention is required for each episode of care and serves as the basic foundation for communication
- Coordination and additional communication will depend on the patient's impairment and home/work/community/leisure situation and requirements. Such services may include:
  - Case management
  - Coordination of care and collaboration with those integral to the patient's rehabilitation program
  - Coordination and monitoring of the delivery of available resources
  - Referrals to other health-care professionals
  - Identification of resources, support groups, or advocacy services
  - Provision of educational or training information
  - Technical assistance
- Specific coordination and communication provisions:
  - Counseling
  - Biofeedback specialist

TMJ/HEADACHE/STRESS | STRESS MANAGEMENT   385

Patient Instruction

Basic Anatomy and Biomechanics
- Spinal anatomy and biomechanics as related to postural stresses
- Lower quarter biomechanical alignment as related to increased postural stresses
- Role of bruxing in onset of headaches and relationship of bruxing to excess stress
- Normal mechanics of diaphragmatic vs. accessory breathing

Handouts
- Home use of thermal modalities
  - Heating pads
  - Hot baths
  - Sauna/whirlpool
- Patient information sheet, *Relaxation and Stress Management*
- Commercially available products, such as:
  - Krames Communications (1100 Grundy Lane, San Bruno, CA 94066):
    - *A Guide to Managing Stress*
    - *A Positive Approach to Balancing Work and Family*
    - *Overcoming Anxiety*
    - *Coping with Change: How to Manage the Stress of Change*
    - *Steps Toward Healthier Living*
- Specific home exercise instruction

Functional Considerations
- Ergonomic workstation adjustment
- Importance of frequent positional changes, preferably at a minimum of every hour
- Proper posture/body mechanics
  - Sitting
  - Lifting
  - Standing
- General recognition of stressors in everyday life

Direct Intervention

Treatment Phase: 6–12 Visits
- Therapeutic exercise and home program
  - Stretching
    - Hamstrings
    - Gluteals
    - Quadriceps
    - Gastrocnemius/soleus
    - Pectorals
    - Muscles of mastication
    - Cervical ROM
    - Side-lying spinal rotation for general trunk ROM
    - Cat/camel
    - Press-ups
  - Strengthening
    - Squats
    - Multidirectional lunges
    - Abdominals
      a. Partial curl up
      b. Abdominal bracing progression
      c. Single-leg stance; posterior overhead reach with arms
    - Spinal extensors
      a. Therapeutic ball exercises
      b. Quadruped opposite arm and leg extension
    - Scapular retractors
      a. Therapeutic ball exercises
      b. Resistive band diagonals
    - Cervical musculature
      a. Cervical isometrics
      b. Gravity/resistive band resisted
  - Cardiovascular conditioning based on patient preference and other existing symptoms
    - Walking/running
    - Swimming
    - Cross-country skiing or ski machine
    - Stair climbing
    - Cycling
  - Stress management drills
    - Visualization/guided imagery
    - Self-relaxation techniques
    - Contract/relax
    - Diaphragmatic breathing
- Manual therapy techniques
  - Soft-tissue techniques
    - Soft-tissue mobilization
    - Trigger-point techniques
  - Assisted ROM and stretching techniques
  - Suboccipital inhibitive distraction
  - Postural isometric techniques for ROM and pain reduction
  - Joint mobilization
    - Oscillatory mobilization to promote relaxation

- Specific joint mobilization to hypomobile spinal segments or joints
- Electrotherapeutic modalities
  - Biofeedback
- Physical agents and mechanical modalities
  - Thermal modalities
  - Ultrasound

Functional Carryover
- Patient should be encouraged to use exercise as a healthy outlet for excess stress
- Patient should be referred to a specialist if substance abuse is suspected
- Patient is aware of incorporating home exercise program into ADLs and vocational activities
- Patient should be referred to a stress management specialist or psychotherapist if significant emotional or psychological overlay is suspected or if patient has difficulty identifying mechanisms for managing everyday stress

DISCHARGE PLANNING AND PATIENT RESPONSIBILITY

Criteria for Discharge
- Understanding that changing stress reaction habits takes time and that the home program must continue for a minimum of 60 days
- All goals/outcomes have been achieved

Circumstances Requiring Additional Visits
- Severe deconditioning
- Special occupational needs requiring extensive fitness/strengthening
- Psychosocial and socioeconomic complicating factors
- Level of patient/client adherence to the intervention program
- Preexisting systemic conditions of diseases

Home Program
- Flexibility
- Strengthening
- Cardiovascular conditioning
- Self-guided relaxation techniques

Monitoring
- Patient is to call for follow-up at 2–4 weeks post-discharge to ensure continued progress toward resuming all previous activities
- Schedule clinic follow-up as needed for home program adjustment or referral to other health care professionals

REFERENCES
1. American Physical Therapy Association. *Guide to Physical Therapist Practice.* Alexandria, VA: APTA; 1997.
2. Arena JE, Bruno GM, Hannah SL, Meador KJ. A comparison of frontal electromyographic biofeedback training, trapezius electromyographic biofeedback training and progressive relaxation therapy in the treatment of tension headache. *Headache.* 1995;35:411-419.
3. Engel JM. Relaxation training: a self-help approach for children with headaches. *Am J Occup Ther.* 1992;46:591-596.
4. Gary WJ, Brunsen J, Branson SJ. The effectiveness of physical therapy in the treatment of chronic daily headaches. *Headache.* 1989;29:156-162.
5. Gray H; Williams PL, ed. *Gray's Anatomy.* 38th ed. New York, NY: Churchill Livingstone; 1995.
6. Hamill JM, Cook TM, Rosecrance JC. Effectiveness of a physical therapy regime in the treatment of tension-type headache. *Headache.* 1996;36:149-153.
7. Lehrer PM, Carr R, Sargunaraj D, Woolfolk RL. Stress management techniques: are they all equivalent, or do they have specific effects? *Biofeedback Self Regul.* 1994;19:353-401.

388   STRESS MANAGEMENT | TMJ/Headache/Stress

TEMPOROMANDIBULAR DYSFUNCTION
SUMMARY OVERVIEW

ICD-9

524.6   526.9   728.9   729.1   784.0   848.1   959.09

APTA Preferred Practice Pattern: 4B, 4C, 4D, 4E, 4F, 4G, 4H, 4I

EXAMINATION

- History and Systems Review
- Tests and Measures
  Systems review per APTA's *Guide to Physical Therapy Practice*
  - Aerobic capacity and endurance
  - Anthropometric characteristics
  - Integumentary integrity
  - Joint integrity and mobility
  - Motor function
  - Muscle performance
  - Pain
  - Posture
  - ROM
  - Reflex integrity
  - Sensory integrity
  - Special tests
- Establish Plan of Care

GOALS/OUTCOMES

- Balanced posture (head position, shoulder position, and spinal curvatures)
- Pain: 2/10 or less
- Normalization of muscle balance (cervical, upper quadrant, and masticatory)
- Normalization of mandibular dynamics to achieve 40–45 mm of pain-free symmetrical mandibular motion
- Effective implementation of stress management skills
- Functional strength and endurance of jaw musculature to allow normal mastication
- Resolution of inflammatory process
- Cervical ROM: A minimum of 80% of AMA guides
- Return to previous functional status for ADLs and vocational, recreational, and sports activities as identified by patient
- Independence in a progressive home exercise program emphasizing function

INTERVENTION
NUMBER OF VISITS: 6–14

- Patient Instruction
  - Basic Anatomy and Biomechanics
  - Handouts
  - Functional Training in Self-Care and Home Management
- Direct Interventions
  - Acute Phase: 4–6 Visits
  - Subacute Phase: 2–8 Visits
- Functional Carryover

DISCHARGE PLANNING AND PATIENT RESPONSIBILITY

- Criteria for Discharge
  - All goals/outcomes have been achieved with the exception of return to recreational and sports activities
  - Patient demonstrates understanding of and compliance with nutritional and food choice guidelines
  - Patient displays understanding of the role of proper posture in decreasing stresses to the cervical spine and temporomandibular region
- Circumstances Requiring Additional Visits
  - Persistent functional motor performance deficit (inability to chew) or 2+/5 on manual muscle test
  - History of previous injury/surgery to the neck or TMJ
  - Persistent radicular symptoms
  - Severe deconditioning
  - Special occupational needs that require extensive fitness/strengthening
  - Craniovertebral instability
  - Head/facial impact in motor vehicle accident
  - Multiple injury sites
  - Psychosocial and socioeconomic complicating factors
  - Level of patient/client adherence to the intervention program
  - Preexisting systemic conditions or diseases

- Home Program
  - Flexibility and strengthening exercises to maintain postural balance
  - Cardiovascular conditioning
  - Use of modalities as needed for flare-ups
  - Self-guided relaxation techniques
- Monitoring

TEMPOROMANDIBULAR DYSFUNCTION

ICD-9

524.6	Temporomandibular joint disorders
526.9	Unspecified disease of the jaws
728.9	Unspecified disorder of muscle, ligament, and fascia
729.1	Myalgia and myositis, unspecified
784.0	Headache
848.1	Jaw sprain
959.09	Other and unspecified injury of face and neck

APTA Preferred Practice Pattern: 4B, 4C, 4D, 4E, 4F, 4G, 4H, 4I

EXAMINATION

History and Systems Review
- History of current condition
  - Location, nature, and behavior of symptoms
    - Headaches, ear, or oral factors
    - Dizziness
    - Other radiating symptoms
    - Aggravating/relieving factors
- Other tests and measures
- Medication
- Past medical/surgical history
- Functional status and activity level (current/prior)
  - Occupation/employment
    - Ergonomic environment
  - ADLs
  - Recreational/sport
- Social history
- Patient's functional goals

Tests and Measures
Systems review per APTA's *Guide to Physical Therapy Practice*
- Aerobic capacity and endurance
  - Respiration, alteration in nasal diaphragmatic breathing
- Anthropometric characteristics
  - Edema
- Integumentary integrity
  - Discoloration
  - Scars

- Joint integrity and mobility
  - Cervical segmental testing, C0–T3
  - Temporomandibular joint (TMJ)
    - Loading for reproduction of pain: Place palms of hands under the mandible and gently apply pressure superiorly up and through the TMJ
    - Joint end feel
      a. Distraction
      b. Anteromedial glide
      c. Lateral glide
- Motor function
  - Tongue rest position
  - Swallowing pattern
  - Lip closure position
  - Mandibular and condylar rest position
  - Presence of tongue thrust
- Muscle performance
  - Key muscle tests, C3–T1
  - Palpation of muscles, tendons, and ligaments Masticatory, cervical, scapular, and chest regions
    - Trigger-points, with or without referral
    - Hyperactivity
    - Hypertrophy
    - Atrophy
- Pain
- Posture
  - General
    - Swayback
    - Lordosis
    - Flatback
  - Forward head posture (see "Objective Measurement of Forward Head Posture" in *Cervical/Thoracic General Pain* guideline)

TMJ/HEADACHE/STRESS | TEMPOROMANDIBULAR DYSFUNCTION   391

- ROM
  - Cervical
    - Flexion
    - Extension
    - Side bending
    - Rotation
  - Mandibular
    Looking for deflection, moment of translation, and available rotation
    - Opening
    - Protrusion
    - Overjet
    - Overbite
    - Laterotrusion
      a. Normal mandibular ROM
      b. Opening: 40–50 mm
      c. Laterotrusion: 8–12 mm
      d. Protrusion: 2–6 mm
    - Auscultation for popping, clicking, and crepitation
  - Seated thoracic rotation
  - Upper-extremity functional ROM
    - Patient demonstrates ability to touch mid-back from a shoulder flexed/externally rotated and extended/internally rotated position
- Reflex integrity
  - Reflexes, C5–C7
- Sensory integrity
  - Sensation, C1–T1
- Special tests
  - Clear cervical spine and upper extremity
  - Craniovertebral stress tests
  - Vertebral artery test
  - Rule out thoracic outlet syndrome (see *Thoracic Outlet Syndrome* guideline)

Establish Plan of Care
- Based on history, tests, and measures

GOALS/OUTCOMES
- Balanced posture (head position, shoulder position, and spinal curvatures)
- Pain: 2/10 or less
- Normalization of muscle balance (cervical, upper quadrant, and masticatory)
- Normalization of mandibular dynamics to achieve 40–45 mm of pain-free symmetrical mandibular motion

- Effective implementation of stress management skills
- Functional strength and endurance of jaw musculature to allow normal mastication
- Resolution of inflammatory process
- Cervical ROM: A minimum of 80% of AMA guides

	Normal	*80%*
Flexion	60°	50°
Extension	75°	60°
Rotation	80°	65°
Side bend	45°	35°

- Return to previous functional status for ADLs and vocational, recreational, and sports activities as identified by patient
- Independence in a progressive home exercise program emphasizing function

INTERVENTION
Number of Visits: 6–14

Coordination, Communication, and Documentation
- Provision of services between admission and discharge that facilitate cost-effective and efficient integration or reintegration to home, community, or work
- Documentation of therapeutic intervention is required for each episode of care and serves as the basic foundation for communication
- Coordination and additional communication will depend on the patient's impairment and home/work/community/leisure situation and requirements. Such services may include:
  - Case management
  - Coordination of care and collaboration with those integral to the patient's rehabilitation program
  - Coordination and monitoring of the delivery of available resources
  - Referrals to other health-care professionals
  - Identification of resources, support groups, or advocacy services
  - Provision of educational or training information
  - Technical assistance
- Specific coordination and communication provisions:
  - Dentist/oral surgeon regarding intraoral appliance
  - Biofeedback specialist
  - Counseling

Patient Instruction

Basic Anatomy and Biomechanics

- Fibrocartilagenous disc, ligaments, capsule, and surrounding musculature
- Pertinent Gray's Anatomy (Gray. 1995. 578–582, 799–805)

Handouts

- Commercially available products, such as:
  - Krames Communications (1100 Grundy Lane, San Bruno, CA 94066)
    - *Poor Posture Hurts*
    - *TM Disorders*
  - Musculoskeletal Approach to Maxillofacial Pain (Rocabado. 1991)
  - Let's Do Lunch: A Handbook of Instructions and Recipes for Patients of Oral Surgery and Others Requiring Soft Foods or Liquid Diets
- Specific home program

Functional Training in Self-Care and Home Management

- Effects of bruxing on TMJ and surrounding soft tissue
- Purpose of intraoral appliance and importance of compliance with use
- Effects of poor posture on temporomandibular dysfunction
- Dietary influences on temporomandibular dysfunction

Direct Interventions

Acute Phase: 4–6 Visits

- Therapeutic exercise and home program
  - Contract/relax jaw opening (performed in pain-free, noise-free range)
  - Self-trigger-point acupressure
  - Soft-tissue stretching
    - Cervical
    - Thoracic
    - Shoulder girdle
    - Masticatory
  - Tongue rest position
  - Controlled mandibular opening
  - Axial extension
  - Initiate a cardiovascular conditioning program

- Manual therapy techniques
  - Soft-tissue techniques to the cervical and masticatory regions
    - Direct and indirect trigger-point techniques
    - Soft-tissue mobilization
    - Muscle energy techniques
    - Intraoral massage
  - Proprioceptive neuromuscular facilitation
  - Joint mobilization
    - Grades I–V to hypomobile spinal segments
    - Grades I–II to the temporomandibular joint for pain relief
- Electrotherapeutic modalities
  - Iontophoresis
  - Biofeedback
  - Microcurrent electrical nerve stimulator
  - Low-power laser
  - Mid-power laser
- Physical agents and mechanical modalities
  - Cryotherapy/thermal
  - Ultrasound
- Goals/outcomes
  - Pain: 5/10 or less
  - Decrease spasm and inflammation
  - Restore functional jaw AROM, achieving a minimum of 30 mm of mandibular opening
  - Cervical ROM: A minimum of 50% of AMA guides
    - Flexion: 30°
    - Extension: 40°
    - Rotation: 40°
    - Side bend: 25°
  - Restore normal joint/tongue rest position and proper mandibular dynamics (rotation/translation)

Subacute Phase: 2–8 Visits

- Therapeutic exercise and home program
  - Self-intraoral massage
  - Rest position of tongue
  - Controlled opening
  - Isometric contraction starting at mid-range, progressing to full ranges
    - Opening
    - Closing
    - Lateral deviation
  - Cervical nodding
  - Axial cervical extension
  - Thoracic extension

TMJ/HEADACHE/STRESS | TEMPOROMANDIBULAR DYSFUNCTION 393

- Specific facilitation
  - Contract/relax
  - Hold/relax
- Postural exercises
  - Stretching
  - Strength
- Spinal stabilization exercises
  - Therapeutic ball
- Cardiovascular conditioning
  - Walking program/treadmill
  - Aquatic therapy/swimming
    a. Avoid use of snorkel
  - Ski machine
  - Upper or lower extremity cycling
- Manual therapy techniques
  - Soft-tissue techniques to the cervical and masticatory regions
    - Soft-tissue mobilization
    - Direct or indirect trigger-point techniques
    - Intraoral massage
  - Proprioceptive neuromuscular facilitation
  - Joint mobilization progressing grade as indicated
    - Vertebral
    - Cranial
    - TMJ
      a. Distraction
      b. Medial and lateral gapping techniques
- Physical agents and mechanical modalities
  - Continue effective modalities as in acute phase, with increased emphasis on use as needed at home
- Goals/outcomes
  - Pain: 2/10 or less
  - Eliminate inflammation
  - Soft-tissue relaxation
  - Destruction of adhesions (adhesive capsulitis)
  - Increase extensibility of fibrous capsule (hypomobility)
  - Stabilize hypermobility
  - Achieve 40–45 mm of pain-free symmetrical mandibular opening
  - Achieve a minimum of 80% of AMA guides for cervical ROM:
    - Flexion: 50°
    - Extension: 60°
    - Rotation: 65°
    - Side bend: 35°

Functional Carryover

- Ergonomic evaluation: Proper sitting and standing posture (critical for reducing abnormal strain on neck and jaw muscles)
- Proper nutrition to promote healing
- Avoid foods that stress the TMJ and surrounding soft tissue
  - Hard foods
  - More textured/chewy foods
  - Gum
- Stress management skills incorporated into ADLs and vocational activities (see Patient Information Sheet *Relaxation and Stress Management*)
- Address sleep disturbances (interferes with management of a chronic condition) and sleep postures

DISCHARGE PLANNING AND PATIENT RESPONSIBILITY

Criteria for Discharge

- All goals/outcomes have been achieved with the exception of return to recreational and sports activities
- Patient demonstrates understanding of and compliance with nutritional and food choice guidelines
- Patient displays understanding of the role of proper posture in decreasing stresses to the cervical spine and temporomandibular region

Circumstances Requiring Additional Visits

- Persistent functional motor performance deficit (inability to chew) or 2+/5 on manual muscle test
- History of previous injury/surgery to the neck or TMJ
- Persistent radicular symptoms
- Severe deconditioning
- Special occupational needs requiring extensive fitness/ strengthening
- Craniovertebral instability
- Head/facial impact in motor vehicle accident
- Multiple injury sites
- Psychosocial and socioeconomic complicating factors
- Level of patient/client adherence to the intervention program
- Preexisting systemic conditions or diseases

Home Program

- Flexibility and strengthening exercises to maintain postural balance
- Cardiovascular conditioning
- Use of modalities as needed for flare-ups
- Self-guided relaxation techniques

Monitoring

- Patient understands that, in most cases, there is not a "cure" but rather that this is a management issue
- Patient is reminded of the importance of dental checkups to monitor proper fit of orthotics, if indicated, and compliance with orthotics to prevent further damage of dentition and surrounding soft tissue
- Patient is to call for follow-up at 2–4 weeks post-discharge to report progress and address difficulties with home program
- Patient is versed in the expectations of slow but continued improvement in symptoms as he/she continues with the home program and management skills and is instructed to call for advice should a negative trend occur

REFERENCES

1. American Physical Therapy Association. *Guide to Physical Therapist Practice*. Alexandria, VA: APTA; 1997.
2. Aspinall W. Clinical testing for cervical mechanical disorders which produce ischemic vertigo. *J Orthop Sports Phys Ther.* 1989;11(5):176-182.
3. Eggleton T, Langton D. *Introduction to Craniomandibular Disorders and Dysfunction of the Temporomandibular Joint.* March 22-24, 1991. Edmonds, WA: Ursa Foundation.
4. Eggleton T, Langton D. *Advanced Physical Therapy Management of Craniomandibular and Vertebral Dysfunction.* October 1-3, 1993. Edmonds, WA: Ursa Foundation.
5. Gray H; Williams PL, ed. *Gray's Anatomy.* 38th ed. New York, NY: Churchill Livingstone; 1995.
6. Gray RJM, Quayle AA, Hall CA, Schofield MA. Physiotherapy in the treatment of temporomandibular joint disorders: a comparative study of four treatment methods. *Br Dent J.* 1994;176:250-261.
7. Hart A, Hopkins C, Ford B. *ICD-9-CM Expert for Physicians, Volume 1&2.* 7th ed. USA: Ingenix; 2005.
8. Helland M. Anatomy and function of the temporomandibular joint. In: Grieve G, ed. *Modern Manual Therapy of the Vertebral Column.* New York, NY: Churchill Livingston; 1986:64-76.
9. Kirk W, Calabrese D. Clinical evaluation of physical therapy in the management of internal derangement of the temporomandibular joint. *J Oral Maxillofac Surg.* 1989;47:113-119.
10. Rocabado M. *Musculoskeletal Approach to Maxillofacial Pain.* Philadelphia, PA: JB Lippincott; 1991.
11. Suvinen TI, Hanes KR, Reade PC. Outcome of therapy in the conservative management of temporomandibular pain dysfunction disorder. *J Oral Rehab.* 1997;24:718-724.
12. Trott P. Examination of the temporomandibular joint. In: Grieve G, ed. *Modern Manual Therapy of the Vertebral Column.* New York, NY: Churchill Livingston; 1986:521-529.
13. Waide FL, Montana J, Bade DM, Dimitroff M. Tolerance of ultrasound over the temporomandibular joint. *J Orthop Sports Phys Ther.* 1992;15(5):206-214.

396   TEMPOROMANDIBULAR DYSFUNCTION | TMJ/HEADACHE/STRESS

Shoulder

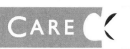

SHOULDER

Adhesive Capsulitis	399
Biceps Tendon Rupture	405
Humerus Fracture	411
Labrum Tear	417
Postop. Rehab. For Shoulder Instability	423
Postop. Rehab. of the Rotator Cuff	429
Postop. Total Shoulder Arthroplasty	435
Shoulder Anterior Dislocation	441
Shoulder Bursitis	447
Shoulder Degenerative Joint Disease	455
Shoulder Fracture	461
Shoulder Joint Pathology	467
Shoulder Sprain/Strain	475
Shoulder Tendinitis	483

398   SHOULDER

ADHESIVE CAPSULITIS
SUMMARY OVERVIEW

ICD-9

716.91　719.41　726.0　726.2

APTA Preferred Practice Pattern: 4D, 4E, 4F, 4G, 4J, 7A

EXAMINATION

- History and Systems Review
- Tests and Measures
  Systems review per APTA's *Guide to Physical Therapy Practice*
  - Joint integrity and mobility
  - Muscle performance
  - Pain
  - Posture
  - ROM
  - Special tests
- Establish Plan of Care

GOALS/OUTCOMES

- Shoulder AROM: 80% of AMA guides
- Functional cervical ROM or a minimum of 80% of AMA guides
- Pain: 2/10 or less with activity, 0/10 at rest
- Strength: 4/5 on manual muscle test or equal to uninvolved extremity
- Self-care and home management
- Return to prior functional status and activity level for ADLs and vocational, recreational, and sports activities as identified by patient
- Independence in a progressive home exercise program emphasizing function

INTERVENTION
NUMBER OF VISITS: 7–16

- Patient Instruction
  - Basic Anatomy and Biomechanics
  - Handouts
  - Functional Considerations
- Direct Interventions
  - Acute Phase: 1–4 Visits
  - Subacute Phase: 6–12 Visits
- Functional Carryover

DISCHARGE PLANNING AND PATIENT RESPONSIBILITY

- Criteria for Discharge
  - Patient is compliant with home program
  - All rehabilitation goals/outcomes achieved except may discharge with less ROM if all other goals/outcomes attained
  - The therapist determines that further progression and attainment of all rehabilitation goals/outcomes will be achieved with patient's continued efforts/compliance with home program outside the clinical environment
- Circumstances Requiring Additional Visits
  - Cervical pathology or radiating signs/symptoms
  - Unable to achieve functional goals
  - Presence of concomitant tendinitis
  - Inability to progress because current vocational demands are exacerbating symptoms
- Home Program
  - Stretching and strengthening
  - Self-mobilization techniques
  - Cardiovascular conditioning
- Monitoring

SUMMARY OVERVIEW | SHOULDER | ADHESIVE CAPSULITIS   399

ADHESIVE CAPSULITIS

ICD-9

716.91	Arthropathy, unspecified, shoulder region
719.41	Pain in joint, shoulder region
726.0	Adhesive capsulitis of shoulder
726.2	Other affections of shoulder region, not elsewhere classified

APTA Preferred Practice Pattern: 4D, 4E, 4F, 4G, 4J, 7A

EXAMINATION

History and Systems Review

- History of current condition
  - Gradual onset
  - Location, nature, and behavior of symptoms
    - Aggravating/relieving factors
- Past history of current condition
  - Injury to upper extremity or cervical spine
  - Surgery
  - Direct intervention
- Other tests and measures
- Functional status and activity level (current/prior)
  - Inability to lift arm overhead or reach behind back
  - Disruption of sleep
- Patient's functional goals/outcomes

Tests and Measures

Systems review per APTA's *Guide to Physical Therapy Practice*

- Joint integrity and mobility
  - Glenohumeral
  - Acromioclavicular
  - Sternoclavicular
  - Scapulothoracic
- Muscle performance
  - Antalgic movement pattern with dressing activities
  - Functional use of upper extremity during gait
  - Scapulohumeral rhythm
    - Arms at side
    - Hands on hips
    - Arms elevated 90° anteriorly
  - Patient demonstrates ability to touch mid-back with the shoulder flexed/externally rotated and extended/internally rotated
- Pain
  - Measured on visual analog scale

- Posture
  - Forward head
  - Rounded shoulders
  - Flattening of the thoracic spine
  - Shoulder girdle asymmetry
    - Winging of the scapula
    - Clavicular position
    - Humeral head position
    - Muscular development/atrophy
  - Ability to actively achieve a more balanced postural position
- ROM
  - Shoulder girdle ROM (differential diagnosis)
    - AROM and PROM display capsular pattern of restriction with the greatest limitation being external rotation, followed by abduction, followed by an equal limitation of flexion and internal rotation
    - Restriction of passive joint ROM in all planes, especially anterior and inferior glides
- Special tests
  - Clear elbow, wrist, and hand
  - Clear cervical spine
    - AROM
    - PROM
    - Overpressure
    - Quadrant compression test

Establish Plan of Care

- Based on history, tests, and measures

GOALS/OUTCOMES

- Shoulder AROM: 80% of AMA guides

	Normal	80%
Flexion	180°	145°
Extension	50°	40°
Abduction	180°	145°
Internal rotation	90°	70°
External rotation	90°	70°

400   ADHESIVE CAPSULITIS | SHOULDER

- Functional cervical ROM or a minimum of 80% of AMA guides:

	Normal	80%
Flexion	60°	50°
Extension	70°	60°
Side bend	45°	35°
Rotation	85°	65°

- Pain: 2/10 or less with activity, 0/10 at rest
- Strength: 4/5 on manual muscle test or equal to uninvolved extremity
- Self-care and home management
  - Able to reach into back pocket or fasten undergarments
  - Able to comb hair
  - Able to reach into cupboard or lift overhead
  - Able to perform work/ADL tasks (weight and repetition specific)
- Return to prior functional status and activity level for ADLs and vocational, recreational, and sports activities as identified by patient
- Independence in a progressive home exercise program emphasizing function

INTERVENTION
NUMBER OF VISITS: 7–16

Coordination, Communication, and Documentation

- Provision of services between admission and discharge that facilitate cost-effective and efficient integration or reintegration to home, community, or work
- Documentation of therapeutic intervention is required for each episode of care and serves as the basic foundation for communication
- Coordination and additional communication will depend on the patient's impairment and home/work/community/leisure situation and requirements. Such services may include:
  - Case management
  - Coordination of care and collaboration with those integral to the patient's rehabilitation program
  - Coordination and monitoring of the delivery of available resources
  - Referrals to other health-care professionals
  - Identification of resources, support groups, or advocacy services
  - Provision of educational or training information
  - Technical assistance

Patient Instruction

Basic Anatomy and Biomechanics
- Explanation of physiological changes of soft-tissue and shoulder capsule
- Pertinent Gray's Anatomy (Gray. 1995. 627–632, 839, 842)
- Mechanism of shoulder joint and related tissues

Handouts
- Specific home program
- Sleeping postures
- Home use of cryotherapy

Functional Considerations
- Role of posture in pathogenesis of condition
- Importance of repetitive movement to allow normal joint mechanics
- Avoidance of forward head or rounded shoulder posture

Direct Interventions

Acute Phase: 1–4 Visits
- Therapeutic exercise and home program
  - Flexibility exercises
    - Codman's exercise
    - Pain-free assisted ROM using wand or home pulley
    - AROM in pain-free range, including scapular retraction/depression
  - Posture
    - Proper sitting posture
    - Sleeping postures to avoid stress to shoulder
  - Neuromuscular/balance/proprioceptive reeducation
    - Modified plantargrade propping on elbows
    - Plantargrade movement in all planes
- Manual therapy techniques
  - Soft-tissue techniques
    - Soft-tissue mobilization to the cervical/thoracic spine and shoulder girdle
  - Joint mobilization
    - Glenohumeral grades I–II with intent of pain relief
    - Grades III–IV to corresponding hypomobilities in the shoulder complex, spine, and elbow
- Physical agents and mechanical modalities
  - Cryotherapy/thermal modalities
  - Athermal/deep thermal modalities to surrounding musculature

SHOULDER | ADHESIVE CAPSULITIS   401

- Goals/outcomes
  - Pain: 5/10 or less
  - Strength: 4/5 on manual muscle test for shoulder girdle musculature
  - Shoulder ROM: 60% of AMA guides
    - Flexion: 110°
    - Extension: 30°
    - Abduction: 110°
    - External rotation: 55°
    - Internal rotation: 55°
  - Functional activity
    - Increased duration of uninterrupted sleep as compared to initial evaluation

Subacute Phase: 6–12 Visits

- Therapeutic exercise and home program
  - Flexibility
    - Wand exercises for external rotation, elevation, circumduction, and diagonal patterns
    - Pulley exercises for elevation and internal rotation
    - Codman's exercise with cuff weights
    - Postural stretches—anterior shoulder/chest muscles
  - Strengthening
    - Isometric exercises
    - ROM exercises through available range
    - Short arc exercises utilizing elastic bands (elevation, abduction, external, and internal rotation)
    - Postural correction exercises
      a. Horizontal abduction
      b. External rotation
  - Neuromuscular/balance/proprioceptive reeducation
    - Quadruped multidirectional rocking
    - Three-point rocking
    - Push-ups
    - Push-ups off therapeutic ball
    - Bodyblade®
  - Cardiovascular conditioning
    - Walking program
    - Ski machine
    - Cycling
- Manual therapy techniques
  - Continue effective soft-tissue mobilization
  - Progressive graded mobilization techniques stressing anterior, inferior, and posterior capsule at the point of restriction
- Physical agents and mechanical modalities
  - Continue effective modalities as in acute phase with increased emphasis on use as needed at home

- Ultrasound prior to mobilization: Shoulder abducted and externally rotated, ultrasound anterior, inferior capsule, posterior capsule as indicated
- Goals/outcomes
  - Pain: 2/10 or less
  - Strength: 4/5 on manual muscle test or equal to uninvolved extremity
  - Shoulder ROM: 75% of uninvolved extremity or a minimum of 80% of AMA guides
  - Functional activities
    - Able to reach into back pocket or fasten undergarments
    - Able to comb hair
    - Able to reach into cupboard or lift overhead
    - Able to perform work/ADL tasks (weight and repetition specific)

Functional Carryover

- Modification of work and home environment as progression dictates to minimize stress on involved extremity
- Dressing without assistive aides including fastening undergarments and buttons behind back

DISCHARGE PLANNING AND PATIENT RESPONSIBILITY

Criteria for Discharge

- Patient is compliant with home program
- All rehabilitation goals/outcomes achieved except may discharge with less ROM if all other goals/outcomes attained
- The therapist determines that further progression and attainment of all rehabilitation goals/outcomes will be achieved with patient's continued efforts/compliance with home program outside the clinical environment

Circumstances Requiring Additional Visits

- Cervical pathology or radiating signs/symptoms
- Unable to achieve functional goals
- Presence of concomitant tendinitis
- Inability to progress because current vocational demands are exacerbating symptoms

Home Program

- Stretching and strengthening
- Self-mobilization techniques
- Cardiovascular conditioning

Monitoring

- Full recovery can take up to a year or longer, so follow-up clinic visits may be indicated on a monthly basis to progress home exercise program and emphasize follow through with instructions
- Patient is instructed to call for advice should progression halt or a negative trend occur

REFERENCES

1. American Physical Therapy Association. *Guide to Physical Therapist Practice.* Alexandria, VA: APTA; 1997.

2. Corrigan B, Maitland GD. *Practical Orthopaedic Medicine: Capsulitis.* London, England: Butterworth; 1983:50-53.

3. Einhorn AR. Shoulder rehabilitation equipment modifications. *J Orthop Sports Phys Ther.* 1985;6(4):247-253.

4. Engelberg AL. *Guides to The Evaluation of Permanent Impairment.* 3rd ed. Chicago, IL: American Medical Association; 1989.

5. Gray H; Williams PL, ed. *Gray's Anatomy.* 38th ed. New York, NY: Churchill Livingstone; 1995.

6. Kronberg M, Nemeth G, Brostrom L. Muscle activity and coordination in the normal shoulder. *Clin Orthop Rel Res.* 1990;257:76-85.

7. Saunders D. *Evaluation, Treatment And Prevention of Musculoskeletal Disorders.* 3rd ed. Bloomington, MN: Saunders Group; 1993.

8. Vermeulen HM, Rozing PM, Obermann WR, le Cessie S, Vliet Vlieland TP. Comparison of high-grade and low-grade mobilization techniques in the management of adhesive capsulitis of the shoulder: randomized controlled trial. *Phys Ther.* 2006;86(3):355-68.

404   ADHESIVE CAPSULITIS | SHOULDER

BICEPS TENDON RUPTURE
SUMMARY OVERVIEW

ICD-9

727.62

APTA Preferred Practice Pattern: **4E, 4I**

EXAMINATION

- History and Systems
- Tests and Measures
  Systems review per APTA's *Guide to Physical Therapy Practice*
  - Joint integrity and mobility
  - Muscle performance
  - Pain
  - Posture
  - ROM
  - Special testing
- Establish Plan of Care

GOALS/OUTCOMES

- Shoulder ROM: 90% of AMA guides or equal to uninvolved extremity
- Functional cervical ROM or a minimum of 80% of AMA Guides
- Pain: 2/10 or less with resisted motion, 0/10 at rest
- Strength: 4/5 on manual muscle test
- Return to prior functional status and activity level for ADLs and vocational, recreational, and sports activities as identified by patient
- Independence in a progressive home exercise program emphasizing function
- Functional activities

INTERVENTION
NUMBER OF VISITS: 6–12

- Patient Instruction
  - Basic Anatomy and Biomechanics
  - Handouts
  - Functional Considerations
- Direct Interventions
  - Acute Phase: 3–6 Visits
  - Subacute Phase: 3–6 Visits
- Functional Carryover

DISCHARGE PLANNING AND PATIENT RESPONSIBILITY

- Criteria for Discharge
  - All rehabilitation goals/outcomes reached except return to vocational or sports activity
  - Patient able to continue to make progress with compliance with home program
  - If continuation of pain and instability prevent patient progression, consider orthopedic consultation
- Circumstances Requiring Additional Visits
  - Severe degenerative changes
  - History of other pathology
  - Presence of other medical conditions
  - Contractures
  - Cognitive limitations
  - Postoperative complications
  - Excessive environmental barriers to discharge
  - Special occupational needs that require extensive strengthening
  - Multiple injury sites (rotator cuff)
  - Presence of ligamentous instability
  - Presence of cervical pathology
- Home Program
  - Motor performance for shoulder and elbow supination/pronation to maximize strength of rotator cuff, scapular stabilizers, and elbow supination/pronation
  - Flexibility
  - Diagonal pattern work for functional overhead work without fatigue or pain
  - Cardiovascular conditioning for better tolerance for work and home vocational activities
- Monitoring

SUMMARY OVERVIEW | SHOULDER | BICEPS TENDON RUPTURE   405

BICEPS TENDON RUPTURE

ICD-9
    727.62   Nontraumatic rupture of tendons of biceps (long head)
APTA Preferred Practice Pattern: 4E, 4I

EXAMINATION

History and Systems

- History of current condition
  - Location, nature, and behavior of symptoms
    - Aggravating /relieving factors
    - a.m./p.m.
- Past history of current condition
  - Cervical/thoracic spine or upper extremity injury
  - Surgery
  - Direct intervention
- Other tests and measures
- Medications
- Past medical/surgical history
- Functional status and activity level (current/prior)
- Patient's functional goals

Tests and Measures

Systems review per APTA's *Guide to Physical Therapy Practice*

- Joint integrity and mobility
  - Glenohumeral
    - Anterior capsule
    - Posterior capsule
    - Inferior capsule
  - Acromioclavicular
  - Sternoclavicular
  - Scapulothoracic
  - Radio-humeral
  - Ulno-humeral
- Muscle performance (including strength, power, and endurance)
  - Resisted testing
    - Glenohumeral
    - Scapular muscles
    - Supraspinatus isolation ("empty can" position)
      a. Shoulder internally rotated, thumb pointed to floor
      b. Abduct the arm to 90°, maintain position 30° anterior to the mid-frontal plane
      c. Radio-humeral
      d. Ulno-humeral

- Antalgic movement pattern with dressing activities
- Functional use of upper extremity during gait
- Scapulohumeral position and rhythm
  - Arms at side
  - Hands on hips
  - Arms elevated 90° anteriorly
- Pain
  - Measured on visual analog scale
- Posture
  - Forward head
  - Rounded shoulders
  - Flattening of the thoracic spine
  - Shoulder girdle asymmetry
    - Winging of the scapula
    - Clavicular position
    - Humeral head position
    - Muscular development/atrophy
  - Ability to actively achieve a more balanced postural position
- ROM (including muscle length)
  - Cervical screening
    - Active/passive ROM
    - Overpressure
    - Quadrant compression test
  - Shoulder girdle mobility
    - AROM flexion/elevation (observe for inability to maintain depressed humeral head)
      a. Abduction
      b. Internal rotation
      c. External rotation
      d. Extension
    - Overpressure and PROM to all motions
    - PROM
    - Elbow screening
      a. Active/passive ROM
      b. Overpressure

406   BICEPS TENDON RUPTURE | SHOULDER

- Special Testing
  - Apprehension Test
    - Patient in supine
    - Involved arm is in abduction and external rotation
    - Push anteriorly on posterior aspect of humeral head
      a. Patient with recurrent dislocation will experience apprehension
      b. Patient with anterior instability (subluxation) will experience pain but not apprehension
      c. Patient with normal shoulder will be asymptomatic
  - Relocation test
    - Administer test with posteriorly directed force on humeral head from apprehension test position
      a. Patient with primary impingement will generally have no change in their pain
      b. Patient with instability (subluxation) and secondary impingement will have pain relief and will tolerate maximal external rotation with the humeral head maintained in a reduced position
  - Clunk Test
    - Patient is supine
    - Move arm into full flexion and caudal glide, then perform circumduction motion
      a. Positive if clunk, pain, or pseudolocking occurs
      b. Implicates labral tear
  - Neer's test
    - Patient is seated or supine
    - Place patient's arm in full flexion with no internal or external rotation, then apply flexion overpressure
      a. Pain implicates supraspinatus and long head of biceps
  - Active compression test
    - Patient seated
    - Forward flexion to 90° with elbow in complete extension. Adduct horizontally 10°.
    - Maximal shoulder internal rotation
    - Apply a downward force while patient resists
    - Repeat test with maximal lateral rotation
      a. Positive test is pain in first position (internal rotation) with relief or no pain in second position (lateral rotation)
  - Yergason test
    - Patient standing, elbow flexed to 90° and palm down (pronation)
    - Resist the patient's attempted supination
    - Pain in the bicipital groove implicates the bicep tendon

Establish Plan of Care
- Based on history, tests, and measures

GOALS/OUTCOMES
- Shoulder ROM: 90% of AMA guides or equal to uninvolved extremity
  - Flexion: 160°
  - Extension: 45°
  - Abduction: 160°
  - Internal rotation: 80°
  - External rotation: 80°
- Functional cervical ROM or a minimum of 80% of AMA guides
  - Flexion: 50°
  - Extension: 60°
  - Rotation: 65°
  - Side bending: 35°
- Pain: 2/10 or less with resisted motion, 0/10 at rest
- Strength: 4/5 on manual muscle test
- Return to prior functional status and activity level for ADLs and vocational, recreational, and sports activities as identified by patient
- Independence in a progressive home exercise program emphasizing function
- Functional Activities
  - Able to reach into back pocket or fasten undergarments
  - Able to comb hair
  - Able to reach into cupboard or lift overhead
  - Perform work/ADL tasks

INTERVENTION
Number of Visits: 6–12

Coordination, Communication, and Documentation

- Provision of services between admission and discharge that facilitate cost-effective and efficient integration or reintegration to home, community, or work
- Documentation of therapeutic intervention is required for each episode of care and serves as the basic foundation for communication
- Coordination and additional communication will depend on the patient's impairment and home/work/community/leisure situation and requirements. Such services may include:
  - Case management
  - Coordination of care and collaboration with those integral to the patient's rehabilitation program
  - Coordination and monitoring of the delivery of available resources
  - Referrals to other health-care professionals
  - Identification of resources, support groups, or advocacy services
  - Provision of educational or training information
  - Technical assistance

Patient Instruction

Basic Anatomy and Biomechanics
- Gray's Anatomy
- Instructions for sports medicine patients

Handouts
- Home program
  - Specific home program for forearm supination/elbow flexion
  - Specific home program for scapular stabilization
  - Specific home program for rotator cuff strength in overhead position

Functional Considerations
- Posture (sitting, standing, sleeping, driving)
- Assistive devices (crutches, canes, walkers, collars, tape, etc.)
- Precautions
- Alteration of ADLs
- Avoidance of prolonged postures

- Positioning for relief of symptoms
- Body mechanic instruction for lifting, pushing, pulling, etc.
- Training recommendations (cross training, periodization, etc.)
- Avoidance of activities that cause exacerbation of symptoms
- Reduction of motions causing overload forces

Direct Interventions

Acute Phase: 3–6 Visits
- Therapeutic exercises and home program
  - PROM
    - Codman's, pulleys, and active assist wand exercises, all planes
  - Pain-free AROM
    - High-repetitions and low-resistance, with purpose of promoting vascularization of healing tissues
    - Internal/external rotation
    - Supraspinatus isolation
      a. Shoulder is internally rotated, thumb pointed to floor
      b. Abduct the arm to 90°, maintaining a position 30° anterior to the mid-frontal plane
- Scapular retraction/depression
- Scapular upward rotation
- Upper body ergometer
  - Postural correction exercises
  - Neuromuscular/balance/proprioception
    - Bodyblade®
  - Cardiovascular conditioning
    - Treadmill or walking
    - Lower-extremity cycling
- Manual therapy techniques
  - Soft-tissue mobilization
    - Friction massage, myofascial release/stretching
  - Joint mobilization
    - Grades I–II to gait pain/guarding
    - Grades III–V to correct hypomobility to glenohumeral, sternoclavicular, or acromioclavicular joints or thoracic spine
  - ROM
    - Within pain-free range specific to rotator cuff musculature/shoulder girdle/pectorals
    - Within pain-free range specific to elbow

- Physical agents and mechanical modalities
  - Cryotherapy
  - Athermal, deep thermal modalities
- Goals/outcomes
  - Pain: 4/10 following activity, 2/10 or less at rest
  - Pain-free ROM: 50% of AMA guides
    - Flexion: 90°
    - Extension: 25°
    - Abduction: 90°
    - Internal rotation: 45°
    - External rotation: 45°
    - Elbow flexion to 120°, supination/pronation to 40°
  - Increased duration of uninterrupted sleep (set specific goal based on number of interruption hours of sleep at initial evaluation)

Subacute Phase: 3–6 Visits

- Therapeutic exercises and home program
  - Progressive strengthening (isometric, pulley, resistive bands, free weights)
    - Exercises should not elicit painful response
    - Use resistive bands, surgical tubing for internal/external rotation, elbow flexed at 90°
    - Isometrics in planes not tolerating banded resistance
    - Internal rotation lying on involved side
    - External rotation lying on uninvolved side
    - Supraspinatus isolation ("empty can" position)
    - Shoulder extension
      a. Prone with arm hanging off table or forward bent at waist in standing
      b. Extend arm to side of trunk (105°)
    - Elbow supination and pronation
  - Flexibility/posture correction
  - Neuromuscluar/balance/proprioceptive reeducation
    - Quadruped multidirectional rocking
    - Three-point rocking
    - Push-ups
    - Push-ups off therapeutic ball
    - Body blade
  - Progression into vocation/sport-specific activity
- Manual therapy techniques
  - Joint mobilization
    - Grades III–IV to persistent hypomobilities of the glenohumeral, sternoclavicular, acromioclavicular, and scapulothoracic regions
    - Grades III–V to cervical/thoracic spine

  - Continue effective soft-tissue techniques
- Physical agents and mechanical modalities
  - Continue effective modalities as in acute phase, with increased emphasis on use as needed at home
- Goals/outcomes
  - Shoulder/elbow ROM: 90% of AMA guides or equal to the uninvolved extremity
    - Flexion: 160°
    - Extension: 45°
    - External rotation: 80°
    - Internal rotation: 80°
    - Abduction: 160°
    - Elbow flexion 120°
    - Elbow supination/pronation 70°
  - Pain: 2/10 following activity, 0/10 at rest
  - Strength: Equal to uninvolved side or 4/5 on manual muscle test
  - Functional activities
    - Able to reach into back pocket or fasten undergarments
    - Able to comb hair
    - Able to reach into cupboard or lift overhead
    - Perform work/ADL tasks (weight and repetition specific)

Functional Carryover

- Integration of home exercise program into vocational environment
- Completion of ergonomic adjustments to home, automobile, and vocational areas
- Incorporation of proper posture and body mechanics to avoid exacerbation of symptoms
- Recognition/avoidance of activities that increase or exacerbate radiating symptoms

DISCHARGE PLANNING AND PATIENT RESPONSIBILITY

Criteria for Discharge

- All rehabilitation goals/outcomes reached except return to vocational or sports activity
- Patient able to continue to make progress with compliance with home program
- If continuation of pain and instability prevent patient progression, consider orthopedic consultation

Circumstances Requiring Additional Visits
- Severe degenerative changes
- History of other pathology
- Presence of other medical conditions
- Contractures
- Cognitive limitations
- Postoperative complications
- Excessive environmental barriers to discharge
- Special occupational needs that require extensive strengthening
- Multiple injury sites (rotator cuff)
- Presence of ligamentous instability
- Presence of cervical pathology

Home Program
- Motor performance for shoulder and elbow supination/pronation to maximize strength of rotator cuff, scapular stabilizers, and elbow supination/pronation
- Flexibility
- Diagonal pattern work for functional overhead work without fatigue or pain
- Cardiovascular conditioning for better tolerance for work and home vocational activities

Monitoring
- Return to physical therapy or physician:
  - If symptoms persist longer than 12 weeks post-injury
  - If supination weakness does not allow return to work/home activities
  - If "cramping" pain persist in biceps area

REFERENCES
1. American Physical Therapy Association. *Guide to Physical Therapist Practice.* Alexandria, VA: APTA; revised 2003.
2. Gray H; Williams PL, ed. *Gray's Anatomy.* 39th ed. New York, NY: Churchill Livingstone; 2005.
3. Safran G, Stone DA, Zachazewski J. *Instructions For Sports Medicine Patients.* Philadelphia, Pennsylvania: Elsevier; 2003.

HUMERUS FRACTURE
SUMMARY OVERVIEW

ICD-9

812.0   812.19   812.21   812.30

APTA Preferred Practice Pattern: 4G, 4H, 4I

EXAMINATION

- History and Systems Review
- Tests and Measures
  Systems review per APTA's *Guide to Physical Therapy Practice*
  - Joint integrity and mobility
  - Muscle performance
  - Pain
  - Posture
  - ROM
- Establish Plan of Care

GOALS/OUTCOMES

- Pain-free glenohumeral and scapulo-thoracic AROM: A minimum of 80% of AMA guides
- Functional cervical ROM or minimum of 80% of AMA guides
- Shoulder complex muscle performance: Equal to uninvolved side
- Elbow muscle performance: Equal to uninvolved side
- Pain: 2/10 or less with activity, 0/10 at rest
- Functional Activities
- Normal glenohumeral rhythm
- Return to prior functional status and activity level for ADLs and vocational, recreational, and sports activities as identified by patient
- Independence in a progressive home exercise program emphasizing function

INTERVENTION
NUMBER OF VISITS: 6–18

- Patient Instruction
  - Basic Anatomy and Biomechanics
  - Handouts
  - Functional Considerations
- Direct Interventions
  - Acute Phase: 3–8 Visits
  - Subacute Phase: 3–10 Visits
- Functional Carryover

DISCHARGE PLANNING AND PATIENT RESPONSIBILITY

- Criteria for Discharge
  - All rehabilitation goals reached except return to vocational or sports activities
  - Patient able to continue to make progress with compliance with home program
  - If continuation of pain and dysfunction prevent patient progression, consider orthopedic consultation
- Circumstances Requiring Additional Visits
  - Severe degenerative changes
  - History of other pathology
  - Presence of other medical conditions
  - Contractures
  - Cognitive limitations
  - Postoperative complications
  - Excessive environmental barriers to discharge
  - Delayed union
  - Pain greater than would be expected for healing time
- Home Program
  - Motor performance for shoulder elevation; elbow flexion; extension, pronation, and supination; and scapular stabilizers. Using free weights and resistance bands.
  - Flexibility to ensure full elevation and reaching up the back
  - Diagonal pattern work for functional overhead activities without fatigue or pain
  - Cardiovascular conditioning for better tolerance for work and home vocational activities
- Monitoring

SUMMARY OVERVIEW | SHOULDER | HUMERUS FRACTURE   411

HUMERUS FRACTURE

ICD-9

812.0	Closed fracture of upper end of humerus
812.19	Other open fracture of upper end of humerus
812.21	Closed fracture of shaft of humerus
812.30	Open fracture of unspecified part of humerus

APTA Preferred Practice Pattern: 4G, 4H, 4I

EXAMINATION

History and Systems Review
- History of current condition
- Past history of current condition
- Other tests and measures
- Medications
- Past medical/surgical history
- Functional status and activity level (current/prior)
- Patient's functional goals

Tests and Measures
Systems review per APTA's *Guide to Physical Therapy Practice*
- Joint integrity and mobility
  - Glenohumeral
    - Anterior capsule
    - Posterior capsule
    - Inferior glide
  - Acromioclaviclar
  - Sternoclavicular
  - Scapulothoracic
  - Radio-humeral
  - Ulno-humeral
- Muscle performance (including strength, power, and endurance)
  - Antalgic movement pattern with dressing activities
  - Functional use of upper extremity during gait
  - Scapulo-humeral rhythm
    - Arm at side
    - Hands on hips
    - Arms elevated 90° anteriorly
  - Resisted testing of shoulder girdle
- Pain
  - Measured on visual analog scale
- Posture
  - Forward head
  - Rounded shoulders
  - Flattening of the thoracic spine
  - Shoulder girdle asymmetry
    - Winging of the scapula
    - Clavicular position
    - Humeral head position
    - Muscular development/atrophy
  - Ability to actively achieve a more balanced postural position
- ROM (including muscle length)
  - Shoulder girdle ROM
    - AROM
    - PROM
    - Shoulder girdle mobility

Establish Plan of Care
- Based on history, tests, and measures

GOALS/OUTCOMES
- Pain-free glenohumeral and scapulo-thoracic AROM: A minimum of 80% of AMA guides
  - Flexion: 145°
  - Extension: 40°
  - Abduction: 145°
  - Internal rotation: 70°
  - External rotation: 70°
- Functional cervical ROM or minimum of 80% of AMA guides
  - Cervical flexion: 50°
  - Extension: 60°
  - Rotation: 65°
  - Side bending: 35°
- Shoulder complex muscle performance: Equal to uninvolved side
- Elbow muscle performance: Equal to uninvolved side
- Pain: 2/10 or less with activity, 0/10 at rest
- Functional Activities:
  - Able to reach into back pocket or fasten undergarments

- Able to comb hair
- Able to reach into cupboard or lift overhead
- Able to perform work/ADL tasks (weight and repetition specific
- Normal glenohumeral rhythm
- Return to prior functional status and activity level for ADLs and vocational, recreational, and sports activities as identified by patient
- Independence in a progressive home exercise program emphasizing function

INTERVENTION
NUMBER OF VISITS: 6–18

Coordination, Communication, and Documentation

- Provision of services between admission and discharge that facilitate cost-effective and efficient integration or reintegration to home, community, or work
- Documentation of therapeutic intervention is required for each episode of care and serves as the basic foundation for communication
- Coordination and additional communication will depend on the patient's impairment and home/work/community/leisure situation and requirements. Such services may include:
  - Case management
  - Coordination of care and collaboration with those integral to the patient's rehabilitation program
  - Coordination and monitoring of the delivery of available resources
  - Referrals to other health-care professionals
  - Identification of resources, support groups, or advocacy services
  - Provision of educational or training information
  - Technical assistance
- Specific coordination and communication provisions

Patient Instruction

Basic Anatomy and Biomechanics
- Pertinent Gray's Anatomy (Gray. 1995. 817–858)
- *Instructions for Sports Medicine Patients*

Handouts
- Home program
  - Home program including all wrist motions to improve upper-extremity and grip strength
  - Home program for shoulder rotator cuff strength to improve overhead motion
  - Home program for scapular strength to improve overhead motion
  - Home program for close-chain upper-extremity work to improve tolerance for weight-bearing activities, such as pushing out of chair or pushing doors open

Functional Considerations
- Posture (sitting, standing, sleeping, driving)
- Assistive devices (crutches, canes, walkers, collars, tape, etc.)
- Precautions: Bone healing time
- Alteration of ADLs
- Avoidance of prolonged postures
- Positioning for relief of symptoms
- Body mechanic instruction for lifting, pushing, pulling, etc.
- Training recommendations (cross training, periodization, etc.)
- Osteoporosis instruction as indicated

Direct Interventions

Acute Phase: 3–8 Visits
- Therapeutic exercises and home program
  - Upper body ergometer for ROM
  - Pain-free passive exercises for vascularization of rotator cuff (unweighting, supported ROM)
  - Strengthening exercises are performed as long as muscle contractions do not stress fracture site
    - Internal/external rotation with arm at the side, elbow flexed to 90°, using surgical tubing for resistance
      a. If external rotation is painful, limit the degree of rotation
      b. If pain continues, begin with isometric exercises in same position
      c. If still painful, move shoulder to loose pack position (i.e. slight abduction and elevation)
      d. As pain decreases and strength increases, progress to free weight
    - Internal rotation lying on involved side

SHOULDER | HUMERUS FRACTURE   413

- External rotation lying on uninvolved side
- Supraspinatus isolation ("empty can" position)
  a. Shoulder is internally rotated, thumb pointed to floor
  b. Abduct the arm to 90°, maintaining a position 30° anterior to the mid-frontal plane
  c. If this exercise cannot be accomplished at this stage, try without internal rotation and emphasize scapular motion
- Shoulder extension in prone with arm hanging off table or forward bent at waist in standing
  a. Extend arm to side of trunk (0°)
  b. Shoulder extensors also function as depressors of humeral head, which decreases the upward migration and likelihood of impingement
- Scapular stabilization program: Depression, retraction
- Manual therapy techniques
  - Soft-tissue techniques
    - Myofascial release
    - Soft-tissue mobilization
    - Acupressure
    - Strain/counterstrain
  - Passive, pain-free ROM emphasizing posterior positioning of the humeral head
  - Joint mobilization
    - Do not stress/mobilize fracture site
    - Grades I–II to inhibit pain
    - Grades III–V to surrounding hypomobile joints of the cervical/thoracic spine, acromioclavicular, sternoclavicular, scapulothoracic, elbow, or wrist
- Physical agents and mechanical modalities
  - Cryotherapy
- Goals/outcomes
  - Pain: 5/10 or less
  - Shoulder ROM: 70% of AMA guides
    - Flexion: 126 °
    - Extension: 35°
    - Abduction: 125°
    - Internal rotation: 65°
    - External rotation: 65°
  - Shoulder girdle strength: 3+/5 on manual muscle test
  - Able to reach to eye level

Subacute Phase: 3–10 Visits
- Therapeutic exercise and home program
  - Strengthening

- Continue tubing exercises
- Continue free-weight and pulley exercises emphasizing eccentric contractions
- Horizontal adduction and military press
- Functional diagonals
- Optional use of isokinetic exercise
  - Neuromuscular/balance/proprioceptive reeducation
    - Quadruped multidirectional rocking
    - Three-point rocking
    - Wall push-ups
    - Push-ups
    - Bodyblade®
  - Plyometrics with compact medicine ball, tossing and catching (1 kg, progressing to 3 kg)
  - Begin throwing program or progression toward sport-specific activity
  - Cardiovascular conditioning
- Manual therapy techniques
  - Continue effective soft-tissue techniques
  - Joint mobilization
    - Grades I–II with intent of pain relief
    - Continue progressive graded mobilization to surrounding areas of hypomobility
    - Progressive grades II–IV to glenohumeral joint, with consideration of healing status and location of fracture
- Physical agents and mechanical modalities
  - Continue effective modalities as in acute phase, with increased emphasis on use as needed at home
- Goals/outcomes
  - Pain: 2/10 or less
  - Shoulder AROM: 80% of AMA guides
  - Strength: 4-/5 on manual muscle test or 80% of uninvolved extremity
  - Improve glenohumeral rhythm to enhance return to previous level of ADLs and vocational, recreational, and sports activities
  - Functional activities
    - Reaching and lifting 5–15 lbs out in front of trunk
    - Lifting small objects

Functional Carryover

- Integration of home exercise program into vocational environment
- Completion of ergonomic adjustments to home, automobile, and vocational areas
- Incorporation of proper posture and body mechanics to avoid exacerbation of symptoms
- Recognition/avoidance of activities that increase or exacerbate radiating symptoms

DISCHARGE PLANNING AND PATIENT RESPONSIBILITY

Criteria for Discharge

- All rehabilitation goals reached except return to vocational or sports activities
- Patient able to continue to make progress with compliance with home program
- If continuation of pain and dysfunction prevent patient progression, consider orthopedic consultation

Circumstances Requiring Additional Visits

- Severe degenerative changes
- History of other pathology
- Presence of other medical conditions
- Contractures
- Cognitive limitations
- Postoperative complications
- Excessive environmental barriers to discharge
- Delayed union
- Pain greater than would be expected for healing time

Home Program

- Motor performance exercise for shoulder elevation, scapular stabilizers, elbow flexion, extension, pronation and supination. May use free weights and or resistance bands.
- Flexibility to ensure full elevation and reaching up the back
- Diagonal pattern work for functional overhead activities without fatigue or pain
- Cardiovascular conditioning for better tolerance for work and home vocational activities

Monitoring

- Return to physical therapy or physician:
  - If symptoms persist longer than 12 weeks post-injury
  - If significant shoulder rotator cuff weakness persists longer than 12 weeks post-injury
  - If sleep is still disturbed greater than 2 hours per night at 12 weeks post-injury

REFERENCES

1. American Physical Therapy Association. *Guide to Physical Therapist Practice*. Alexandria, VA: APTA; revised 2003.
2. Gray H; Williams PL, ed. *Gray's Anatomy*. 39th ed. New York, NY: Churchill Livingstone; 2005.
3. Safran G, Stone DA, Zachazewski J. *Instructions For Sports Medicine Patients*. Philadelphia, Pennsylvania: Elsvier; 2003.

416   HUMERUS FRACTURE | SHOULDER

LABRUM TEAR
SUMMARY OVERVIEW

ICD-9

840.7

APTA Preferred Practice Pattern: **4D, 4E, 4I**

EXAMINATION

- History and Systems Review
- Tests and Measures
  Systems review per APTA's *Guide to Physical Therapy Practice*
  - Joint integrity and mobility
  - Muscle performance
  - Pain
  - Posture
  - ROM
  - Special testing
  - Self-care and home management
  - Sensory integrity
  - Ventilation and respiration/gas exchange
  - Work (job/school/play), community, and leisure integration or reintegration
- Establish Plan of Care

GOALS/OUTCOMES

- Shoulder ROM: 90% of AMA guides or equal to uninvolved extremity
- Functional cervical ROM or a minimum of 80% of AMA guides
- Pain: 2/10 or less with resisted motion, 0/10 at rest
- Strength: 4/5 on manual muscle test
- Return to prior functional status and activity level for ADLs and vocational, recreational, and sports activities as identified by patient
- Independence in a progressive home exercise program that emphasizes function
- Functional Activities

INTERVENTION
NUMBER OF VISITS: 7–16

- Patient Instruction
  - Basic Anatomy and Biomechanics
  - Handouts
  - Functional considerations
- Direct Interventions
  - Acute Phase: 3–8 Visits
  - Subacute Phase: 4–8 Visits
- Functional Carryover

DISCHARGE PLANNING AND PATIENT RESPONSIBILITY

- Criteria for Discharge
  - All goals/outcomes have been achieved (may not be dependent upon return to previous recreational and sports activities)
- Circumstances Requiring Additional Visits
  - Severe degenerative changes
  - History of other pathology
  - Presence of other medical conditions
  - Contractures
  - Cognitive limitations
  - Postoperative complications
  - Excessive environmental barriers to discharge
  - Multiple injury sites (rotator cuff or ligaments)
  - Special occupational needs that require extensive strengthening
  - Presence of cervical pathology
  - Special occupational needs that require weight bearing of the upper extremity
- Home Program
  - Motor performance for glenohumeral and scapular stabilizers
  - Flexibility for glenohumeral joint and scapulo-thoracic motion
  - Cardiovascular conditioning for better tolerance for work and home activities
  - Diagonal pattern exercises for functional overhead work without fatigue or pain
- Monitoring

SUMMARY OVERVIEW | SHOULDER | LABRUM TEAR   417

LABRUM TEAR

ICD-9
    840.7   Superior glenoid labrum lesion
APTA Preferred Practice Pattern: **4D, 4E, 4I**

EXAMINATION

History and Systems Review
- History of current condition
- Past history of current condition
- Other tests and measures
- Medications
- Past medical/surgical history
  - Injury to upper extremity or cervical/thoracic spine
  - Surgery
  - Therapeutic intervention
- Functional status and activity level (current/prior)
- Patient's functional goals

Tests and Measures
Systems review per APTA's *Guide to Physical Therapy Practice*
- Joint integrity and mobility
  - Glenohumeral
    - Anterior capsule
    - Posterior capsule
    - Inferior capsule
  - Acromioclavicular
  - Sternoclavicular
  - Scapulo-thoracic
  - Radio-humeral
  - Ulno-humeral
  - First/second rib costo-transverse
- Muscle performance (including strength, power, and endurance)
  - Resisted testing
    - Glenohumeral
    - Scapular
    - Supraspinatus isolation ("empty can" position)
      a. Shoulder internally rotated, thumb pointed to floor
      b. Abduct the arm to 90°, maintain a position 30° anterior to the mid-frontal plane
    - Radio-humeral
    - Ulno-humeral
  - Antalgic movement pattern with dressing activities

- Functional use of upper extremity during gait and with overhead motion
  - Scapulohumeral rhythm
    - Arms at side
    - Hands on hips
    - Arms elevated 90° anteriorly
- Pain
  - Measured on visual analog scale
- Posture
  - Forward head
  - Rounded shoulders
  - Flattening of the thoracic spine
  - Shoulder girdle asymmetry
    - Winging of the scapula
    - Clavicular position
    - Humeral head position
    - Muscular development/atrophy
  - Ability to actively achieve a more balanced postural position
- ROM (including muscle length)
  - Cervical spine screening
    - Active/passive ROM
    - Overpressure
    - Quadrant compression test
  - Shoulder girdle mobility
    - AROM
      a. Flexion/elevation
        - Observe for inability to maintain depressed humeral head
    - Abduction
    - Internal rotation
    - External rotation
    - Extension
  - Overpressure
  - PROM
  - Elbow Screening
    - Active/Passive ROM
    - Overpressure

418   LABRUM TEAR | SHOULDER

- Special testing
  - Apprehension test
    - Patient in supine
    - Involved arm is in abduction and external rotation
    - Push anterior on posterior aspect of humeral head
      a. Patient with recurrent dislocation with experience apprehension
      b. Patient with anterior instability will experience pain but not apprehension
      c. Patient with normal shoulder will be asymptomatic
  - Relocation test
    - Administer test with posterior directed force on humeral head from apprehension test position
      a. Patient with primary impingement will generally have no change in their pain
      b. Patient with instability and secondary impingement will have pain relief and will tolerate maximal external rotation with the humeral head maintained in the reduced position
  - Clunk test
    - Patient is supine
    - Move arm into full flexion and caudal glide, then perform circumduction motion
      a. Positive if clunk, pain, or pseudolocking occurs
      b. Implicates labral tear
  - Active Compression test
    - Patient seated
    - Forward flexion to 90° with elbow in complete extension. Adduct horizontally 10°.
    - Maximal shoulder internal rotation
    - Apply a downward force while the patient resists
    - Repeat test with maximal lateral rotation
      a. Positive test is pain in first position (internal rotation) with relief or no pain in the second position (lateral rotation)
- Self-care and home management (including ADLs and instrumental ADLs)
- Sensory integrity
- Ventilation and respiration/gas exchange
- Work (job/school/play), community, and leisure integration or reintegration (including instrumental ADLs)

Establish Plan of Care
- Based on history, tests, and measures

GOALS/OUTCOMES
- Shoulder ROM: 90% of AMA guides or equal to uninvolved extremity

	Normal	90%
Flexion	180°	160°
Extension	50°	45°
Abduction	180°	160°
Internal rotation	90°	80°
External rotation	90°	80°

- Functional cervical ROM or a minimum of 80% of AMA guides

	Normal	80%
Flexion	60°	50°
Extension	75°	60°
Rotation	80°	65°
Side bending	45°	35°

- Pain: 2/10 or less with resisted motion, 0/10 at rest
- Strength: 4/5 on manual muscle test
- Return to prior functional status and activity level for ADLs and vocational, recreational, and sports activities as identified by patient
- Independence in a progressive home exercise program that emphasizes function
- Functional activities:
  - Able to reach into back pocket or fasten undergarments
  - Able to comb hair
  - Able to reach into a cupboard or lift overhead
  - Perform work/ADL tasks

INTERVENTION
NUMBER OF VISITS: 7–16

Coordination, Communication, and Documentation
- Provision of services between admission and discharge that facilitate cost-effective and efficient integration or reintegration to home, community, or work
- Documentation of therapeutic intervention is required for each episode of care and serves as the basic foundation for communication
- Coordination and additional communication will depend on the patient's impairment and home/work/

community/leisure situation and requirements. Such services may include:

- ○ Case management
- ○ Coordination of care and collaboration with those integral to the patient's rehabilitation program
- ○ Coordination and monitoring of the delivery of available resources
- ○ Referrals to other health-care professionals
- ○ Identification of resources, support groups, or advocacy services
- ○ Provision of educational or training information
- ○ Technical assistance
- Specific coordination and communication provisions

Patient Instruction

Basic Anatomy and Biomechanics
- Pertinent Gray's Anatomy (Gray. 1995. 817–849)
- Instructions for Sports Medicine Patients (Safran, Stone. 2003. 762–768)

Handouts
- Home program
  - ○ Specific home program for scapular stabilization
  - ○ Specific home program for rotator cuff strength in neutral and overhead position
  - ○ Specific home program for close-chain strengthening
  - ○ Specific home exercises for thoracic motion

Functional Considerations
- Posture (sitting, standing, sleeping, driving)
- Assistive devices (crutches, canes, walkers, collars, tape)
- Precautions
- Alteration of ADLs
- Avoidance of prolonged postures
- Positioning for relief of symptoms
- Body mechanic instruction for lifting, pushing, pulling, etc.
- Training recommendations (cross training, periodization, etc.)

Direct Interventions

Acute Phase: 3–8 Visits
- Therapeutic exercise and home program
  - ○ Assisted stretching in pain-free ROM
    - ▪ Cervical/thoracic spine

- ▪ Shoulder girdle
- ▪ Elbow
- ○ Initiate manually resisted exercises in pain-free ROM
- ○ PROM
  - ▪ Pulley
  - ▪ Wand
- ○ Pain-free AROM
  - ▪ High-repetition and low-resistance, with purpose of promoting vascularization in healing tissues
  - ▪ Internal/external rotation
    - a. May need to use apparatus to support elbow for pain-free ROM
  - ▪ Supraspinatus isolation ("empty can" position)
    - a. Shoulder is internally rotated, thumb pointed to floor
    - b. Abduct the arm to 90°, maintaining position 30° anterior to the midfrontal plan
  - ▪ Scapular retraction/depression
  - ▪ Upper body ergometry
- ○ Postural correction exercises
- ○ Neuromuscular/balance/proprioceptive reeducation
  - ▪ Pain-free modified plantargrade position for elbow propping
  - ▪ Bodyblade®
- ○ Cardiovascular conditioning
  - ▪ Walking program
  - ▪ Lower-extremity cycling
- Manual therapy
  - ○ Soft-tissue techniques
    - ▪ Soft-tissue mobilization to the scapular stabilizer and rotator cuff musculature
    - ▪ Friction massage within pain tolerance
    - ▪ Myofascial release
  - ○ Joint mobilization
    - ▪ Joint mobilization to restore proper joint mechanics to the shoulder girdle, including acromioclavicular, sternoclavicular, and scapulothoracic regions; ensure that posterior capsule mobility is normal (away from area of injury)
    - ▪ Grades III–IV to cervical/thoracic spinal hypomobilities
- Electrotherapeutic modalities
  - ○ Iontophoresis

- Physical agents and mechanical modalities
- Cryotherapy
- Athermal, deep thermal modalities
- Goals
  - Pain: 5/10 with resistive motion, 2/10 at rest
  - Pain free ROM: 50% AMA guides
    - Flexion 90°
    - Extension: 25°
    - Abduction: 90°
    - Internal rotation: 45°
    - External rotation: 45°
  - Patient utilizes scapular stabilization with static posture

Subacute Phase: 4–8 Visits

- Therapeutic exercise and home program
  - Manual resistive exercises: Isometric
  - Progress passive stretches in pain-free ROM
    - Glide hand forward and horizontally on table, hold at end point
    - Pectorals
    - Shoulder complex
    - Cervical/thoracic spine
  - Cardiovascular conditioning
    - Walking program
    - Ski machine
  - Progressive strengthening utilizing isometric, pulley, resistive bands, or free-weight resistance
    - As patient accomplishes pain-free, high-repetitive, low-load exercises (1 set of 30 reps), progress to strengthening with moderate load (3 sets of 10 reps)
    - Rotator cuff with emphasis on involved tendon
    - Scapular retraction/depression
    - Diagonal and functional patterns
  - Flexibility exercises
    - Pectorals
    - Internal rotators
  - Neuromuscular/balance/proprioceptive reeducation
    - Hands-knees
    - Three-point rocking
    - Push-ups (on wall initially)
    - Push-ups off therapeutic ball
    - Bodyblade®

- Plyometrics
  - Underhand
  - Two-handed
  - Overhand
- Sport or activity specific training (see *Upper Extremity Injury Return to Throwing* and *Elbow/Shoulder Injury Return to Tennis* in "Return to Sport" section later in this book)
- Manual therapy
  - Joint mobilization
    - Grades II–IV to restore glenohumeral capsular mobility
    - Progressive mobilization to persistent hypomobilities in the shoulder complex or spinal region
  - Continue effective soft-tissue techniques
    - Friction massage
- Physical agents and mechanical modalities
  - Continue effective modalities as in acute phase, with increased emphasis on use as needed at home
- Goals
  - Pain: 2/10 with resisted motion, 0/10 at rest
  - Functional activities
    - Able to reach into back pocket or fasten undergarments
    - Able to comb hair
    - Able to reach into cupboard or lift overhead
    - Perform work/ADL tasks (weight and repetition specific)
  - Shoulder ROM: 90% of AMA guides
    - Flexion: 160°
    - Extension: 45°
    - Abduction: 160°
    - External rotation: 80°
    - Internal rotation: 80°
  - Strength: 4/5 on a manual muscle test for shoulder girdle musculature

Functional Carryover

- Integration of home exercise program into vocational environment
- Completion of ergonomic adjustments to home, automobile, and vocational areas
- Incorporation of proper posture and body mechanics to avoid exacerbation of symptoms
- Recognition/avoidance of activities that increase or exacerbate radiating symptoms

DISCHARGE PLANNING AND PATIENT RESPONSIBILITY

Criteria for Discharge

- All goals/outcomes have been achieved (may not be dependent upon return to previous recreational and sports activities)

Circumstances Requiring Additional Visits

- Severe degenerative changes
- History of other pathology
- Presence of other medical conditions
- Contractures
- Cognitive limitations
- Postoperative complications
- Excessive environmental barriers to discharge
- Multiple injury sites (rotator cuff or ligaments)
- Special occupational needs that require extensive strengthening
- Presence of cervical pathology
- Special occupational needs requiring weight bearing of the upper extremity

Home Program

- Motor performance for glenohumeral and scapular stabilizers
- Flexibility for glenohumeral joint and scapulo-thoracic motion
- Cardiovascular conditioning for better tolerance for work and home activities
- Diagonal pattern exercises for functional overhead work without fatigue or pain

Monitoring

- Consult physical therapist:
  - If painful popping with active or resisted motion after 3–4 weeks
  - If sleep is still disturbed more than 2 hours per night after 6 weeks
  - If unable to advance resisted exercises after 4 weeks

REFERENCES

1. American Physical Therapy Association. *Guide to Physical Therapist Practice.* Alexandria, VA: APTA; revised 2003.

2. Gray H; Williams PL, ed. *Gray's Anatomy.* 39th ed. New York, NY: Churchill Livingstone; 2005.

3. Safran G, Stone DA, Zachazewski J. *Instruction For Sports Medicine Patients.* Philadelphia, Pennsylvania: Elsevier, 2003.

4. Brotzman BS, Wilk KE. *Clinical Orthopaedic Rehabilitation.* 2nd ed. Philadelphia, Pennsylvania: Mosby, 2003.

POSTOP. REHAB. FOR SHOULDER INSTABILITY
SUMMARY OVERVIEW

ICD-9

718.21   718.31   718.81   831.0   831.1

APTA Preferred Practice Pattern: **4B, 4D, 4E, 4F, 4G, 4J**

EXAMINATION

- History and Systems Review
- Tests and Measures
  Systems review per APTA's *Guide to Physical Therapy Practice*
  - Integumentary integrity
  - Joint integrity and mobility
  - Muscle performance
  - Pain
  - Posture
  - ROM
- Establish Plan of Care

GOALS/OUTCOMES

- Shoulder ROM: 90% of AMA guides with the exception of internal/external rotation dependant upon location of surgical repair
- Functional cervical ROM or a minimum of 80% of AMA guides
- Pain: 2/10 with activity, 0/10 at rest
- Strength: Equal to uninvolved side, 4/5 on a manual muscle test, or as demonstrated functionally
- Normal glenohumeral rhythm (timing of scapular and glenohumeral joint movement)
- Return to functional status and activity level (current/prior) for ADLs and vocational, recreational, and sports activities as identified by patient
- Independence in a progressive home exercise program emphasizing function

INTERVENTION
NUMBER OF VISITS: 6–14

- Patient Instruction
  - Basic Anatomy and Biomechanics
  - Handouts
  - Functional Considerations
  - Description of Surgical Procedure
- Direct Interventions
  - Phase I: 1–4 Visits, Weeks 1–5
  - Phase II: 5–10 Visits, Weeks 6+
- Functional Carryover

DISCHARGE PLANNING AND PATIENT RESPONSIBILITY

- Criteria for Discharge
  - All rehabilitation goals/outcomes achieved except may discharge at 80% of shoulder AROM if all other goals/outcomes achieved
  - Patient is compliant with home program
  - Patient understands progressions for continued motor performance and ROM over the next 3–6 months
- Circumstances Requiring Additional Visits
  - Cervical pathology or radiating signs/symptoms
  - Inability to depress humeral head during elevation
  - Postoperative infection/complications
  - Severe postoperative scarring
  - Multiple injury sites
  - Special occupational needs that require extensive strengthening
- Home Program
  - Muscle performance
  - Flexibility
  - Cardiovascular conditioning
- Monitoring

POSTOP. REHAB. FOR SHOULDER INSTABILITY

ICD-9

718.21	Pathological dislocation, shoulder region
718.31	Recurrent dislocation of joint, shoulder region
718.81	Other joint derangement, not elsewhere classified, shoulder region
831.0	Closed dislocation of shoulder
831.1	Open dislocation of shoulder

APTA Preferred Practice Pattern: 4B, 4D, 4E, 4F, 4G, 4J

EXAMINATION

History and Systems Review

- History of current condition
  - Surgical procedure and postoperative limitations
  - Location, nature, and behavior of symptoms
    - Aggravating/relieving factors
- Past history of current condition
  - Injury to cervical/thoracic spine or upper extremity
  - Additional surgeries
  - Direct intervention
- Functional status and activity level (current/prior)
- Patient's functional goals/outcomes

Tests and Measures

Systems review per APTA's *Guide to Physical Therapy Practice*

If the initial evaluation is performed after the 6th week postoperatively, also perform shoulder AROM and resisted tests.

- Integumentary integrity
  - Observation/palpation of incision
  - Edema/tenderness
  - Integrity of scar tissue
  - Skin/scar mobility
- Joint integrity and mobility
  - Shoulder girdle musculature
  - Tendons
  - Ligaments
- Muscle performance
  - Resisted testing
- Pain
  - Measured on visual analog scale
- Posture
- ROM
  - AROM
  - Overpressure

- Shoulder girdle passive ROM
  - Caution with external rotation for repair of anterior instability
  - Caution with internal rotation for repair of posterior instability
  - With repair of anterior instability, avoid stressing the anterior/inferior capsule
  - With repair of posterior instability, avoid stressing the posterior capsule

Establish Plan of Care

- Based on history, tests, and measures

GOALS/OUTCOMES

- Shoulder ROM: 90% of AMA guides with the exception of internal/external rotation dependent upon location of surgical repair

	Normal	90%
Flexion	180°	160°
Extension	50°	45°
Abduction	180°	160°
Internal rotation	90°	80°*
External rotation	90°	80°†

*With repair for posterior instability, goal is 50°
†With repair for anterior instability, goal is 50°

- Functional cervical ROM or a minimum of 80% of AMA guides:

	Normal	80%
Flexion	60°	50°
Extension	75°	60°
Rotation	80°	65°
Side bend	45°	35°

424   POSTOP REHAB FOR SHOULDER INSTABILITY | SHOULDER

- Pain: 2/10 with activity, 0/10 at rest
- Strength: Equal to uninvolved side, 4/5 on a manual muscle test or as demonstrated functionally, as in
  - Able to reach into back pocket or fasten undergarments
  - Able to comb hair
  - Able to reach into cupboard or lift overhead
  - Perform work/ADL tasks (weight and repetition specific)
- Normal glenohumeral rhythm (timing of scapular and glenohumeral joint movement)
- Return to functional status and activity level (current/prior) for ADLs and vocational, recreational, and sports activities as identified by patient
- Independence in a progressive home exercise program emphasizing function

INTERVENTION
NUMBER OF VISITS: 6–14

Coordination, Communication, and Documentation
- Provision of services between admission and discharge that facilitate cost-effective and efficient integration or reintegration to home, community, or work
- Documentation of therapeutic intervention is required for each episode of care and serves as the basic foundation for communication
- Coordination and additional communication will depend on the patient's impairment and home/work/community/leisure situation and requirements. Such services may include:
  - Case management
  - Coordination of care and collaboration with those integral to the patient's rehabilitation program
  - Coordination and monitoring of the delivery of available resources
  - Referrals to other health-care professionals
  - Identification of resources, support groups, or advocacy services
  - Provision of educational or training information
  - Technical assistance
- Specific coordination and communication provisions:
  - Referral to physician for any surgical complications

Patient Instruction

Basic Anatomy and Biomechanics
- Review of bony, muscular, ligamentous, and joint dynamics of the glenohumeral, sternoclavicular, acromioclavicular, and scapulothoracic regions
- Importance of adequate motor performance, postural alignment, and ROM of the cervical/thoracic spine to promote postoperative healing
- Pertinent Gray's Anatomy (Gray. 1995. 627–632, 839–842, 1537)

Handouts
- Specific home program
- Commercially available products, such as:
  - Krames Communications (1100 Grundy Lane, San Bruno, CA 94066):
    - *Shoulder Instability*

Functional Considerations
- Review of immobilization guides as determined by physician
- Avoidance of aggravating activities or positions
  - Sleeping posture
  - Driving
- Recognition of inappropriate substitution patterns with exercises, such as shoulder shrug with attempted elevation
- Restrictions from contact activities
- Avoidance of dislocation mechanism
  - With anterior repair, avoid external rotation and horizontal abduction

Description of Surgical Procedure
- Review of operative procedure and relation to joint biomechanics, rehabilitation, and function

Direct Interventions

Phase I: 1–4 Visits, Weeks 1–5
- Therapeutic exercise and home program
  - Active ROM
    - Elbow, wrist, hand
    - Cervical/thoracic spine
  - Passive shoulder ROM including wand, Codman's, and pulley exercises

- Upper body ergometry for ROM with passive participation of the involved extremity
- Initiate cardiovascular conditioning
  - Walking program
  - Lower-extremity cycling
- Postural correction activities
- Manual therapy techniques
  - Soft-tissue techniques
    - Soft-tissue mobilization
    - Myofascial release
    - Trigger-point techniques
  - Joint mobilization
    - Grades I–II with intent of pain relief
    - Grades III–V to specific areas of hypomobility in the cervical/thoracic spine
  - ROM
    - Shoulder: Pain-free range on all planes
      a. Avoid stressing external rotation for anterior repair
      b. Avoid stressing internal rotation for posterior repair
- Electrotherapeutic modalities
- Physical agents and mechanical modalities
  - Cryotherapy
  - Athermal, deep thermal modalities
- Goals/outcomes
  - Pain: 3/10 or less
  - Compliance with postoperative restrictions
  - Pain-free shoulder PROM: 60% of AMA guides with the exception of internal/external rotation dependent upon location of surgical repair
    - Flexion: 110°
    - Extension: 30°
    - Abduction: 110°
    - Internal rotation: 55° (with repair for posterior instability, goal is 35°)
    - External rotation: 55° (with repair for anterior instability, goal is 35°)

Phase II: 5–10 Visits, Weeks 6+
- Therapeutic exercise and home program
  - Manual resistive exercise
    - Diagonal or functional patterns, with special consideration for internal and external rotation within surgical limitations
  - Progressive cardiovascular conditioning
  - Progressive active assistive to resistive exercises

  - Internal/external rotation
  - Supraspinatus isolation ("empty can" position)
    a. Shoulder is internally rotated, thumb pointed to floor
    b. Abduct the arm to 90°, maintaining a position 30° anterior to the mid-frontal plane
  - Horizontal abduction/adduction
  - Elbow and wrist
  - Scapular
  - Neuromuscular/balance/proprioceptive reeducation
    - Bodyblade®
      Precautions must be taken with glenohumeral weight-bearing following a repair for posterior instability
    - Hands and knees rocking
    - Three-point rocking
    - Push-up progression
      a. Wall
      b. Modified hands and knees
      c. Hands and toes
  - Plyometrics
    Caution: Avoid movement posteriorly beyond mid-frontal plane
    - Underhand toss
    - Two-hand toss
    - Overhand toss
  - Activity specific progression for vocational, racquet, or throwing demands per physician's restrictions
- Manual therapy techniques
  - Continue effective soft-tissue techniques
  - Joint mobilization
    - Progressive grades of mobilization in all planes of glenohumeral motion utilizing caution when stressing location of surgical repair
    - Grades III–V to persistent areas of hypomobility in the cervical/thoracic spine
  - Assisted stretching to the shoulder complex, with emphasis on the subscapularis and latissimus dorsi
- Goals/outcomes
  - Shoulder AROM: 90% of AMA guides, with the exception of internal/external rotation limitation secondary to surgical procedure

○ Muscle strength: Equal to uninvolved shoulder, 4/5 on manual muscle test, or achieve a predetermined functional motor performance parameter, such as:
  ▪ Reaching and lifting 5–15 lbs in front of trunk
  ▪ Lifting 5–20 lbs overhead
  ▪ Reaching into kitchen cabinets and lowering dishes
○ Normal glenohumeral rhythm (timing of scapular and glenohumeral joint movement)

Functional Carryover
• Avoid activities requiring excessive rotation or movement posteriorly beyond the frontal plane that may stress the surgical repair
• Importance of maintaining proper posture of the cervical/thoracic spine to optimize glenohumeral positioning
• Ergonomic modifications to work and home environment

DISCHARGE PLANNING AND PATIENT RESPONSIBILITY

Criteria for Discharge
• All rehabilitation goals/outcomes achieved except may discharge at 80% of shoulder AROM if all other goals/ outcomes achieved
• Patient is compliant with home program
• Patient understands progressions for continued motor performance and ROM over the next 3–6 months

Circumstances Requiring Additional Visits
• Cervical pathology or radiating signs/symptoms
• Inability to depress humeral head during elevation
• Postoperative infection/complications
• Severe postoperative scarring
• Multiple injury sites
• Special occupational needs that require extensive strengthening

Home Program
• Muscle performance
  ○ Rotator cuff
  ○ Biceps/triceps
  ○ Scapular stabilizers
• Flexibility
• Cardiovascular conditioning

Monitoring
• Instruct patient to call for advice should progression halt or a negative trend occur
• Follow up with phone call in 2–4 weeks to ensure return to previous functional level

REFERENCES
1. American Physical Therapy Association. *Guide to Physical Therapist Practice*. Alexandria, VA: APTA; 1997.
2. Engelberg AL. *Guides to The Evaluation of Permanent Impairment*. 3rd ed. Chicago, IL: American Medical Association; 1989.
3. Gray H; Williams PL, ed. *Gray's Anatomy*. 38th ed. New York, NY: Churchill Livingstone; 1995.
4. Matsen FA, Harryman DT, Sidles JA. Mechanics of glenohumeral instability. *Clin Sports Med*. 1992;10:783-788.
5. Neer CS, Foster CR. Inferior capsular shift for involuntary inferior and multidirectional instability of the shoulder. *J Bone Joint Surg*. 1980;62A:897-908.
6. O'Brien SJ, Neves MC, Arnoczsky SP, et al. The anatomy and histology of the inferior glenohumeral ligament complex of the shoulder. *Am J Sports Med*. 1990;18:449-456.
7. Rodosky MW, Hamer CD, Fu FH. The role of the long head of the biceps muscle and superior glenoid labrum in anterior stability of the shoulder. *Am J Sports Med*. 1994;22:121-130.
8. Warner JJP, Deng X, Warren RF, Torzilli PA, O'Brien SJ. Superioinferior translation in the intact and vented glenohumeral joint. *J Shoulder Elbow Surg*. 1993;2:99-105.
9. Warner JJ, Deng XH, Warren RF, Torzilli PA. Static capsuloligamentous restraints to superior-inferior translation of the glenohumeral joint. *Am J Sports Med*. 1992;20:675-685.

POSTOP. REHAB. OF THE ROTATOR CUFF
SUMMARY OVERVIEW

ICD-9

726.1   727.61

APTA Preferred Practice Pattern: 4B, 4C, 4D, 4E, 4F, 4J

EXAMINATION

- History and Systems Review
- Tests and Measures
  Systems review per APTA's *Guide to Physical Therapy Practice*
  - Integumentary integrity
  - Joint integrity and mobility
  - Muscle performance
  - Pain
  - Posture
  - ROM
  - Special tests
- Establish Plan of Care

GOALS/OUTCOMES

- Pain-free ROM: 90% of AMA guides for glenohumeral and scapulothoracic joint motion or 90% of uninvolved extremity
- Functional cervical ROM or a minimum of 80% of AMA guides
- Strength: Equal to uninvolved side, 4/5 on manual muscle test, or as demonstrated functionally
- Pain: 0/10 with all activity, including throwing
- Normal glenohumeral rhythm (timing of scapular and glenohumeral joint movements)
- Return to functional status and activity level (current/ prior) for ADLs and vocational, recreational, and sports activities as identified by patient
- Independence in a progressive home exercise program emphasizing function

INTERVENTION
NUMBER OF VISITS: 6–15

- Patient Instruction
  - Basic Anatomy and Biomechanics
  - Handouts
  - Functional Considerations
- Direct Interventions
  - Phase I: 1–4 Visits, Weeks 1–5
  - Phase II: 4–7 Visits, Weeks 6–10
  - Phase III: 1–4 Visits, Weeks 11–12
- Functional Carryover

DISCHARGE PLANNING AND PATIENT RESPONSIBILITY

- Criteria for Discharge
  - All rehabilitation goals/outcomes achieved with possible exceptions listed in the guidelines
- Circumstances Requiring Additional Visits
  - Cervical pathology or radiating signs/symptoms
  - Inability to depress humeral head during elevation
  - Postoperative infection/complications
  - Severe postoperative scarring
  - Multiple injury sites
  - Special occupational needs that require extensive strengthening
- Home Program
  - Continue exercise program until motor performance, pain-free ROM, and functional activity level has returned
  - Cardiovascular conditioning
  - Pain management techniques
  - Advanced functional diagonals incorporating stretch/ shortening, or speed training exercise program related to activity or sport-specific needs
  - Progress to "Return to Sport" guidelines as indicated
- Monitoring

SUMMARY OVERVIEW | SHOULDER | POSTOP. REHAB. OF THE ROTATOR CUFF   429

POSTOP. REHAB. OF THE ROTATOR CUFF

ICD-9

    726.1   Rotator cuff syndrome of shoulder and allied disorders
    727.61   Complete rupture of rotator cuff

APTA Preferred Practice Pattern: 4B, 4C, 4D, 4E, 4F, 4J

EXAMINATION

History and Systems Review

- History of current condition
  - Surgical procedure and postoperative limitations
    - Use of immobilizer
  - Location, nature, and behavior of symptoms
    - Aggravating/relieving factors
- Past history of current condition
  - Injury to cervical/thoracic spine or upper extremity
  - Additional surgeries
  - Direct intervention
- Functional status and activity level (current/prior)
- Patient's functional goals/outcomes

Tests and Measures

Systems review per APTA's *Guide to Physical Therapy Practice*

If initial evaluation is performed beyond 6 weeks postoperatively, also include AROM, resisted testing, and special tests depending on surgical procedure performed and postoperative restrictions (see *Shoulder Strain/Sprain* guideline).

- Integumentary integrity
  - Observation/palpation of incision
    - Edema/tenderness
    - Integrity of scar tissue
    - Skin/scar mobility
- Joint integrity and mobility
  - Glenohumeral
    - Anterior capsule
    - Posterior capsule
    - Inferior capsule
  - Acromioclavicular
  - Sternoclavicular
  - Scapulothoracic
- Muscle performance
  - Palpation of muscles, tendons, and ligaments
- Pain
  - Measured on visual analog scale

- Posture
- ROM
  - Within postoperative limitations
  - Impingement/painful arc assessment
  - Passive only until week 5 postoperative or per specific physician preference
  - Passive joint ROM
    - Dependent upon SIN (severity/irritability/nature)
  - AROM
    - Flexion/elevation
      a. Observe for inability to maintain depressed humeral head
    - Abduction
    - Internal rotation
    - External rotation
    - Extension
- Special tests
  - Clear cervical spine
    - Quadrant compression test
    - Overpressure

Establish Plan of Care

- Based on history, tests, and measures

GOALS/OUTCOMES

- Pain-free ROM: 90% of AMA guides for glenohumeral and scapulothoracic joint motion or 90% of uninvolved extremity

	Normal	*90%*
Flexion	180°	160°
Extension	50°	45°
Abduction	180°	160°
Internal rotation	90°	80°
External rotation	90°	80°

- Functional cervical ROM or a minimum of 80% of AMA guides:

	Normal	*80%*
Flexion	60°	50°
Extension	75°	60°
Rotation	80°	65°
Side bend	45°	35°

- Strength: Equal to uninvolved side, 4/5 on manual muscle test, or as demonstrated functionally
  - Able to reach into back pocket or fasten undergarments
  - Able to comb hair
  - Able to reach into cupboard or lift overhead
  - Perform work/ADL tasks (weight and repetition specific)
- Pain: 0/10 with all activity, including throwing
- Normal glenohumeral rhythm (timing of scapular and glenohumeral joint movements)
- Return to functional status and activity level (current/prior) for ADLs and vocational, recreational, and sports activities as identified by patient
- Independence in a progressive home exercise program emphasizing function

INTERVENTION
NUMBER OF VISITS: 6–15

Coordination, Communication, and Documentation
- Provision of services between admission and discharge that facilitate cost-effective and efficient integration or reintegration to home, community, or work
- Documentation of therapeutic intervention is required for each episode of care and serves as the basic foundation for communication
- Coordination and additional communication will depend on the patient's impairment and home/work/community/leisure situation and requirements. Such services may include:
  - Case management
  - Coordination of care and collaboration with those integral to the patient's rehabilitation program
  - Coordination and monitoring of the delivery of available resources
  - Referrals to other health-care professionals
  - Identification of resources, support groups, or advocacy services
  - Provision of educational or training information
  - Technical assistance

Patient Instruction

Basic Anatomy and Biomechanics
- Review of bony, muscular, ligamentous, and joint dynamics for the glenohumeral, sternoclavicular, acromioclavicular, and scapulothoracic regions
- Pertinent Gray's Anatomy (Gray. 1995. 627–632, 839–842)
- Importance of adequate motor performance, postural alignment, and ROM of the cervical/thoracic spine to promote postoperative healing

Handouts
- Commercially available products, such as:
  - Krames Communications (1100 Grundy Lane, San Bruno, CA 94066):
    - *Shoulder Arthroscopy*
    - *Rotator Cuff Injuries*
    - *Shoulder Owner's Manual*
- Specific home program

Functional Considerations
- Long term strengthening options
- Avoidance of contraction of rotator cuff musculature for 5–6 weeks postoperatively
- Avoidance of reaching or lifting until active Phase II is initiated
- Review of immobilization guidelines as determined by physician
- Avoidance of aggravating activities or positions
  - Sleeping posture
  - Driving
- Recognition of inappropriate substitution patterns with exercises, such as shoulder shrug with attempted elevation
- Description of surgical procedure
  - Review of operative report
  - Discussion of specific procedure and its relation to the biomechanics of the shoulder complex
  - Ellman "Rotator Cuff Surgery"

Direct Interventions

Phase I: 1–4 Visits, Weeks 1–5
- Therapeutic exercise and home program
  - Passive shoulder ROM, including wand, Codman's, and pulley exercise

SHOULDER | POSTOP REHAB OF THE ROTATOR CUFF   431

- Upper body ergometer for ROM
  - Passive participation of the involved extremity
- Initiate cardiovascular conditioning
  - Walking program
  - Stationary cycling
- Manual therapy techniques
  - Soft-tissue techniques
    - Soft-tissue mobilization
    - Trigger-point techniques
  - Manually assisted ROM
    - Elevation
    - Internal rotation
    - External rotation
    - Cervical spine
  - Joint mobilization
    - Grades I–II to the involved shoulder for pain relief
    - Grades III–IV to areas of hypomobility, including the cervical/thoracic spine
- Electrotherapeutic modalities
- Physical agents and mechanical modalities
  - Cryotherapy
  - Athermal, deep thermal modalities
- Goals/outcomes
  - Pain: 5/10 or less
  - Shoulder PROM: 50% of AMA guides
    - Flexion: 90°
    - Extension: 25°
    - Abduction: 90°
    - Internal rotation: 45°
    - External rotation: 45°

Phase II: 4–7 Visits, Weeks 6–10

- Therapeutic exercise and home program
  - Progress active/assistive to resistive exercises using pulleys, tubing, or free-weights
    - Internal/external rotation performed with arm at side, elbow flexed to 90°
    - Shoulder extension
    - Supraspinatus isolation ("empty can" position)
      a. Shoulder is internally rotated, thumb pointed to floor
      b. Abduct the arm to 90°, maintaining a position 30° anterior to the mid-frontal plane
    - Horizontal adduction in supine
    - Progress to horizontal abduction
    - Shoulder shrugs
    - Scapular retraction/depression

- Elbow and wrist strengthening
- Upper body ergometer
  - Cardiovascular conditioning
  - Neuromuscular/balance/proprioceptive reeducation
    - Quadruped multidirectional rocking
    - Three-point rocking
    - Push-up progression
      a. Wall
      b. Modified hands/knees
      c. Hands/toes
    - Bodyblade®
      a. Working all planes of motion, especially transverse
- Manual therapy techniques
  - Continue effective soft-tissue techniques
  - Joint mobilization
    - Joint mobilization to stretch glenohumeral joint capsule and inhibit pain and guarding through receptor facilitation
    - Mobilization techniques to other shoulder complex joints if necessary, including sternoclavicular, acromioclavicular, and scapulothoracic
    - Progressive graded mobilization to cervical/thoracic spine
  - Assisted stretching to the shoulder complex and cervical/thoracic spine
  - Manually resisted functional or diagonal patterns
- Goals/outcomes
  - Pain: 2/10 or less
  - PROM: 80% of AMA guides
    - Flexion: 145°
    - Extension: 40°
    - Abduction: 145°
    - Internal rotation: 70°
    - External rotation: 70°
  - Functional activities
    - Pain-free driving
    - Dressing
    - Increased duration of uninterrupted sleep as compared to initial evaluation

Phase III: 1–4 Visits, Weeks 11–12

- Therapeutic exercise and home program
  - Continue isotonic exercise, emphasizing eccentric contractions

432   POSTOP REHAB OF THE ROTATOR CUFF | SHOULDER

- ○ Neuromuscular/balance/proprioceptive reeducation
  - ▪ Bodyblade® for contraction throughout ROM
  - ▪ Push-ups with scapular protraction
  - ▪ Dynamic stabilization prone over therapeutic ball
  - ▪ Push-ups off therapeutic ball
- ○ Military press
- ○ Elbow and wrist strengthening
- ○ Plyometrics with compact medicine ball, tossing and catching (1–3 kg)
  - ▪ Underhand
  - ▪ Two-handed
  - ▪ Overhand
- ○ Begin gradual progression into sport-specific activities
- ○ Cardiovascular conditioning
  - ▪ Walking/running
  - ▪ Upper or lower body cycling
  - ▪ Ski machine
- Goals/outcomes
  - ○ Pain-free AROM: 90% of AMA guides or uninvolved extremity
    - ▪ Flexion: 160°
    - ▪ Extension: 45°
    - ▪ Abduction: 160°
    - ▪ Internal rotation: 80°
    - ▪ External rotation: 80°
  - ○ Strength: Equal to uninvolved shoulder, 4/5 on manual muscle test, or achieve a predetermined functional motor performance parameter, such as
    - ▪ Reaching and lifting 5–15 lbs out in front of trunk
    - ▪ Lifting 5–20 lbs overhead
    - ▪ Reaching into kitchen cabinets and lowering dishes
  - ○ Proper shoulder mechanics for ADLs and vocational tasks
  - ○ Return to independent function in household, occupational, and recreational activities
  - ○ Pain: 0/10 at rest, 2/10 or less with activity

Functional Carryover

- Importance of proper lifting techniques, keeping objects close to trunk, and using lower extremities to generate force
- Activity modification if less than optimal recovery
- Importance of maintaining proper posture of the cervical/thoracic spine to optimize glenohumeral positioning
- Ergonomic modification to work and home environments

DISCHARGE PLANNING AND PATIENT RESPONSIBILITY

Criteria for Discharge

- All rehabilitation goals/outcomes achieved except:
  - ○ May not achieve pain-free recreational/sports activities but shows signs of progression
  - ○ Strength: May discharge at less than 90% if patient displays appropriate motor performance for their specific needs
  - ○ May discharge at 80% ROM

Circumstances Requiring Additional Visits

- Cervical pathology or radiating signs/symptoms
- Inability to depress humeral head during elevation
- Postoperative infection/complications
- Severe postoperative scarring
- Multiple injury sites
- Special occupational needs that require extensive strengthening

Home Program

- Continue exercise program until motor performance, pain-free ROM, and functional activity level has returned
  - ○ Flexibility
  - ○ Motor performance
    - ▪ Resistance exercises with pulley or tubing
    - ▪ Proper progression for weight training activities in health club
- Cardiovascular conditioning
- Pain management techniques
- Advanced functional diagonals incorporating stretch/shortening, or speed training exercise program related to activity or sport-specific needs
- Progress to "Return to Sport" guidelines as indicated

Monitoring

- Instruct patient to call for advice should progression halt or a negative trend occur
- Patient to recheck/call at 4 weeks post-discharge to ensure expected return to function and attainment of rehabilitation goals/outcomes

SHOULDER | POSTOP REHAB OF THE ROTATOR CUFF   433

REFERENCES

1. American Physical Therapy Association. *Guide to Physical Therapist Practice*. Alexandria, VA: APTA; 1997.

2. Brewster C, Schwab DR. Rehabilitation of the shoulder following rotator cuff injury or surgery. *J Orthop Sports Phys Ther.* 1993;18(2):422-426.

3. Cordasco FA, Wolfe IN, Wootten ME, Bigliani LU. An electromyographic analysis of the shoulder during a medicine ball rehabilitation program. *Am J Sports Med.* 1996;24(3):386-392.

4. Einhorn AR. Shoulder rehabilitation equipment modifications. *J Orthop Sports Phys Ther.* 1985;6(4):247-253.

5. Ellman H. Rotator cuff surgery: what is it good for and how good is it? In: Rockwood, CA, Matson FA, eds. *The Shoulder.* Philadelphia, PA: WB Saunders; 1990.

6. Engelberg AL. *Guides to The Evaluation of Permanent Impairment.* 3rd ed. Chicago, IL: American Medical Association; 1989.

7. Gray H; Williams PL, ed. *Gray's Anatomy.* 38th ed. New York, NY: Churchill Livingstone; 1995.

8. Kronberg M, Nemeth G, Brostrom L. Muscle activity and coordination in the normal shoulder. *Clin Orthop Rel Res.* 1990;257:76-85.

9. Mulligan E. Conservative management of shoulder impingement syndrome. *Athl Train.* 1988;23:348-353.

10. Rockwood CA; Matson FA, ed. *The Shoulder.* Philadelphia, PA: WB Saunders; 1990.

11. Thein LA. Impingement syndrome and its conservative management. *J Orthop Sports Phys Ther.* 1989;11(5):183-191.

12. Warner JP, Micheli LJ, Arslanian LE, Kennedy J, Kennedy R. Patterns of flexibility, laxity and strength in normal shoulders and shoulders with instability and impingement. *Am J Sports Med.* 1990;18:366-375.

POSTOP. TOTAL SHOULDER ARTHROPLASTY
SUMMARY OVERVIEW

ICD-9

812.00   812.20   V43.61

APTA Preferred Practice Pattern: 4D, 4H, 4I, 4J

EXAMINATION

- History and Systems Review
- Tests and Measures
  Systems review per APTA's *Guide to Physical Therapy Practice*
  - Anthropometric characteristics
  - Motor function
  - Pain
  - ROM
- Establish Plan of Care

GOALS/OUTCOMES

- Pain-free dressing
- Pain-free glenohumeral, scapulothoracic, sternoclavicular, and acromioclavicular joint motion exhibiting proper scapulohumeral rhythm
- Glenohumeral and scapulothoracic ROM: At least 80% of AMA guides or equal to uninvolved extremity
- Functional cervical ROM or a minimum of 80% of AMA guides
- Strengthen shoulder complex musculature to equal uninvolved side
- Proper shoulder mechanics to enable return to functional status and activity level (current/prior) for ADLs and vocational and recreational activities
- Independence in a progressive home exercise program emphasizing function

INTERVENTION
NUMBER OF VISITS: 4–16

- Patient Instruction
  - Basic Anatomy and Biomechanics
  - Handouts
  - Functional Considerations
  - Description of Surgical Procedure
- Direct Intervention
  - Acute Phase: 2–4 Visits, Postoperative Weeks 1–2
  - Subacute Phase: 2–12 Visits, Postoperative Weeks 2–12
- Functional Carryover

DISCHARGE PLANNING AND PATIENT RESPONSIBILITY

- Criteria for Discharge
  - All rehabilitation goals/outcomes achieved with the possible exception of return to previous vocational status
  - Patient demonstrates compliance with home program
- Circumstances Requiring Additional Visits
  - Cervical pathology or radiating signs/symptoms
  - Inability to depress humeral head during elevation
  - Postoperative infection/complications
  - Severe postoperative scarring
  - Multiple injury sites
  - Special occupational needs that require extensive strengthening
- Home Program
  - Motor performance
  - Flexibility
  - Cardiovascular conditioning
- Monitoring

POSTOP. TOTAL SHOULDER ARTHROPLASTY

ICD-9

812.00   Closed fracture of unspecified part of upper end of humerus
812.20   Closed fracture of unspecified part of humerus
V43.61   Shoulder joint replacement

APTA Preferred Practice Pattern: 4D, 4H, 4I, 4J

EXAMINATION

History and Systems Review

- History of current condition
  - Date and type of procedure
    - Obtain surgical report or communicate with surgeon regarding:
      a. Was deltoid released? (Delay active exercise)
      b. Was anterior capsule lengthened? (Delay passive external rotation)
      c. Was the greater tuberosity salvaged? (Delay eccentric loading)
  - Location, nature, and behavior of symptoms
    - Aggravating/relieving factors
    - a.m./p.m.
  - Postoperative progression/complications
    - Dependent edema of forearm or hand
- Past history of current condition
  - Upper extremity or cervical injury
  - Surgery
  - Therapeutic intervention
- Functional status and activity level (current/prior)
  - Feeding self with surgical hand
  - Performing basic hygiene with surgical hand
  - Avoiding bearing weight on surgical arm; no active shoulder motion
- Patient's functional goals/outcomes

Tests and Measures

Systems review per APTA's *Guide to Physical Therapy Practice*

- Anthropometric characteristics
  - Comparative girth measurements
    - Circumferential measurement of brachium, forearm, and hand if necessary
- Motor function
  - Check for brachial plexus damage (use as baseline, knowing nervous degeneration may be delayed)
- Pain
  - Measured on visual analog scale

- ROM
  - Cervical
    - Active and passive
    - Overpressure
  - Active/ROM shoulder
    - The four planes of shoulder ROM activity
      a. Elevation (scapular plane): The plane of the long axis of the humerus lies in the same plane as the body of the scapula. This is approximately 30° anterior to the frontal plane of the body.
      b. External rotation: With humerus parallel to the body of the scapula (elbow on folded towel), central axis of glenoid perpendicular to long axis of humerus (humerus passively abducted 4–6 in. from patient's side)
      c. Functional internal rotation: Furthest up back tip of thumb excursion reaches, noting spinous process level
      d. Horizontal adduction: Delay until Phase II stretching (see following)
  - PROM
    - Avoid passive flexion and abduction secondary to intrinsic anatomic barriers

Establish Plan of Care

- Based on history, tests, and measures

GOALS/OUTCOMES

- Pain-free dressing
- Pain-free glenohumeral, scapulothoracic, sternoclavicular, and acromioclavicular joint motion exhibiting proper scapulohumeral rhythm
- Glenohumeral and scapulothoracic ROM: at least 80% of the AMA guides or equal to uninvolved extremity

	Normal	80%
Flexion/elevation	180°	145°
Extension	50°	40°
Internal rotation	90°	70°
External rotation	90°	70°

436   POSTOP TOTAL SHOULDER ARTHROPLASTY | SHOULDER

- ROM goals/outcomes will need modification in the presence of concomitant rotator cuff tear, severe osteoarthritis, rheumatoid arthritis, or traumatic arthritis
- Functional cervical ROM or minimum of 80% of AMA guides:

	Normal	*80%*
Flexion	60°	50°
Extension	75°	60°
Rotation	80°	65°
Side bend	45°	35°

- Strengthen shoulder complex musculature to equal uninvolved side
- Proper shoulder mechanics to enable return to functional status and activity level (current/prior) for ADLs and vocational and recreational activities
- Independence in a progressive home exercise program emphasizing function

INTERVENTION
NUMBER OF VISITS: 4–16

Coordination, Communication, and Documentation

- Provision of services between admission and discharge that facilitate cost-effective and efficient integration or reintegration to home, community, or work
- Documentation of therapeutic intervention is required for each episode of care and serves as the basic foundation for communication
- Coordination and additional communication will depend on the patient's impairment and home/work/community/leisure situation and requirements. Such services may include:
  ○ Case management
  ○ Coordination of care and collaboration with those integral to the patient's rehabilitation program
  ○ Coordination and monitoring of the delivery of available resources
  ○ Referrals to other health-care professionals
  ○ Identification of resources, support groups, or advocacy services
  ○ Provision of educational or training information
  ○ Technical assistance
- Specific coordination and communication provisions:
  ○ Neurologist

Patient Instruction

Basic Anatomy and Biomechanics
- Pertinent Gray's Anatomy (Gray. 1995. 627–634)
- Biomechanics of shoulder motion in relation to specific surgical procedure

Handouts
- Specific home exercise program
- Commercially available products, such as:
  ○ Krames Communications (1100 Grundy Lane, San Bruno, CA 94066):
    - *Shoulder Replacement Surgery*

Functional Considerations
- Review of postoperative limitations as determined by physician
- Instruction on avoidance of muscle contracture if applicable
- Timeline for initiation of active movement

Description of Surgical Procedure
- Review operative report

Direct Intervention

Acute Phase: 2–4 Visits, Postoperative Weeks 1–2
Initiated 24–48 hours after joint replacement; continue until elevation 140°, external rotation 40°; treatment twice daily.
- Therapeutic exercise and home program
  ○ Codman's exercises
    - T-spine parallel to floor
    - Utilizing positions of forearm pronation and supination to create shoulder internal/external rotation
    - Perform circumduction in clockwise and counterclockwise directions
    - 30–60 seconds duration for each position
  ○ Assisted supine elevation in scapular plane
    - Apply gentle pressure for 3–5 seconds
    - Repeat 3–5 times
  ○ Assisted external rotation
    - Supine with folded towel under humerus, shoulder slightly abducted
    - Dowel assisted motion with proper orientation to rotate humerus, not extend elbow

SHOULDER | POSTOP TOTAL SHOULDER ARTHROPLASTY   437

- 5–10 repetitions with 30–60 second hold
  - Assisted elevation with pulley
    - Pulley positioned one foot higher than reach of normal shoulder
    - Beware of unwanted eccentric deltoid and supraspinatus contraction
    - 60–90 seconds duration
  - Assisted abduction supine
    - Use uninvolved arm to assist elevation of affected arm, fingers intertwined, hands brought overhead, then clasped behind neck
    - Elbows brought gently down to the table actively horizontally abducting, followed by horizontal adduction bringing elbows together
    - 30–60 seconds duration
  - Assisted shoulder flexion and abduction/adduction using unaffected arm for assistance
    - "Burp the Baby" and "Rock the Baby"
  - Seated table slides for passive flexion and abduction
  - Perform hand and elbow AROM exercises
  - Initiate cardiovascular conditioning
    - Walking program
    - Lower-extremity cycling
- Manual therapy techniques
- Physical agents and mechanical modalities
  - Cryotherapy/thermal modalities
  - PROM in pain-free range
- Goals/outcomes
  - Pain: 5/10 or less with motion, 2/10 or less at rest
  - Shoulder PROM: 70% of uninvolved side

Subacute Phase: 2–12 Visits, Postoperative Weeks 2–12

Continue until elevation 160°, external rotation 60°
- Therapeutic exercise and home program
  - Postural balancing activities
  - Assisted internal rotation
    - Both hands placed behind back, uninvolved arm grasps affected arm
    - Affected arm is pulled into extension, keeping humerus in sagittal plane, while affected wrist is assisted further up the back
  - Assisted external rotation
    - Standing in a doorway, affected arm at side, elbow flexed to 90°, palm of hand braced in doorway
    - Torso turns away, to externally rotate shoulder

- Stretching (postoperative weeks 3–6) Designed to attain last 20° of motion in all directions, or to anatomic maximum
  - Assisted elevation
    a. Corner stretch in scapular plane
  - Assisted external rotation
    a. Bilateral arms elevated to near 90°, arms span doorway with elbows flexed to 90°, torso leans forward
  - Assisted internal rotation
    a. Use a towel in uninvolved hand to assist involved hand further up the back
  - Assisted adduction
    a. Unaffected arm pulls affected arm across torso under chin, stretching posterior capsule
- Motor performance (postoperative weeks 4–6) Patients with shoulder replacement for primary osteoarthritis may start strengthening 10–14 days postoperatively, and stretching may be unnecessary. If the greater tuberosity is salvaged and reattached to the prosthesis, confer with physician prior to implementing eccentric loading.
  - Active assisted elevation followed by eccentric anterior deltoid, supraspinatus with lowering of affected arm from 90–0° in supine
  - When able to perform this with 5 lbs, may progress to strengthening performed standing or sitting
    a. Active assisted scapular plane elevation
    b. Deltoid strengthening, 3 parts, using resistive tubing
    c. Internal rotation using tubing
    d. External rotation using tubing
  - Neuromuscular/balance/proprioceptive reeducation
    - Push-ups off wall with progression to modified quadruped for dynamic scapular stabilization
  - Cardiovascular conditioning
- Goals/outcomes
  - ROM: 80% of AMA guides
  - Pain: 2/10 or less for ADLs
  - Muscle strength: 3+/5 on manual muscle test for shoulder girdle musculature
  - Functional activities
    - Able to comb hair
    - Able to reach into cupboard or lift light items above shoulder height

438   POSTOP TOTAL SHOULDER ARTHROPLASTY | SHOULDER

Functional Carryover

- Importance of proper lifting techniques with objects close to trunk
- Activity modification if less than optimal recovery
- Importance of maintaining proper posture of the cervical/thoracic spine to optimize glenohumeral positioning
- Ergonomic modification to vocational and home environments

DISCHARGE PLANNING AND PATIENT RESPONSIBILITY

Criteria for Discharge

- All rehabilitation goals/outcomes achieved with the possible exception of return to previous vocational status
- Patient demonstrates compliance with home program

Circumstances Requiring Additional Visits

- Cervical pathology or radiating signs/symptoms
- Inability to depress humeral head during elevation
- Postoperative infection/complications
- Severe postoperative scarring
- Multiple injury sites
- Special occupational needs that require extensive strengthening

Home Program

- Motor performance
- Flexibility
- Cardiovascular conditioning

Monitoring

- Return to full functional activities may take up to 6 months postoperatively
- Follow up with phone call at 2 weeks and 6 weeks post-discharge to ensure expected return to function
- Patient is instructed to call for advice should progression halt or a negative trend occur

REFERENCES

1. American Physical Therapy Association. *Guide to Physical Therapist Practice*. Alexandria, VA: APTA; 1997.
2. Arntz CT, Jackins S, Matsen III FA. Prosthetic replacement of the shoulder for the treatment of defects in the rotator cuff and the surface of the glenohumeral joint. *J Bone Joint Surg*. 1993;75:485-491.
3. Brems JJ. Rehabilitation following total shoulder arthroplasty. *Clin Orthop Rel Res*. October 1994:70-85.
4. Comito CA, Self EB, Bigliani LU. Arthroplasty and acute shoulder trauma: reasons for success and failure. *Clin Orthop Rel Res*. 1994:27-36.
5. Engelberg AL. *Guides To The Evaluation Of Permanent Impairment*. 3rd ed. Chicago, IL: American Medical Association; 1989.
6. Gray H; Williams PL, ed. *Gray's Anatomy*. 38th ed. New York, NY: Churchill Livingstone; 1995.
7. Johnson RL. Total shoulder arthroplasty. *Orthop Nurs*. 1993;12(1):14-22.
8. Laurence M. Replacement arthroplasty of the rotator cuff deficient shoulder. *J Bone Joint Surg*. 1991;73:916-919.
9. Lee DH, Niemann KM. Bipolar shoulder arthroplasty. *Clin Orthop Rel Res*. July 1994:97-107.
10. Viadero A, Harrison B, Farbent J. Postoperative care of the TSR patient. *Clin Manage Phys Ther*. 1987;7(4):14-15.
11. Wilcox III R, Arslanian L, Millett P. Rehabilitation following total shoulder arthroplasty. *J Ortho Sports Phys Ther*. 2005; 35(12).

440   PostOp Total Shoulder Arthroplasty | Shoulder

SHOULDER ANTERIOR DISLOCATION
SUMMARY OVERVIEW

ICD-9

    718.31   718.81   831.00   831.01

APTA Preferred Practice Pattern: **4B, 4D, 4E, 4F, 4G, 4J**

EXAMINATION

- History and Systems Review
- Tests and Measures
  Systems review per APTA's *Guide to Physical Therapy Practice*
  - Joint integrity and mobility
  - Muscle performance
  - Pain
  - Posture
  - ROM
  - Special tests
- Establish Plan of Care

GOALS/OUTCOMES

- Shoulder ROM: Equal to uninvolved extremity or 90% of AMA guides
- Functional cervical ROM or a minimum of 80% of AMA guides
- Pain: 0/10
- Strength: Equal to uninvolved side or 4/5 on manual muscle test
- Self-care and home management
- Return to prior functional status and activity level for ADLs and vocational, recreational, and sports activities as identified by patient
- Independence in a progressive home exercise program emphasizing function

INTERVENTION
NUMBER OF VISITS: 4–14

- Patient Instruction
  - Basic Anatomy and Biomechanics
  - Handouts
  - Functional Considerations
- Direct Interventions
  - Acute Phase: 1–4 Visits
  - Subacute Phase: 3–10 Visits
- Functional Carryover

DISCHARGE PLANNING AND PATIENT RESPONSIBILITY

- Criteria for Discharge
  - All rehabilitation goals/outcomes achieved with possible exceptions listed in the guidelines
- Circumstances Requiring Additional Visits
  - Cervical pathology or radiating signs/symptoms
  - Surgery is indicated, however patient is not a surgical candidate due to risk factors
  - Persistent functional/occupational deficits
  - Special occupational needs that require extensive strengthening
  - Inability to progress because current vocational demands are exacerbating symptoms
  - Concomitant contractile lesion
- Home Program
  - Flexibility and strengthening for postural balance
  - Strengthening
  - Progression to sport-specific activities
  - Cardiovascular conditioning
- Monitoring

SUMMARY OVERVIEW | SHOULDER | SHOULDER ANTERIOR DISLOCATION   441

SHOULDER ANTERIOR DISLOCATION

ICD-9

718.31	Recurrent dislocation of joint, shoulder region
718.81	Other joint derangement, not elsewhere classified, shoulder region
831.00	Closed dislocation of shoulder, unspecified
831.01	Anterior dislocation of humerus, closed

APTA Preferred Practice Pattern: 4B, 4D, 4E, 4F, 4G, 4J

EXAMINATION

History and Systems Review

- History of current condition
  - Pattern and number of dislocations
  - Location, nature, and behavior of symptoms
    - Aggravating/relieving factors
- Past history of current condition
  - Upper extremity or cervical/thoracic spine injury
  - Surgery
  - Therapy intervention
- Other tests and measures
- Functional status and activity level (current/prior)
- Patient's functional goals/outcomes

Tests and Measures

Systems review per APTA's *Guide to Physical Therapy Practice*

The appropriateness of the objective tests will be determined by elapsed time from the most recent dislocation and the therapist's clinical judgment.

- Joint integrity and mobility
  - Avoid stressing the anterior capsule
  - Glenohumeral
    - Anterior capsule
    - Posterior capsule
    - Inferior capsule
  - Acromioclavicular
  - Sternoclavicular
  - Scapulothoracic
- Muscle performance
  - Resisted
    - Glenohumeral
    - Scapular
    - Supraspinatus isolation ("empty can" position)
      a. Shoulder is internally rotated, thumb pointed to floor
      b. Abduct the arm to 90°, maintaining a position 30° anterior to the mid-frontal plane

- Antalgic movement pattern with dressing activities
- Functional use of upper extremity during gait
- Scapulohumeral rhythm
  - Arms at side
  - Hands on hips
  - Arms elevated 90° anteriorly
- Patient demonstrates ability to touch mid-back with the shoulder flexed/externally rotated and extended/internally rotated
- Pain
  - Measured on visual analog scale
- Posture
  - Forward head
  - Rounded shoulders
  - Flattening of the thoracic spine
  - Shoulder girdle asymmetry
    - Winging of the scapula
    - Clavicular position
    - Humeral head position
    - Muscular development/atrophy
  - Ability to actively achieve a more balanced postural position
- ROM
  - Shoulder girdle ROM
    - AROM
      a. Flexion/elevation
      b. Observe for inability to maintain depressed humeral head
      c. Abduction
      d. Internal rotation
      e. External rotation
      f. Extension
    - Overpressure
    - PROM
      a. Glenohumeral
      b. Acromioclavicular
      c. Sternoclavicular
      d. Scapulothoracic

442   SHOULDER ANTERIOR DISLOCATION | SHOULDER

- Special tests
  - Clear cervical spine
    - AROM
    - PROM
    - Overpressure
    - Quadrant compression test
  - Apprehension test—*Avoid this test if physician provides ROM limitations*
    - Patient supine
    - Involved arm in abduction and external rotation
    - Push anteriorly on posterior aspect of humeral head
      a. Patient with recurrent dislocation will experience apprehension
      b. Patient with anterior instability (subluxation) will experience pain, but not apprehension
      c. Patient with normal shoulder will be asymptomatic
  - Relocation test
    - Administer test with posteriorly directed force on humeral head from apprehension test position
      a. Patient with primary impingement will generally have no change in their pain
      b. Patient with instability (subluxation) and secondary impingement will have pain relief and will tolerate maximal external rotation with the humeral head maintained in a reduced position
  - Clunk test
    - Patient supine
    - Move arm into full flexion and caudal glide, then perform circumduction motion
      a. Positive if clunk, pain, or pseudolocking occurs
      b. Implicates labral tear
  - Neer's test
    - Patient seated or supine
    - Place patient's arm in full flexion with no internal or external rotation, then apply flexion overpressure
      a. Pain implicates supraspinatus and long head of biceps
  - Crossover test
    - Patient is seated or supine
    - Move patient's arm into full horizontal adduction and apply overpressure
    - Implications:

      a. Subscapularis, supraspinatus, and long head of biceps if pain is anterior
      b. Acromioclavicular joint if pain is superior
      c. Infraspinatus, teres minor, posterior capsule of pain is posterior
  - Sulcus sign
    - Patient is seated, arm relaxed at side. Apply inferior distraction.
      a. Excessive translation of humeral head with sulcus inferior to acromion is positive test and implicates multidirectional instability
    - Patient is seated, arm abducted to 90° and resting on examiner's shoulder. Apply caudally directed force.
      a. Excessive translation of humeral head with sulcus at acromion is positive test and implicates multidirectional instability

Establish Plan of Care
- Based on history, tests, and measures

GOALS/OUTCOMES
- Shoulder ROM: Equal to uninvolved extremity or 90% of AMA guides

	Normal	*90%*
Flexion	180°	160°
Extension	50°	45°
External rotation	90°	80°
Internal rotation	90°	80°
Abduction	180°	160°

- Functional cervical ROM or a minimum of 80% of AMA guides:

	Normal	*80%*
Flexion	60°	50°
Extension	70°	60°
Rotation	85°	65°
Side bend	45°	35°

- Pain: 0/10
- Strength: Equal to uninvolved side or 4/5 on manual muscle test
- Self-care and home management
  - Able to reach into back pocket or fasten undergarments
  - Able to comb hair
  - Able to reach into cupboard or lift overhead
  - Perform work/ADL tasks (weight and repetition specific)

SHOULDER | SHOULDER ANTERIOR DISLOCATION   443

- Return to prior functional status and activity level for ADLs and vocational, recreational, and sports activities as identified by patient
- Independence in a progressive home exercise program emphasizing function

INTERVENTION
NUMBER OF VISITS: 4–14

Coordination, Communication, and Documentation
- Provision of services between admission and discharge that facilitate cost-effective and efficient integration or reintegration to home, community, or work
- Documentation of therapeutic intervention is required for each episode of care and serves as the basic foundation for communication
- Coordination and additional communication will depend on the patient's impairment and home/work/community/leisure situation and requirements. Such services may include:
  - Case management
  - Coordination of care and collaboration with those integral to the patient's rehabilitation program
  - Coordination and monitoring of the delivery of available resources
  - Referrals to other health-care professionals
  - Identification of resources, support groups, or advocacy services
  - Provision of educational or training information
  - Technical assistance

Patient Instruction

Basic Anatomy and Biomechanics
- Review of bony, muscular, ligamentous, and joint dynamics of the glenohumeral, sternoclavicular, acromioclavicular, and scapulothoracic regions
- Importance of adequate motor performance, postural alignment, and ROM of the cervical/thoracic spine to promote healing
- Pertinent Gray's Anatomy (Gray. 1995. 627–632, 839, 842, 1537)

Handouts
- Specific home program
- Commercially available products, such as:
  - Krames Communications (1100 Grundy Lane, San Bruno, CA 94066):
    - *Shoulder Owner's Manual*
    - *Shoulder Instability*

Functional Considerations
- Importance of movement and active motion on repetitive basis to allow normal capsular motion
- Avoidance of activities involving extreme external rotation with abduction, such as throwing or reaching above or behind body
- Recognition of inappropriate substitution patterns with exercises, such as shoulder shrug with attempted elevation
- Restrictions from contact activities

Direct Interventions

Acute Phase: 1–4 Visits
- Therapeutic exercise and home program
  - Manual resisted exercises
    - Shoulder
    - Elbow
    - Wrist
    - Hand
  - Posture correction activities
  - AROM: Hand, wrist, elbow
  - Strengthening
    - Isometrics in pain-free range up to 50° external rotation
  - Neuromuscular/balance/proprioceptive reeducation
    - Pain-free modified plantargrade position for elbow propping
    - Bodyblade®
- Manual therapy techniques
  - Soft-tissue mobilization and manipulation
  - Joint mobilization
    - Grade I oscillation in resting position, abduction 55°, horizontal adduction 30°
    - Grade II traction with glenohumeral joint in resting position, abduction 55°, horizontal adduction 30°
    - Grades III–V mobilization to hypomobilities of the cervical/thoracic spines, acromioclavicular, sternoclavicular, and scapulothoracic regions

444 SHOULDER ANTERIOR DISLOCATION | SHOULDER

- Assisted stretching
  - Cervical spine
  - Latissimus dorsi
  - Subscapularis
- Electrotherapeutic modalities
- Physical agents and mechanical modalities
  - Cryotherapy/thermal modalities
  - Ultrasound to surrounding musculature
- Goals/outcomes
  - Pain: 2/10 or less
  - Pain-free AROM
  - Strength: 70% of uninvolved side
  - Functional activities
    - Increased duration of uninterrupted sleep (as compared to initial evaluation)
    - Pain-free personal hygiene

Subacute Phase: 3–10 Visits

- Therapeutic exercise and home program
  - Continue flexibility exercises to restore a balanced postural relationship
  - ROM exercises with elbow at side
  - Strengthening
    - Progress isometric exercises in varying ranges up to 50° external rotation
    - Tubing, pulley, or free-weight exercise
      a. Internal rotation with elbow at side
      b. Progress to dynamic strengthening with arm no longer adducted at side
      c. External rotation strengthening added to centralize humerus in glenoid
      d. Abduction/adduction with arm elevated up to 90° with internal rotation
      e. Overhead flexion/extension
  - Neuromuscular/balance/proprioceptive reeducation
    - Hands-knees
    - Three-point rocking
    - Push-ups
    - Push-ups off therapeutic ball
    - Bodyblade®

- Manual therapy techniques
  - Continue effective soft-tissue techniques
  - Joint mobilization
    - Grade III traction with glenohumeral joint in 55° abduction, 30° horizontal adduction, and slight external rotation (external rotation necessary for functional elevation of humerus)
      a. Make sure to limit external rotation to 50°
    - Progressive graded mobilization to surrounding hypomobilities
- Physical agents and mechanical modalities
  - Continue effective modalities as in acute phase, with increased emphasis on as-needed home use
- Goals/outcomes
  - Pain: 0/10
  - Strength: 4/5 on manual muscle test for shoulder girdle musculature
  - Normal scapulohumeral biomechanical motion
  - Shoulder ROM: 80% of AMA guides
    - Flexion: 145°
    - Extension: 40°
    - Abduction: 145°
    - Internal rotation: 70°
    - External rotation: 70°

Functional Carryover

- Avoid activities that may stress the anterior capsule; excessive external rotation or movement beyond the mid-frontal plane
- Avoid behind-head military presses, latissimus dorsi pull-downs, or similar activities
- Importance of maintaining proper posture of the cervical/thoracic spine to optimize glenohumeral positioning
- Importance of adequate strength and ROM of the lower extremity to generate and attenuate forces at the shoulder

DISCHARGE PLANNING AND PATIENT RESPONSIBILITY

Criteria for Discharge
- All rehabilitation goals/outcomes achieved, except may discharge:
  - With 80% of shoulder AROM
  - Prior to return to previous recreational/sports activities

Circumstances Requiring Additional Visits
- Cervical pathology or radiating signs/symptoms
- Surgery is indicated, however patient is not a surgical candidate due to risk factors
- Persistent functional/occupational deficits
- Special occupational needs that require extensive strengthening
- Inability to progress because current vocational demands are exacerbating symptoms
- Concomitant contractile lesion

Home Program
- Flexibility and strengthening for postural balance
  - Stretch pectorals in neutral rotation position
  - Scapular retractor/depressor strengthening
- Strengthening
  - Rotator cuff, especially internal rotation
  - Horizontal adductors
  - Biceps/triceps
  - Scapular stabilizers
- Progression to sport-specific activities
- Cardiovascular conditioning

Monitoring
- Patient is instructed to call for advice should progression halt or a negative trend occur
- Follow up at 4–8 weeks post-discharge to ensure expected return to function and progression toward attaining all rehabilitation goals/outcomes

REFERENCES

1. American Physical Therapy Association. *Guide to Physical Therapist Practice.* Alexandria, VA: APTA; 1997.
2. Aronen JG, Rega K. Decreasing the incidence of recurrence of first time anterior shoulder dislocations with rehabilitation. *Am J Sports Med.* 1984;12:283-291.
3. Burkhead WZ, Rockwood CA. Treatment of instability of the shoulder with an exercise program. *J Bone Joint Surg.* 1992;74A:890-896.
4. Engelberg AL. *Guides to The Evaluation of Permanent Impairment.* 3rd ed. Chicago, IL: American Medical Association; 1989.
5. Gould JA. *Orthopaedic and Sports Physical Therapy.* 2nd ed. St Louis, MO: CV Mosby; 1990.
6. Gray H; Williams PL, ed. *Gray's Anatomy.* 38th ed. New York, NY: Churchill Livingstone; 1995.
7. Kisner C, Colby LA. *Therapeutic Exercise Foundations and Techniques.* Philadelphia, PA: FA Davis; 1985.
8. Matsen FA, Harryman DT, Sidles JA. Mechanics of glenohumeral instability. *Clin Sports Med.* 1992;10:783-788.
9. Moseley JB, Jobe FW, Pink M, et al. EMG analysis of the scapular muscles during a shoulder rehabilitation program. *Am J Sports Med.* 1992;20:128-134.
10. O'Connell PW, Nuber GW, Mileski RA, et al. The contribution of the glenohumeral ligaments to anterior stability of the shoulder joint. *Am J Sports Med.* 1990;18:579-584.
11. Simonet WT, Cofield RA. Prognosis in anterior shoulder dislocation. *Am J Sports Med.* 1984;12:19-24.
12. Smith RH, Brunolti J. Shoulder kinesthesia after anterior glenohumeral dislocation. *Phys Ther.* 1989;69:106-112.
13. Terry GC, Hammon D, France P, et al. The stabilizing function of passive shoulder restraints. *Am J Sports Med.* 1991;19:26-34.
14. Turkel S, Panio MW, Marshall JL, et al. Stabilizing mechanisms preventing anterior dislocations of the glenohumeral joint. *J Shoulder Elbow Surg.* 1981;63A:1208-1217.
15. Warren RF. Subluxation of the shoulder in athletes. *Clin Sports Med.* 1983;2:339-354.

SHOULDER BURSITIS
SUMMARY OVERVIEW

ICD-9

716.91   726.1   727.3

APTA Preferred Practice Pattern: **4D, 4E, 4F, 4G, 4J**

EXAMINATION

- History and Systems Review
- Tests and Measures
  Systems review per APTA's *Guide to Physical Therapy Practice*
  - Joint integrity and mobility
  - Muscle performance
  - Pain
  - Posture
  - ROM
  - Special tests
- Establish Plan of Care

GOALS/OUTCOMES

- Pain: 2/10 or less
- ROM
- Muscle performance: Shoulder complex musculature equal to uninvolved side or 4/5 on a manual muscle test
- Functional activities
- Return to previous functional status and activity level for ADLs and vocational, recreational, and sports activities as identified by patient
- Independence in a progressive home exercise program emphasizing function

INTERVENTION
NUMBER OF VISITS: 4–14

- Patient Instruction
  - Basic Anatomy and Biomechanics
  - Handouts
  - Functional Considerations
- Direct Interventions
  - Acute Phase: 2–6 Visits
  - Subacute Phase: 2–8 Visits
- Functional Carryover

DISCHARGE PLANNING AND PATIENT RESPONSIBILITY

- Criteria for Discharge
  - All subacute goals/outcomes achieved
  - Patient returns to prior functional status and activity level for ADLs and vocational activities
  - Patient is independent in a progressive home exercise program emphasizing function
- Circumstances Requiring Additional Visits
  - Cervical pathology or radiating signs/symptoms
  - Inability to progress because current vocational demands are exacerbating symptoms
  - Multiple injury site or concomitant shoulder pathology
- Home Program
  - Advanced functional diagonals with stretch/shortening, strengthening, or speed training exercise program related to functional needs
  - Plyometrics with compact medicine ball, tossing and catching 1–3 kg ball
  - Gradual throwing, swinging program for sports activities or progression into sport-specific or function-specific activity for individual patient
  - Pain-free sleeping and reaching
  - Continued flexibility techniques for postural balance
  - Use of cryotherapy to manage occasional flare-ups
- Monitoring

SUMMARY OVERVIEW | SHOULDER | SHOULDER BURSITIS   **447**

SHOULDER BURSITIS

ICD-9

716.91	Arthropathy, unspecified, shoulder region
726.1	Rotator cuff syndrome of shoulder and allied disorders
727.3	Other bursitis

APTA Preferred Practice Pattern: 4D, 4E, 4F, 4G, 4J

EXAMINATION

History and Systems Review

- History of current condition
  - Mechanism and date of injury/onset
    - Rapid onset without injury
  - Location, nature, and behavior of symptoms
    - Aggravating/relieving factors
    - Pain is greater with abduction than other movements
- Past history of current condition
  - Upper extremity or cervical injury
  - Surgery
  - Direct intervention
- Other tests and measures
- Functional status and activity level (current/prior)
- Patient's functional goals/outcomes

Tests and Measures

Systems review per APTA's *Guide to Physical Therapy Practice*

- Joint integrity and mobility
  - Glenohumeral
  - Acromioclavicular
  - Sternoclavicular
  - Scapulothoracic
- Muscle performance

  Can be used for differential diagnosis. Patient may be unwilling to attempt due to pain with movement as opposed to limited ROM.
  - Patient demonstrates ability to touch mid-back with the shoulder flexed/externally rotated and extended/internally rotated
  - Antalgic movement pattern with dressing activities
  - Functional use of upper extremity during gait
  - Scapulohumeral rhythm
    - Arms at side
    - Hands on hips
    - Arms elevated 90° anteriorly
    - Arms elevated to 180°

- Resisted
  - Pain with all movements, especially abduction and flexion
  - Pain is reduced with the addition of long axis distraction during resisted testing
- Palpation
  - The subacromial bursa is palpated with the humerus in passive extension
  - Inferior to the acromion, lateral to the bicipital groove, and beneath the deltoid muscle
  - Tenderness is obvious when compared to the uninvolved extremity
  - Unilateral thickening may be noted
  - Generally minimal muscle spasm noted
- Pain
  - Measured on visual analog scale
- Posture
  - Forward head
  - Rounded shoulders
  - Flattening of the thoracic spine
  - Shoulder girdle asymmetry
    - Winging of the scapula
    - Clavicular position
    - Humeral head position
    - Muscular development/atrophy
  - Ability to actively achieve a more balanced postural position
- ROM
  - Shoulder girdle ROM
    - AROM
      a. Marked limitation of abduction due to pain
      b. Patient hesitant to move in all other planes
    - PROM
      a. Non-capsular pattern
      b. 30–45° of abduction with minimal restriction of internal or external rotation
- Special tests
  - Clear elbow, wrist, hand
  - Clear cervical spine
    - AROM

- PROM
- Overpressure
- Quadrant compression tests
○ Painful arc
  - Usually unable to detect with acute bursitis due to limited ROM
  - However, as abduction range improves, the painful arc may appear
○ Apprehension test: Patient is supine, involved arm in abduction and external rotation, push anteriorly on posterior aspect of humeral head
  - Patient with recurrent dislocation will experience apprehension
  - Patient with anterior instability (subluxation) will experience pain, but not apprehension
  - Patient with normal shoulder will be asymptomatic
○ Relocation test: Administer test with posteriorly directed force on humeral head from apprehension test position
  - Patient with primary impingement will generally have no change in their pain
  - Patient with instability (subluxation) and secondary impingement will have pain relief and will tolerate maximal external rotation with the humeral head maintained in a reduced position
○ Clunk test: Patient supine, move arm into full flexion and caudal glide, then perform circumduction motion
  - Positive if clunk, pain, or pseudolocking occurs
  - Implicates labral tear
○ Neer's test: Patient seated or supine, place patient's arm in full flexion with no internal or external rotation, then apply flexion overpressure. Pain implicates supraspinatus and long head of biceps.
○ Crossover test: Patient is seated or supine, move patient's arm into full horizontal adduction and apply overpressure
  Implications:
  a. Subscapularis, supraspinatus, and long head of biceps if pain is anterior
  b. Acromioclavicular joint if pain is superior
  c. Infraspinatus, teres minor, posterior capsule of pain is posterior
○ Drop test: Patient is seated, passively abduct patient's arm to 90°, patient is asked to hold arm stationary, administer pressure inferiorly on lateral arm. If arm drops, test implicates rotator cuff rupture.

○ Sulcus sign
  - Patient is seated, arm relaxed at side. Apply inferior distraction. Excessive translation of humeral head with sulcus inferior to acromion is positive test and implicates multidirectional instability.
  - Patient is seated, arm abducted to 90° and resting on examiner's shoulder. Apply caudally directed force. Excessive translation of humeral head with sulcus at acromion is positive test and implicates multidirectional instability.
○ Labral Test
  - Compression rotation test: Patient supine, glenohumeral joint manually compressed through the long axis of the humerus while humerus is passively rotated through internal and external rotation in an attempt to trap the labrum.
  - Pronated load test: Patient supine, the glenohumeral joint is abducted to 90° and externally rotated, forearm pronated. When max external rotation is achieved, patient is instructed to perform isometric biceps contraction.
○ Upper limb tension tests (ULTTs)
  - ULTT 1 (median nerve dominant)
    a. Patient supine, depress shoulder, abduct to approximately 110°, supinate forearm, extend elbow, wrist, and fingers
    b. Side bend head/neck both toward and away
    c. Assess normal vs. abnormal response (see Butler. 1991)
  - ULTT 2 (radial nerve dominant)
    a. Patient supine, depress shoulder, shoulder abducted and internally rotated, pronate forearm, extend elbow, and flex the wrist
    b. Side bend head/neck both toward and away
    c. Assess normal vs. abnormal response (see Butler. 1991)
  - ULTT 3 (ulnar nerve dominant)
    a. Patient supine, extend wrist, supinate forearm, fully flex elbow, depress and abduct shoulder
    b. Side bend head/neck both toward and away
    c. Assess normal vs. abnormal response (see Butler. 1991)

A positive response to any of the special tests may lead the clinician to the specific guideline for the implicated structure.

Establish Plan of Care

- Based on history, tests, and measures

GOALS/OUTCOMES

- Pain: 2/10 or less
- ROM:
  - Rhythm: Pain-free glenohumeral and scapulothoracic joint motion exhibiting proper scapulohumeral rhythm
  - Shoulder AROM: 90% of AMA guides or equal to uninvolved extremity

	Normal	90%
Flexion	180°	160°
Extension	50°	45°
Abduction	180°	160°
Internal rotation	90°	80°
External rotation	90°	80°

  - Functional cervical ROM or a minimum of 80% of AMA guides:

	Normal	80%
Flexion	60°	50°
Extension	75°	60°
Rotation	80°	65°
Side bend	45°	35°

- Muscle performance: shoulder complex musculature equal to uninvolved side or 4/5 on a manual muscle test
- Functional activities
  - Able to reach into back pocket or fasten undergarments
  - Able to comb hair
  - Able to reach into cupboard or lift overhead
  - Able to perform work/ADL tasks (weight and repetition specific)
- Return to previous functional status and activity level for ADLs and vocational, recreational, and sports activities as identified by patient
- Independence in a progressive home exercise program emphasizing function

INTERVENTION
NUMBER OF VISITS: 4–14

Coordination, Communication, and Documentation

- Provision of services between admission and discharge that facilitate cost-effective and efficient integration or reintegration to home, community, or work
- Documentation of therapeutic intervention is required for each episode of care and serves as the basic foundation for communication
- Coordination and additional communication will depend on the patient's impairment and home/work/community/leisure situation and requirements. Such services may include:
  - Case management
  - Coordination of care and collaboration with those integral to the patient's rehabilitation program
  - Coordination and monitoring of the delivery of available resources
  - Referrals to other health-care professionals
  - Identification of resources, support groups, or advocacy services
  - Provision of educational or training information
  - Technical assistance

Patient Instruction

Basic Anatomy and Biomechanics

- Description, location, and function of the subdeltoid bursa
- Shoulder mechanics, musculature, and motion
- Pertinent Gray's Anatomy (Gray. 1995. 627–632, 839, 842)

Handouts

- Specific home program
- Commercially available products, such as:
  - Krames Communications (1100 Grundy Lane, San Bruno, CA 94066):
    - *Shoulder Owner's Manual*

Functional Considerations

- Activities and positions to reduce subacromial compression
  - Avoid sidelying
  - Avoid weight-bearing on upper extremity
- Appropriate use of cryotherapy

450   SHOULDER BURSITIS | SHOULDER

Direct Interventions

Acute Phase: 2–6 Visits

- Therapeutic exercise and home program
  - Active assistive or AROM in pain-free range
  - Rest
  - Cryotherapy
  - Performed in pain-free ROM with low-load, high-repetition format, inhibiting deltoid co-contraction to decrease excessive subacromial compression
- Manual therapy techniques
  - Soft-tissue techniques
    - Soft-tissue mobilization to shoulder complex musculature
  - Joint mobilization
    - Mobilization techniques as patient presentation dictates to cervical/thoracic spine, sternoclavicular, acromioclavicular, and scapulothoracic joints
    - Grades I–II glenohumeral joint mobilization to inhibit pain
  - ROM
    - Pain-free ROM emphasizing subacromial decompression with long-axis distraction
- Electrotherapeutic modalities
  - Iontophoresis
- Physical agents and mechanical modalities
  - Cryotherapy
  - Athermal and thermal modalities
- Goals/outcomes
  - Pain: 5/10 or less with activity, 3/10 or less at rest
  - Functional activity:
    - Increased duration of uninterrupted sleep
  - Shoulder PROM: 80% of AMA guides
    - Flexion: 145°
    - Extension: 40°
    - Abduction: 145°
    - Internal rotation: 70°
    - External rotation: 70°

Subacute Phase: 2–8 Visits

- Therapeutic exercise and home program
  - Flexibility
    - Stretch soft-tissue tightness
    - Pectorals
    - Latissimus dorsi
    - Upper trapezius
    - Levator scapulae

- Subscapularis
- Address cervical/thoracic spine postural dysfunctions
  - Progressive strengthening in pain-free ROM to inhibit humeral head anterior/superior translation during functional tasks; active-assisted, active, isometric, pulley, tubing, or free-weights
    - Scapular rotators
    - Scapular elevators/depressors
    - Internal/external rotation
      a. Motor performance exercises for internal and external glenohumeral rotation are performed with arm at the side, elbow flexed at 90° using surgical tubing or Isoflex™ for resistance
      b. If painful, humerus should be placed in 15° of abduction, well supported to inhibit deltoid co-contraction. Axis of rotation should be placed at 30–45° from horizontal plane.
      c. If pain continues, restrict arc of motion and begin with isometric exercise in same position
    - Supraspinatus isolation ("empty can" position): Shoulder is internally rotated, thumb pointed to floor. Abduct the arm to 90°, maintaining a position 30° anterior to the mid-frontal plane
    - Flexion
    - Abduction
      a. Emphasize rhomboids by having ulnar portion of the arm lead the motion
      b. Emphasize lower trapezius by having the thumb lead the motion
  - Firing of long head of biceps to depress the humeral head
  - Functional or diagonal progressions
  - Neuromuscular/balance/proprioceptive reeducation
    - Wall press-ups
    - Scapular protraction in quadruped
    - Push-ups with scapular protraction
    - Dynamic stabilization prone over therapeutic ball with hands on floor
    - Push-ups off therapeutic ball
  - Cardiovascular conditioning
- Manual therapy techniques
  - Continue effective soft-tissue techniques to improve shoulder girdle posture and scapulohumeral rhythm
  - Joint mobilization
    - Progress graded mobilization as tolerated to areas of persistent hypomobility

SHOULDER | SHOULDER BURSITIS 451

- Physical agents and mechanical modalities
  - Continue effective modalities as in acute phase, with increased emphasis on use as needed at home
- Goals/outcomes
  - Pain: 2/10 or less with activity, 0/10 at rest
  - ROM: 90% of AMA guides or equal to uninvolved extremity
  - Functional activities
    - Able to reach into back pocket or fasten undergarments
    - Able to comb hair
    - Able to reach into cupboard or lift overhead
    - Able to perform work/ADL tasks (weight and repetition specific)
  - Strength: 4-/5 on manual muscle tests or 90% of uninvolved extremity

Functional Carryover
- Proper postures for pain-free activities
  - Sleeping
  - Driving
  - Working
- Ergonomic modifications to avoid exacerbation of symptoms
- Proper lifting mechanics emphasizing the use of lower extremities and trunk to generate and attenuate force at the shoulder

DISCHARGE PLANNING AND PATIENT RESPONSIBILITY

Criteria for Discharge
- All subacute goals/outcomes achieved
- Patient returns to prior functional status and activity level for ADLs and vocational activities
- Patient is independent in a progressive home exercise program emphasizing function

Circumstances Requiring Additional Visits
- Cervical pathology or radiating signs/symptoms
- Inability to progress because current vocational demands are exacerbating symptoms
- Multiple injury site or concomitant shoulder pathology

Home Program
- Advanced functional diagonals with stretch/shortening, strengthening, or speed training exercise program related to functional needs
- Plyometrics with compact medicine ball, tossing and catching 1–3 kg ball
- Gradual throwing, swinging program for sports activities or progression into sport-specific or function-specific activity for individual patient
- Pain-free sleeping and reaching
- Continued flexibility techniques for postural balance
- Use of cryotherapy to manage occasional flare-ups

Monitoring
- Follow-up clinic visits as needed to address difficulties with return to previous recreational/sports activities
- Patient is instructed to call for advice should progression halt or a negative trend occur
- Follow up at 4–8 weeks post-discharge to ensure expected return to function and progression toward attaining all rehabilitation goals/outcomes

REFERENCES

1. American Physical Therapy Association. *Guide To Physical Therapist Practice*. Alexandria, VA: APTA; 1997.

2. Butler DS. *Mobilization of The Nervous System*. Melbourne, Australia: Churchill Livingstone; 1991.

3. Culham E, Peat M. Functional anatomy of the shoulder complex. *J Orthop Sports Phys Ther*. 1993;18(1):342-350.

4. Engelberg AL. *Guides to The Evaluation of Permanent Impairment*. 3rd ed. Chicago, IL: American Medical Association; 1989.

5. Gray H; Williams PL, ed. *Gray's Anatomy*. 38th ed. New York, NY: Churchill Livingstone; 1995.

6. Harryman DT, Sidles JA, Clarck JM, et al. Translation of the humeral head on the glenoid with passive glenohumeral motion. *J Bone Joint Surg*. 1990;72A:1334-1343.

7. Jobe FW, Kitne RS. Shoulder pain in the overhand or throwing athlete. *Orthop Rev*. 1989;18:963-975.

8. Paine RM, Voight M. The role of the scapula. *J Orthop Sports Phys Ther*. 1993;18(1):386-391.

9. Saha AK. Dynamic stability of the glenohumeral joint. *Acta Orthop Scand*. 1971;42:491-505.

10. Saha AK. Mechanism of shoulder movements and a plea for the recognition of "zero position" of the glenohumeral joint. *Clin Orthop Rel Res*. 1983;173:3-10.

11. Wilk KE, Arrigo CA. An integrated approach to upper extremity exercises. *Orthop Clin North Am*. 1992;23:337-360.

12. Wilk KE, et al. Current concepts in the recognition and treatment of superior labral (SLAP) lesions. *J Orthop Sports Phys Ther*. May 2005;35(5): 273-291.

SHOULDER DEGENERATIVE JOINT DISEASE
SUMMARY OVERVIEW

ICD-9

716.91   719.41

APTA Preferred Practice Pattern: 4F, 4D, 4G, 7A

EXAMINATION

- History and Systems Review
- Tests and Measures
  Systems review per APTA's *Guide to Physical Therapy Practice*
  - Joint integrity and mobility
  - Muscle performance
  - Pain
  - Posture
  - ROM
  - Special tests
- Establish Plan of Care

GOALS/OUTCOMES

- Pain: 2/10 or less
- Pain-free glenohumeral and scapulothoracic joint motion to 90% of uninvolved side or 80% of the AMA guides
- Functional cervical ROM or a minimum of 80% of AMA guides
- Proper scapulohumeral rhythm
- Shoulder girdle motor performance: Equal to uninvolved side
- Functional activities
- Return to functional status and activity level (current/ prior) for ADLs and vocational activities as identified by patient
- Independence in a progressive home exercise program emphasizing function

INTERVENTION
NUMBER OF VISITS: 4-12

- Patient Instruction
  - Basic Anatomy and Biomechanics
  - Handouts
  - Functional Considerations
- Direct Interventions
  - Acute Phase: 1–4 Visits
  - Subacute Phase: 3–8 Visits
- Functional Carryover

DISCHARGE PLANNING AND PATIENT RESPONSIBILITY

- Criteria for Discharge
  - All rehabilitation goals/outcomes achieved with possible exceptions listed in the guidelines
  - Patient demonstrates compliance with home program and avoidance of activities that could exacerbate symptoms
- Circumstances Requiring Additional Visits
  - Cervical pathology or radiating signs/symptoms
  - Presence of concomitant tendinitis or adhesive capsulitis
  - Inability to progress because current vocational demands are exacerbating symptoms
  - Special occupational needs that require extensive strengthening
  - Multiple injury sites
  - Presence of ligamentous laxity
  - Presence of capsular pattern of restriction
  - Presence of contractile lesion
- Home Program
  - Self-stretch without impingement
  - Motor performance
- Monitoring

SHOULDER DEGENERATIVE JOINT DISEASE

ICD-9

716.91   Arthropathy, unspecified, shoulder region
719.41   Pain in joint, shoulder region

APTA Preferred Practice Pattern: 4F, 4D, 4G, 7A

EXAMINATION

History and Systems Review

- History of current condition
  - Location, nature, and behavior of symptoms
    - Aggravating/relieving factors
    - a.m./p.m.
- Past history of current condition
  - Upper extremity or cervical/thoracic injury
  - Surgery
  - Direct intervention
- Other tests and measures
- Functional status and activity level (current/prior)
- Patient's functional goals/outcomes

Tests and Measures

Systems review per APTA's *Guide to Physical Therapy Practice*

- Joint integrity and mobility
  - Glenohumeral (passive)
    - Anterior capsule
    - Posterior capsule
    - Inferior capsule
  - Acromioclavicular
  - Sternoclavicular
  - Scapulothoracic
- Muscle performance
  - Antalgic movement pattern with dressing activities
  - Functional use of upper extremity during gait
  - Scapulohumeral rhythm
    - Arms at side
    - Hands on hips
    - Arms elevated 90° anteriorly
  - Patient demonstrates ability to touch mid-back with the shoulder flexed/externally rotated and extended/internally rotated
  - Resisted testing
    - Glenohumeral

- Scapular
- Supraspinatus isolation ("empty can" position)
  - a. Shoulder is internally rotated, thumb pointed to floor
  - b. Abduct the arm to 90°, maintaining a position 30° anterior to the mid-frontal plane
- Pain
  - Measured on visual analog scale
- Posture
  - Forward head
  - Rounded shoulders
  - Flattening of the thoracic spine
  - Shoulder girdle asymmetry
    - Winging of the scapula
    - Clavicular position
    - Humeral head position
    - Muscular development/atrophy
  - Ability to actively achieve a more balanced postural position
- ROM
  - AROM: Shoulder
    - Flexion/elevation
      - a. Observe for inability to maintain depressed humeral head
    - Abduction
    - Internal rotation
    - External rotation
    - Extension
  - PROM: Shoulder
- Special tests
  - Clear cervical spine
    - Active/passive ROM
    - Overpressure
    - Quadrant compression test

Establish Plan of Care

- Based on history, tests, and measures

456   SHOULDER DEGENERATIVE JOINT DISEASE | SHOULDER

GOALS/OUTCOMES

- Pain: 2/10 or less
- Pain-free glenohumeral and scapulothoracic joint motion to 90% of uninvolved side or 80% of the AMA guides:

	Normal	80%
Flexion	180°	145°
Extension	50°	40°
Abduction	180°	145°
Internal rotation	90°	70°
External rotation	90°	70°

- Functional cervical ROM or a minimum of 80% of AMA guides:

	Normal	80%
Flexion	60°	50°
Extension	75°	60°
Rotation	80°	65°
Side bend	45°	35°

- Proper scapulohumeral rhythm
- Shoulder girdle motor performance: Equal to uninvolved side
- Functional activities
  - Able to reach into back pocket
  - Able to hook brassiere in front and twist it around for proper wear
  - Able to comb hair
  - Able to reach into cupboard
- Return to functional status and activity level (current/prior) for ADLs and vocational activities as identified by patient
- Independence in a progressive home exercise program emphasizing function

INTERVENTION
NUMBER OF VISITS: 4–12

Coordination, Communication, and Documentation

- Provision of services between admission and discharge that facilitate cost-effective and efficient integration or reintegration to home, community, or work
- Documentation of therapeutic intervention is required for each episode of care and serves as the basic foundation for communication
- Coordination and additional communication will depend on the patient's impairment and home/work/community/leisure situation and requirements. Such services may include:
  - Case management
  - Coordination of care and collaboration with those integral to the patient's rehabilitation program
  - Coordination and monitoring of the delivery of available resources
  - Referrals to other health-care professionals
  - Identification of resources, support groups, or advocacy services
  - Provision of educational or training information
  - Technical assistance

Patient Instruction

Basic Anatomy and Biomechanics
- Shoulder girdle anatomical review
- Pertinent Gray's Anatomy (Gray. 1995. 627–632, 839, 842)
- Importance of adequate motor performance, postural alignment, and ROM of the cervical/thoracic spine to optimize shoulder function

Handouts
- Specific home program
- Commercially available products, such as:
  - Krames Communications (1100 Grundy Lane, San Bruno, CA 94066)
    - *Shoulder Owner's Manual*

Functional Considerations
- Avoid positions of subacromial compression
  - Sidelying
  - Weight bearing on upper extremity
- Reduction of motions/activities causing overload to the shoulder complex
- Role of proper posture in ADL/vocational activities
- Importance of proper body mechanics, emphasizing use of lower extremities and trunk to generate and attenuate force at the shoulder joint

Direct Interventions

Acute Phase: 1–4 Visits

- Therapeutic exercise and home program
  - Performed in pain-free ROM with low-load and high-repetition format, inhibiting deltoid co-contraction to decrease excessive subacromial compression
    - Internal and external glenohumeral rotation are performed with arm at the side, elbow flexed at 90° using pulley system, resistive band, or tubing
      a. If painful, humerus should be placed in 15° of abduction, well supported to inhibit deltoid co-contraction
  - Isometric strengthening
    - Shoulder flexion, extension, internal/external rotation, abduction
  - Postural correction activities
    - Pectoral stretching
    - Latissimus dorsi stretching
    - Scapular retractor/depressor strengthening
- Manual therapy techniques
  - Soft-tissue techniques
    - Soft-tissue mobilization to the shoulder girdle
    - Trigger-point techniques
    - Myofascial release
  - Joint mobilization
    - Glenohumeral joint mobilization Grades I–II to inhibit pain
    - Posterior capsular stretching to emphasize posterior positioning of the humeral head in glenoid
    - Mobilization techniques as patient presentation dictates to sternoclavicular, acromioclavicular, scapulothoracic joints
    - Grades III–V to cervical/thoracic hypomobilities
  - Pain-free ROM emphasizing subacromial decompression with long axis distraction
  - Assisted stretching techniques
    - Shoulder girdle
    - Cervical/thoracic spine
- Electrotherapeutic modalities
- Physical agents and mechanical modalities
  - Cryotherapy/thermal modalities
  - Athermal and deep thermal modalities
- Goals/outcomes
  - Shoulder girdle strength: 70% of uninvolved side
  - Shoulder ROM: 70% of uninvolved side or 50% of AMA guides

- Flexion: 90°
- Extension: 25°
- Abduction: 90°
- Internal rotation: 45°
- External rotation: 45°
  - Pain: 4/10 or less with activity, 0/10 at rest

Subacute Phase: 3–8 Visits

- Therapeutic exercise and home program
  - Muscle balance
    - Stretch soft-tissue tightness
  - Strengthening
    - Scapular upward/downward rotators, elevators/depressors
    - Resisted abduction
      a. Emphasize rhomboids by having the ulnar portion of the arm lead the motion
      b. Emphasize the lower trapezii by having the thumb lead the motion
  - Motor performance
    - Functional patterns of motion using surgical tubing, free weights, or wall pulley for resistance
  - Neuromuscular/balance/proprioceptive reeducation
    - Scapular protraction in quadruped
    - Press-ups off wall
    - Push-ups with scapular protraction
    - Dynamic stabilization while prone over ball
    - Hands on floor, progressing to push-ups off therapeutic ball
    - Bodyblade®
  - Plyometrics
    - Underhand toss
    - Two-handed throw
    - Overhand throw
- Manual therapy techniques
  - Soft-tissue mobilization to promote normalizing scapulohumeral rhythm
  - Progressive joint mobilization
    - Maximize glenohumeral movement
      a. Emphasize stretch to anterior and inferior capsule
    - Continue mobilization as indicated to surrounding joints
- Physical agents and mechanical modalities
  - Continue effective modalities as in acute phase with increased emphasis on as-needed home use

- Goals/outcomes
  - Strength: 90% of uninvolved extremity
  - ROM: 80% of uninvolved side or 70% of AMA guides
    - Flexion: 125°
    - Extension: 35°
    - Abduction: 125°
    - Internal rotation: 65°
    - External rotation: 65°
  - Pain: 2/10

Functional Carryover

- Integration of proper postural positions for ADLs and vocational and recreational activities
- Importance of proper lifting technique, keeping objects close to trunk
- Ergonomic modifications to home and vocational environments

DISCHARGE PLANNING AND PATIENT RESPONSIBILITY

Criteria for Discharge

- All rehabilitation goals/outcomes achieved, except may be discharged:
  - With 70% of shoulder ROM
  - With 4/5 on a manual muscle test if all other rehabilitation goals/outcomes achieved
  - Prior to attaining previous level of participation in sports or recreational activities
  - If the therapist determines that further progression and attainment of all rehabilitation goals/outcomes will be achieved with patient's continued efforts/compliance with home program outside the clinical environment
- Patient demonstrates compliance with home program and avoidance of activities that could exacerbate symptoms

Circumstances Requiring Additional Visits

- Cervical pathology or radiating signs/symptoms
- Presence of concomitant tendinitis or adhesive capsulitis
- Inability to progress because current vocational demands exacerbate symptoms
- Special occupational needs that require extensive strengthening

- Multiple injury sites
- Presence of ligamentous laxity
- Presence of capsular pattern of restriction
- Presence of contractile lesion

Home Program

- Self-stretch without impingement
- Motor performance
  - Gradual throwing/swinging program or progression into sport-specific or function-specific activity for individual patient

Monitoring

- Patient is instructed to call for advice should progression halt or a negative trend occur
- Follow up at 4–8 weeks post-discharge to ensure expected return to function and progression toward attaining all rehabilitation goals/outcomes

REFERENCES

1. American Physical Therapy Association. *Guide to Physical Therapist Practice.* Alexandria, VA: APTA; 1997.
2. Culham E, Peat M. Functional anatomy of the shoulder complex. *J Orthop Sports Phys Ther.* 1993;18:342-350.
3. Engelberg AL. *Guides to The Evaluation of Permanent Impairment,* 3rd ed. Chicago: American Medical Association. 1989.
4. Gray H; Williams PL, ed. *Gray's Anatomy.* 38th ed. New York, NY: Churchill Livingstone; 1995.
5. Howell SM, Galinat BJ, Renzi AJ, et al. Normal and abnormal mechanics of the glenohumeral joint in the horizontal plane. *J Bone Joint Surg.* 1988;70A:230-235.
6. Paine RM, Voight M. The role of the scapula. *J Orthop Sports Phys Ther.* 1993;18(1):386-391.
7. Wilk KE, Arrigo CA. An integrated approach to upper extremity exercises. *Orthop Clin North Am.* 1992;1(2):337-360.

SHOULDER FRACTURE
SUMMARY OVERVIEW

ICD-9

810   812

APTA Preferred Practice Pattern: **4D, 4H, 4I, 4J**

EXAMINATION

- History and Systems Review
- Tests and Measures
  Systems review per APTA's *Guide to Physical Therapy Practice*
  - Joint integrity and mobility
  - Muscle performance
  - Pain
  - Posture
  - ROM
  - Special tests
- Establish Plan of Care

GOALS/OUTCOMES

- ROM
- Shoulder complex muscle performance: Equal to uninvolved side
- Pain: 2/10 or less with activity, 0/10 at rest
- Functional activities
- Normal glenohumeral rhythm (timing of scapular and glenohumeral joint movements)
- Return to prior functional status and activity level for ADLs and vocational, recreational, and sports activities as identified by patient
- Independence in a progressive home exercise program emphasizing function

INTERVENTION
NUMBER OF VISITS: 6–18

- Patient Instruction
  - Basic Anatomy and Biomechanics
  - Handouts
  - Functional Considerations
- Direct Interventions
  - Acute Phase: 1–6 Visits, 1–5 Weeks Post-Fracture
  - Subacute Phase: 5–12 Visits, 6–12 Weeks Post-Fracture
- Functional Carryover

DISCHARGE PLANNING AND PATIENT RESPONSIBILITY

- Criteria for Discharge
  - All rehabilitation goals/outcomes have been met, except may discharge with strength of 4-/5 if all other goals/outcomes achieved
  - Patient demonstrates compliance with home program
- Circumstances Requiring Additional Visits
  - Cervical pathology or radiating signs/symptoms
  - Unable to achieve functional goals
  - Presence of concomitant adhesive capsulitis or tendinitis
  - Delayed union
- Home Program
  - Continue exercise program until strength, pain-free ROM, and functional activity level have returned to pre-injury status
  - Cardiovascular conditioning
- Monitoring

SUMMARY OVERVIEW | SHOULDER | SHOULDER FRACTURE   461

SHOULDER FRACTURE

ICD-9

810	Fracture of clavicle
812	Fracture of humerus

APTA Preferred Practice Pattern: 4D, 4H, 4I, 4J

EXAMINATION

History and Systems Review

- History of current condition
  - Location, nature, and behavior of symptoms
    - Aggravating/relieving factors
- Past history of current condition
  - Upper extremity or thoracic/cervical spine injury
  - Surgery
  - Direct intervention
- Other tests and measures
- Functional status and activity level (current/prior)
- Patient's functional goals/outcomes

Tests and Measures

Systems review per APTA's *Guide to Physical Therapy Practice*

Objective assessment will be based on the healing status and severity of the fracture. Communication with the physician is recommended.

- Joint integrity and mobility
  - Glenohumeral
  - Acromioclavicular
  - Sternoclavicular
  - Scapulothoracic
- Muscle performance
  - Antalgic movement pattern with dressing activities
  - Functional use of upper extremity during gait
  - Scapulohumeral rhythm
    - Arms at side
    - Hands on hips
    - Arms elevated 90° anteriorly
  - Resisted testing of the shoulder girdle
- Pain
  - Measured on visual analog scale
- Posture
  - Forward head
  - Rounded shoulders
  - Flattening of the thoracic spine
  - Shoulder girdle asymmetry

- Winging of the scapula
- Clavicular position
- Humeral head position
- Muscular development/atrophy
  - Ability to actively achieve a more balanced postural position
- ROM
  - Shoulder girdle ROM
    - AROM
    - PROM
- Special tests

At 6 weeks post-fracture, consult physician regarding healing status prior to performing special tests.

- Clear elbow, wrist, and hand
- Clear cervical spine
  - AROM
  - PROM
  - Overpressure
  - Quadrant compression test
- Apprehension test: Patient supine, involved arm in abduction and external rotation, push anteriorly on posterior aspect of humeral head
  - Patient with recurrent dislocation will experience apprehension
  - Patient with anterior instability (subluxation) will experience pain, but not apprehension
  - Patient with normal shoulder will be asymptomatic
- Relocation test: Administer test with posteriorly directed force on humeral head from apprehension test position
  - Patient with primary impingement will generally have no change in their pain
  - Patient with instability (subluxation) and secondary impingement will have pain relief and will tolerate maximal external rotation with the humeral head maintained in a reduced position
- Clunk test: Patient supine, move arm into full flexion and caudal glide, then perform circumduction motion. Positive if clunk, pain, or pseudolocking occurs.

○ Neer's test: Patient seated or supine, place patient's arm in full flexion with no internal or external rotation, then apply flexion overpressure. Pain implicates supraspinatus and long head of biceps.

○ Crossover test: Patient is seated or supine, move patient's arm into full horizontal adduction and apply overpressure

Implications:

   a. Subscapularis, supraspinatus, and long head of biceps if pain is anterior

   b. Acromioclavicular joint if pain is superior

   c. Infraspinatus, teres minor, posterior capsule of pain is posterior

○ Drop test: Patient is seated, passively abduct patient's arm to 90°, patient is asked to hold arm stationary, administer pressure inferiorly on lateral arm. If arm drops, test implicates rotator cuff rupture.

○ Sulcus sign

   ▪ Patient is seated, arm relaxed at side. Apply inferior distraction. Excessive translation of humeral head with sulcus inferior to acromion is positive test and implicates multidirectional instability.

   ▪ Patient is seated. Arm abducted to 90° and resting on examiner's shoulder. Apply caudally directed force. Excessive translation of humeral head with sulcus at acromion is positive test and implicates multidirectional instability.

○ Upper limb tension tests (ULTTs)

   ▪ ULTT 1 (median nerve dominant)

     a. Patient supine, depress shoulder, abduct to approximately 110°, supinate forearm, extend elbow, wrist, and fingers

     b. Side bend head/neck both toward and away

     c. Assess normal vs. abnormal response (see Butler. 1991)

   ▪ ULTT 2 (radial nerve dominant)

     a. Patient supine, depress shoulder, shoulder abducted and internally rotated, pronate forearm, extend elbow, and flex the wrist

     b. Side bend head/neck both toward and away

     c. Assess normal vs. abnormal response (see Butler. 1991)

   ▪ ULTT 3 (ulnar nerve dominant)

     a. Patient supine, extend wrist, supinate forearm, fully flex elbow, depress and abduct shoulder

     b. Side bend head/neck both toward and away

     c. Assess normal vs. abnormal response (see Butler. 1991)

A positive response to any of the special tests may lead the clinician to the specific guideline for the implicated structure.

Establish Plan of Care

• Based on history, tests, and measures

GOALS/OUTCOMES

• ROM

  ○ Shoulder—pain free glenohumeral and scapulothoracic AROM: A minimum of 80% of AMA guides

Flexion	145°
Extension	40°
Abduction	145°
Internal rotation	70°
External rotation	70°

  ○ Functional cervical ROM or a minimum of 80% of AMA guides:

Flexion	50°
Extension	60°
Rotation	65°
Side bend	35°

• Shoulder complex muscle performance: Equal to uninvolved side

• Pain: 2/10 or less with activity, 0/10 at rest

• Functional activities:

  ○ Able to reach into back pocket or fasten undergarments

  ○ Able to comb hair

  ○ Able to reach into cupboard or lift overhead

  ○ Able to perform work/ADL tasks (weight and repetition specific)

• Normal glenohumeral rhythm (timing of scapular and glenohumeral joint movements)

• Return to prior functional status and activity level for ADLs and vocational, recreational, and sports activities as identified by patient

• Independence in a progressive home exercise program emphasizing function

SHOULDER | SHOULDER FRACTURE   463

INTERVENTION
NUMBER OF VISITS: 6–18

Coordination, Communication, and Documentation

- Provision of services between admission and discharge that facilitate cost-effective and efficient integration or reintegration to home, community, or work
- Documentation of therapeutic intervention is required for each episode of care and serves as the basic foundation for communication
- Coordination and additional communication will depend on the patient's impairment and home/work/community/leisure situation and requirements. Such services may include:
  - Case management
  - Coordination of care and collaboration with those integral to the patient's rehabilitation program
  - Coordination and monitoring of the delivery of available resources
  - Referrals to other health-care professionals
  - Identification of resources, support groups, or advocacy services
  - Provision of educational or training information
  - Technical assistance

Patient Instruction

Basic Anatomy and Biomechanics
- Review the nature of fracture and correlation to anatomical structures
- Biomechanics of proper glenohumeral rhythm and role of posture in influencing motor performance and ROM
- Pertinent Gray's Anatomy (Gray. 1995. 619, 623–624, 627–632, 839, 842)

Handouts
- Postfracture precautions
- Specific home program

Functional Considerations

- Long term strengthening options
- Guidance in postures/positions to avoid exacerbation of shoulder symptoms
- Proper lifting techniques, keeping the weight close to the trunk and utilizing the lower extremities to generate force
- Immobilization implications if appropriate

Direct Interventions

Acute Phase: 1–6 Visits, 1–5 Weeks Post-Fracture
- Therapeutic exercise and home program
  - Upper body ergometer for ROM
  - High-repetition pain-free passive exercises for vascularization of rotator cuff (unweighting, supported ROM)
  - Strengthening exercises are performed as long as muscle contractions do not stress fracture site.
    - Internal/external rotation with arm at the side, elbow flexed to 90° using surgical tubing for resistance:
      a. If external rotation is painful, limit the degree of rotation
      b. If pain continues, begin with isometric exercise in same position
      c. If still painful, move shoulder to loose pack position (i.e. slight abduction and elevation)
      d. As pain decreases and strength increases, progress to free weights
    - Internal rotation lying on involved side
    - External rotation lying on uninvolved side
    - Supraspinatus isolation ("empty can" position)
      a. Shoulder is internally rotated, thumb pointed to floor
      b. Abduct the arm to 90°, maintaining a position 30° anterior to the mid-frontal plane
      c. If this exercise cannot be accomplished at this stage, try without internal rotation and emphasize scapular motion
    - Shoulder extension in prone with arm hanging off table or forward bent at waist in standing
      a. Extend arm to side of trunk (0°)
      b. Shoulder extensors also function as depressors of humeral head, which decreases the upward migration and likelihood of impingement
    - Scapular stabilization program: Depression, retraction

464　SHOULDER FRACTURE | SHOULDER

- Manual therapy techniques
  - Soft-tissue techniques
    - Myofascial release
    - Soft-tissue mobilization
    - Acupressure
    - Strain/counterstrain
  - Passive, pain-free ROM emphasizing posterior positioning of the humeral head
  - Joint mobilization
    - Do not stress/mobilize fracture site
    - Grades I–II to inhibit pain
    - Grades III–V to surrounding hypomobile joints of the cervical/thoracic spine, acromioclavicular, sternoclavicular, scapulothoracic, elbow, or wrist
- Physical agents and mechanical modalities
  - Cryotherapy
- Goals/outcomes
  - Pain: 5/10 or less
  - Shoulder ROM: 70% of AMA guides
    - Flexion: 125°
    - Extension: 35°
    - Abduction: 125°
    - Internal rotation: 65°
    - External rotation: 65°
  - Shoulder girdle strength: 3+/5 on manual muscle test
  - Able to reach to eye level

Subacute Phase: 5–12 Visits, 6–12 Weeks Post-Fracture

- Therapeutic exercise and home program
  - Strengthening
    - Continue tubing exercise
    - Continue free-weight and pulley exercises, emphasizing eccentric contractions
    - Horizontal adduction and military press
    - Functional diagonals
    - Optional use of isokinetic exercise

- Neuromuscular/balance/proprioceptive reeducation
    - Quadruped multidirectional rocking
    - Three-point rocking
    - Wall push-ups
    - Push-ups
    - Bodyblade®
  - Plyometrics with compact medicine ball, tossing and catching (1 kg, progress to 3 kg)
  - Begin throwing program or progression toward sport-specific activity
  - Cardiovascular conditioning
- Manual therapy techniques
  - Continue effective soft-tissue techniques
  - Joint mobilization
    - Grades I–II with intent of pain relief
    - Continue progressive graded mobilization to surrounding areas of hypomobility
    - Progressive Grades II–IV to glenohumeral joint, with consideration of healing status and location of fracture
- Physical agents and mechanical modalities
  - Continue effective modalities as in acute phase with increased emphasis on use as needed at home
- Goals/outcomes
  - Pain: 2/10 or less
  - Shoulder AROM: 80% of AMA guides
  - Strength: 4-/5 on manual muscle test or 80% of uninvolved extremity
  - Improve glenohumeral rhythm to enhance return to previous level of ADLs and vocational, recreational, and sports activities
  - Functional activities:
    - Reaching and lifting 5–15 lbs out in front of trunk
    - Lifting small objects

Functional Carryover

- Proper lifting techniques and body mechanics
- Ergonomic modifications to prevent overuse of shoulder girdle and promote normal postural relationship
- Activity modification if less than optimal recovery

SHOULDER | SHOULDER FRACTURE 465

DISCHARGE PLANNING AND PATIENT RESPONSIBILITY

Criteria for Discharge
- All rehabilitation goals/outcomes have been met except may discharge with strength of 4-/5 if all other goals/outcomes achieved
- Patient demonstrates compliance with home program

Circumstances Requiring Additional Visits
- Cervical pathology or radiating signs/symptoms
- Unable to achieve functional goals
- Presence of concomitant adhesive capsulitis or tendinitis
- Delayed union

Home Program
- Continue exercise program until strength, pain-free ROM, and functional activity level have returned to pre-injury status
- Cardiovascular conditioning

Monitoring
- Patient is instructed to call for advice should progression halt or a negative trend occur
- Follow up at 4-8 weeks post-discharge to ensure expected return to function and progression toward attaining all rehabilitation goals/outcomes

REFERENCES

1. American Physical Therapy Association. *Guide to Physical Therapist Practice.* Alexandria, VA: APTA; 1997.
2. Brewster C, Schwab DR. Rehabilitation of the shoulder following rotator cuff injury or surgery. *J Orthop Sports Phys Ther.* 1993;18(2):422-426.
3. Butler DS. *Mobilization of the Nervous System.* Melbourne, Australia: Churchill Livingstone; 1991.
4. Culham E, Peat M. Functional anatomy of the shoulder complex. *J Orthop Sports Phys Ther.* 1993;18(1):342-350.
5. Einhorn AR. Shoulder rehabilitation equipment modifications. *J Orthop Sports Physical Ther.* 1985;6(4):247-253.
6. Engelberg AL. *Guides to the Evaluation of Permanent Impairment.* 3rd ed. Chicago, IL: American Medical Association; 1989.
7. Gray H; Williams PL, ed. *Gray's Anatomy.* 38th ed. New York, NY: Churchill Livingstone; 1995.
8. Kronberg M, Nemeth G, Brostrom L. Muscle activity and coordination in the normal shoulder. *Clin Orthop Rel Res.* 1990;257:76-85.
9. McClure PW, Flowers KR. Treatment of limited shoulder motion: a case study based on biomechanical considerations. *Phys Ther.* 1992;72:929-936.
10. Mulligan E. Conservative management of shoulder impingement syndrome. *Athl Train.* 1988;23:348-353.
11. Sillman JF, Dean MJ. Neurovascular injuries to the shoulder complex. *J Orthop Sports Phys Ther.* 1993;18(2):442-448.
12. Thein LA. Impingement syndrome and its conservative management. *J Orthop Sports Phys Ther.* 1989;11(5):183-191.
13. Warner JP, Micheli LJ, Arslanian LE, Kennedy J, Kennedy R. Patterns of flexibility, laxity, and strength in normal shoulders and shoulders with instability and impingement. *Am J Sports Med.* 1990;18:366-375.
14. Wilk KE, Arrigo CA. An integrated approach to upper extremity exercises. *Orthop Clin North Am.* 1992;23:337-360.

SHOULDER JOINT PATHOLOGY
SUMMARY OVERVIEW

ICD-9

718.91   719.51   719.52   719.91

APTA Preferred Practice Pattern: **4F, 4H, 4I**

EXAMINATION

- History and Systems Review
- Tests and Measures
  Systems review per APTA's *Guide to Physical Therapy Practice*
  - Anthropometric characteristics
  - Arousal, attention, and cognition
  - Assistive and adaptive devices
  - Circulation
  - Environmental, home, and work (job/school/play) barriers
  - Ergonomics and body mechanics
  - Integumentary integrity
  - Joint integrity and mobility
  - Motor function
  - Muscle performance
  - Pain
  - Peripheral nerve integrity
  - Posture
  - ROM
  - Reflex integrity
  - Special tests
- Establish Plan of Care

GOALS/OUTCOMES

- Shoulder ROM: 90% of AMA guides or equal to the uninvolved extremity
- Functional cervical ROM or a minimum of 80% of AMA guides
- Pain: 2/10 following activity, 0/10 at rest
- Strength: Equal to uninvolved side or 4/5 on manual muscle test for shoulder girdle musculature
- Functional activities
- Return to functional status and activity level (current/prior) for ADLs and vocational, recreational, and sports activities as identified by patient
- Independence in a progressive home exercise program emphasizing function

INTERVENTION
NUMBER OF VISITS: 6–12

- Patient Instruction
  - Basic Anatomy and Biomechanics
  - Handouts
- Direct Interventions
  - Acute Phase: 3–6 Visits
  - Subacute Phase: 3–6 Visits
- Functional Carryover

DISCHARGE PLANNING AND PATIENT RESPONSIBILITY

- Criteria for Discharge
  - All rehabilitation goals/outcomes achieved with possible exception of return to pain-free function for vocational or sports activities
  - The therapist determines that further progression and attainment of all rehabilitation goals/outcomes will be achieved with patient's continued efforts/compliance with home program outside the clinical environment
  - If continuing pain and instability prevents patient progression, consider orthopedic consultation
- Circumstances Requiring Additional Visits
  - Cervical pathology or radiating signs/symptoms
  - Inability to progress because current vocational demands are exacerbating symptoms
  - Special occupational/athletic needs that require extensive strengthening
  - Multiple injury sites
  - Presence of ligamentous laxity
  - Cognitive limitations
  - Postoperative complications
- Home Program
  - Motor performance for progressive proximodistal strengthening
  - Flexibility, especially of posterior shoulder structures
  - Advanced functional diagonals with stretch/shortening (plyometric), strengthening, or speed

SUMMARY OVERVIEW | SHOULDER | SHOULDER JOINT PATHOLOGY   467

training exercise program related to functional/athletic needs
- o Cardiovascular conditioning
- o Throwing program for return to athletic performance
- Monitoring

SHOULDER JOINT PATHOLOGY

ICD-9

718.91	Unspecified derangement of joint, shoulder region
719.51	Stiffness of joint, not elsewhere classified, shoulder region
719.52	Stiffness of joint, not elsewhere classified, upper arm
719.91	Unspecified disorder of joint, shoulder region

APTA Preferred Practice Pattern: 4F, 4H, 4I

EXAMINATION

History and Systems Review

- History of current condition
  - Age
  - Medications
  - Mechanism of injury
  - Date of injury, including repeat injuries suggesting instability
  - Location, nature, and behavior of symptoms
    - Lateral brachial pain
    - Vascular symptoms
    - Radicular symptoms
    - Peripheral nerve entrapment symptoms
- Past history of current condition
  - Functional status and activity level (prior)
  - Patient's functional goals/outcomes
  - Injections
  - Surgical intervention
  - Systemic pathology
    - Cardiac
    - Respiratory
    - Cervical spine
    - Thoracic spine
- Other tests and measures
  - Functional status and activity level (current)
  - Occupational demands
- Medications
- Past medical/surgical history

Tests and Measures

Systems review per APTA's *Guide to Physical Therapy Practice*

- Anthropometric characteristics
  - General muscular definition
- Arousal, attention, and cognition
  - As it relates to complexity of home exercise program planning

- Assistive and adaptive devices
- Circulation (arterial, venous, lymphatic)
  - Swelling
  - Thoracic inlet/outlet testing
- Environmental, home, and work (job/school/play) barriers
  - Occupational, recreational demands
- Ergonomics and body mechanics
  - Work site analysis, repetitive movement analysis
- Integumentary integrity
  - Incision healing
  - Adhesive allergies
- Joint integrity and mobility
- Motor function (motor control and motor learning)
  - Muscle performance
    - Antalgic movement pattern with dressing activities
    - Functional use of upper extremity during gait
    - Proximodistal movement patterning
  - Scapulohumeral rhythm
    - Arms at side
    - Hands on hips
    - Arms elevated 90° anteriorly
- Muscle performance (including strength, power, and endurance)
  - Resisted
    - Glenohumeral
    - Scapular
    - Supraspinatus isolation ("empty can" position)
      a. Shoulder is internally rotated, thumb pointed to floor
      b. Abduct the arm to 90°, maintaining a position in the scapular plane
- Pain
  - Measured on visual analog scale
- Peripheral nerve integrity
  - Radial nerve entrapment
  - Median nerve integrity

SHOULDER | SHOULDER JOINT PATHOLOGY   469

- o Upper limb tension tests with radial, median, and ulnar bias
- Posture
  - o Forward head
  - o Rounded shoulders
  - o Flattening of the thoracic spine
  - o Shoulder girdle asymmetry
    - Winging of the scapula/scapular plane
    - Clavicular position
    - Humeral head position
    - Muscular development/atrophy
- ROM (including muscle length)
  - o AROM
    - Flexion/elevation
      a. Observe for inability to maintain depressed humeral head
    - Abduction
    - Internal rotation
      a. Reach behind back
      b. 90° abduction
    - External rotation
      a. Neutral abduction
      b. 90° abduction
    - Extension
  - o Overpressure
  - o PROM
    - Glenohumeral
      a. Anterior capsule
      b. Posterior capsule
      c. Inferior capsule
      d. Anterior glenohumeral ligament
      e. Inferior glenohumeral ligament
    - Acromioclavicular
    - Sternoclavicular
    - Scapulothoracic
- Reflex integrity
  - o Deltoid (C5)
  - o Brachioradialis (C5/6)
  - o Biceps (C6)
  - o Triceps (C7)
  - o Rule out upper motor neuron lesion
    - Clonus
    - Dysdiadokokinesis
- Special tests
  - o Apprehension test
    - Patient supine
    - Involved arm in abduction and external rotation

- Push anteriorly on posterior aspect of humeral head
  a. Patient with recurrent dislocation will experience apprehension
  b. Patient with anterior instability (subluxation) will experience pain, but not apprehension
  c. Patient with normal shoulder will be asymptomatic
- o Relocation test
  - Administer test with posteriorly directed force on humeral head from apprehension test position
    a. Patient with primary impingement will generally have no change in their pain
    b. Patient with instability (subluxation) and secondary impingement will have pain relief and will tolerate maximal external rotation with the humeral head maintained in a reduced position
- o Clunk test
  - Patient supine
  - Move arm into full flexion and caudal glide, then perform circumduction motion
    a. Positive if clunk, pain, or pseudolocking occurs
    b. Implicates labral tear
- o Neer's test
  - Patient seated or supine
  - Place patient's arm in full flexion with no internal or external rotation, then apply flexion overpressure
    a. Pain implicates supraspinatus and long head of biceps
- o Crossover test
  - Patient is seated or supine
  - Move patient's arm into full horizontal adduction and apply overpressure
  - Implications:
    a. Subscapularis, supraspinatus, and long head of biceps if pain is anterior
    b. Acromioclavicular joint if pain is superior
    c. Infraspinatus, teres minor, posterior capsule of pain is posterior
- o Drop test
  - Patient is seated
  - Passively abduct patient's arm to 90°
  - Patient is asked to hold arm stationary
  - Administer pressure inferiorly on lateral arm
    a. If arm drops, test implicates rotator cuff rupture

- Sulcus sign
  - Patient is seated, arm relaxed at side. Apply inferior distraction.
    a. Excessive translation of humeral head with sulcus inferior to acromion is positive test and implicates multidirectional instability
  - Patient is seated, arm abducted to 90° and resting on examiner's shoulder. Apply caudally directed force.
    a. Excessive translation of humeral head with sulcus at acromion is positive test and implicates multidirectional instability
- Labral test
  - Compression Rotation Test: Patient supine, glenohumeral joint manually compressed through the long axis of the humerus while humerus is passively rotated through internal and external rotation in an attempt to trap the labrum
  - Pronated Load Test: Patient supine, the glenohumeral joint is abducted to 90° and externally rotated, forearm pronated. When max external rotation is achieved, the patient is instructed to perform isometric biceps contraction.
- Upper limb tension tests (ULTTs)
  - ULTT 1 (median nerve dominant)
    a. Patient supine, depress shoulder, abduct to approximately 110°, supinate forearm, extend elbow, wrist, and fingers
    b. Side bend head/neck both toward and away
    c. Assess normal vs. abnormal response (see Butler. 1991)
  - ULTT 2 (radial nerve dominant)
    a. Patient supine, depress shoulder, shoulder abducted and internally rotated, pronate forearm, extend elbow, flex the wrist and thumb
    b. Side bend head/neck both toward and away
    c. Assess normal vs. abnormal response (see Butler. 1991)
  - ULTT 3 (ulnar nerve dominant)
    a. Patient supine, extend wrist, supinate forearm, fully flex elbow, depress and abduct shoulder
    b. Side bend head/neck both toward and away
    c. Assess normal vs. abnormal response (see Butler. 1991)
- A positive response to any of the special tests may lead the clinician to the specific guideline for the implicated structure

Establish Plan of Care
- Based on history, tests, and measures

GOALS/OUTCOMES
- Shoulder ROM: 90% of AMA guides or equal to the uninvolved extremity

	Normal	*90%*
Flexion	180°	160°
Extension	50	45°
Abduction	180°	160°
External rotation	90°	80°
Internal rotation	90°	80°

- Functional cervical ROM or a minimum of 80% of AMA guides:

	Normal	*80%*
Flexion	60°	50°
Extension	75°	60°
Rotation	80°	65°
Side bend	45°	35°

- Pain: 2/10 following activity, 0/10 at rest
- Strength: Equal to uninvolved side or 4/5 on manual muscle test for shoulder girdle musculature
- Functional activities
  - Able to reach into back pocket or fasten undergarments
  - Able to comb hair
  - Able to reach into cupboard or lift overhead
  - Perform work/ADL tasks (weight and repetition specific)
- Return to functional status and activity level (current/prior) for ADLs and vocational, recreational, and sports activities as identified by patient
- Independence in a progressive home exercise program emphasizing function

INTERVENTION
NUMBER OF VISITS: 6–12

Coordination, Communication, and Documentation
- Provision of services between admission and discharge that facilitate cost-effective and efficient integration or reintegration to home, community, work, or athletic

team. May require direct communication to coaching staff of athlete.

- Documentation of therapeutic intervention is required for each episode of care and serves as the basic foundation for communication
- Coordination and additional communication will depend on the patient's impairment and home/work/community/leisure situation and requirements. Such services may include:
  - Case management
  - Coordination of care and collaboration with those integral to the patient's rehabilitation program
  - Coordination and monitoring of the delivery of available resources
  - Referrals to other health-care professionals
  - Identification of resources, support groups, or advocacy services
  - Provision of educational or training information
  - Technical assistance

Patient Instruction

Basic Anatomy and Biomechanics
- Musculature, ligaments, and joint structure in relation to shoulder motion
- Mechanism of supraspinatus in relation to depression of humeral head to avoid impingement
- Mechanism of long head of biceps in relation to anterior sling of head of humerus
- Mechanism of first two thoracic segments for shoulder elevation
- Mechanics of labrum for static stability
- Pertinent Gray's Anatomy (Gray. 1995. 621–622, 627–632, 839–842)

Handouts
- Commercially available products
- Specific home program
- Proper body mechanics for lifting, carrying, pushing, and pulling
- Commercially available products, such as:
  - Krames Communications (100 Grundy Lane, San Bruno, CA 94066):
    - *Shoulder Owner's Manual*
    - *Rotator Cuff Injuries*
- Home program
  - Initiated with proximodistal stabilization awareness, initiating with axial thoracic extension, abdominal

stabilization, and scapular stabilization, progressing to distal mobility on proximal base. Progress to work-site-specific or sport-specific training regimen.

- Functional considerations
  - Posture (sitting, standing, sleeping, driving)
  - Assistive devices (crutches, canes, walkers, collars, tape)
  - Precautions
  - Alteration of ADLs
  - Avoidance of prolonged postures
  - Positioning for relief of symptoms
  - Body mechanic instruction for lifting, pushing, pulling, etc.
  - Training recommendations (cross training, periodization, etc.)
  - Optimal positions of rest
- Body mechanics to avoid unnecessary stress on shoulder complex
- Avoidance of activities which cause exacerbation of symptoms

Direct Interventions

Acute Phase: 3–6 Visits
- Therapeutic exercise and home program
  - PROM
    - Codman's
    - Pulley
    - Wand
  - Pain-free AROM
    - High-repetition and low-resistance with purpose of promoting vascularization of healing tissues
    - Internal/external rotation
    - Supraspinatus isolation ("empty can" position)
      a. Shoulder is internally rotated, thumb pointed to floor
      b. Abduct the arm to 90°, maintaining a position 30° anterior to the mid-frontal plane
    - Scapular retraction/depression
    - Upper body ergometry
  - Postural correction exercises
  - Neuromuscular/balance/proprioceptive reeducation
    - Pain-free modified plantargrade position for elbow propping
    - Bodyblade®
  - Cardiovascular conditioning
    - Walking program
    - Lower-extremity cycling

472   SHOULDER JOINT PATHOLOGY | SHOULDER

- Manual therapy techniques
  - Soft-tissue techniques
    - Soft-tissue mobilization
    - Myofascial release/stretching
    - Ischemic compression to trigger-points
    - Friction massage
  - Joint mobilization
    - Grades I–II to inhibit pain and guarding
    - Grades III–V to hypomobilities of the glenohumeral, sternoclavicular, acromioclavicular, or cervical/thoracic spine
  - ROM
    - Within pain-free range specific to rotator cuff musculature
    - Shoulder girdle
    - Pectorals
    - Cervical/thoracic musculature
- Physical agents and mechanical modalities
  - Cryotherapy/thermal modalities
  - Athermal, deep thermal modalities
- Goals/outcomes
  - Pain: 4/10 following activity, 2/10 or less at rest
  - Pain-free ROM: 50% of AMA guides
    - Flexion: 90°
    - Extension: 25°
    - Abduction: 90°
    - Internal rotation: 45°
    - External rotation: 45°
  - Increased duration of uninterrupted sleep (set specific goal based on number of interrupted hours of sleep at initial evaluation)

Subacute Phase: 3–6 Visits

- Therapeutic exercise and home program
  - Progressive strengthening (isometric, pulley, resistive bands, free-weight)
    - Exercises should not elicit painful response
    - Use resistive bands, surgical tubing for internal/external rotation, elbow flexed at 90°
    - Isometrics in planes not tolerating banded resistance
    - Internal rotation lying on involved side
    - External rotation lying on uninvolved side
    - Supraspinatus isolation ("empty can" position)
    - Shoulder extension
      a. Prone with arm hanging off table or forward bent at waist in standing
      b. Extend arm to side of trunk (0°)

- Flexibility/posture correction
- Neuromuscular/balance/proprioceptive reeducation
  - Quadruped multidirectional rocking
  - Three-point rocking
  - Push-ups
  - Push-ups off therapeutic ball
  - Bodyblade®
- Progression into vocational/sport-specific activity
- Manual therapy techniques
  - Joint mobilization
    - Grades III–IV to persistent hypomobilities of the glenohumeral, sternoclavicular, acromioclavicular, and scapulothoracic regions
    - Grades III–V to cervical/thoracic spine
  - Continue effective soft-tissue techniques
- Physical agents and mechanical modalities
  - Continue effective modalities as in acute phase with increased emphasis on use as needed at home
- Goals/outcomes
  - Shoulder ROM: 90% of AMA guides or equal to the uninvolved extremity
    Flexion: 160°
    Extension: 45°
    External rotation: 80°
    Internal rotation: 80°
    Abduction: 160°
  - Pain: 2/10 following activity, 0/10 at rest
  - Strength: Equal to uninvolved side or 4/5 on manual muscle test
  - Functional activities
    - Able to reach into back pocket or fasten undergarments
    - Able to comb hair
    - Able to reach into cupboard or lift overhead
    - Perform work/ADL tasks (weight and repetition specific)

Functional Carryover

- Integration of home exercise program into vocational environment
- Completion of ergonomic adjustments to home, automobile, and vocational areas
- Incorporation of proper posture and body mechanics to avoid exacerbation of symptoms
- Recognition/avoidance of activities that increase or exacerbate radiating symptoms
- Importance of maintaining proper posture of the cervical/thoracic spine to optimize glenohumeral positioning

- Ergonomic modification to work and home environments
- Avoidance of activities which increase pain
- Pain-free sleeping positions
- Proper lifting/throwing mechanics emphasizing the use of lower extremities and trunk to generate and attenuate force at the shoulder

DISCHARGE PLANNING AND PATIENT RESPONSIBILITY

Criteria for Discharge
- All rehabilitation goals/outcomes achieved with possible exception of return to pain-free function for vocational or sports activities
- The therapist determines that further progression and attainment of all rehabilitation goals/outcomes will be achieved with patient's continued efforts/compliance with home program outside the clinical environment
- If continuing pain and instability prevents patient progression, consider orthopedic consultation

Circumstances Requiring Additional Visits
- Cervical pathology or radiating signs/symptoms
- Inability to progress because current vocational demands are exacerbating symptoms
- Special occupational/athletic needs that require extensive strengthening
- Multiple injury sites
- Presence of ligamentous laxity
- Cognitive limitations
- Postoperative complications

Home Program
- Motor performance for progressive proximodistal strengthening
- Flexibility, especially of posterior shoulder structures
- Advanced functional diagonals with stretch/shortening (plyometric), strengthening, or speed training exercise program related to functional/athletic needs
- Cardiovascular conditioning
- Throwing program for return to athletic performance

Monitoring
- Follow-up contact by patient to report progress or exacerbation of symptoms
- Instruct patient to call should progression halt or a negative trend occur
- Return to physician

REFERENCES
1. American Physical Therapy Association. *Guide to Physical Therapist Practice.* Alexandria, VA: APTA; revised 2003.
2. Butler DS. *Mobilization of the Nervous System.* Melbourne, Australia: Churchill Livingstone; 1991.
3. Brewster C, Schwab DR. Rehabilitation of the shoulder following rotator cuff injury or surgery. *J Orthop Sports Phys Ther.* 1993;18(2):422-426.
4. Gray H; Williams PL, ed. *Gray's Anatomy.* 38th ed. New York, NY: Churchill Livingstone; 1995.
5. Litchfield R, Hawkings R, Dillman CJ, Atkins J, Hagerman G. Rehabilitation for the overhead athlete. *J Orthop Sports Phys Ther.* 1993;18(2):433-441.
6. Lo IK, Nonweiler B, Woolfrey M, Litchfield R, Kirkley A. An evaluation of the apprehension, relocation and surprise tests for anterior shoulder instability. *Am J Sports Med.* 2004;32:301-307.
7. Matsen III FA, Lippitt SB, Sidles JA, Harryman DT. *Practical Evaluation and Management of the Shoulder.* Philadelphia: W.B. Saunders; 1994.
8. Wilk KE, Reinold MM, Dugas JR. Current concepts in the recognition and treatment of superior labral (SLAP) lesions. *J Orthop Sports Phys Ther.* May 2005;35(5):273-291.

SHOULDER SPRAIN/STRAIN
SUMMARY OVERVIEW

ICD-9

716.91   718.81   719.41   726.1   726.2   840   959.2

APTA Preferred Practice Pattern: 4B, 4D, 4E, 4F, 4G, 4H, 4J, 7A

EXAMINATION

- History and Systems Review
- Tests and Measures
  Systems review per APTA's *Guide to Physical Therapy Practice*
  - Muscle performance
  - Pain
  - Posture
  - ROM
  - Special tests
- Establish Plan of Care

GOALS/OUTCOMES

- ROM
- Pain: 2/10 following activity, 0/10 at rest
- Strength: Equal to uninvolved side or 4/5 on manual muscle test for shoulder girdle musculature
- Functional activities
- Return to functional status and activity level (current/prior) for ADLs and vocational, recreational, and sports activities as identified by patient
- Independence in a progressive home exercise program emphasizing function

INTERVENTION
NUMBER OF VISITS: 6–16

- Patient Instruction
  - Basic Anatomy and Biomechanics
  - Handouts
  - Functional Considerations
- Direct Interventions
  - Acute Phase: 2–4 Visits
  - Subacute Phase: 4–12 Visits
- Functional Carryover

DISCHARGE PLANNING AND PATIENT RESPONSIBILITY

- Criteria for Discharge
  - All rehabilitation goals/outcomes achieved with possible exception of return to pain-free function for vocational or sports activities
  - The therapist determines that further progression and attainment of all rehabilitation goals/outcomes will be achieved with patient's continued efforts/compliance with home program outside the clinical environment
  - If continuing pain and instability prevents patient progression, consider orthopedic consultation
- Circumstances Requiring Additional Visits
  - Cervical pathology or radiating signs/symptoms
  - Inability to progress because current vocational demands are exacerbating symptoms
  - Special occupational needs that require extensive strengthening
  - Multiple injury sites
  - Presence of ligamentous laxity
- Home Program
  - Motor performance
  - Flexibility
  - Advanced functional diagonals with stretch/shortening, strengthening, or speed training exercise program related to functional needs
  - Cardiovascular conditioning
- Monitoring

SUMMARY OVERVIEW | SHOULDER | SHOULDER SPRAIN/STRAIN   475

SHOULDER SPRAIN/STRAIN

ICD-9

716.91	Arthropathy, unspecified, shoulder region
718.81	Other joint derangement, not elsewhere classified, shoulder region
719.41	Pain in joint, shoulder region
726.1	Rotator cuff syndrome of shoulder and allied disorders
726.2	Other affections of shoulder region, not elsewhere classified
840	Sprains and strains of shoulder and upper arm
959.2	Other and unspecified injury to shoulder and upper arm

APTA Preferred Practice Pattern: 4B, 4D, 4E, 4F, 4G, 4H, 4J, 7A

EXAMINATION

History and Systems Review

- History of current condition
  - Location, nature, and behavior of symptoms
    - Aggravating/relieving factors
- Past history of current condition
  - Cervical/thoracic spine or upper extremity injury
  - Surgery
  - Direct intervention
- Other tests and measures
- Functional status and activity level (current/prior)
- Patient's functional goals/outcomes

Tests and Measures

Systems review per APTA's *Guide to Physical Therapy Practice*

- Muscle performance
  - Antalgic movement pattern with dressing activities
  - Functional use of upper extremity during gait
  - Scapulohumeral rhythm
    - Arms at side
    - Hands on hips
    - Arms elevated 90° anteriorly
  - Resisted
    - Glenohumeral
    - Scapular
    - Supraspinatus isolation ("empty can" position)
      a. Shoulder is internally rotated, thumb pointed to floor
      b. Abduct the arm to 90°, maintaining a position 30° anterior to the mid-frontal plane
- Pain
  - Measured on visual analog scale

- Posture
  - Forward head
  - Rounded shoulders
  - Flattening of the thoracic spine
  - Shoulder girdle asymmetry
    - Winging of the scapula
    - Clavicular position
    - Humeral head position
    - Muscular development/atrophy
  - Ability to actively achieve a more balanced postural position
- ROM
  - AROM
    - Flexion/elevation: Observe for inability to maintain depressed humeral head
    - Abduction
    - Internal rotation
    - External rotation
    - Extension
  - Overpressure
  - PROM
    - Glenohumeral
      a. Anterior capsule: Superior/inferior, anterior/posterior
      b. Posterior capsule: Superior/inferior, anterior/posterior
      c. Inferior capsule: Upward, downward rotation, lateral
    - Acromioclavicular
    - Sternoclavicular
    - Scapulothoracic

476 SHOULDER SPRAIN/STRAIN | SHOULDER

- Special tests
  - Apprehension test: Patient supine, involved arm in abduction and external rotation, push anteriorly on posterior aspect of humeral head
    - Patient with recurrent dislocation will experience apprehension
    - Patient with anterior instability (subluxation) will experience pain, but not apprehension
    - Patient with normal shoulder will be asymptomatic
  - Relocation test: Administer test with posteriorly directed force on humeral head from apprehension test position
    - Patient with primary impingement will generally have no change in their pain
    - Patient with instability (subluxation) and secondary impingement will have pain relief and will tolerate maximal external rotation with the humeral head maintained in a reduced position
  - Clunk test: Patient supine, move arm into full flexion and caudal glide, then perform circumduction motion. Positive if clunk, pain, or pseudolocking occurs. Implicates labral tear.
  - Neer's test: Patient seated or supine, place patient's arm in full flexion with no internal or external rotation, then apply flexion overpressure. Pain implicates supraspinatus and long head of biceps
  - Crossover test: Patient is seated or supine, move patient's arm into full horizontal adduction and apply overpressure. Implications:
    - Subscapularis, supraspinatus, and long head of biceps if pain is anterior
    - Acromioclavicular joint if pain is superior
    - Infraspinatus, teres minor, posterior capsule of pain is posterior
  - Drop test: Patient is seated, passively abduct patient's arm to 90°. Patient is asked to hold arm stationary while examiner administers pressure inferiorly on lateral arm. If arm drops, test implicates rotator cuff rupture.
  - Sulcus sign
    - Patient is seated, arm relaxed at side. Apply inferior distraction. Excessive translation of humeral head with sulcus inferior to acromion is positive test and implicates multidirectional instability.
    - Patient is seated, arm abducted to 90° and resting on examiner's shoulder. Apply caudally directed force. Excessive translation of humeral head with sulcus at acromion is positive test and implicates multidirectional instability
  - Labral Test
    - Compression Rotation Test: Patient supine, glenohumeral joint manually compressed through the long axis of the humerus while humerus is passively rotated through internal and external rotation in an attempt to trap the labrum
    - Pronated Load Test: Patient supine, the glenohumeral joint is abducted to 90° and externally rotated, forearm pronated. When maximum external rotation is achieved, the patient is instructed to perform isometric biceps contraction.
  - Upper limb tension tests (ULTTs)
    - ULTT 1 (median nerve dominant)
      a. Patient supine, depress shoulder, abduct to approximately 110°, supinate forearm, extend elbow, wrist, and fingers
      b. Side bend head/neck both toward and away
      c. Assess normal vs. abnormal response (see Butler. 1991)
    - ULTT 2 (radial nerve dominant)
      a. Patient supine, depress shoulder, shoulder abducted and internally rotated, pronate forearm, extend elbow, and flex the wrist
      b. Side bend head/neck both toward and away
      c. Assess normal vs. abnormal response (see Butler. 1991)
    - ULTT 3 (ulnar nerve dominant)
      a. Patient supine, extend wrist, supinate forearm, fully flex elbow, depress and abduct shoulder
      b. Side bend head/neck both toward and away
      c. Assess normal vs. abnormal response (see Butler. 1991)

A positive response to any of the special tests may lead the clinician to the specific guideline for the implicated structure.

Establish Plan of Care

- Based on history, tests, and measures

GOALS/OUTCOMES
- ROM
  - Shoulder ROM: 90% of AMA guides or equal to the uninvolved extremity

	Normal	90%
Flexion	180°	160°
Extension	50	45°
Abduction	180°	160°
External rotation	90°	80°
Internal rotation	90°	80°

  - Functional cervical ROM or a minimum of 80% of AMA guides:

	Normal	80%
Flexion	60°	50°
Extension	75°	60°
Rotation	80°	65°
Side bend	45°	35°

- Pain: 2/10 following activity, 0/10 at rest
- Strength: Equal to uninvolved side or 4/5 on manual muscle test for shoulder girdle musculature
- Functional activities
  - Able to reach into back pocket or fasten undergarments
  - Able to comb hair
  - Able to reach into cupboard or lift overhead
  - Perform work/ADL tasks (weight and repetition specific)
- Return to functional status and activity level (current/prior) for ADLs and vocational, recreational, and sports activities as identified by patient
- Independence in a progressive home exercise program emphasizing function

INTERVENTION
NUMBER OF VISITS: 6–16

Coordination, Communication, and Documentation
- Provision of services between admission and discharge that facilitate cost-effective and efficient integration or reintegration to home, community, or work
- Documentation of therapeutic intervention is required for each episode of care and serves as the basic foundation for communication
- Coordination and additional communication will depend on the patient's impairment and home/work/

community/leisure situation and requirements. Such services may include:
  - Case management
  - Coordination of care and collaboration with those integral to the patient's rehabilitation program
  - Coordination and monitoring of the delivery of available resources
  - Referrals to other health-care professionals
  - Identification of resources, support groups, or advocacy services
  - Provision of educational or training information
  - Technical assistance

Patient Instruction

Basic Anatomy and Biomechanics
- Musculature, ligaments, and joint structure in relation to shoulder motion
- Mechanism of supraspinatus in relation to depression of humeral head to avoid impingement
- Pertinent Gray's Anatomy (Gray. 1995. 621–622, 627–632, 839–842)

Handouts
- Specific home program
- Proper body mechanics for lifting, carrying, pushing, and pulling
- Commercially available products, such as:
  - Krames Communications (100 Grundy Lane, San Bruno, CA 94066):
    - *Shoulder Owner's Manual*
    - *Rotator Cuff Injuries*

Functional Considerations
- Optimal positions of rest
- Body mechanics to avoid unnecessary stress on shoulder complex
- Avoidance of activities that cause exacerbation of symptoms

Direct Interventions

Acute Phase: 2–4 Visits
- Therapeutic exercise and home program
  - PROM
    - Codman's
    - Pulley
    - Wand

478   SHOULDER SPRAIN/STRAIN | SHOULDER

- Pain-free AROM
- High-repetition and low-resistance with purpose of promoting vascularization of healing tissues
  - Internal/external rotation
  - Supraspinatus isolation ("empty can" position)
    a. Shoulder is internally rotated, thumb pointed to floor
    b. Abduct the arm to 90°, maintaining a position 30° anterior to the mid-frontal plane
  - Scapular retraction/depression
  - Upper body ergometry
- Postural correction exercises
- Neuromuscular/balance/proprioceptive reeducation
  - Pain-free modified plantargrade position for elbow propping
  - Bodyblade®
- Cardiovascular conditioning
  - Walking program
  - Lower-extremity cycling
- Manual therapy techniques
  - Soft-tissue techniques
    - Soft-tissue mobilization
    - Myofascial release/stretching
    - Ischemic compression to trigger-points
    - Friction massage
  - Joint mobilization
    - Grades I–II to inhibit pain and guarding
    - Grades III–V to hypomobilities of the glenohumeral, sternoclavicular, acromioclavicular, or cervical/thoracic spine
  - ROM
    - Within pain-free range specific to rotator cuff musculature
    - Shoulder girdle
    - Pectorals
    - Cervical/thoracic musculature
- Physical agents and mechanical modalities
  - Cryotherapy/thermal modalities
  - Athermal, deep thermal modalities
- Goals/outcomes
  - Pain: 4/10 following activity, 2/10 or less at rest
  - Pain-free ROM: 50% of AMA guides
    - Flexion: 90°
    - Extension: 25°
    - Abduction: 90°

- Internal rotation: 45°
- External rotation: 45°
- Increased duration of uninterrupted sleep (set specific goal based on number of interrupted hours of sleep at initial evaluation)

Subacute Phase: 4–12 Visits

- Therapeutic exercise and home program
  - Progressive strengthening (isometric, pulley, resistive bands, free-weight)
    - Exercises should not elicit painful response
    - Use resistive bands, surgical tubing for internal/external rotation, elbow flexed at 90°
    - Isometrics in planes not tolerating banded resistance
    - Internal rotation lying on involved side
    - External rotation lying on uninvolved side
    - Supraspinatus isolation ("empty can" position)
    - Shoulder extension
      a. Prone with arm hanging off table or forward bent at waist in standing
      b. Extend arm to side of trunk (0°)
  - Flexibility/posture correction
  - Neuromuscular/balance/proprioceptive reeducation
    - Quadruped multidirectional rocking
    - Three-point rocking
    - Push-ups
    - Push-ups off therapeutic ball
    - Bodyblade®
  - Progression into vocational/sport-specific activity
- Manual therapy techniques
  - Joint mobilization
    - Grades III–IV to persistent hypomobilities of the glenohumeral, sternoclavicular, acromioclavicular, and scapulothoracic regions
    - Grades III–V to cervical/thoracic spine
  - Continue effective soft-tissue techniques
- Physical agents and mechanical modalities
  - Continue effective modalities as in acute phase with increased emphasis on use as needed at home

- Goals/outcomes
  - Shoulder ROM: 90% of AMA guides or equal to the uninvolved extremity
    - Flexion: 160°
    - Extension: 45°
    - External rotation: 80°
    - Internal rotation: 80°
    - Abduction: 160°
  - Pain: 2/10 following activity, 0/10 at rest
  - Strength: Equal to uninvolved side or 4/5 on manual muscle test
  - Functional activities
    - Able to reach into back pocket or fasten undergarments
    - Able to comb hair
    - Able to reach into cupboard or lift overhead
    - Perform work/ADL tasks (weight and repetition specific)

Functional Carryover

- Importance of maintaining proper posture of the cervical/thoracic spine to optimize glenohumeral positioning
- Ergonomic modification to work and home environments
- Avoidance of activities that increase pain
- Pain-free sleeping positions
- Proper lifting/throwing mechanics emphasizing the use of lower extremities and trunk to generate and attenuate force at the shoulder

DISCHARGE PLANNING AND PATIENT RESPONSIBILITY

Criteria for Discharge

- All rehabilitation goals/outcomes achieved with possible exception of return to pain-free function for vocational or sports activities
- The therapist determines that further progression and attainment of all rehabilitation goals/outcomes will be achieved with patient's continued efforts/compliance with home program outside the clinical environment
- If continuing pain and instability prevents patient progression, consider orthopedic consultation

Circumstances Requiring Additional Visits

- Cervical pathology or radiating signs/symptoms
- Inability to progress because current vocational demands are exacerbating symptoms
- Special occupational needs that require extensive strengthening
- Multiple injury sites
- Presence of ligamentous laxity

Home Program

- Motor performance
- Flexibility
- Advanced functional diagonals with stretch/shortening, strengthening, or speed training exercise program related to functional needs
- Cardiovascular conditioning

Monitoring

- Follow-up contact by patient to report progress or exacerbation of symptoms

REFERENCES

1. American Physical Therapy Association. *Guide to Physical Therapist Practice.* Alexandria, VA: APTA; 1997.
2. Brewster C, Schwab DR. Rehabilitation of the shoulder following rotator cuff injury or surgery. *J Orthop Sports Phys Ther.* 1993;18(2):422-426.
3. Butler DS. *Mobilization of the Nervous System.* Melbourne, Australia: Churchill Livingstone; 1991.
4. Einhorn AR. Shoulder rehabilitation equipment modifications. *J Orthop Sports Phys Ther.* 1985;6(4):247-253.
5. Engelberg AL. *Guides to the Evaluation of Permanent Impairment.* 3rd ed. Chicago, IL: American Medical Association; 1989.
6. Gray H; Williams PL, ed. *Gray's Anatomy.* 38th ed. New York, NY: Churchill Livingstone; 1995.
7. Kronberg M, Nemeth G, Brostrom L. Muscle activity and coordination in the normal shoulder. *Clin Orthop Rel Res.* 1990;257:76-85.
8. Litchfield R, Hawkings R, Dillman CJ, Atkins J, Hagerman G. Rehabilitation for the overhead athlete. *J Orthop Sports Phys Ther.* 1993;18(2):433-441.
9. Lo IKY et al, An evaluation of the apprehension, relocation and surprise tests for anterior shoulder instability. *Am J Sports Med.* 2004;32:301-307.

10. Moynes DR. Prevention of injury to the shoulder through exercises and therapy. *Clin Sports Med.* 1983;2:414-422.

11. Wilk KE, Arrigos C. Current concepts in the rehabilitation of the athletic shoulder. *J Orthop Sports Phys Ther.* 1993;18(1):365-378.

12. Wilk KE, Voight ML, Keirns MA, et al. Stretch-shortening drills for the upper extremities: theory and clinical application. *J Orthop Sports Phys Ther.* 1993;17(5):225-239.

13. Wilk KE, Reinold MM, Dugas JR. Current concepts in the recognition and treatment of superior labral (SLAP) lesions. *J Orthop Sports Phys Ther.* May 2005;35(5): 273-291.

482   SHOULDER SPRAIN/STRAIN | SHOULDER

SHOULDER TENDINITIS
SUMMARY OVERVIEW

ICD-9

716.91   719.41   726.1   726.91   840.3   959.2

APTA Preferred Practice Pattern: **4D, 4E, 4F, 4G, 4J, 7A**

EXAMINATION

- History and Systems Review
- Tests and Measures
  Systems review per APTA's *Guide to Physical Therapy Practice*
  - Joint integrity and mobility
  - Muscle performance
  - Pain
  - Posture
  - ROM
  - Special tests
- Establish Plan of Care

GOALS/OUTCOMES

- ROM
- Pain: 2/10 with resisted motion or following activity, 0/10 at rest
- Strength: Equal to uninvolved side or 4/5 on manual muscle test
- Proper upper extremity motion during gait
- Return to prior functional status and activity level for ADLs and vocational, recreational, and sports activities as identified by patient
- Independence in a progressive home exercise program emphasizing function
- Normal glenohumeral rhythm (timing of scapular and glenohumeral joint movement)
- Functional activities

INTERVENTION
NUMBER OF VISITS: 5–13

- Patient Instruction
  - Basic Anatomy and Biomechanics
  - Handouts
  - Functional Considerations
- Direct Interventions
  - Acute Phase: 2–4 Visits
  - Subacute Phase: 3–9 Visits
- Functional Carryover

DISCHARGE PLANNING AND PATIENT RESPONSIBILITY

- Criteria for Discharge
  - All rehabilitation goals achieved with the possible exceptions listed in the guidelines
- Circumstances Requiring Additional Visits
  - Cervical pathology or radiating signs/symptoms
  - Concomitant presence of adhesive capsulitis
  - Inability to progress because current vocational demands are exacerbating symptoms
  - Special occupational needs that require extensive strengthening
  - Multiple injury sites
  - Presence of ligamentous laxity or labral insufficiency
- Home Program
  - Stretching to regain full mobility
  - Rotator cuff strengthening
  - Home program for strengthening of scapular stabilizers
  - Progression for specific sports or activities
- Monitoring

SHOULDER TENDINITIS

ICD-9

716.91	Arthropathy, unspecified, shoulder region
719.41	Pain in joint, shoulder region
726.1	Rotator cuff syndrome of shoulder and allied disorders
726.91	Exostosis of unspecified site
840.3	Infraspinatus (muscle) (tendon) sprain
959.2	Other and unspecified injury to shoulder and upper arm

APTA Preferred Practice Pattern: 4D, 4E, 4F, 4G, 4J, 7A

EXAMINATION

History and Systems Review

- History of current condition
  - Location, nature, and behavior of symptoms
    - Aggravating/relieving factors
- Other tests and measures
- Past history of current condition
  - Injury to upper extremity or cervical/thoracic spine
  - Surgery
  - Therapeutic intervention
  - Cardiac pathology
- Functional status and activity level (current/prior)
  - Inability to lie on shoulder during sleeping
- Patient's functional goals

Tests and Measures

Systems review per APTA's *Guide to Physical Therapy Practice*

- Joint integrity and mobility
  - Glenohumeral
    - Anterior, posterior, inferior capsule
    - Inferior glenohumeral ligament
  - Acromioclavicular
  - Sternoclavicular
  - Scapulothoracic
- Muscle performance
  - Resisted testing
    - Glenohumeral
    - Scapular
    - Supraspinatus isolation ("empty can" position)
      a. Shoulder is internally rotated, thumb pointed to floor
      b. Abduct the arm to 90°, maintaining a position 30° anterior to the mid-frontal plane
  - Antalgic movement pattern with dressing activities
  - Functional use of upper extremity during gait

- Scapulohumeral rhythm
  - Arms at side
  - Hands on hips
  - Arms elevated 90° in scapular plane
  - Arms elevated, full allowable motion in scapular plane
- Pain
  - Measured on visual analog scale
- Posture
  - Forward head
  - Scapular position
  - Flattening/kyphosis/scoliosis of the thoracic spine
  - Shoulder girdle asymmetry
    - Winging of the scapula
    - Clavicular position
    - Humeral head position
    - Muscular development/atrophy
  - Ability to actively achieve a more balanced postural position
- ROM
  - Cervical screening
    - Active/passive ROM
    - Overpressure
    - Quadrant compression test
  - Shoulder girdle mobility
    - AROM
      a. Flexion/elevation
      b. Observe for inability to maintain depressed humeral head
      c. Abduction
      d. Internal rotation in neutral abduction and 90° of abduction
      e. External rotation in neutral abduction and 90° of abduction
      f. Extension
    - Overpressure
    - PROM

484   SHOULDER TENDINITIS | SHOULDER

- Special tests
  - Apprehension test: Patient supine, involved arm in abduction and external rotation. Push anteriorly on posterior aspect of humeral head.
    - Patient with recurrent dislocation will experience apprehension
    - Patient with anterior instability (subluxation) will experience pain, but not apprehension
    - Patient with normal shoulder will be asymptomatic
  - Relocation test: Administer test with posteriorly directed force on humeral head from apprehension test position
    - Patient with primary impingement will generally have no change in their pain
    - Patient with instability (subluxation) and secondary impingement will have pain relief and will tolerate maximal external rotation with the humeral head maintained in a reduced position
  - Surprise test: Sudden release of posteriorly directed pressure from Relocation test is administered
  - Clunk test: Patient supine, move arm into full flexion and caudal glide, then perform circumduction motion. Positive if clunk, pain, or pseudolocking occurs. Implicates labral tear.
  - Neer's test: Patient seated or supine, place patient's arm in full flexion with no internal or external rotation, then apply flexion overpressure. Pain implicates supraspinatus and long head of biceps.
  - Crossover test: Patient is seated or supine, move patient's arm into full horizontal adduction and apply overpressure. Implications:
    - Subscapularis, supraspinatus, and long head of biceps if pain is anterior
    - Acromioclavicular joint if pain is superior
    - Infraspinatus, teres minor, posterior capsule of pain is posterior
  - Drop test: Patient is seated, passively abduct patient's arm to 90°. Patient is asked to hold arm stationary while examiner administers pressure inferiorly on lateral arm. If arm drops, test implicates rotator cuff rupture.
  - Sulcus sign
    - Patient is seated, arm relaxed at side. Apply inferior distraction. Excessive translation of humeral head with sulcus inferior to acromion is positive test and implicates multidirectional instability.

- Patient is seated, arm abducted to 90° and resting on examiner's shoulder. Apply caudally directed force. Excessive translation of humeral head with sulcus at acromion is positive test and implicates multidirectional instability.
  - Labral Test
    - Compression Rotation Test: Patient supine, glenohumeral joint manually compressed through the long axis of the humerus while humerus is passively rotated through internal and external rotation in an attempt to trap the labrum
    - Pronated Load Test: Patient supine, the glenohumeral joint is abducted to 90° and externally rotated, forearm pronated. When maximum external rotation is achieved, the patient is instructed to perform isometric biceps contraction.
  - Upper limb tension tests (ULTTs)
    - ULTT 1 (median nerve dominant)
      a. Patient supine, depress shoulder, abduct to approximately 110°, supinate forearm, extend elbow, wrist, and fingers
      b. Side bend head/neck both toward and away
      c. Assess normal vs. abnormal response (see Butler. 1991)
    - ULTT 2 (radial nerve dominant)
      a. Patient supine, depress shoulder, shoulder abducted and internally rotated, pronate forearm, extend elbow, and flex the wrist
      b. Side bend head/neck both toward and away
      c. Assess normal vs. abnormal response (see Butler. 1991)
    - ULTT 3 (ulnar nerve dominant)
      a. Patient supine, extend wrist, supinate forearm, fully flex elbow, depress and abduct shoulder
      b. Side bend head/neck both toward and away
      c. Assess normal vs. abnormal response (see Butler. 1991)

A positive response to any of the special tests may lead the clinician to the specific guideline for the implicated structure.

Establish Plan of Care
- Based on history, tests, and measures

GOALS/OUTCOMES

- ROM
  - Shoulder: 90% of AMA guides or equal to uninvolved extremity

	Normal	90%
Flexion	180°	160°
Extension	50°	45°
Abduction	180°	160°
Internal rotation	90°	80°
External rotation	90°	80°

  - Functional cervical ROM or a minimum of 80% of AMA guides:

	Normal	80%
Flexion	60°	50°
Extension	75°	60°
Rotation	80°	65°
Side bend	45°	35°

- Pain: 2/10 with resisted motion or following activity, 0/10 at rest
- Strength: Equal to uninvolved side or 4/5 on manual muscle test
- Proper upper-extremity motion during gait
- Return to prior functional status and activity level for ADLs and vocational, recreational, and sports activities as identified by patient
- Independence in a progressive home exercise program emphasizing function
- Normal glenohumeral rhythm (timing of scapular and glenohumeral joint movement)
- Functional activities
  - Able to reach into back pocket or fasten undergarments
  - Able to comb hair
  - Able to reach into cupboard or lift overhead
  - Perform work/ADL tasks (weight and repetition specific)

INTERVENTION
NUMBER OF VISITS: 5–13

Coordination, Communication, and Documentation

- Provision of services between admission and discharge that facilitate cost-effective and efficient integration or reintegration to home, community, or work
- Documentation of therapeutic intervention is required for each episode of care and serves as the basic foundation for communication
- Coordination and additional communication will depend on the patient's impairment and home/work/community/leisure situation and requirements. Such services may include:
  - Case management
  - Coordination of care and collaboration with those integral to the patient's rehabilitation program
  - Coordination and monitoring of the delivery of available resources
  - Referrals to other health-care professionals
  - Identification of resources, support groups, or advocacy services
  - Provision of educational or training information
  - Technical assistance
- Specific coordination and communication provisions
  - Orthopedic surgeon
  - Rheumatologist

Patient Instruction

Basic Anatomy and Biomechanics
- Musculature and tendon attachments, ligaments, and joint structure in relation to shoulder motion
- Pertinent Gray's Anatomy (Gray. 1995. 627–632, 839–842)
- Pathology of tendinitis
- Relationship of posture to onset of symptoms
- Role of adequate lower-extremity and trunk motor performance to generate force at the glenohumeral joint

Handouts
- Specific home program
  - Use of cryotherapy
  - Self-friction massage

486   SHOULDER TENDINITIS | SHOULDER

- Commercially available products, such as:
  - Krames Communications (1100 Grundy Lane, San Bruno, CA 94066):
    - *Shoulder Owner's Manual*
    - *Rotator Cuff Injuries*

Functional Considerations
- Reduction of motions causing overload forces
- Proper shoulder mechanics in daily activity
- Avoidance of repetitive motions

Direct Interventions

Acute Phase: 2–4 Visits
- Therapeutic exercise and home program
  - Assisted stretching in pain-free ROM
    - Cervical/thoracic spine
    - Shoulder girdle
    - Elbow
  - Initiate manually resisted exercises in pain-free ROM
  - PROM
    - Pulley
    - Wand
  - Pain-free AROM
  - High-repetition and low-resistance with purpose of promoting vascularization in healing tissues
    - Internal/external rotation
      a. May need to use apparatus to support elbow for pain-free ROM
    - Supraspinatus isolation ("empty can" position)
      a. Shoulder is internally rotated, thumb pointed to floor
      b. Abduct the arm to 90°, maintaining a position 30° anterior to the mid-frontal plane
    - Scapular retraction/depression
    - Upper body ergometry
  - Postural correction exercises
  - Neuromuscular/balance/proprioceptive reeducation
    - Pain-free modified plantargrade position for elbow propping
    - Bodyblade®
  - Cardiovascular conditioning
    - Walking program
    - Lower-extremity cycling
- Manual therapy
  - Soft-tissue techniques
    - Soft-tissue mobilization to the scapular stabilizer and rotator cuff musculature
    - Friction massage within pain tolerance
    - Myofascial release
  - Joint mobilization
    - Joint mobilization to restore proper joint mechanics to the shoulder girdle, including acromioclavicular, sternoclavicular, scapulothoracic regions, and first and second rings of thoracic spine; ensure posterior capsule mobility is normal
    - Grades III–V to cervical/thoracic spinal hypomobilities
- Electrotherapeutic modalities
  - Iontophoresis
- Physical agents and mechanical modalities
  - Cryotherapy
  - Athermal, deep thermal modalities
- Goals
  - Pain: 5/10 with resistive motion, 2/10 at rest
  - Pain-free ROM: 50% AMA guides
    - Flexion: 90°
    - Extension: 25°
    - Abduction: 90°
    - Internal rotation: 45°
    - External rotation: 45°
  - Patient utilizes scapular stabilization with static posture

Subacute Phase: 3–9 Visits
- Therapeutic exercise and home program
  - Manual resistive exercises: Isometric, isotonic
  - Progress passive stretches in pain-free ROM
    - Glide hand forward and horizontally on table, hold at end point
    - Pectorals
    - Shoulder complex
    - Cervical/thoracic spine
  - Cardiovascular conditioning
    - Walking program
    - Ski machine
  - Progressive strengthening utilizing isometric, pulley, resistive bands, or free-weight resistance
  - As patient accomplishes pain-free, high-repetition, low-load exercises (1 set of 30 reps), progress to strengthening with moderate load (3 sets of 10 reps)
    - Rotator cuff with emphasis on involved tendon
    - Scapular retraction/depression

- Diagonal and functional patterns
  - Flexibility exercises
    - Pectorals
    - Internal rotators
  - Neuromuscular/balance/proprioceptive reeducation
    - Hands-knees
    - Three-point rocking
    - Push-ups
    - Push-ups off therapeutic ball
    - Bodyblade®
  - Plyometrics
    - Underhand
    - Two-handed
    - Overhand
  - Sport- or activity-specific training
- Manual therapy
  - Joint mobilization
    - Grades II–IV to restore glenohumeral capsular mobility
    - Progressive mobilization to persistent hypomobilities in the shoulder complex or spinal region
  - Continue effective soft-tissue techniques
    - Friction massage
- Physical agents and mechanical modalities
  - Continue effective modalities as in acute phase with increased emphasis on use as needed at home
- Goals
  - Pain: 2/10 with resisted motion, 0/10 at rest
  - Functional activities
    - Able to reach into back pocket or fasten undergarments
    - Able to comb hair
    - Able to reach into cupboard or lift overhead
    - Perform work/ADL tasks (weight and repetition specific)
  - Shoulder ROM: 90% AMA guides
    - Flexion: 160°
    - Extension: 45°
    - Abduction: 160°
    - External rotation: 80°
    - Internal rotation: 80°
  - Strength: 4/5 on a manual muscle test for shoulder girdle musculature

Functional Carryover
- Modification of activity to reduce load on bicipital or supraspinatus tendon
- Avoidance of repetitive motion that aggravates symptoms
- To avoid symptoms: Warm-up prior to activity; cryotherapy and stretching after activity

DISCHARGE PLANNING AND PATIENT RESPONSIBILITY

Criteria for Discharge
- All rehabilitation goals achieved, except may be discharged
  - With 90% of shoulder ROM
  - With 4/5 on a manual muscle test if all other rehabilitation goals achieved
  - Prior to attaining previous level of participation in sports or recreational activities
  - If the therapist determines that further progression and attainment of all rehabilitation goals will be achieved with patient's continued efforts/compliance with home program outside the clinical environment

Circumstances Requiring Additional Visits
- Cervical pathology or radiating signs/symptoms
- Concomitant presence of adhesive capsulitis
- Inability to progress because current vocational demands are exacerbating symptoms
- Special occupational needs that require extensive strengthening
- Multiple injury sites
- Presence of ligamentous laxity or labral insufficiency

Home Program
- Stretching to regain full mobility
- Rotator cuff strengthening
- Home program for strengthening of scapular stabilizers
- Progression for specific sport or activities

Monitoring
- Instruct patient to call for advice should progression halt or a negative trend occur
- Instruct patient to recheck/call at 2–4 weeks post-discharge to ensure expected return to function, healing, and progression to attaining all rehabilitation goals

REFERENCES

1. American Physical Therapy Association. *Guide to Physical Therapist Practice.* Alexandria, VA: APTA; 1997.

2. Butler DS. *Mobilization of the Nervous System.* Melbourne, Australia: Churchill Livingstone; 1991.

3. Cyriax, J. *Textbook of Orthopedic Medicine. Vol I. Diagnosis of Soft Tissue Lesion.* Baltimore, MD: Williams & Wilkins; 1969.

4. Engelberg AL. *Guides to the Evaluation of Permanent Impairment.* 3rd ed. Chicago, IL: American Medical Association; 1989.

5. Gerber C, Terrier S, Ganz R. The role of the corocoid process in the chronic impingement syndrome. *J Bone Joint Surg.* 1985;67B:703-708.

6. Gray H; Williams PL, ed. *Gray's Anatomy.* 38th ed. New York, NY: Churchill Livingstone; 1995.

7. Haskins RJ, Abrams JS. Impingement syndrome in the absence of rotator cuff tear (stages 1 and 2). *Orthop Clin North Am.* 1987;18:373-382.

8. Kamar A, Irrgang JJ, Whitney SL. Nonoperative management of secondary shoulder impingement syndrome. *J Orthop Sports Phys Ther.* 1993;17(5):212-224.

9. Kessler RM, Hertling D. *Management of Common Musculoskeletal Disorders.* 2nd ed. Philadelphia, PA: JB Lippincott; 1990.

10. Kronberg M, Nemeth G, Brostrom L. Muscle activity and coordination in the normal shoulder. *Clin Orthop Rel Res.* 1990;257:76-85.

11. Mulligan E. Conservative management of shoulder impingement syndrome. *Athl Train.* 1988;23:348-353.

12. Reid DC. *Sports Injury Assessment and Rehabilitation.* New York, NY: Churchill Livingstone; 1992.

13. Saunders D. *Evaluation, Treatment and Prevention of Musculoskeletal Disorders.* 3rd ed. Bloomington, MN: Saunders Group; 1993.

14. Thein LA. Impingement syndrome and its conservative management. *J Orthop Sports Phys Ther.* 1989;11(5):183-191.

15. Warner JP, Micheli LJ, Arslanian IE, Kennedy J, Kennedy R. Patterns of flexibility, laxity, and strength in normal shoulders and shoulders with instability and impingement. *Am J Sports Med.* 1990;18:366-375.

16. Wilk KE, Reinold MM, Dugas JR. Current concepts in the recognition and treatment of superior labral (SLAP) lesions. *J Orthop Sports Phys Ther.* May 2005;35(5): 273-291.

490   SHOULDER TENDINITIS | SHOULDER

Elbow

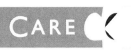

Elbow

Elbow Fracture (Closed)	493
Elbow/Hand Enthesopathy (Other Disorders of the Synovium, Tendon, and Bursa)	498
Elbow Joint Pathology	506
Elbow Sprain/Strain	511
Lateral Epicondylitis	517
Medial Epicondylitis	523
Ulnar Nerve Lesion	530

492   ELBOW

ELBOW FRACTURE (CLOSED)
SUMMARY OVERVIEW

ICD-9

813.0

APTA Preferred Practice Pattern: 4G, 4I

EXAMINATION

- History and Systems Review
- Tests and Measures

  Systems review per APTA's *Guide to Physical Therapy Practice*
  - Anthropometric characteristics
  - Integumentary integrity
  - Joint integrity and mobility
  - Muscle performance
  - Neural integrity
  - Orthotic, protective, and supportive devices
  - Pain
  - Posture
  - ROM
  - Reflex Integrity
  - Self-care and home management
  - Sensory integrity
  - Work (job/school/play), community, and leisure integration or reintegration (including instrumental ADLs)
- Establish Plan of Care

GOALS/OUTCOMES

- ROM
- Muscle performance
- Return to prior functional status and activity level for ADLs and vocational, recreational, and sports activities as identified by patient
- Pain: 2/10 or less on the visual analog scale

INTERVENTION
NUMBER OF VISITS: 6–16

- Patient Instruction
  - Basic Anatomy and Biomechanics
  - Handouts
  - Functional Considerations
- Direct Interventions
  - Acute Phase: 3–8 Visits
  - Subacute Phase: 3–8 Visits
- Functional Carryover

DISCHARGE PLANNING AND PATIENT RESPONSIBILITY

- Criteria for Discharge
  - ROM and strength approach the 80% range of normal parameters in the involved joints
  - Return to normal work duties
  - Pain: 2/10 on visual analog scale
- Circumstances Requiring Additional Visits
  - Postoperative complications such as neuropathy, contracture, open wounds, etc.
  - Environmental barriers in home or work that prevent effective or safe return to full function
  - Multiple areas of injury and dysfunction
  - Presence of other medical conditions, such as severe arthritis, cardiopulmonary disease limiting rehabilitation progression, osteopenia or osteoporosis, cognitive impairments, etc.
  - Transportation restrictions limiting access to physical therapy care
- Home Program
  - Wearing schedule and maintenance of splint, brace, and cast when appropriate
  - Use of home modalities to control pain and swelling
  - Ergonomic instructions relative to physical limitations
  - Home exercise program provided in clear hard copy form for clarity. The program should facilitate full return in ROM and strength and progress to more complex tasks involving lifting, reaching, and work readiness when appropriate.
- Monitoring

SUMMARY OVERVIEW | ELBOW | ELBOW FRACTURE (CLOSED)   493

ELBOW FRACTURE (CLOSED)

ICD-9
>   813.0   Closed fracture of upper end of radius and ulna

APTA Preferred Practice Pattern: **4G, 4I**

EXAMINATION

History and Systems Review

- History of current condition, including mechanism of injury, date of onset, and nature of symptoms (somatic, radicular, vascular)
- Medical reports: Radiology, surgical, etc.
- Medications
- Past medical/surgical history
- Functional status and activity level (current/prior)
- Patient's functional goals

Tests and Measures

Systems review per APTA's *Guide to Physical Therapy Practice*

- Anthropometric characteristics
  Note: Displaced fractures, anatomic neck fractures in a child, as well as supracondylar fractures, with or without displacement, require emergency orthopedic consult. Forearm fractures require thorough wrist exam due to the high incidence of distal radioulnar joint injuries.
  ○ Circulation (arterial, venous, lymphatic) of the entire upper extremity relative to norms and the other upper extremity
- Integumentary integrity of the upper extremity
- Joint integrity and mobility
  ○ Glenhoumeral motion
    ▪ Stress tests
    ▪ Articular motion: Anterior, posterior, inferior, superior, lateral glides
  ○ Elbow motion
    ▪ Stress tests
    ▪ Articular glides
      a. Humeral ulnar
      b. Humeral radial
      c. Proximal radioulnar
      d. Distal radioulnar
- Muscle performance (including strength, power, and endurance) of the shoulder, elbow, wrist, and hand
- Neural integrity (peripheral): Radial, median, ulnar, etc.
- Orthotic, protective, and supportive devices

- Pain
  ○ Measured on visual analog scale
- Posture assessment in the way the arm is held along with an assessment of scapula, cervical, and thoracic spine position
- ROM (including muscle length)
  ○ Shoulder: Angular motion of flexion, extension, abduction, adduction, horizontal abduction, horizontal adduction, internal rotation, external rotation
  ○ Elbow: Angular motion of flexion (pronation), flexion (supination), extension (pronation), extension (supination)
  ○ Wrist and hand motion
- Reflex Integrity: C5 deltoid, C6 biceps, C7 triceps
- Self-care and home management (including ADLs and instrumental ADLs)
- Sensory integrity of the upper extremity
- Work (job/school/play), community, and leisure integration or reintegration (including instrumental ADLs)

Establish Plan of Care

- Based on history, tests, and measures

GOALS/OUTCOMES

- ROM
  ○ Elbow 0–140°, forearm 80° of supination and pronation, wrist 60° of flexion and extension, and full closure (fist) of the hand
  ○ Full ROM of the shoulder to include 160° of elevation or within 10% of uninvolved extremity, external rotation to 60°, and functional reach up back to upper lumbar level
- Muscle performance
  ○ Full strength and endurance, including 5/5 manual muscle test of the functional hand, grip strength within 90% of uninvolved hand or within normal parameters of age/gender norms. Full strength 5/5 of the major shoulder muscles.

- Return to prior functional status and activity level for ADLs and vocational, recreational, and sports activities as identified by patient
- Pain: 2/10 or less on visual analog scale

INTERVENTION
NUMBER OF VISITS: 6–16

Coordination, Communication, and Documentation
- Provision of services between admission and discharge that facilitate cost-effective and efficient integration or reintegration to home, community, or work
- Documentation of therapeutic intervention is required for each episode of care and serves as the basic foundation for communication
- Coordination and additional communication will depend on the patient's impairment and home/work/community/leisure situation and requirements. Such services may include:
  - Case management
  - Coordination of care and collaboration with those integral to the patient's rehabilitation program
  - Coordination and monitoring of the delivery of available resources
  - Referrals to other health-care professionals
  - Identification of resources, support groups, or advocacy services
  - Provision of educational or training information
  - Technical assistance

Patient Instruction

Basic Anatomy and Biomechanics
- Gray's Anatomy

Handouts
- Home program for regaining functional reach, carry, lift, and fine motor skills for ADLs, work, and recreation. Consider VHI program or other like diagrams for clarity and prescription.

Functional Considerations
- Posture (sitting, standing, sleeping, and driving)
- Precautions: Relating to use of splints or braces during daytime and nighttime periods regarding neurovascular compromise, skin changes, etc.

- Alteration of ADLs
- Positioning for relief of symptoms: Loose packed position of shoulder, elbow, forearm, and wrist
- Body mechanics instruction should include protection of fracture regions to avoid premature stress and re-injury
- Training recommendations (cross training, periodization, etc.). Maintain aerobic activity and dynamic exercise to opposite and remote extremities for crossover training benefits.

Direct Interventions

Acute Phase: 3–8 Visits
- Pain modulation and decreasing inflammatory state via use of appropriate modalities, positioning of involved extremity, and activities to avoid in the fracture regions
- Appropriate exercise dosage, intensity, and monitoring
- Scar management using deep transverse friction when indicated
- Joint mobilization for pain modulation (Maitland Grade I–II mobilizations where pain barrier precedes or meets the physiological barrier)
- Endurance training with upper body ergometer light loading to emphasize duration and early mobilization
- Splint management when indicated for early scar mobilization and return of motion

Subacute Phase: 3–8 Visits
- Joint mobilization progression to Maitland Grade III–IV mobilizations when indicated (pain barrier meets or exceeds physiological barrier)
- Appropriate exercise dosage, intensity, and monitoring to assure continued gains in strength, ROM, and coordination
- Neuromuscular reeducation training (proprioceptive neuromuscular facilitation, Bodyblade®, ball toss, etc.)
- Continued endurance training upper body ergometer with gradual increase in resistance, etc.
- Scar management with deep transverse friction massage for improved elasticity and ROM
- Splint management with progression in settings, wear time, and positions to maximize ROM
- Modalities for post-exercise pain, inflammation, and stiffness

Functional Carryover

- Integration of home exercise program into vocational environment
- Completion of ergonomic adjustments to home, automobile, and vocational areas
- Incorporation of proper posture and body mechanics to avoid exacerbation of symptoms
- Recognition/avoidance of activities that increase or exacerbate radiating symptoms

DISCHARGE PLANNING AND PATIENT RESPONSIBILITY

Criteria for Discharge

- ROM and strength approach the 80% range of normal parameters in the involved joints
- Return to normal work duties
- Pain: 2/10 on visual analog scale

Circumstances Requiring Additional Visits

- Postoperative complications, such as neuropathy, contracture, open wounds, etc.
- Environmental barriers in home or work that prevent effective or safe return to full function
- Multiple areas of injury and dysfunction
- Presence of other medical conditions, such as severe arthritis, cardiopulmonary disease limiting rehabilitation progression, osteopenia or osteoporosis, cognitive impairments, etc.
- Transportation restrictions limiting access to physical therapy care

Home Program

- Wearing schedule and maintenance of splint, brace, cast when appropriate
- Use of home modalities to control pain and swelling
- Ergonomic instructions relative to physical limitations
- Home exercise program provided in clear hard copy form for clarity. The program should facilitate full return in ROM and strength and progress to more complex tasks involving lifting, reaching, and work readiness when appropriate.

Monitoring

- Consider follow physical therapy 1–2 months after discharge to check status of elbow ROM, strength, and function. Home exercise program may be progressed or reviewed.
- Follow-up with physician should be encouraged when appropriate regarding fracture healing, open wound management, testing for complications of neurovascular compromise, etc.

REFERENCES

1. American Physical Therapy Association. *Guide to Physical Therapist Practice.* Alexandria, VA: APTA; 2003.
2. Cyriax J. *Textbook of Orthopaedic Medicine.* 8th ed. Tindall, England: Bailliere; 1982.
3. Gray H; Williams PL, ed. *Gray's Anatomy.* 38th ed. New York, NY: Churchill Livingstone; 1995.
4. Richardson J, Iglarsh Z. *Clinical Orthopaedic Physical Therapy.* WB Sanders; 1993.

ELBOW/HAND ENTHESOPATHY (OTHER DISORDERS OF THE SYNOVIUM, TENDON, AND BURSA)

SUMMARY OVERVIEW

ICD-9

> 726.3   726.4   727.0

APTA Preferred Practice Pattern: 4D, 4E, 4F, 4I

EXAMINATION

- History and Systems Review
- Tests and Measures
  - Anthropometric characteristics
  - Ergonomics and body mechanics
  - Joint and integumentary integrity
  - Muscle performance
  - Mobility
  - Pain
  - Posture
  - Self-care and home management (including ADLs and instrumental ADLs)
  - Special tests
- Establish Plan of Care

GOALS/OUTCOMES

- Pain: Less than 2/10 with activity, 0/10 at rest
- Restoration of flexibility/extensibility of the forearm muscle tendon complex to restore functional use equal to the uninvolved side or 100% of the AMA guidelines
- ROM

INTERVENTION
NUMBER OF VISITS: 5–11

- Patient Instruction
  - Basic Anatomy and Biomechanics
  - Handouts
  - Functional Considerations
- Direct Interventions
  - Acute Phase: 1–5 Visits
  - Subacute Phase: 4–6 Visits
- Functional Carryover

DISCHARGE PLANNING AND PATIENT RESPONSIBILITY

- Criteria for Discharge
  - All goals/outcomes achieved, except may discharge at 80% grip strength or 4+/5 manual muscle test
  - Demonstrates understanding of guidelines to prevent exacerbation of symptoms
- Circumstances Requiring Additional Visits
  - Severe degenerative changes
  - History of other pathology
  - Presence of other medical conditions
  - Contractures
  - Cognitive limitations
  - Postoperative complications
  - Excessive environmental barriers to discharge
- Home Program
  - Written exercise program as well as splint wearing and home modality instructions
- Monitoring

SUMMARY OVERVIEW | ELBOW | ELBOW/HAND ENTHESOPATHY   497

ELBOW/HAND ENTHESOPATHY (OTHER DISORDERS OF THE SYNOVIUM, TENDON, AND BURSA)

ICD-9

726.3	Enthesopathy of elbow region
726.4	Enthesopathy of wrist and carpus
727.0	Synovitis and tenosynovitis

APTA Preferred Practice Pattern: 4D, 4E, 4F, 4I

EXAMINATION

History and Systems Review

- History of current condition
  - Date and mechanism of injury/onset
  - Location, nature, and behavior of symptoms
    - Aggravating/relieving symptoms
    - a.m./p.m.
  - Direct intervention
    - Splints/orthotics
- Past history of current condition
  - Cervical spine or upper-extremity injury
  - Surgery
  - Therapeutic intervention
- Other tests and measures
- Medications
- Past medical/surgical history
  - Metabolic or autoimmune diseases
- Functional status and activity level (current/prior)
  - Job duties
  - ADLs
  - Leisure and sports activities
- Patient's functional goals

Tests and Measures

Systems review per APTA's *Guide to Physical Therapy Practice*

- Anthropometric characteristics
  - Comparative circumferential measurement for edema
    - Distal metacarpal heads 2–5 cm
    - Distal palmar crease
    - Wrist creases
    - 10 cm proximal to wrist crease
    - 10 cm distal to lateral/medial epicondyle
    - Lateral/medial epicondyle
    - 10 cm proximal to epicondyle
  - Volumetric measurement for edema
  - Atrophy

- Ergonomics and body mechanics
  - Description of movements and positioning required for job duties and leisure/sports activities
  - Current and prior modifications made to work/leisure/sports activities
- Joint and integumentary integrity
  - Palpation
    - Extensor pollicis longus
    - Abductor pollicis longus
    - Extensor carpi radialis longus
    - Extensor carpi radialis brevis
    - Common extensor origin
    - Common flexor origin
    - Extensor carpi ulnaris
    - Flexor carpi ulnaris
    - Dorsum of 5th metacarpal
    - Radial styloid
  - Deformities
  - Atrophy
  - Skin color and temperature
- Mobility
  - Active/passive ROM, overpressure
    - Elbow flexion/extension
    - Forearm supination/pronation
    - Wrist flexion/extension
    - Radial/ulnar deviation
    - Thumb flexion/extension/abduction/adduction/opposition/circumduction
    - Humeroradial
    - Proximal radioulnar
    - Distal radioulnar
- Muscle performance (including strength, power, and endurance)
  - Manual muscle test
    - C6–7 nerve root
    - Forearm, wrist, and digits
  - Functional use of arm during gait

498   ELBOW/HAND ENTHESOPATHY | ELBOW

- Resisted testing
  - Grip strength
  - Lateral, tip, and palmar pinch
- Pain
  - Measured on visual analog scale
- Posture
  - Forward head posture
  - Shoulder position
  - Shoulder height
  - Carrying angle
  - Guarded/protective posture of hand/wrist/elbow
- Self-care and home management (including ADLs and instrumental ADLs)
  - Limitations
  - Current and prior modifications
- Special tests
  - Clear cervical spine
    - AROM
    - Overpressure
    - Quadrant compression test
  - Contractile tissue assessment in neutral and lengthened position
    - Specific length test for the extensor mechanism (wrist flexion, elbow extension, forearm pronation)
    - Specific length test for the flexor mechanism (wrist extension, elbow extension, supination, finger extension)
  - Upper limb tension tests (ULTTs)
    - ULTT 1 (median nerve bias)
      a. Patient supine, depress shoulder, abduct to approximately 110°, supinate forearm, and extend elbow, wrist, and fingers
      b. Side bend head/neck both toward and away
      c. Assess normal vs. abnormal response (see Butler. 1991)
    - ULTT 2 (radial nerve bias)
      a. Patient supine; depress, abduct, and internally rotate shoulder; pronate forearm, extend elbow, flex the wrist and thumb
      b. Side bend head/neck both toward and away
      c. Assess normal vs. abnormal response (see Butler. 1991)
    - ULTT 3 (ulnar nerve bias)
      a. Patient supine; extend wrist, supinate forearm, fully flex elbow, depress and abduct shoulder
      b. Side bend head/neck both toward and away
      c. Assess normal vs. abnormal response (see Butler. 1991)

- Finkelstein's test
  - Patient flexes thumb into palm, making fist over thumb
  - Wrist is passively deviated ulnarly
  - Positive test produces localized pain over abductor pollicis longus and extensor pollicis longus
- Subluxation of the extensor carpi ulnaris tendon
  - With forearm pronated, palpate extensor carpi ulnaris tendon at the ulnar styloid
  - Patient supinates forearm
  - Positive test produces movement of the extensor carpi ulnaris tendon dorsally over the ulnar styloid
- Grind test
  - With the forearm in neutral position, thumb relaxed, examiner stabilizes the wrist and forearm
  - Mild axial compression and gentle rotation is applied to the 1st metacarpal
  - A positive test produces pain in the trapezial metacarpal joint and indicates osteoarthritis of the trapezial metacarpal joint
- Middle finger test
  - With the shoulder flexed to 75–90°, elbow extended, wrist neutral, fingers extended and abducted, the examiner presses down on the middle finger while the patient attempts to keep the middle finger from flexing
  - A positive test produces pain at the common extensor origin or in the extensor muscle mass

Establish Plan of Care

- Based on history, tests, and measures

GOALS/OUTCOMES

- Pain: less than 2/10 with activity, 0/10 at rest
- Restoration of flexibility/extensibility of the forearm muscle tendon complex to restore functional use equal to the uninvolved side or 100% of the AMA guidelines
- ROM
  - Hand: Ability to form a full fist
  - Fingers
    - Metacarpal phalangeal: 0–90°
    - Proximal interphalangeal: 0–100°
    - Distal Interphalangeal: Full opposition of thumb

- Thumb
  - Metacarpal phalangeal: 0–60°
  - Interphalangeal: 0–80°
  - Radial abduction: 50°
  - Adduction: 0 cm
  - Opposition: 0 cm thumb tip to small finger tip when thumbnail is parallel to the plane of the palm
- Wrist
  - Flexion: 80°
  - Extension: 70°
  - Ulnar deviation: 30°
  - Radial deviation: 20°
- Forearm
  - Supination: 80°+
  - Pronation: 80°+
- Elbow
  - Flexion: 140°+
  - Extension: 0°
- Composite motions
  - Achieve pain-free simultaneous/composite motion of digits, wrist, forearm, and elbow
    a. Composite/simultaneous extension: Finger extension, wrist extension, forearm supination, elbow extension
    b. Composite/simultaneous flexion: Finger flexion, wrist flexion, forearm pronation, elbow extension
    c. Composite/simultaneous radial deviation: Thumb flexion, wrist ulnar deviation, elbow extension (Finkelstein's position)
- Strength
  - 5/5 elbow, wrist, forearm, hand manual muscle test
  - Grip and pinch strength equal to the uninvolved extremity (*if bilateral involvement grip and pinch strength 75% of Mathiowitz norms*)
  - Return to prior functional status and activity level for ADLs and vocational, recreational, and sports activities as identified by the patient.
  - Independence in a progressive home exercise program emphasizing function

INTERVENTION
NUMBER OF VISITS: 5–11

Coordination, Communication, and Documentation

- Provision of services between admission and discharge that facilitate cost-effective and efficient integration or reintegration to home, community, or work
- Documentation of therapeutic intervention is required for each episode of care and serves as the basic foundation for communication
- Coordination and additional communication will depend on the patient's impairment and home/work/community/leisure situation and requirements. Such services may include:
  - Case management
  - Coordination of care and collaboration with those integral to the patient's rehabilitation program
  - Coordination and monitoring of the delivery of available resources
  - Referrals to other health-care professionals
  - Identification of resources, support groups, or advocacy services
  - Provision of educational or training information
  - Technical assistance
- Specific coordination and communication provisions

Patient Instruction

Basic Anatomy and Biomechanics

- Instruction regarding the biomechanics and the positional stress placed on the extensor mechanism when performing simultaneous grip, wrist flexion, forearm pronation, and full elbow extension
- Etiology of repetitive trauma
- Pathology of tendinitis/tendinosis and the tissue response to fatigue that results in micro trauma
- Strategies and techniques to avoid positional stress

Handouts

- Commercially available products, such as:
  - Krames Communications (1100 Grundy Lane, San Bruno, CA 94066)
    - *Preventing Repetitive Motion Injuries*
    - *Elbow Owner's Manual*
    - *Exercises at Your Work Station*
    - *Preventing Repetitive Strain at the Keyboard*

○ Specific home program
- Taping techniques
- Exercise
- Cryotherapy
- Self-friction
- Use of orthotics

Functional Considerations
- Posture of upper extremity
- Modification or avoidance of provocative postures, positions, or activities
- Assistive devices
  ○ Extensor tendon band
  ○ Thumb immobilization splints
  ○ Wrist immobilization splints
- Alteration of ADLs or sport and leisure activities
- Avoidance of prolonged postures
- Positioning for relief of symptoms
- Body mechanic instruction for lifting, pushing, pulling, etc.
- Training recommendations (cross training, periodization, etc.)

Direct Interventions

Acute Phase: 1–5 Visits
- Therapeutic exercise and home program to be performed 6 times per day. Pain is indicator of overload.
  ○ Finger and thumb abduction/adduction
  ○ Metacarpal phalangeal flexion, proximal interphalangeal/distal interphalangeal extension
  ○ Thumb held in protected abduction position initially, progress to full thumb flexion as tolerated
  ○ Thumb radial and palmar abduction
  ○ Opposition initiated to index finger only, progress to middle finger, ring finger, and small finger as tolerated
  ○ Wrist flexion/extension initiated with elbow bent, progress to elbow extended as tolerated
  ○ Wrist radial and ulnar deviation initiated with wrist in neutral position, progress to full ulnar deviation with elbow extended as tolerated
  ○ Forearm pronation/supination
- Manual therapy techniques
  ○ Soft-tissue mobilization
    - Cross-friction massage
    - Dorsal and volar forearm

- Common extensor and flexor origins
- Therapeutic devices and equipment
  ○ Forearm-based thumb spica splint
    - Wrist extended 15–20°
    - Thumb in position of functional prehension—to allow opposition of thumb to index finger
    - Thumb interphalangeal joint is free
    - Initially worn at all times. Progress to wear while sleeping, driving, or times when thumb/hand motion cannot be protected.
  ○ Resting wrist splint
    - Wrist extended 15–20°
    - Finger metacarpal phalangeals free
    - Thumb free if not symptomatic
  ○ Elbow compression band
- Electrotherapeutic modalities
  ○ Iontophoresis
  ○ TENS
  ○ Electrotherapy
- Physical agents and mechanical modalities
  ○ Cryotherapy
  ○ Athermal and thermal modalities
- Goals/outcomes
  ○ Pain: 5/10 or less with activity, 2/10 or less at rest
  ○ Decreased inflammation as noted by reduced edema and tenderness to palpation
  ○ Improved ROM to achieve full AROM of hand, wrist, forearm, and elbow
  ○ Pain-free ability to make a fist

Subacute Phase: 4–6 Visits
- Therapeutic exercise and home program
  ○ Begin limited, gradual resumption of functional activities with explicit parameters for level and type of activity that may be performed
    - Instruction regarding postures and positions that load or unload the affected tissues
  ○ Continue muscle flexibility and lengthening exercises
    - Composite/simultaneous motion of finger extension, wrist extension, forearm supination, elbow extension
    - Composite/simultaneous motion of finger flexion, wrist flexion, forearm pronation, elbow extension

- Composite/simultaneous motion of thumb flexion, wrist ulnar deviation, and elbow extension (Finkelstein's position)
  - Shoulder girdle
  - Cervical spine
- Strengthening exercises
  - Concentric and eccentric contraction
  - Manual resistance, resistive band, resistive therapy putty, and grip strengthening devices
  - Progressive resistive exercises in all planes for hand, wrist, forearm, and elbow
  - Initiate exercises with elbow flexed to 90° and progress to elbow extended with shoulder at 60–90°
  - Initiate hand, wrist, and forearm with ½ lb weight or light resistance
  - Initiate elbow with 1 lb weight or medium resistance
  - Progress to minimum of 5 lbs or heavy resistance
- Upper-extremity conditioning program
  - Upper body ergometry
  - Multi-planar strengthening of the shoulder and upper quarter
- Plyometrics with weighted ball
- Sport, work, and/or activity-specific training
  - Work task simulation
- Cardiovascular endurance
  - Continue bike, swim; may add treadmill, elliptical as tolerated
- Postural correction techniques
- Manual therapy techniques
  - Joint mobilization
    - Progress graded mobilization to persistent areas of hypomobility
  - Soft-tissue techniques
    - Cross-friction massage
    - Myofascial release
    - Soft-tissue mobilization
  - Passive stretches
    - Composite/simultaneous motion of finger extension, wrist extension, forearm supination, and elbow extension
    - Composite/simultaneous motion of finger flexion, wrist flexion, forearm pronation, and elbow extension
    - Composite/simultaneous motion of thumb flexion, wrist ulnar deviation, and elbow extension (Finkelstein's position)

- Shoulder girdle
- Cervical spine
- Physical agents and mechanical modalities
  - Continue effective modalities as in acute phase with emphasis on use as needed at home
- Goals/outcomes
  - Pain: 2/10 or less during activity, 0/10 at rest
  - Increased ROM: Achieve pain-free simultaneous/composite motion of digits, wrist, forearm, and elbow
    - Composite/simultaneous extension: Finger extension, wrist extension, forearm supination, and elbow extension
    - Composite/simultaneous flexion: Finger flexion, wrist flexion, forearm pronation, and elbow extension
    - Composite/simultaneous radial deviation: Thumb flexion, wrist ulnar deviation, and elbow extension (Finkelstein's position)
  - Increased muscle performance to achieve manual muscle test of 5/5 for wrist, forearm, and elbow in all planes
  - Grip strength: 90% of mean for age/gender norms

Functional Carryover

- Gradual resumption of activities as tolerated, including work, sport, leisure, and ADL activities
- Recognition/avoidance of activities and postures that increase or exacerbate symptoms
- Recognition/incorporation of activities and postures that decrease or relieve symptoms
- Incorporate proper posture, body mechanics, activities, and work practices to reduce loads on muscles of shoulder girdle, elbow, forearm, wrist, and digits
- Use of natural breaks in work activity to incorporate stretches from home exercise program
- Use of micro-breaks to promote muscle relaxation for improved circulation and nerve conduction to affected tissues
- Completion of ergonomic modifications and alterations to home, sports, leisure, and vocational tools, equipment, and environment

DISCHARGE PLANNING AND PATIENT RESPONSIBILITY

Criteria for Discharge
- All goals/outcomes achieved, except may discharge at 80% grip strength or 4+/5 manual muscle test
- Demonstrates understanding of guidelines to prevent exacerbation of symptoms, including:
  - Early recognition of signs of injury or exacerbation
  - Postures, positioning, and techniques/practices that promote tissue recovery
  - Modifications to vocational, recreational, and sports tools, equipment, and environment
  - Composite/simultaneous stretching techniques

Circumstances Requiring Additional Visits
- Severe degenerative changes
- History of other pathology
- Presence of other medical conditions
- Contractures
- Cognitive limitations
- Postoperative complications
- Excessive environmental barriers to discharge

Home Program
- Written exercise program as well as splint wearing and home modality instructions

Monitoring
- Patient may phone the clinic or be scheduled for a recheck at 2–4 weeks post-discharge to ensure progression toward achieving all goals and outcomes

REFERENCES

1. American Physical Therapy Association. *Guide to Physical Therapist Practice*. Alexandria, VA: APTA; revised 2003.
2. American Academy of Orthopedic Surgeons. *Joint Motion: Method of Measuring and Recording*. Chicago, IL: AAOS; 1965.
3. Butler DS. *Mobilization of the Nervous System*. Melbourne, Australia: Churchill Livingstone; 1991.
4. Danda D, Shyam Kumar NK, Cherian R, Cherian AM. Enthesopathy: clinical recognition and significance. *Natl Med J India*. Mar-Apr 2001;14(2):90-2.
5. Elvey RL. The investigation of arm pain. In: Grieve GP, ed. *Modern manual of therapy of the vertebral column*. Edinburgh: Churchill Livingstone; 1986.
6. Grundberg AB, Reagan DS. Pathologic anatomy of the forearm: intersection syndrome. *J Hand Surg*. Mar 1985;10(2):299-302.
7. Hunter J, Mackin E, Callahan A, ed. *Rehabilitation of the Hand*. St Louis, MO: CV Mosby; 2002.
8. Hertling D, Kessler RM. *Management of Common Musculoskeletal Disorders*. 2nd ed. Philadelphia, PA: JB Lippincott; 1990.
9. Mathiowetz V, Kashman N, Volland G, et al. Grip and pinch strength: normative data for adults. *Arch Phys Med Rehab*. 1985;66:69-74.

504   Elbow/Hand Enthesopathy | Elbow

ELBOW JOINT PATHOLOGY
SUMMARY OVERVIEW

ICD-9

719.43

APTA Preferred Practice Pattern: **4D, 7A**

EXAMINATION

- History and Systems Review
- Tests and Measures
  Systems review per APTA's *Guide to Physical Therapy Practice*
  - Joint integrity and mobility
  - Muscle performance
  - Pain
  - Posture
  - ROM
  - Sensory integrity
  - Special tests
- Establish Plan of Care

GOALS/OUTCOMES

- Pain: 2/10 or less
- Restoration of flexibility/extensibility of the forearm muscle/tendon complex to restore functional use equal to the uninvolved side or 100% of the AMA guides
- Functional cervical ROM or a minimum of 80% of AMA guides
- Restoration of normal articular mobility
- Restoration of muscle performance/endurance of the forearm muscle/tendon complex to restore functional use of involved extremity
- Return to prior functional status and activity level for ADLs and vocational, recreational, and sports activities as identified by patient
- Independence in a progressive home exercise program emphasizing function

INTERVENTION
NUMBER OF VISITS 5–11

- Patient Instruction
  - Basic Anatomy and Biomechanics
  - Handouts
  - Functional Considerations
- Direct Interventions
  - Acute Phase: 2–4 Visits
  - Subacute Phase: 3–7 Visits
- Functional Carryover

DISCHARGE PLANNING AND PATIENT RESPONSIBILITY

- Criteria for Discharge
  - All goals/outcomes achieved with the possible exception of return to previous level for recreational and sports activities
  - Patient demonstrates understanding of preventive measures, including use of orthotics and adjustments to vocational/recreational/sports environment
- Circumstances Requiring Additional Visits
  - Cervical pathology or radiating signs/symptoms
  - Inability to progress due to current vocational demands exacerbating symptoms
  - Special occupational needs that require extensive strengthening
  - Multiple injury sites
  - Presence of ligamentous laxity
  - Suspicion of returning joint restrictions because of positioning or existing dysfunction at discharge
- Home Program
  - Continue exercise and stretching program until full strength, pain-free ROM, and functional activity level have returned to previous status
  - Avoid overuse activities that stress elbow
- Monitoring

SUMMARY OVERVIEW | ELBOW | ELBOW JOINT PATHOLOGY

ELBOW JOINT PATHOLOGY

ICD-9

719.43   Pain in joint, forearm

APTA Preferred Practice Pattern: **4D, 7A**

EXAMINATION

History and Systems Review

- History of current condition
  - Trauma
  - Location, nature, and behavior of symptoms
    - Aggravating/relieving factors
    - Presence of clicking or popping in the joint
- Past history of current condition
  - Upper-extremity or cervical injury
  - Surgery
  - Direct intervention
- Medical history
  - Medication
  - Previous surgery
  - Review imaging
- Functional status and activity level (current/prior)
- Patient's functional goals/outcomes

Tests and Measures

Systems review per APTA's *Guide to Physical Therapy Practice*

- Joint integrity and mobility
  - Glenohumeral articular mobility assessment (anterior, posterior, inferior, lateral, and superior glide)
  - Glenohumeral ligament stress tests (superior, inferior, and middle glenohumeral ligament)
  - Elbow articular assessment
    - Capsular pattern: Flexion limitation > extension
    - Radial deviation of ulna and radius on humerus
    - Ulnar deviation of the ulna and radius on the humerus
    - Distraction of the olecranon process on the humerus
    - Anterior posterior glide of the radius on the humerus
  - End range scour test in flex/supination, flex/pronation, extension/supination, and extension/pronation

- Elbow stress tests:
  - Radial collateral in extension, 10° and 90° of flexion
  - Ulnar collateral in extension, 10° and 90° of flexion
- Muscle performance
  - Manual muscle test, especially C6–7 nerve root
  - Resisted
  - Grip and pinch strength measurement with dynamometer
  - Palpation of muscles, tendons, and ligaments
- Pain
  - Measured on visual analog scale
- Posture
  - Forward head posture
  - Shoulders rounded
  - Shoulder height
  - Carrying angle
  - Soft-tissue mass comparison, right to left
  - Color and hair pattern consistency
  - Functional use of arm during gait
  - Clear cervical spine
    - AROM
    - Overpressure
    - Quadrant compression test
- ROM
  - Shoulder motion
  - Active/passive/overpressure of elbow
    - Flexion: 140–150°
    - Extension: 0–10°
    - Supination: 90°
    - Pronation: 80–90°
    - Combined motion end feels
  - Wrist motions
- Sensory integrity
  - Two-point discrimination
  - Dermatome patterns
- Special tests
  - Contractile tissue assessment for length and pain
    - Specific length test for extensor mechanism (wrist flexion, elbow extension, forearm pronation)

506   ELBOW JOINT PATHOLOGY | ELBOW

- Specific length test for flexor mechanism (wrist extension, elbow extension, forearm supination)
  o Ability of the radius and ulna to adduct on the humerus (assess for an abduction lesion of the ulna)
  o Screen for tennis elbow, Tinel's sign (at elbow), medial epicondylitis
  o Upper limb tension tests (ULTTs)
    - ULTT 1 (median nerve dominant)
      a. Patient supine, depress shoulder, abduct to approximately 110°, supinate forearm, extend elbow, wrist, and fingers
      b. Side bend head/neck both toward and away
      c. Assess normal vs. abnormal response (see Butler. 1991)
    - ULTT 2 (radial nerve dominant)
      a. Patient supine, depress shoulder, shoulder abducted and internally rotated, pronate forearm, extend elbow, flex the wrist and thumb
      b. Side bend head/neck both toward and away
      c. Assess normal vs. abnormal response (see Butler. 1991)
    - ULTT 3 (ulnar nerve dominant)
      a. Patient supine, extend wrist, supinate forearm, fully flex elbow, depress and abduct shoulder
      b. Side bend head/neck both toward and away
      c. Assess normal vs. abnormal response (see Butler. 1991)

Establish Plan of Care
- Based on history, tests, and measures

GOALS/OUTCOMES
- Pain: 2/10 or less
- Restoration of flexibility/extensibility of the forearm muscle/tendon complex to restore functional use equal to the uninvolved side or 100% of the AMA guides
  o Hand
    - Ability to form full fist
  o Wrist
    - Flexion: 60°+
    - Extension: 60°+
  o Elbow
    - Flexion: 140°+
    - Extension: 0°
    - Supination: 80°+
    - Pronation: 80°+
  o Functional shoulder ROM
    - Flexion: 160°
    - External rotation: 60°

- Functional cervical ROM or a minimum of 80% of AMA guides:

	Normal	80%
Flexion	60°	50°
Extension	75°	60°
Rotation	80°	65°
Side bend	45°	35°

- Restoration of normal articular mobility
- Restoration of muscle performance/endurance of the forearm muscle/tendon complex to restore functional use of involved extremity
  o Grip strength: 90% of uninvolved hand or mean for age/gender norms
  o 5/5 on manual muscle test for wrist, elbow, and forearm
- Return to prior functional status and activity level for ADLs and vocational, recreational, and sports activities as identified by patient
- Independence in a progressive home exercise program emphasizing function

INTERVENTION
NUMBER OF VISITS 5–11

Coordination, Communication, and Documentation
- Provision of services between admission and discharge that facilitate cost-effective and efficient integration or reintegration to home, community, or work
- Documentation of therapeutic intervention is required for each episode of care and serves as the basic foundation for communication
- Coordination and additional communication will depend on the patient's impairment and home/work/community/leisure situation and requirements. Such services may include:
  o Case management
  o Coordination of care and collaboration with those integral to the patient's rehabilitation program
  o Coordination and monitoring of the delivery of available resources
  o Referrals to other health-care professionals
  o Identification of resources, support groups, or advocacy services
  o Provision of educational or training information
  o Technical assistance

ELBOW | ELBOW JOINT PATHOLOGY

Patient Instruction

Basic Anatomy and Biomechanics
- Pertinent Gray's Anatomy (Gray. 1995. 640–643, 645, 844–852)
- Review of elbow joint structure and surrounding soft tissue

Handouts
- Commercially available products, such as:
  - Krames Communications (1100 Grundy Lane, San Bruno, CA 94066):
    - *Elbow Owner's Manual*
- Specific home program
- Primal pictures (http://www.primalpictures.com)

Functional Considerations
- Educate patient to recognize and avoid positions that may lead to recurrent pathology based on the mechanism and degree of injury, namely pushing, pulling, or lifting
- Preventive care and long-term strengthening options

Direct Interventions

Acute Phase: 2–4 Visits
- Therapeutic exercise and home program
  - Explicit advice regarding appropriate level and type of activity that may be performed
  - Pain-free hand, wrist, and shoulder AROM performed three times per day with splint removed
  - Postural correction exercises
- Manual therapy techniques
  - Soft-tissue techniques
    - Soft-tissue mobilization
    - Myofascial release
    - Trigger-point techniques
    - Friction massage
  - Joint mobilization
    - Grades I–II with intent of pain relief
    - Grades III–IV as tolerated to areas of hypomobility identified in evaluation
  - Assisted stretching techniques to the shoulder girdle, elbow, wrist, or hand
- Therapeutic devices and equipment
  - Resting splint (wrist, hand, and fingers)
  - Neoprene elbow sleeve

- Electrotherapeutic modalities
  - IFC to decrease pain and inflammation
  - Ultrasound to increase blood flow to surface soft tissue
  - Iontophoresis to decrease inflammation and pain
- Physical agents and mechanical modalities
  - Cryotherapy
  - Athermal, deep thermal modalities
- Goals/outcomes
  - Pain: 5/10 or less
  - AROM: 70% of AMA guides
    - Wrist
      a. Flexion: 40°
      b. Extension: 40°
    - Elbow
      a. Flexion: 100°
      b. Extension: 20° (short of neutral)
      c. Pronation: 55°
      d. Supination: 55°
    - Decrease inflammation as noted by reduced edema (circumference) and tenderness to palpation

Subacute Phase: 3–7 Visits
- Therapeutic exercise and home program
  - Restore strength, endurance, and ROM of all upper quadrant structures (stretching, isometric, isotonic, and tubing exercises)
    - Perform slow gentle stretch to extensor mechanism and flexor mechanism several times a day
    - Start with high repetitive ROM exercises to upper quadrant
    - Wrist extensor strengthening: "Broom handle exercise"
      a. Tie weight to rope or string 3 ft long that is attached to broom handle or dowel
      b. Broom handle is held in front of patient who then rolls string around handle to raise and lower weight
    - Exercises for concentric and eccentric training using surgical tubing, resistive band, or other elasticized tension cord
    - Ball squeezing exercise or resistance putty to increase grip strength
    - Flies with weight in each hand
    - Biceps: Elbow flexion with free weights or machine
    - Triceps: Elbow extension with free weights or machine

- Upper body ergometer
  - Wrist flexion, extension, radial deviation, ulnar deviation, pronation, and supination with free weights
    - Postural correction activities
- Manual therapy techniques
  - Continue effective soft-tissue techniques
  - Joint mobilization to restore proper joint mechanics
- Physical agents and mechanical modalities
  - Continue effective modalities as in acute phase with increased emphasis on use as needed at home

Functional Carryover
- Guidance on gradual resumption of activities as tolerated, including normal ADLs and recreational and sports activities as symptoms permit
- Assess patients activity for ways to reduce loads imposed on upper quadrant and elbow
  - Sports—racquet sports, golf
  - Vocational—hand tools, lifting
  - Recreational—needlework, gardening, woodwork

DISCHARGE PLANNING AND PATIENT RESPONSIBILITY

Criteria for Discharge
- All goals/outcomes achieved with the possible exception of return to previous level for recreational and sports activities
- Patient demonstrates understanding of preventive measures including use of orthosis and adjustments to vocational/recreational/sports environment

Circumstances Requiring Additional Visits
- Cervical pathology or radiating signs/symptoms
- Inability to progress due to current vocational demands exacerbating symptoms
- Special occupational needs that require extensive strengthening
- Multiple injury sites
- Presence of ligamentous laxity
- Suspicion of returning joint restrictions because of positioning or existing dysfunction at discharge

Home Program
- Continue exercise and stretching program until full strength, pain-free ROM, and functional activity level have returned to previous status
- Avoid overuse activities that stress elbow

Monitoring
- Instruct patient to call for advice should progression halt or a negative trend occur
- Follow-up call in 2–4 weeks to ensure return to full vocational, recreational, and sports activities
- Schedule clinic visit as needed to adjust or progress home program and address return to sport issues

REFERENCES
1. American Physical Therapy Association. *Guide to Physical Therapist Practice.* Alexandria, VA: APTA; 2003.
2. Butler DS. *Mobilization of the Nervous System.* Melbourne, Australia: Churchill Livingstone; 1991.
3. Donatelli R, Wooden M. *Orthopaedic Physical Therapy.* Melbourne, Australia: Churchill Livingstone; 1989.
4. Engelberg AL. *Guides to the Evaluation of Permanent Impairment.* 3rd ed. Chicago, IL: American Medical Association; 1989.
5. Gray H; Williams PL, ed. *Gray's Anatomy.* 38th ed. New York, NY: Churchill Livingstone; 1995.
6. Hertling D, Kessler RM. *Management of Common Musculoskeletal Disorders.* 2nd ed. Philadelphia, PA: JB Lippincott; 1990.
7. Litchfield R, Hawkings R, Dillman CJ, Atkins J, Hagerman G. Rehabilitation for the overhead athlete. *J Orthop Sports Phys Ther.* 1993;18(2):433-441.
8. Mathiowetz V, Kashman N, Volland G, et al. Grip and pinch strength: normative data for adults. *Arch of Phys Med Rehab.* 1985;66:69-74.
9. Richardson JK, Iglarsh ZA. *Clinical Orthopedic Physical Therapy.* Philadelphia, PA: WB Saunders; 1994:232-242.
10. Roy S, Irvin R. *Sports Medicine: Prevention, Evaluation, Management, and Rehabilitation.* Englewood Cliffs, NJ: Prentice-Hall, 1983.
11. Wilk KE, Arrigo C, Andrews JR. Rehabilitation of the elbow in the throwing athlete. *J Orthop Sports Phys Ther.* 1993;17(6):305-317.
12. Wilk KE, Voight ML, Keirns MA, et al. Stretch-shortening drills for the upper extremities: theory and clinical application. *J Orthop Sports Phys Ther.* 1993;17(5):225-239.

ELBOW SPRAIN/STRAIN
SUMMARY OVERVIEW

ICD-9

719.42   841.2   841.3   841.8   841.9

APTA Preferred Practice Pattern: **4D, 4E, 4J, 7A**

EXAMINATION

- History and Systems Review
- Tests and Measures
  Systems review per APTA's *Guide to Physical Therapy Practice*
  - Joint integrity and mobility
  - Muscle performance
  - Pain
  - Posture
  - ROM
  - Special tests
- Establish Plan of Care

GOALS/OUTCOMES

- Pain: 2/10 or less
- Restoration of flexibility/extensibility of the forearm muscle/tendon complex to restore functional use equal to the uninvolved side or 100% of the AMA guides
- Functional cervical ROM or a minimum of 80% of AMA guides
- Restoration of muscle performance/endurance of the forearm muscle/tendon complex to restore functional use of involved extremity
- Return to prior functional status and activity level for ADLs and vocational, recreational, and sports activities as identified by patient
- Independence in a progressive home exercise program emphasizing function

INTERVENTION
NUMBER OF VISITS: 5–12

- Patient Instruction
  - Basic Anatomy and Biomechanics
  - Handouts
  - Functional Considerations
- Direct Interventions
  - Acute Phase: 2–4 Visits
  - Subacute Phase: 3–8 Visits
- Functional Carryover

DISCHARGE PLANNING AND PATIENT RESPONSIBILITY

- Criteria for Discharge
  - All goals/outcomes achieved with the possible exception of return to previous level for recreational and sports activities
  - Patient demonstrates understanding of preventive measures, including use of orthotics and adjustments to vocational/recreational/sports environment
- Circumstances Requiring Additional Visits
  - Cervical pathology or radiating signs/symptoms
  - Inability to progress due to current vocational demands exacerbating symptoms
  - Special occupational needs that require extensive strengthening
  - Multiple injury sites
  - Presence of ligamentous laxity
- Home Program
  - Continue exercise and stretching program until full strength, pain-free ROM, and functional activity level have returned to previous status
  - Avoid overuse activities that stress elbow
- Monitoring

SUMMARY OVERVIEW | ELBOW | ELBOW SPRAIN/STRAIN   511

ELBOW SPRAIN/STRAIN

ICD-9

719.42	Pain in joint, upper arm
841.2	Radiohumeral (joint) sprain
841.3	Ulnohumeral (joint) sprain
841.8	Sprain of other specified sites of elbow and forearm
841.9	Sprain of unspecified site of elbow and forearm

APTA Preferred Practice Pattern: **4D, 4E, 4J, 7A**

EXAMINATION

History and Systems Review

- History of current condition
  - Location, nature, and behavior of symptoms
    - Aggravating/relieving factors
    - a.m./p.m.
- Past history of current condition
  - Upper-extremity or cervical injury
  - Surgery
  - Direct intervention
- Functional status and activity level (current/prior)
- Patient's functional goals/outcomes

Tests and Measures

Systems review per APTA's *Guide to Physical Therapy Practice*

- Joint integrity and mobility
  - Radial collateral—in extension
  - Ulnar collateral—in extension and at 90° flexion
- Muscle performance
  - Manual muscle test, especially C6–7 nerve root
  - Resisted testing
    - Grip strength
  - Palpation of muscles, tendons, and ligaments
- Pain
  - Measured on visual analog scale
- Posture
  - Forward head posture
  - Shoulders rounded
  - Shoulder height
  - Carrying angle
  - Functional use of arm during gait
  - Clear cervical spine
    - AROM
    - Overpressure
    - Quadrant compression test

- ROM
  - Active/passive/overpressure
    - Elbow/wrist ROM (elbow flexion/extension, forearm pronation/supination, wrist flexion/extension)
  - Humeroradial
  - Proximal radioulnar
  - Humeroulnar
- Special tests
  - Contractile tissue assessment for length and pain
    - Specific length test for extensor mechanism (wrist flexion, elbow extension, forearm pronation)
    - Specific length test for flexor mechanism (wrist extension, elbow extension, forearm supination)
  - Upper limb tension tests (ULTTs)
    - ULTT 1 (median nerve dominant)
      a. Patient supine, depress shoulder, abduct to approximately 110°, supinate forearm, extend elbow, wrist, and fingers
      b. Side bend head/neck both toward and away
      c. Assess normal vs. abnormal response (see Butler. 1991)
    - ULTT 2 (radial nerve dominant)
      a. Patient supine, depress shoulder, shoulder abducted and internally rotated, pronate forearm, extend elbow, flex the wrist and thumb
      b. Side bend head/neck both toward and away
      c. Assess normal vs. abnormal response (see Butler. 1991)
    - ULTT 3 (ulnar nerve dominant)
      a. Patient supine, extend wrist, supinate forearm, fully flex elbow, depress and abduct shoulder
      b. Side bend head/neck both toward and away
      c. Assess normal vs. abnormal response (see Butler. 1991)

Establish Plan of Care

- Based on history, tests, and measures

GOALS/OUTCOMES

- Pain: 2/10 or less
- Restoration of flexibility/extensibility of the forearm muscle/tendon complex to restore functional use equal to the uninvolved side or 100% of the AMA guides
  - Hand
    - Ability to form full fist
  - Wrist
    - Flexion: 60°+
    - Extension: 60°+
  - Elbow
    - Flexion: 140°+
    - Extension: 0°
    - Supination: 80°+
    - Pronation: 80°+
  - Functional shoulder ROM
    - Flexion: 162°
    - External Rotation: 60°
- Functional cervical ROM or a minimum of 80% of AMA guides:

	Normal	*80%*
Flexion	60°	50°
Extension	75°	60°
Rotation	80°	65°
Side bend	45°	35°

- Restoration of muscle performance/endurance of the forearm muscle/tendon complex to restore functional use of involved extremity
  - Grip strength: 90% of uninvolved hand or mean for age/gender norms
  - 5/5 on manual muscle test for wrist, elbow, and forearm
- Return to prior functional status and activity level for ADLs and vocational, recreational, and sports activities as identified by patient
- Independence in a progressive home exercise program emphasizing function

INTERVENTION
NUMBER OF VISITS: 5–12

Coordination, Communication, and Documentation

- Provision of services between admission and discharge that facilitate cost-effective and efficient integration or reintegration to home, community, or work
- Documentation of therapeutic intervention is required for each episode of care and serves as the basic foundation for communication
- Coordination and additional communication will depend on the patient's impairment and home/work/community/leisure situation and requirements. Such services may include:
  - Case management
  - Coordination of care and collaboration with those integral to the patient's rehabilitation program
  - Coordination and monitoring of the delivery of available resources
  - Referrals to other health-care professionals
  - Identification of resources, support groups, or advocacy services
  - Provision of educational or training information
  - Technical assistance

Patient Instruction

Basic Anatomy and Biomechanics

- Pertinent Gray's Anatomy (Gray. 1995. 640–643, 645, 844–852)
- Review of elbow joint structure and surrounding soft tissue

Handouts

- Commercially available products, such as:
  - Krames Communications (1100 Grundy Lane, San Bruno, CA 94066):
    - *Elbow Owner's Manual*
- Specific home program

Functional Considerations

- Educate patient to recognize and avoid positions that may lead to recurrent pathology based on the mechanism and degree of injury, such as pushing, pulling, or lifting
- Preventive care and long-term strengthening options

ELBOW | ELBOW SPRAIN/STRAIN   513

Direct Interventions

Acute Phase: 2–4 Visits

- Therapeutic exercise and home program
  - Explicit advice regarding appropriate level and type of activity that may be performed
  - Pain-free hand, wrist, and shoulder AROM performed three times per day with splint removed
  - Postural correction exercises
- Manual therapy techniques
  - Soft-tissue techniques
    - Soft-tissue mobilization
    - Myofascial release
    - Trigger-point techniques
    - Friction massage
  - Joint mobilization
    - Grades I–II with intent of pain relief
    - Grades III–IV as tolerated to areas of hypomobility identified in evaluation
  - Assisted stretching techniques to the shoulder girdle, elbow, wrist, or hand
- Therapeutic devices and equipment
  - Resting splint (wrist, hand, and fingers)
  - Neoprene elbow sleeve
- Electrotherapeutic modalities
  - Iontophoresis
- Physical agents and mechanical modalities
  - Cryotherapy
  - Athermal, deep thermal modalities
- Goals/outcomes
  - Pain: 5/10 or less
  - AROM: 70% of AMA guides
    - Wrist
      a. Flexion: 40°
      b. Extension: 40°
    - Elbow
      a. Flexion: 100°
      b. Extension: 20° (short of neutral)
      c. Pronation: 55°
      d. Supination: 55°
  - Decrease inflammation as noted by reduced edema (circumference) and tenderness to palpation

Subacute Phase: 3–8 Visits

- Therapeutic exercise and home program
  - Restore strength, endurance, and ROM of all upper quadrant structures (stretching, isometric, isotonic, and tubing exercises)
    - Perform slow, gentle stretch to extensor mechanism and flexor mechanism several times a day
    - Start with high-repetitive ROM exercises to upper quadrant
    - Wrist extensor strengthening: "Broom handle exercise"
      a. Tie weight to rope or string 3 ft long that is attached to broom handle or dowel
      b. Broom handle is held in front of patient who then rolls string around handle to raise and lower weight
    - Exercises for concentric and eccentric training using surgical tubing, resistive bands, or other elasticized tension cord
    - Ball squeezing exercise or resistance putty to increase grip strength
    - Flies with weight in each hand
    - Biceps: Elbow flexion with free weights or machine
    - Triceps: Elbow extension with free weights or machine
    - Upper body ergometer
    - Wrist flexion, extension, radial deviation, ulnar deviation, pronation, and supination with free weights
  - Postural correction activities
- Manual therapy techniques
  - Continue effective soft-tissue techniques
  - Joint mobilization to restore proper joint mechanics
- Physical agents and mechanical modalities
  - Continue effective modalities as in acute phase with increased emphasis on use as needed at home
- Goals/outcomes
  - Pain: 2/10 or less
  - AROM to achieve at least 90% of AMA guides
    - Wrist
      a. Flexion: 55°+
      b. Extension: 55°+

514   ELBOW SPRAIN/STRAIN | ELBOW

- Elbow
  a. Flexion: 125°
  b. Extension: 0°
  c. Pronation: 70°+
  d. Supination: 70°+
  ○ Muscle performance: 4/5 on manual muscle test to enhance return to full ADLs and vocational, recreational, and sports activities as tolerated
  ○ Grip strength: 80% of mean for age/gender norms

Functional Carryover

- Guidance on gradual resumption of activities as tolerated, including normal ADLs and recreational and sports activities as symptoms permit
- Assess patient's activity for ways to reduce loads imposed on upper quadrant and elbow
  ○ Sports: Racquet sports, golf
  ○ Vocational: Hand tools, lifting
  ○ Recreational: Needlework, gardening, woodwork

DISCHARGE PLANNING AND PATIENT RESPONSIBILITY

Criteria for Discharge

- All goals/outcomes achieved with the possible exception of return to previous level for recreational and sports activities
- Patient demonstrates understanding of preventive measures, including use of orthotics and adjustments to vocational/recreational/sports environment

Circumstances Requiring Additional Visits

- Cervical pathology or radiating signs/symptoms
- Inability to progress due to current vocational demands exacerbating symptoms
- Special occupational needs that require extensive strengthening
- Multiple injury sites
- Presence of ligamentous laxity

Home Program

- Continue exercise and stretching program until full strength, pain-free ROM, and functional activity level have returned to previous status
- Avoid overuse activities that stress elbow

Monitoring

- Instruct patient to call for advice should progression halt or a negative trend occur
- Follow-up call in 2–4 weeks to ensure return to full vocational, recreational, and sports activities
- Schedule clinic visit as needed to adjust or progress home program and address return to sport issues

REFERENCES

1. American Physical Therapy Association. *Guide to Physical Therapist Practice*. Alexandria, VA: APTA; 1997.
2. Butler DS. *Mobilization of the Nervous System*. Melbourne, Australia: Churchill Livingstone; 1991.
3. Donatelli R, Wooden M. *Orthopaedic Physical Therapy*. Melbourne, Australia: Churchill Livingstone; 1989.
4. Engelberg AL. *Guides to the Evaluation of Permanent Impairment*. 3rd ed. Chicago, IL: American Medical Association; 1989.
5. Gray H; Williams PL, ed. *Gray's Anatomy*. 38th ed. New York, NY: Churchill Livingstone; 1995.
6. Hertling D, Kessler RM. *Management of Common Musculoskeletal Disorders*. 2nd ed. Philadelphia, PA: JB Lippincott; 1990.
7. Litchfield R, Hawkings R, Dillman CJ, Atkins J, Hagerman G. Rehabilitation for the overhead athlete. *J Orthop Sports Phys Ther*. 1993;18(2):433-441.
8. Mathiowetz V, Kashman N, Volland G, et al. Grip and pinch strength: normative data for adults. *Arch of Phys Med Rehab*. 1985;66:69-74.
9. Retting AC, Sherrill C, Shead DS, Mendler JC, Mieling P. Non-operative treatment of ulnar collateral ligament injuries in throwing athletes. *Am J Sports Med* 2001;29(1):15-7.
10. Richardson JK, Iglarsh ZA. *Clinical Orthopedic Physical Therapy*. Philadelphia, PA: WB Saunders; 1994:232-242.
11. Roy S, Irvin R. *Sports Medicine: Prevention, Evaluation, Management, and Rehabilitation*. Englewood Cliffs, NJ: Prentice-Hall; 1983.
12. Wilk KE, Arrigo C, Andrews JR. Rehabilitation of the elbow in the throwing athlete. *J Orthop Sports Phys Ther*. 1993;17(6):305-317.
13. Wilk KE, Voight ML, Keirns MA, et al. Stretch-shortening drills for the upper extremities: theory and clinical application. *J Orthop Sports Phys Ther*. 1993;17(5):225-239.

516   ELBOW SPRAIN/STRAIN | ELBOW

LATERAL EPICONDYLITIS
SUMMARY OVERVIEW

ICD-9

719.42   726.32   841.9

APTA Preferred Practice Pattern: 4E, 4F, 4J, 4D, 7A

EXAMINATION

- History and Systems Review
- Tests and Measures
  Systems review per APTA's *Guide to Physical Therapy Practice*
  - Joint integrity and mobility
  - Muscle performance
  - Pain
  - Posture
  - ROM
  - Special tests
- Establish Plan of Care

GOALS/OUTCOMES

- Pain: Less than 2/10 with use, 0/10 at rest
- Restoration of flexibility/extensibility of the forearm muscle tendon complex to restore functional use equal to the uninvolved side or 100% of the AMA guides
- Functional shoulder ROM
- Functional cervical ROM or a minimum of 80% of AMA guides
- Restoration of muscle performance/endurance of muscle/tendon complex to restore functional use of involved extremity
- Reduction of overload forces to prevent recurrence
- Return to prior functional status and activity level for ADLs and vocational, recreational, and sports activities as identified by patient
- Independence in a progressive home exercise program emphasizing function

INTERVENTION
NUMBER OF VISITS: 6–12

- Patient Instruction
  - Basic Anatomy and Biomechanics
  - Handouts
  - Functional Considerations
- Direct Interventions
  - Acute Phase: 1–3 Visits
  - Subacute Phase: 5–9 Visits
- Functional Carryover

DISCHARGE PLANNING AND PATIENT RESPONSIBILITY

- Criteria for Discharge
  - All goals/outcomes achieved, except may discharge at 80% grip strength or 4/5 on manual muscle test
  - Demonstrates understanding of preventive measures, such as splinting, early intervention, adjustments to vocational/recreational/sports environment
- Circumstances Requiring Additional Visits
  - Cervical pathology or radiating signs/symptoms
  - Inability to progress due to current vocational demands exacerbating symptoms
  - Special occupational needs that require extensive strengthening
  - Multiple injury sites
- Home Program
  - Continue strengthening and stretching program until full, pain-free motor performance, ROM, and functional activity level have returned
  - Gradual weaning from orthotics
  - Progression to "Return to Sport" guideline
- Monitoring

SUMMARY OVERVIEW | ELBOW | LATERAL EPICONDYLITIS   517

LATERAL EPICONDYLITIS

ICD-9

719.42	Pain in joint, upper arm
726.32	Lateral epicondylitis
841.9	Sprain of unspecified site of elbow and forearm

APTA Preferred Practice Pattern: 4E, 4F, 4J, 4D, 7A

EXAMINATION

History and Systems Review

- History of current condition
  - Location, nature, and behavior of symptoms
    - Aggravating/relieving factors
    - a.m./p.m.
- Past history of current condition
  - Cervical spine or upper-extremity injury
  - Surgery
  - Direct intervention
- Other tests and measures
- Functional status and activity level (current/prior)
  - Occupational activities
  - Recreational activities
- Patient's functional goals/outcomes

Tests and Measures

Systems review per APTA's *Guide to Physical Therapy Practice*

- Joint integrity and mobility
  - Palpation of muscles, tendons, and ligaments
- Muscle performance
  - Manual muscle test, especially C6–7 nerve root
  - Functional use of arm during gait
  - Resisted testing
    - Including grip strength
- Pain
  - Measured on visual analog scale
- Posture
  - Forward head posture
  - Shoulders rounded
  - Shoulder height
  - Carrying angle

- ROM
  - Active/passive/overpressure
    - Elbow/wrist ROM (elbow flexion/extension, forearm pronation/supination, wrist flexion/extension)
  - Humeroradial
  - Proximal radioulnar
- Special tests
  - Clear cervical spine
    - AROM
    - Overpressure
    - Quadrant compression test
  - Contractile tissue assessment in neutral and lengthened position
    - Specific length test for the extensor mechanism (wrist flexion, elbow extension, forearm pronation)
    - Specific length test for flexor mechanism (wrist extension, elbow extension, supination, finger extension)
  - Upper limb tension tests (ULTTs)
    - ULTT 1 (median nerve dominant)
      a. Patient supine, depress shoulder, abduct to approximately 110°, supinate forearm, extend elbow, wrist, and fingers
      b. Side bend head/neck both toward and away
      c. Assess normal vs. abnormal response (see Butler. 1991)
    - ULTT 2 (radial nerve dominant)
      a. Patient supine, depress shoulder, shoulder abducted and internally rotated, pronate forearm, extend elbow, flex the wrist and thumb
      b. Side bend head/neck both toward and away
      c. Assess normal vs. abnormal response (see Butler. 1991)
    - ULTT 3 (ulnar nerve dominant)
      a. Patient supine, extend wrist, supinate forearm, fully flex elbow, depress and abduct shoulder
      b. Side bend head/neck both toward and away
      c. Assess normal vs. abnormal response (see Butler. 1991)

518 LATERAL EPICONDYLITIS | ELBOW

Establish Plan of Care
- Based on history, tests, and measures

GOALS/OUTCOMES
- Pain: Less than 2/10 with use, 0/10 at rest
- Restoration of flexibility/extensibility of the forearm muscle tendon complex to restore functional use equal to the uninvolved side or 100% of the AMA guides
  - Hand
    - Ability to form full fist
  - Wrist
    - Flexion: 60°+
    - Extension: 60°+
  - Elbow
    - Flexion: 140°+
    - Extension: 0°
    - Supination: 80°+
    - Pronation: 80°+
- Functional shoulder ROM:
  - Flexion: 162°
  - External rotation: 60°
- Functional cervical ROM or a minimum of 80% of AMA guides:

	Normal	80%
Flexion	60°	50°
Extension	75°	60°
Rotation	80°	65°
Side bend	45°	35°

- Restoration of muscle performance/endurance of muscle/tendon complex to restore functional use of involved extremity
  - Grip strength: 90% of uninvolved hand or mean for age/gender norms
  - Wrist, forearm, elbow: 5/5 on manual muscle test
- Reduction of overload forces to prevent recurrence
- Return to prior functional status and activity level for ADLs and vocational, recreational, and sports activities as identified by patient
- Independence in a progressive home exercise program emphasizing function

INTERVENTION
NUMBER OF VISITS: 6–12

Coordination, Communication, and Documentation
- Provision of services between admission and discharge that facilitate cost-effective and efficient integration or reintegration to home, community, or work
- Documentation of therapeutic intervention is required for each episode of care and serves as the basic foundation for communication
- Coordination and additional communication will depend on the patient's impairment and home/work/ community/leisure situation and requirements. Such services may include:
  - Case management
  - Coordination of care and collaboration with those integral to the patient's rehabilitation program
  - Coordination and monitoring of the delivery of available resources
  - Referrals to other health-care professionals
  - Identification of resources, support groups, or advocacy services
  - Provision of educational or training information
  - Technical assistance

Patient Instruction

Basic Anatomy and Biomechanics
- Pertinent Gray's Anatomy (Gray. 1995. 640–643, 848–852)
- Instruction regarding the biomechanics and the positional stress placed on the extensor mechanism when performing simultaneous grip, wrist flexion, forearm pronation, and full elbow extension
- Etiology of repetitive trauma injury

Handouts
- Commercially available products, such as:
  - Krames Communications (1100 Grundy Lane, San Bruno, CA 94066):
    - *Exercises at Your Station*
    - *Preventing Repetitive Strain at the Keyboard*
    - *Elbow Owner's Manual*
    - *Preventing Repetitive Motion Injuries*

ELBOW | LATERAL EPICONDYLITIS   519

- Specific home program
  - Exercise
  - Cryotherapy
  - Self-friction
  - Use of orthotics

Functional Considerations

- Utilize a supinated position to facilitate biceps and wrist flexors while lifting
- If injury is racquet related, encourage patient to pursue professional guidance in grip and stroke dynamics from a reputable professional
- Advise patient regarding activities requiring grasping, pinching, or fine finger movements, such as needlework or woodworking
- Importance of proper ergonomic adjustments in home and vocational environments
- Importance of utilizing proper body mechanics and posture, especially with lifting and reaching activities

Direct Interventions

Acute Phase: 1–3 Visits

- Therapeutic exercise and home program
  - Submaximal resisted isometrics to wrist extensors in pain-free ROM following friction massage
  - AROM exercises 3 times per day
    If wearing orthotics, remove for exercises
    - Simultaneous wrist flexion, forearm pronation, elbow extension to promote extensibility of muscle and tendon
    - High repetition, pain-free active wrist flexion/ extension to help vascularize involved tendon and to promote alignment of collagen fibers
  - Instruction on resting positions and avoidance of aggravating activities
  - Home cryotherapy
- Manual therapy techniques
  - Soft-tissue techniques
    - Friction massage to induce hyperemia to specific location of pain over myotendinous junction, tendon, or periosteal junction
    - Soft-tissue mobilization to patient tolerance
    - Acupressure
    - Myofascial release
  - Passive stretching to the wrist flexors and extensors in pain-free ROM

- Joint mobilization to hypomobilities in the cervical spine, shoulder, elbow, or wrist
- Therapeutic devices and equipment
  - Resting splint/wrist splint/compression band
- Electrotherapeutic modalities
  - Iontophoresis
- Physical agents and mechanical modalities
  - Cryotherapy
  - Athermal and thermal modalities
- Goals/outcomes
  - Pain: 5/10 or less with activity, 2/10 or less at rest
  - Decrease inflammation as noted by reduced edema and tenderness to palpation
  - Improve ROM to achieve full AROM of hand, wrist, forearm, and elbow
  - Pain-free ability to make a fist

Subacute Phase: 5–9 Visits

- Therapeutic exercise and home program
  - Explicit parameters for level and type of activity that may be performed
  - Restore strength, endurance, and ROM utilizing stretching, isometric, isotonic, or tubing exercises
    - Perform slow, gentle stretch to extensor mechanism several times a day
      a. Wrist flexion, ulnar deviation, forearm pronation, and elbow extension
    - Continue with high-repetitive ROM exercises for wrist and fingers into extension
    - Wrist extensor strengthening: "Broom handle exercise"
      a. Tie weight to rope or string 3 ft long that is attached to broom handle or dowel
      b. Broom handle is held in front of patient who then rolls string around handle to raise and lower weight
    - Concentric and eccentric training using surgical tubing, resistive bands, or other elasticized tension cord
    - Squeezing resistance putty or bags of rice/beans to increase grip strength
    - Horizontal abduction with weight in each hand
    - Elbow extension
    - Wrist flexion/extension/pronation/supination with weight
    - Upper body ergometry
    - Latissimus pulls

520　LATERAL EPICONDYLITIS | ELBOW

- Manual therapy techniques
  - Continue effective soft-tissue techniques
  - Joint mobilization
    - Progress graded mobilization to persistent hypomobilities
    - Manipulation: Stoddard
      a. Indication: Chronic cases with pain on gripping
      b. Shoulder abducted 90°: Pronate and supinate to identify maximum tension in extensor digitorum communis. Varus thrust at elbow by forearm adduction.
      c. Contraindicated with elbow osteoarthritis and loss of full elbow extension
  - Assisted stretching
    - Muscle bellies of extensor mechanism to decrease muscular tension of involved tendons
    - Shoulder girdle
    - Cervical spine
  - Joint mobilization to restore proper joint mechanics
- Physical agents and mechanical modalities
  - Continue effective modalities as in acute phase with increased emphasis on use as needed at home
- Goals/outcomes
  - Pain: 2/10 or less with activity, 0/10 at rest
  - Increase ROM to achieve pain-free simultaneous full flexion of wrist/hand with pronation of forearm and extension of elbow
  - Increase muscle performance to achieve manual muscle test of 4/5 for all muscle groups
  - Grip strength: 80% of mean for age/gender norms

Functional Carryover

- Gradual resumption of activities with use of orthotics as needed, such as inelastic cuff formed around proximal forearm extensors or tennis elbow splint
- Ergonomic instruction and alteration of equipment used: Larger grip, Hemlock hammer, decrease string tension in tennis racquet
- Assess patient's activity for ways to reduce loads imposed on wrist extensor group

DISCHARGE PLANNING AND PATIENT RESPONSIBILITY

Criteria for Discharge

- All goals/outcomes achieved, except may discharge at 80% grip strength or 4/5 on manual muscle test
- Demonstrates understanding of preventive measures, such as splinting, early intervention, adjustments to vocational/recreational/sports environment

Circumstances Requiring Additional Visits

- Cervical pathology or radiating signs/symptoms
- Inability to progress due to current vocational demands exacerbating symptoms
- Special occupational needs that require extensive strengthening
- Multiple injury sites

Home Program

- Continue strengthening and stretching program until full, pain-free motor performance, ROM, and functional activity level have returned
- Gradual weaning from orthotics
- Progression to "Return to Sport" guideline

Monitoring

- Instruct patient to call for advice should progression halt or a negative trend occur
- Follow-up call in 2–4 weeks to ensure return to previous functional level
- Schedule clinic visit as needed to progress home program or address return to work/sport issues

REFERENCES

1. American Physical Therapy Association. *Guide to Physical Therapist Practice.* Alexandria, VA: APTA; 1997.
2. Binder A, Hodge G, Greeenwood AM, Hazleman BL, Page-Thomas DP. Is therapeutic ultrasound effective in treating soft tissue lesions? *Br Med J (Clin Res Ed).* 1985;290(6467):512-514.
3. Butler DS. *Mobilization of the Nervous System.* Melbourne, Australia: Churchill Livingstone; 1991.
4. Engelberg AL. *Guides to the Evaluation of Permanent Impairment.* 3rd ed. Chicago, IL: American Medical Association; 1989.
5. Gray H; Williams PL, ed. *Gray's Anatomy.* 38th ed. New York, NY: Churchill Livingstone; 1995.

ELBOW | LATERAL EPICONDYLITIS **521**

6. Klaiman MD, Shrader JA, Danoff JV, et al. Phonophoresis versus ultrasound in the treatment of common musculoskeletal conditions. *Med Sci Sports Exerc.* 1998;30(9):1349-1355.

7. Mathiowetz V, Kashman N, Volland G, et al. Grip and pinch strength: normative data for adults. *Arch Phys Med Rehab.* 1985;66:69-74.

8. Nirschi RP, Sobel J. Conservative treatment of tennis elbow. *Physician Sports Med.* 1981;9(6):43-53.

9. Reid DC. *Sports Injury Assessment and Rehabilitation.* New York, NY; Churchill Livingstone; 1992.

10. Richardson JK, Iglarsh ZA. *Clinical Orthopedic Physical Therapy.* Philadelphia, PA: WB Saunders; 1994:232-242.

11. Roy S, Irvin R. *Sports Medicine: Prevention, Evaluation, Management, and Rehabilitation.* Englewood Cliffs, NJ: Prentice-Hall, 1983.

12. Stasinopoulos D, Johnson MI. Cyriax physiotherapy for tennis elbow/lateral epicondylitis. *Br J Sports Med.* 2004:38(6):675-7.

13. Wilk KE, Arrigo C, Andrews JR. Rehabilitation of the elbow in the throwing athlete. *J Orthop Sports Phys Ther.* 1993;17(6):305-317.

14. Wilk KE, Voight ML, Kelms MA, et al. Stretch-shortening drills for the upper extremities: theory and clinical application. *J Orthop Sports Phys Ther.* 1993;17(5):225-239.

MEDIAL EPICONDYLITIS
SUMMARY OVERVIEW

ICD-9

719.42   726.31   813.00   841.9

APTA Preferred Practice Pattern: **4D, 4E, 4F, 4H, 4J, 7A**

EXAMINATION

- History and Systems Review
- Tests and Measures
  Systems review per APTA's *Guide to Physical Therapy Practice*
  - Joint integrity and mobility
  - Muscle performance
  - Pain
  - Posture
  - ROM
  - Special tests
- Establish Plan of Care

GOALS/OUTCOMES

- Restoration of flexibility/extensibility of the forearm muscle tendon complex to restore functional use equal to the uninvolved side or 100% of the AMA guides
- Functional shoulder ROM
- Functional cervical ROM or a minimum of 80% of AMA guides
- Pain: 2/10 with activity, 0/10 at rest
- Grip strength: Mean for age/gender norms
- Return to prior functional status and activity level for ADLs and vocational, recreational, and sports activities as previously identified by patient
- Independence in a progressive home exercise program emphasizing function and pacing

INTERVENTION
NUMBER OF VISITS: 6–12

- Patient Instruction
  - Basic Anatomy and Biomechanics
  - Handouts
  - Functional Considerations
- Direct Interventions
  - Acute Phase: 1–3 Visits
  - Subacute Phase: 5–9 Visits
- Functional Carryover

DISCHARGE PLANNING AND PATIENT RESPONSIBILITY

- Criteria for Discharge
  - All rehabilitation goals/outcomes achieved except may discharge at 80% grip motor performance if all other goals/outcomes achieved
- Circumstances Requiring Additional Visits
  - Cervical pathology or radiating signs/symptoms
  - Inability to progress due to current vocational demands exacerbating symptoms
  - Special occupational needs that require extensive strengthening
  - Multiple injury sites
  - Overuse injury while patient remains in occupation that requires repetitive activity
- Home Program
  - Continue strengthening and stretching exercises until previous pain-free functional activity levels are achieved
  - Cryotherapy for periodic flare-ups
  - Self-friction massage
  - Progression to "Return to Sport" guideline
- Monitoring

MEDIAL EPICONDYLITIS

ICD-9

719.42	Pain in joint, upper arm
726.31	Medial epicondylitis
813.00	Closed fracture of upper end of forearm, unspecified
841.9	Sprain of unspecified site of elbow and forearm

APTA Preferred Practice Pattern: 4D, 4E, 4F, 4H, 4J, 7A

EXAMINATION

History and Systems Review

- History of current condition
  - Location, nature, and behavior of symptoms
    - Aggravating/relieving symptoms
    - a.m./p.m.
- Past history of current condition
  - Cervical spine or upper-extremity injury
  - Surgery
  - Direct intervention
- Other tests and measures
- Functional status and activity level (current/prior)
  - Occupational activities
  - Recreational activities
- Patient's functional goals/outcomes

Tests and Measures

Systems review per APTA's *Guide to Physical Therapy Practice*

- Joint integrity and mobility
  - Palpations of muscles, tendons, and ligaments
- Muscle performance
  - Resisted testing
    - Including grip strength
  - Manual muscle tests, especially C6–7 nerve root
  - Functional use of arm during gait
- Pain
  - Measured on visual analog scale
- Posture
  - Forward head posture
  - Shoulders rounded
  - Shoulder height
  - Carrying angle
- ROM
  - Active/passive/overpressure
    - Elbow/wrist ROM (elbow flexion/extension, forearm pronation/supination, wrist flexion/extension)

- Passive joint ROM
  - Humeroradial
  - Proximal radioulnar
- Special tests
  - Clear cervical spine
    - AROM
    - Overpressure
    - Quadrant compression test
  - Contractile tissue assessment in neutral and lengthened position
    - Length test for flexor mechanism
      a. Elbow extension, wrist extension, supination, finger extension
    - Resisted test for flexor mechanism
    - Length test for extensor mechanism, wrist flexion, elbow extension, pronation, and finger flexion
  - Upper limb tension tests (ULTTs)
    - ULTT 1 (median nerve dominant)
      a. Patient supine, depress shoulder, abduct to approximately 110°, supinate forearm, extend elbow, wrist, and fingers
      b. Side bend head/neck both toward and away
      c. Assess normal vs. abnormal response (see Butler. 1991)
    - ULTT 2 (radial nerve dominant)
      a. Patient supine, depress shoulder, shoulder abducted and internally rotated, pronate forearm, extend elbow, flex the wrist and thumb
      b. Side bend head/neck both toward and away
      c. Assess normal vs. abnormal response (see Butler. 1991)
    - ULTT 3 (ulnar nerve dominant)
      a. Patient supine, extend wrist, supinate forearm, fully flex elbow, depress and abduct shoulder
      b. Side bend head/neck both toward and away
      c. Assess normal vs. abnormal response (see Butler. 1991)

Establish Plan of Care

- Based on history, tests, and measures

GOALS/OUTCOMES

- Restoration of flexibility/extensibility of the forearm muscle tendon complex to restore functional use equal to the uninvolved side or 100% of the AMA guides
  - Hand
    - Ability to form full fist
  - Wrist
    - Flexion: 60°+
    - Extension: 60°+
  - Elbow
    - Flexion: 140°+
    - Extension: 0°
    - Supination: 80°+
    - Pronation: 80°+
- Functional shoulder ROM:
  - Flexion: 160°
  - External rotation: 60°
- Functional cervical ROM or a minimum of 80% of AMA guides:

	Normal	*80%*
Flexion	60°	50°
Extension	75°	60°
Rotation	80°	65°
Side bend	45°	35°

- Pain: 2/10 with activity, 0/10 at rest
- Grip strength: Mean for age/gender norms
- Return to prior functional status and activity level for ADLs and vocational, recreational, and sports activities as previously identified by patient
- Independence in a progressive home exercise program emphasizing function and pacing

INTERVENTION

NUMBER OF VISITS: 6–12

Coordination, Communication, and Documentation

- Provision of services between admission and discharge that facilitate cost-effective and efficient integration or reintegration to home, community, or work
- Documentation of therapeutic intervention is required for each episode of care and serves as the basic foundation for communication
- Coordination and additional communication will depend on the patient's impairment and home/work/community/leisure situation and requirements. Such services may include:
  - Case management
  - Coordination of care and collaboration with those integral to the patient's rehabilitation program
  - Coordination and monitoring of the delivery of available resources
  - Referrals to other health-care professionals
  - Identification of resources, support groups, or advocacy services
  - Provision of educational or training information
  - Technical assistance

Patient Instruction

Basic Anatomy and Biomechanics

- Anatomy of the elbow, forearm, and wrist and its relationship to gripping activities
- Pertinent Gray's Anatomy (Gray. 1995. 640–643, 844–848)
- Pathology of tendinitis and the tissue response to fatigue causing microdamage

Handouts

- Specific home program
- Taping techniques
- Commercially available products, such as:
  - Krames Communications (1100 Grundy Lane, San Bruno, CA 94066):
    - *Preventing Repetitive Motion Injuries*
    - *Elbow Owner's Manual*

- If injury is golf related, encourage patient to pursue professional guidance in grip and swing dynamics from a reputable golf professional

Functional Considerations
- Avoidance of activities aggravating symptoms
- Cryotherapy before and after activity
- Use of orthotics
  - Extensor tendon band
  - Wrist splint
  - Taping during ADLs/sports activity

Direct Interventions

Acute Phase: 1–3 Visits
- Therapeutic exercise and home program
  - Pain-free submaximally resisted isometrics to wrist flexors following friction massage
  - High-repetition, pain-free, active wrist flexion/extension
  - Active wrist extension to inhibit flexors
  - Submaximal resistive wrist flexion concentric and eccentric in pain-free range
  - Rest position instruction for day and sleeping
  - Instruction on activity precautions and modifications
- Manual therapy techniques
  - Soft-tissue techniques
    - Friction massage without imposing longitudinal stress to healing tissue
    - Myofascial release
    - Soft-tissue mobilization
    - Acupressure
  - Joint mobilization (as indicated per evaluation)
    - Mid-carpal, radiocarpal, proximal/distal radioulnar, humeroulnar, humeroradial joints
    - Shoulder, wrist, and cervical spine
  - Passive ROM to the wrist flexors and extensors in pain-free ROM
- Therapeutic devices and equipment
  - Resting splint/wrist splint/compression band
- Electrotherapeutic modalities
  - Iontophoresis
- Physical agents and mechanical modalities
  - Cryotherapy
  - Athermal, thermal modalities
- Goals/outcomes
  - Pain: 3/10 or less at rest

- Pain-free ROM: Pain-free wrist flexion/extension
- Grip strength: 50–75% of mean for age/gender norms

Subacute Phase: 5–9 Visits
- Therapeutic exercise and home program
  - Manual resistive exercise
  - Implementation of pacing techniques when condition is related to repetitive motion
  - Flexibility exercises
    - Simultaneous motion of wrist extension, forearm supination, elbow extension
  - Strengthening exercises
    - High repetition exercise for wrist and fingers into flexion and extension
    - Wrist flexor: "Broom handle exercise"
      a. Tie weight to rope or string 3 ft long that is attached to broom handle or dowel
      b. Broom handle is held in front of patient who then rolls string around handle to raise and lower weight
    - Concentric and eccentric training using surgical tubing
    - Grip strength
    - Wrist flexion/extension and pronation/supination with weight
    - Upper-extremity diagonals and functional patterns
  - Upper-extremity conditioning program
    - Upper body ergometry
    - Latissimus dorsi pull downs
    - Pulley program
  - Plyometrics with ball
  - Sport- or activity-specific training
  - Cardiovascular conditioning
- Manual therapy techniques
  - Joint mobilization
    - Progress graded mobilization to persistent areas of hypomobility
  - Soft-tissue techniques
    - Friction massage
    - Myofascial release
    - Soft-tissue mobilization
  - Passive stretches
    - Wrist flexor mechanism into wrist extension, radial deviation, forearm supination, and elbow extension
    - Shoulder girdle
    - Cervical spine

- Physical agents and mechanical modalities
  - Continue effective modalities as in acute phase with increased emphasis on use as needed at home
- Goals/outcomes
  - Grip strength: 80% of mean for age/gender norms
  - Increase ROM to achieve pain-free simultaneous wrist extension, forearm supination, and elbow extension
  - Pain: 0/10 at rest, 2/10 or less with activity

Functional Carryover
- Gradual resumption of activities with use of orthotics as needed
- Alteration of equipment used or grip (such as larger grip, change of golf grip)
- Assess patient's activity for ways to reduce loads imposed on wrist flexor group
- Avoid overuse activities that stress wrist flexors

Criteria for Discharge
- All rehabilitation goals/outcomes achieved except may discharge at 80% grip motor performance if all other goals/outcomes achieved

Circumstances Requiring Additional Visits
- Cervical pathology or radiating signs/symptoms
- Inability to progress due to current vocational demands exacerbating symptoms
- Special occupational needs that require extensive strengthening
- Multiple injury sites
- Overuse injury while patient remains in occupation that requires repetitive activity

Home Program
- Continue strengthening and stretching exercises until previous pain-free functional activity levels are achieved
- Cryotherapy for periodic flare-ups
- Self-friction massage
- Progression to "Return to Sport" guideline

Monitoring
- If symptoms consistently recur, consideration of reassessment for direct intervention or potential as surgical candidate
- Patient is instructed to call for advice should progression halt or a negative trend occur
- Follow-up at 4–8 weeks post-discharge to ensure expected return to function and progression toward attaining all rehabilitation goals/outcomes

REFERENCES
1. American Physical Therapy Association. *Guide to Physical Therapist Practice.* Alexandria, VA: APTA; 1997.
2. Butler DS. *Mobilization of the Nervous System.* Melbourne, Australia: Churchill Livingstone; 1991.
3. Ciccotti MC, Schwartz MA, Ciccotti MG. Diagnosis and treatment of medial epicondylitis of elbow. *Clin Sports Med.* 2004;23(4):693-705, xi.
4. Engelberg AL. *Guides to the Evaluation of Permanent Impairment.* 3rd ed. Chicago, IL: American Medical Association; 1989.
5. Gray H; Williams PL, ed. *Gray's Anatomy.* 38th ed. New York, NY: Churchill Livingstone; 1995.
6. Hoppenfeld S. *Physical Examination of the Spine & Extremities.* Norwalk, CT: Appleton-Century-Crofts; 1976:35-58.
7. Mathiowitz V, Kashman N, Volland G, et al. Grip and pinch strength: normative data for adults. *Arch Phys Med Rehab.* 1985;66:69-74.

528   MEDIAL EPICONDYLITIS | ELBOW

ULNAR NERVE LESION
SUMMARY OVERVIEW

ICD-9

   354.2

APTA Preferred Practice Pattern: **4E, 5F**

EXAMINATION

- History and Systems Review
- Tests and Measures
  Systems review per APTA's *Guide to Physical Therapy Practice*
  - Anthropometric characteristics
  - Joint integrity and mobility
  - Muscle performance
  - Pain
  - Posture
  - ROM
  - Sensory integrity
  - Special tests
- Establish Plan of Care

GOALS/OUTCOMES

- Pain: 2/10 or less
- Restoration of flexibility/extensibility of the forearm muscle/tendon complex to restore functional use equal to the uninvolved side or 100% of the AMA guides
- Functional cervical ROM or a minimum of 80% of AMA guides
- Restoration of normal articular and neural mobility
- Restoration of muscle performance/endurance of the forearm muscle/tendon complex to restore functional use of involved extremity
- Return to prior functional status and activity level for ADLs and vocational, recreational, and sports activities as identified by patient
- Independence in a progressive home exercise program emphasizing function

INTERVENTION
NUMBER OF VISITS 5–12

- Patient Instruction
  - Basic Anatomy and Biomechanics
  - Handouts
  - Functional Considerations
- Direct Interventions
  - Acute Phase: 2–4 Visits
  - Subacute Phase: 3–8 Visits
- Functional Carryover

DISCHARGE PLANNING AND PATIENT RESPONSIBILITY

- Criteria for Discharge
  - All goals/outcomes achieved with the possible exception of return to previous level for recreational and sports activities
  - Patient demonstrates understanding of preventive measures including use of orthotics and adjustments to vocational/recreational/sports environment
- Circumstances Requiring Additional Visits
  - Continued nerve pain not allowing progression of exercise program
  - Cervical pathology or radiating signs/symptoms
  - Inability to progress due to current vocational demands exacerbating symptoms
  - Special occupational needs that require extensive strengthening
  - Multiple injury sites
  - Presence of ligamentous laxity
- Home Program
  - Continue home program until full strength, pain-free ROM, and functional activity level have returned to previous status
  - Avoid overuse activities that stress elbow
- Monitoring

SUMMARY OVERVIEW | ELBOW | ULNAR NERVE LESION   **529**

ULNAR NERVE LESION

ICD-9

> 354.2   Lesion of ulnar nerve

APTA Preferred Practice Pattern: **4E, 5F**

EXAMINATION

History and Systems Review

- History of current condition
  - Trauma: Dislocation, repeated blow, or resting elbows on a hard surface while sitting
  - Location, nature, and behavior of symptoms
- Past history of current condition
  - Upper-extremity or cervical injury
  - Supracondylar or epicondylar fracture
  - Direct intervention
- Medical History
  - Medication
  - Previous surgery: Reposition
  - Review imaging: Osteophyte, ganglion, lipoma
- Functional status and activity level (current/prior)
- Patient's functional goals/outcomes

Tests and Measures

Systems review per APTA's *Guide to Physical Therapy Practice*

- Anthropometric characteristics
  - Callus formation
  - Wasting of intrinsic muscle of the hand
- Joint integrity and mobility
  - Cervical scan
  - Shoulder scan
  - Elbow articular assessment
    - Capsular pattern: Flexion limitation > extension
    - Radial deviation of ulna and radius on humerus
    - Ulnar deviation of the ulna and radius on the humerus
    - Distraction of the olecranon process on the humerus
    - Anterior posterior glide of the radius on the humerus
  - End range scour test in flex/supination, flex/pronation, extension/supination, extension/pronation
  - Elbow stress tests:
    - Radial collateral in extension, 10° and 90° of flexion
    - Ulnar collateral in extension, 10° and 90° of flexion
- Muscle performance
  - Adductor pollicis
  - Manual muscle test cervical roots, especially C6-7
  - Resisted
    - Grip and pinch strength measurement with dynamometer
  - Palpation of triceps and other muscles, tendons, and ligaments
- Pain
  - Measured on visual analog scale
- Posture
  - Forward head posture
  - Shoulders rounded
  - Shoulder height
  - Carrying angle
  - Soft-tissue mass comparison, right to left
  - Color and hair pattern consistency
  - Functional use of arm during sitting and sleeping
- ROM
  - Active/passive/overpressure of elbow
    - Flexion: 140–150°
    - Extension: 0–10°
    - Supination: 90°
    - Pronation: 80–90°
    - Combined motion end feels
  - Wrist motions
- Sensory integrity
  - Two-point discrimination
  - Dermatome patterns
- Special tests
  - Contractile tissue assessment for length and pain
    - Specific length test for extensor mechanism (wrist flexion, elbow extension, forearm pronation)
    - Specific length test for flexor mechanism (wrist extension, elbow extension, forearm supination)
  - Elbow flexion test: Reproduction of symptoms after 5 minutes of flexion
  - Tinel's sign
  - Froment's sign: Flexion of thumb tip as gripped paper is pulled away
  - Medial and lateral epicondylitis tests

○ Upper limb tension tests (ULTTs)
- ULTT 1 (median nerve dominant)
  a. Patient supine, depress shoulder, abduct to approximately 110°, supinate forearm, extend elbow, wrist, and fingers
  b. Side bend head/neck both toward and away
  c. Assess normal vs. abnormal response (see Butler. 1991)
- ULTT 2 (radial nerve dominant)
  a. Patient supine, depress shoulder, shoulder abducted and internally rotated, pronate forearm, extend elbow, flex the wrist and thumb
  b. Side bend head/neck both toward and away
  c. Assess normal vs. abnormal response (see Butler. 1991)
- ULTT 3 (ulnar nerve dominant)
  a. Patient supine, extend wrist, supinate forearm, fully flex elbow, depress and abduct shoulder
  b. Side bend head/neck both toward and away
  c. Assess normal vs. abnormal response (see Butler. 1991)

Establish Plan of Care

- Based on history, tests, and measures

GOALS/OUTCOMES

- Pain: 2/10 or less
- Restoration of flexibility/extensibility of the forearm muscle/tendon complex to restore functional use equal to the uninvolved side or 100% of the AMA guides
  ○ Hand
    - Ability to form full fist
  ○ Wrist
    - Flexion: 60°+
    - Extension: 60°+
  ○ Elbow
    - Flexion: 140°+
    - Extension: 0°
    - Supination: 80°+
    - Pronation: 80°+
  ○ Functional shoulder ROM:
    - Flexion: 162°
    - External Rotation: 60°

- Functional cervical ROM or a minimum of 80% of AMA guides:

	Normal	*80%*
Flexion	60°	50°
Extension	75°	60°
Rotation	80°	65°
Side bend	45°	35°

- Restoration of normal articular and neural mobility
- Restoration of muscle performance/endurance of the forearm muscle/tendon complex to restore functional use of involved extremity
  ○ Grip strength: 90% of uninvolved hand or mean for age/gender norms
  ○ 5/5 on manual muscle test for wrist, elbow, and forearm
- Return to prior functional status and activity level for ADLs and vocational, recreational, and sports activities as identified by patient
- Independence in a progressive home exercise program emphasizing function

INTERVENTION
NUMBER OF VISITS 5–12

Coordination, Communication, and Documentation

- Provision of services between admission and discharge that facilitate cost-effective and efficient integration or reintegration to home, community, or work
- Documentation of therapeutic intervention is required for each episode of care and serves as the basic foundation for communication
- Coordination and additional communication will depend on the patient's impairment and home/work/community/leisure situation and requirements. Such services may include:
  ○ Case management
  ○ Coordination of care and collaboration with those integral to the patient's rehabilitation program
  ○ Coordination and monitoring of the delivery of available resources
  ○ Referrals to other health-care professionals
  ○ Identification of resources, support groups, or advocacy services
  ○ Provision of educational or training information
  ○ Technical assistance

ELBOW | ULNAR NERVE LESION   531

Patient Instruction

Basic Anatomy and Biomechanics
- Pertinent Gray's Anatomy (Gray. 1995. 640–643, 645, 844–852)
- Review of elbow joint structure and surrounding soft tissue

Handouts
- Commercially available products, such as:
  - Krames Communications (1100 Grundy Lane, San Bruno, CA 94066):
    - *Elbow Owner's Manual*
- Specific home program
- Primal pictures (http://www.primalpictures.com)

Functional Considerations
- Educate patient to recognize and avoid positions that may lead to recurrent pathology based on the mechanism and degree of injury, namely pushing, pulling, or lifting
- Preventive care and long-term strengthening options

Direct Interventions

Acute Phase: 2–4 Visits
- Complete rest of aggravating positions
- Therapeutic exercise and home program
  - Explicit advice regarding appropriate level and type of activity that may be performed
  - Pain-free hand, wrist, and shoulder AROM performed three times per day with splint removed
  - Postural correction exercises
- Manual therapy techniques (most important for postoperative cases)
  - Soft-tissue techniques
    - Soft-tissue mobilization
    - Myofascial release
    - Trigger-point techniques
    - Friction massage
  - Joint mobilization if surrounding joint restrictions are detected
    - Grades I–II with intent of pain relief
    - Grades III–IV as tolerated to areas of hypomobility identified in evaluation
  - Assisted stretching techniques to the shoulder girdle, elbow, wrist, or hand

- Electrotherapeutic modalities
  - IFC to decrease pain and inflammation
  - Ultrasound to increase blood flow to surface soft tissue
  - Iontophoresis to decrease inflammation and pain
- Physical agents and mechanical modalities
  - Cryotherapy
  - Athermal, deep thermal modalities
- Goals/outcomes
  - Pain: 5/10 or less
  - AROM: 70% of AMA guides
    - Wrist
      a. Flexion: 40°
      b. Extension: 40°
    - Elbow
      a. Flexion: 100°
      b. Extension: 20° (short of neutral)
      c. Pronation: 55°
      d. Supination: 55°
  - Decrease inflammation as noted by reduced edema (circumference) and tenderness to palpation

Subacute Phase: 3–8 Visits
- Continue to monitor avoidance of aggravating positions
- Therapeutic exercise and home program
  - Restore strength, endurance, and ROM of all upper quadrant structures (stretching, isometric, isotonic, and tubing exercises) as condition becomes pain free
    - Exercises for concentric and eccentric training using surgical tubing, resistive bands, or other elasticized tension cord
    - Ball squeezing exercise or resistance putty to increase grip strength
    - Flies with weight in each hand
    - Biceps: Elbow flexion with free weights or machine
    - Triceps: Elbow extension with free weights or machine
    - Upper body ergometer
    - Wrist flexion, extension, radial deviation, ulnar deviation, pronation, and supination with free weights
  - Postural correction activities
- Manual therapy techniques
  - Continue effective soft-tissue techniques
  - Joint mobilization to restore proper joint mechanics

532   ULNAR NERVE LESION | ELBOW

- Physical agents and mechanical modalities
  - Continue effective modalities as in acute phase with increased emphasis on use as needed at home
- Goals/outcomes
  - Pain: 2/10 or less
  - AROM to achieve at least 90% of AMA guides
    - Wrist
      a. Flexion: 55°+
      b. Extension: 55°+
    - Elbow
      a. Flexion: 125°
      b. Extension: 0°
      c. Pronation: 70°+
      d. Supination: 70°+
  - Muscle performance: 4/5 on manual muscle test to enhance return to full ADLs and vocational, recreational, and sports activities as tolerated
  - Grip strength: 80% of mean for age/gender norms

Functional Carryover

- Guidance on gradual resumption of activities as tolerated, including normal ADLs and recreational and sports activities as symptoms permit
- Assess patient's activity for ways to reduce loads imposed on upper quadrant and elbow
  - Sports: Racquet sports, golf
  - Vocational: Hand tools, lifting
  - Recreational: Needlework, gardening, woodwork

DISCHARGE PLANNING AND PATIENT RESPONSIBILITY

Criteria for Discharge

- All goals/outcomes achieved with the possible exception of return to previous level for recreational and sports activities
- Patient demonstrates understanding of preventive measures, including use of orthotics and adjustments to vocational/recreational/sports environment

Circumstances Requiring Additional Visits

- Continued nerve pain not allowing progression of exercise program
- Cervical pathology or radiating signs/symptoms
- Inability to progress due to current vocational demands exacerbating symptoms

- Special occupational needs that require extensive strengthening
- Multiple injury sites
- Presence of ligamentous laxity

Home Program

- Continue home until full strength, pain-free ROM, and functional activity level have returned to previous status
- Avoid overuse activities that stress elbow

Monitoring

- Instruct patient to call for advice should progression halt or a negative trend occur
- Follow-up call in 2–4 weeks to ensure return to full vocational, recreational, and sports activities
- Schedule clinic visit as needed to adjust or progress home program and address return to sport issues

REFERENCES

1. American Physical Therapy Association. *Guide to Physical Therapist Practice.* Alexandria, VA: APTA; 1997.
2. Butler DS. *Mobilization of the Nervous System.* Melbourne, Australia: Churchill Livingstone; 1991.
3. Donatelli R, Wooden M. *Orthopaedic Physical Therapy.* Melbourne, Australia: Churchill Livingstone; 1989.
4. Engelberg AL. *Guides to the Evaluation of Permanent Impairment.* 3rd ed. Chicago, IL: American Medical Association; 1989.
5. Gray H; Williams PL, ed. *Gray's Anatomy.* 38th ed. New York, NY: Churchill Livingstone; 1995.
6. Hertling D, Kessler RM. *Management of Common Musculoskeletal Disorders.* 2nd ed. Philadelphia, PA: JB Lippincott; 1990.
7. Litchfield R, Hawkings R, Dillman CJ, Atkins J, Hagerman G. Rehabilitation for the overhead athlete. *J Orthop Sports Phys Ther.* 1993;18(2):433-441.
8. Mathiowetz V, Kashman N, Volland G, et al. Grip and pinch strength: normative data for adults. *Arch of Phys Med Rehab.* 1985;66:69-74.
9. Reid DC. *Sports Injury Assessment and Rehabilitation.* New York, NY: Churchill Livingstone; 1992.
10. Richardson JK, Iglarsh ZA. *Clinical Orthopedic Physical Therapy.* Philadelphia, PA: WB Saunders; 1994:232-242.
11. Roy S, Irvin R. *Sports Medicine: Prevention, Evaluation, Management, and Rehabilitation.* Englewood Cliffs, NJ: Prentice-Hall; 1983.

12. Wilk KE, Arrigo C, Andrews JR. Rehabilitation of the elbow in the throwing athlete. *J Orthop Sports Phys Ther.* 1993;17(6):305-317.

13. Wilk KE, Voight ML, Keirns MA, et al. Stretch-shortening drills for the upper extremities: theory and clinical application. *J Orthop Sports Phys Ther.* 1993;17(5):225-239.

Wrist/Hand

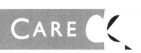

WRIST/HAND

Carpal Tunnel Syndrome	537
Dequervain's Tendinitis	543
Flexor Tendon Repair	549
Hand Arthropathy	557
Hand Fracture	561
Postoperative Carpal Tunnel Release	565
Postoperative Dequervain's Syndrome	571
Postoperative Dupuytren's Fasciectomy	577
Proximal Interphalangeal Joint Injuries Collateral Ligament Sprain	583
Proximal Interphalangeal Joint Injuries Dorsal Dislocation	589
Reflex Sympathetic Dystrophy of the Upper Extremity	593
Wrist Fracture	599
Wrist Sprain/Strain	605

536   WRIST/HAND

CARPAL TUNNEL SYNDROME
SUMMARY OVERVIEW

ICD-9

354.0

APTA Preferred Practice Pattern: **4F**

EXAMINATION

- History and Systems Review
- Tests and Measures
  Systems review per APTA's *Guide to Physical Therapy Practice*
  - Anthropometric characteristics
  - Integumentary integrity
  - Muscle performance
  - Pain
  - ROM
  - Sensory integrity
  - Special tests
- Establish Plan of Care

GOALS/OUTCOMES

- Pain-free wrist and forearm AROM: 100% of AMA guides
- Pain-free thumb AROM: 100% of American Academy of Orthopædic Surgeons norms
- Pain: 3/10 or less with activity, 0/10 at rest
- Restoration of strength/endurance of forearm/wrist complex to restore functional use of involved extremity
- Sensory: 6 mm or less on two-point discrimination test
- Return to prior functional status and activity level (current/prior) for ADLs and vocational, recreational, and sports activities as identified by patient
- Independence in a progressive home exercise program emphasizing function

INTERVENTION
NUMBER OF VISITS: 5–12

- Patient Instruction
  - Basic Anatomy and Biomechanics
  - Handouts
  - Functional Considerations
- Direct Interventions
  - Acute Phase: 3–6 Visits
  - Subacute Phase: 2–6 Visits
- Functional Carryover

DISCHARGE PLANNING AND PATIENT RESPONSIBILITY

- Criteria for Discharge
  - All rehabilitation goals/outcomes achieved except may experience intermittent recurrence of symptoms
- Circumstances Requiring Additional Visits
  - Exacerbation of volar edema
  - Job tasks of a forceful or repetitive nature that exacerbate symptoms
  - Need for modification or replacement of splints
- Home Program
  - Stretching exercises
  - Tendon/nerve gliding
  - Use of splint if recurrence of symptoms
  - Anti-vibration pad/gloves/tool handles
- Monitoring

CARPAL TUNNEL SYNDROME

ICD-9
    354.0   Carpal tunnel syndrome
APTA Preferred Practice Pattern: **4F**

EXAMINATION

History and Systems Review
- History of current condition
  - Date and mechanism of injury/onset
  - Location, nature, and behavior of symptoms
    - Aggravating/relieving factors
    - Sensory changes
    - a.m./p.m.
- Past history of current condition
  - Upper extremity or cervical spine injuries
  - Surgery
    - Ganglion cysts
  - Direct intervention
- Other tests and measures
  - Diagnostic procedures
- Functional status and activity level (current/prior)
  - Occupational activities and work status
  - ADLs
  - Leisure activities
- Growth and development
  - Hand dominance
- Patient's functional goals/outcomes

Tests and Measures
Systems review per APTA's *Guide to Physical Therapy Practice*
- Anthropometric characteristics
  - Atrophy of intrinsics
  - Deformity
- Integumentary integrity
  - Scars
- Muscle performance
  - Strength
    - Elbow, wrist, digits, and thumb
    - Grip and pinch, retest every 2 weeks
  - Palpation
    - Mid-palm, thumb, and wrist
- Pain
  - Measured on visual analog scale

- ROM
  - Upper extremity functional ROM
  - Active ROM
    - Forearm
    - Wrist
    - Digits
- Sensory integrity
  - Two-point discrimination
  - Semmes-Weinstein monofilament
- Special tests
  - Cervical scan
  - Reverse Phalen's
    - Replication of symptoms by wrist hyperextension
    - Hold 30–60 seconds
  - Phalen's
    - Palmar pinch with maximal active wrist flexion
    - Hold 60 seconds
  - Tinel's
    - Tap along nerve at wrist flexion creases
    - Symptoms will occur along distribution of nerve distally
  - Upper limb tension test (ULTTs)
    - ULTT 1 (median nerve dominant)
      a. With patient supine, depress shoulder, abduct to approximately 110°, supinate forearm, extend wrist, fingers, and elbow
      b. Side bend head both toward and away
      c. Assess normal vs. abnormal responses (see Butler. 1991)
    - ULTT 2 (radial nerve dominant)
      a. Patient is supine; shoulder abducted and internally rotated, pronate forearm, extend the elbow, and flex the wrist
      b. Side bend head both toward and away
      c. Assess normal vs. abnormal responses (see Butler. 1991)
    - ULTT 3 (ulnar nerve dominant)
      a. Patient is supine; extend wrist, supinate forearm, fully flex elbow, depress shoulder, and abduct shoulder
      b. Side bend head both toward and away
      c. Assess normal vs. abnormal responses (see Butler. 1991)

Establish Plan of Care
- Based on history, tests, and measures

GOALS/OUTCOMES
- Pain-free wrist and forearm AROM: 100% of AMA guides
  - Wrist
    - Flexion: 60°
    - Extension: 60°
    - Ulnar deviation: 30°
    - Radial deviation: 20°
  - Forearm
    - Pronation: 80°
    - Supination: 80°
- Pain-free thumb AROM: 100% of American Academy of Orthopædic Surgeons (AAOS) norms
  - Metacarpal phalangeal: 0–60°
  - Interphalangeal: 0–80°
  - Radial abduction: 50°
  - Adduction: 0 cm
- Pain: 3/10 or less with activity, 0/10 at rest
- Restoration of strength/endurance of forearm/wrist complex to restore functional use of involved extremity
  - Grip strength: 90% of uninvolved hand or mean for age/gender norms
  - 5/5 on manual muscle test for wrist, forearm, and elbow
- Sensory: 6 mm or less on two-point discrimination test
- Return to prior functional status and activity level (current/prior) for ADLs and vocational, recreational, and sports activities as identified by patient
- Independence in a progressive home exercise program emphasizing function

INTERVENTION
NUMBER OF VISITS: 5–12

Coordination, Communication, Documentation
- Provision of services between admission and discharge that facilitate cost-effective and efficient integration or reintegration to home, community, or work
- Documentation of therapeutic intervention is required for each episode of care and serves as the basic foundation for communication
- Coordination and additional communication will depend on the patient's impairment and home/work/community/leisure situation and requirements. Such services may include:
  - Case management
  - Coordination of care and collaboration with those integral to the patient's rehabilitation program
  - Coordination and monitoring of the delivery of available resources
  - Referrals to other health-care professionals
  - Identification of resources, support groups, or advocacy services
  - Provision of educational or training information
  - Technical assistance

Patient Instruction

Basic Anatomy and Biomechanics
- Refer to anatomical chart, focusing on relation of movement and posture to nerves and tendons in carpal tunnel
- Pertinent Gray's Anatomy (Gray. 1995. 649–654, 852, 1272)
- Netter
- Commercially available products, such as:
  - Krames Communications (1100 Grundy Lane, San Bruno, CA 94066):
    - *Carpal Tunnel Syndrome: Relieving the Pressure in Your Wrist*
  - *Cumulative Trauma: Reducing the Risk*

Handouts
- Home exercise program for stretching
- Hydrotherapy or thermal modalities
- Soft-tissue massage
- Splinting instructions

Functional Considerations
- Ergonomic consultation or job site visit
- Advise patient regarding activities requiring grasping, pinching, or fine finger movements, such as needlework or woodworking

Direct Interventions

Acute Phase: 3–6 Visits
- Therapeutic exercise and home program
  - Cervical/thoracic postural exercise instructions

WRIST/HAND | CARPAL TUNNEL SYNDROME

- Manual therapy techniques
  - Soft-tissue mobilization and manipulation
    - Soft-tissue mobilization of thenar eminence muscle group and carpal tunnel region
  - Manual lymphatic drainage
  - Joint mobilization—Grades I–III
    - Long axis extension
    - Anterior/posterior glide of proximal carpal bones on distal radius
    - Anterior glide of distal carpal bones on proximal carpal bones
    - Distal radio-ulnar joint
    - Thumb
      a. Carpo-metacarpal long axis extension
      b. Anterior/posterior tilt
      c. Lateral tilt and rotation
- Therapeutic devices and equipment
  - Neutral wrist support (custom or prefabricated)
  - Or may splint in slight dorsiflexion
  - Wear routinely for approximately 4–6 weeks
- Electrotherapeutic modalities
  - Iontophoresis
  - TENS
- Physical agents and mechanical modalities
  - Thermal modalities in elevated position
  - Contact particles for desensitization, Fluidotherapy®
  - Hydrotherapy
- Goals/outcomes
  - Pain: 5/10 with activity, 3/10 at rest
  - Sensory: 7 mm on two-point discrimination test
  - Increase in functional activity to include light work, activity

Subacute Phase: 2–6 Visits
- Therapeutic exercise and home program
  - Cardiovascular
  - Musculoskeletal
    - Cervical spine
    - Shoulder girdle
    - Elbow
    - Wrist
    - Hand
  - Strengthening
    Progress exercises in pain-free, symptom-free range
    - Elbow flexion/extension
    - Forearm pronation/supination
    - Wrist extension
    - Wrist flexion
    - Grip

- Manual therapy techniques
  - Joint mobilization—Grades III–V
    - Anterior/posterior glide of proximal carpal bones on distal radius
    - Distal radioulnar joint
- Therapeutic devices and equipment
  - Worn at work and at rest if symptoms persist
- Electrotherapeutic modalities
  - Iontophoresis
  - TENS
- Physical agents and mechanical modalities
  - Continue effective modalities as in acute phase, with increased emphasis on use as needed at home
- Goals/outcomes
  - Pain-free ROM: 100% of AMA guides for wrist and forearm and 100% AAOS norms for thumb
  - Pain: 3/10 or less during day, 0/10 at rest
  - Grip strength: 90% of mean for age/gender norms
  - Tolerance for repetitive functional activities
  - Sensory: 6 mm or less on two-point discrimination test

Functional Carryover
- Patient is to implement micro-work breaks and perform appropriate stretching exercise
- Avoidance of wrist and hand posture that aggravates symptoms
  - Ulnar deviation
  - Wrist flexion with digit flexion
  - Contact palm pressures, such as firm or prolonged grip or restrictive circumferential wrist band
  - Contact vibration
- Ergonomic modifications to work site as appropriate

DISCHARGE PLANNING AND PATIENT RESPONSIBILITY

Criteria for Discharge
- All rehabilitation goals/outcomes achieved except may experience intermittent recurrence of symptoms

Circumstances Requiring Additional Visits
- Exacerbation of volar edema
- Job tasks of a forceful or repetitive nature that exacerbate symptoms
- Need for modification or replacement of splints

540   CARPAL TUNNEL SYNDROME | WRIST/HAND

Home Program

- Stretching exercises
- Tendon/nerve gliding
- Use of splint if recurrence of symptoms
- Anti-vibration pad/gloves/tool handles

Monitoring

- Patient is instructed to call for advice should progression halt or a negative trend occur
- Follow up at 4–8 weeks post-discharge to ensure expected return to function and progression toward attaining all rehabilitation goals/outcomes

REFERENCES

1. Alfonso MI, Dzwierzynski W. Hoffman-Tinel sign: the realities. *Phys Med Rehabil Clin North Am.* 1998;9:721-736.
2. American Academy of Orthopædic Surgeons. *Joint Motion: Method of Measuring and Recording.* Chicago, IL: AAOS; 1965.
3. American Physical Therapy Association. *Guide to Physical Therapist Practice.* Alexandria, VA: APTA; 1997.
4. Armstrong T. *An Ergonomics Guide to Carpal Tunnel Syndrome.* Akron, OH: American Industrial Hygiene Association; 1983.
5. Armstrong T, Castelli W, Evans F, et al. Some histological changes in carpal tunnel contents and their biomechanical implications. *J Occup Med.* 1984;26:197-201.
6. Armstrong TJ, Fine LJ, Silverstein BA. *Occupational Risk Factors of Cumulative Trauma Disorders of the Hand and Wrist: A Final Report.* Cincinnati, OH: National Institutes for Occupational Safety and Health; 1985 (contract no. 200-82-2507).
7. Banta CA. A prospective, nonrandomized study of iontophoresis, wrist splinting, and anti-inflammatory medication in the treatment of early-mild carpal tunnel syndrome. *J Occup Med.* 1994;36:166-168.
8. Barrer S. Gaining the upper hand on carpal tunnel syndrome. *Occup Health Safety.* January 1991;60(1):38-43.
9. Boninger ML, Cooper RA, Baldwin MA, et al. Wheelchair pushrim kinetics: bodyweight and median nerve function. *Arch Phys Med Rehabil.* 1999;80:910-915.
10. Butler DS. *Mobilization of the Nervous System.* Melbourne, Australia: Churchill Livingstone; 1991.

11. Chao E, Opgrande J, Axmear F. Three-dimensional force analysis of finger joints in selected isometric hand function. *J Biomech.* 1976;9:387-396.
12. Durken J. A new diagnostic test for carpal tunnel syndrome. *J Bone Joint Surg.* 1991;73A:535-538.
13. Engelberg AL. *Guides to the Evaluation of Permanent Impairment.* 3rd ed. Chicago, IL: American Medical Association; 1989.
14. Engenbichler GR, Resch KL, Nicolakis P, et al. Ultrasound treatment for treating the carpal tunnel syndrome: randomized "sham" controlled trial. *Br Med J.* 1998;316:731-735.
15. Gelberman R, Szabo R, Williamson R, Dimick M. Sensibility testing in peripheral-nerve compression syndromes. *J Bone Joint Surg.* 1983;65A:632-638.
16. Ghavanini MR. Carpal tunnel syndrome: reappraisal of five clinical tests. *Electromyogr Clin Neurophysiol.* 1998;38:437-441.
17. Gray H; Williams PL, ed. *Gray's Anatomy.* 38th ed. New York, NY: Churchill Livingstone; 1995.
18. Hurley R, ed. *Rehabilitation of the Hand.* St Louis, MO: CV Mosby; 1995.
19. Mathiowetz V, Kashman N, Volland G, et al. Grip and pinch strength: normative data for adults. *Arch Phys Med Rehabil.* 1985;66:69-74.
20. Ozatas O, Turan B, Bora I, et al. Ultrasound therapy effect in carpal tunnel syndrome. *Arch Phys Med Rehabil.* 1998;79:1540-1544.
21. Pecina M, Krmpotic-Nemanic J, Markiewitz AD. *Tunnel Syndromes.* Boca Raton, FL: CRC Press; 1991:55-67.
22. Phalens G. The carpal tunnel syndrome. *J Bone Joint Surg.* 1966;48A:211-228.
23. Rempel D, Harrison R, Barnhart S. Work-related cumulative trauma disorders of the upper extremity. *JAMA.* 1992;267:838-842.
24. Robbins H. Anatomical study of the median nerve in the carpal tunnel and etiologies of the carpal tunnel syndrome. *J Bone Joint Surg.* 1963;45A:953-966.
25. Rozmaryn LM, Dovelle S, Rothman ER, et al. Nerve and tendon gliding exercises and the conservative management of carpal tunnel syndrome. *J Hand Ther.* 1998;11:171-179.
26. Saunders HD. *Cumulative Trauma: Reducing the Risk.* Chaska, MN: Saunders Group; 1990.
27. Silverstein BA, Fine LJ. Occupational factors and carpal tunnel syndrome. *Am J Ind Med.* 1987;23:343-358.

28. Stolp-Smith KA, Pascoe MK, Ogburn PL Jr. Carpal tunnel syndrome in pregnancy: frequency, severity, and prognosis. *Arch Phys Med Rehabil.* 1998;79:1285-1287.

29. Sucher BM, Hinrichs RN. Manipulative treatment of carpal tunnel syndrome: biomechanical and osteopathic intervention to increase the length of the transverse carpal ligament. *J Am Osteopath Assoc.* 1998;98:679-686.

30. Tittiranonda P, Rempel D, Armstrong T, et al. Effect of four computer keyboards in computer users with upper extremity musculoskeletal disorders. *Am J Ind Med.* 1999;35:647-661.

DEQUERVAIN'S TENDINITIS
SUMMARY OVERVIEW

ICD-9

727.04

APTA Preferred Practice Pattern: **4F**

EXAMINATION

- History and systems review
- Tests and Measures
  Systems review per APTA's *Guide to Physical Therapy Practice*
  - Anthropometric characteristics
  - Muscle performance
  - Pain
  - Posture
  - ROM
  - Special tests
- Establish Plan of Care

GOALS/OUTCOMES

- Pain-free thumb and digit ROM: 100% of American Academy of Orthopædic Surgeons norms
- Wrist ROM: 100% of AMA guides
- Pain: 0/10
- Strength: 5/5 on wrist/hand manual muscle test and grip motor performance equal to uninvolved extremity
- Return to prior functional status and activity level (current/prior) for ADLs and vocational, recreational, and sports activities as identified by patient
- Independence in a progressive home exercise program emphasizing function

INTERVENTION
NUMBER OF VISITS: 6–12

- Patient Instruction
  - Basic Anatomy and Biomechanics
  - Handouts
  - Functional Considerations
- Direct Interventions
  - Acute Phase: 3–6 Visits
  - Subacute Phase: 3–6 Visits
- Functional Carryover

DISCHARGE PLANNING AND PATIENT RESPONSIBILITY

- Criteria for Discharge
  - All rehabilitation goals/outcomes achieved with exception of ability to perform heavy repetitious tasks
- Circumstances Requiring Additional Visits
  - Reflex sympathetic dystrophy
  - Persistent inflammation
  - Job tasks of a forceful or repetitive nature that exacerbate symptoms
  - Need for modification or replacement of splints
- Home Program
  - Motor performance and flexibility exercises to increase tolerance and endurance for repetitive tasks
  - Self-friction massage
- Monitoring

DEQUERVAIN'S TENDINITIS

ICD-9

727.04   Radial styloid tenosynovitis

APTA Preferred Practice Pattern: 4F

EXAMINATION

DeQuervain's is an inflammation of a tendon sheath (tenosynovitis) that commonly involves the tendons that straighten or span the thumb away from the hand (abductor pollicis longus and extensor pollicis brevis tendons), producing a constricture of their sheaths in their common osteofibrous canal.

History and systems review

- History of current condition
  - Date and mechanism of injury/onset
  - Location, nature, and behavior of symptoms
    - Aggravating/relieving factors
    - a.m./p.m.
- Past history of current condition
  - Upper extremity or cervical spine injury
  - Surgery
    - Ganglion cysts
  - Therapeutic intervention
- Functional status and activity level (current/prior)
  - Occupational situation
  - ADLs
- Growth and development
  - Hand dominance
- Patient's functional goals/outcomes

Tests and Measures

Systems review per APTA's *Guide to Physical Therapy Practice*

- Anthropometric characteristics
  - Comparative circumferential measurement for edema
    - Distal palmar crease
    - Wrist flexion creases
    - 10 cm proximal to wrist
  - Atrophy
- Muscle performance
  - Strength
    - Wrist, digits, and thumb
    - Grip and pinch

- Palpation
  - Abductor pollicis longus
  - Extensor pollicis brevis
  - Extensor carpi radialis
- Pain
  - Measured on visual analog scale
- Posture
  - Observation
    - Deformity
    - Extremity position
- ROM
  - Active/passive ROM
    - Forearm
    - Wrist
    - Thumb
- Special tests
  - Finkelstein's Test
    - Patient flexes thumb into palm, making fist over thumb
    - Wrist is passively deviated ulnarly
    - Positive test produces localized pain over abductor pollicis longus tendon

Establish Plan of Care

- Based on history, tests, and measures

GOALS/OUTCOMES

- Pain-free thumb and digit ROM: 100% of American Academy of Orthopædic Surgeons (AAOS) norms
  - Digits
    - Metacarpal phalangeal (MP): 0–90°
    - Proximal interphalangeal (PIP): 0–100°
    - Distal interphalangeal (DIP): 0–70°
  - Thumb
    - MP: 0–60°
    - Interphalangeal (IP): 0–80°
    - Radial abduction: 50°
    - Adduction: 0 cm
    - Opposition: 8 cm

544   DEQUERVAIN'S TENDINITIS | WRIST/HAND

- Wrist ROM: 100% of AMA guides
  - Flexion: 60°
  - Extension: 60°
  - Ulnar deviation: 30°
  - Radial deviation: 20°
- Pain: 0/10
- Strength: 5/5 on wrist/hand manual muscle test and grip motor performance equal to uninvolved extremity
- Return to prior functional status and activity level (current/prior) for ADLs and vocational, recreational, and sports activities as identified by patient
- Independence in a progressive home exercise program emphasizing function

INTERVENTION
NUMBER OF VISITS: 6–12

Coordination, Communication, and Documentation
- Provision of services between admission and discharge that facilitate cost-effective and efficient integration or reintegration to home, community, or work
- Documentation of therapeutic intervention is required for each episode of care and serves as the basic foundation for communication
- Coordination and additional communication will depend on the patient's impairment and home/work/community/leisure situation and requirements. Such services may include:
  - Case management
  - Coordination of care and collaboration with those integral to the patient's rehabilitation program
  - Coordination and monitoring of the delivery of available resources
  - Referrals to other health-care professionals
  - Identification of resources, support groups, or advocacy services
  - Provision of educational or training information
  - Technical assistance

Patient Instruction

Basic Anatomy and Biomechanics
- Refer to anatomical chart with focus on tendon location and first dorsal component
- Pertinent Gray's Anatomy (Gray. 1995. 649–654, 851–852, 1927)
- Therapist's management of DeQuervain's disease (Totten. 1990)

Handouts
- Home exercise program
- Cryotherapy or thermal modalities in elevated position
- Friction massage or vibration massager
- Hydrotherapy
  - Contrast baths

Functional Considerations
- Avoidance of ulnar deviation and thumb flexion
- Use of assistive devices to maintain independence in ADLs

Direct Interventions

Acute Phase: 3–6 Visits
- Therapeutic exercise and home program
  To be performed 6 times per day. Pain is indicator of overload.
  - Digit abduction/adduction
  - Intrinsic-plus position
    - MP flexion, PIP, and DIP extension
  - Fisting
  - Guarded-thumb MP and IP flexion
    - Thumb held in protected abduction position initially
    - Progress to full thumb flexion as tolerated
  - Thumb radial and palmar abduction
  - Opposition
    - Initiated to index finger only
    - Progress to the middle, ring, and small finger as tolerated
  - Wrist flexion/extension
  - Wrist radial and ulnar deviation to neutral only, progressing to full ulnar deviation as tolerated
  - Forearm pronation/supination

WRIST/HAND | DEQUERVAIN'S TENDINITIS 545

- Manual therapy techniques
  - Soft-tissue techniques
    - Friction massage
    - Soft-tissue mobilization to dorsal forearm
- Therapeutic devices and equipment
  - Forearm-based thumb spica splint
  - Wrist: 15–20° extension
  - Thumb: Mid position to allow opposition of thumb to index finger
  - Thumb IP joint is free
  - Worn at all times except for exercises or hygiene
- Electrotherapeutic modalities
  - TENS
  - Electrotherapy
  - Iontophoresis
- Physical agents and mechanical modalities
  - Cryotherapy/thermal modalities
  - Ultrasound
- Goals/outcomes
  - Pain: 2/10 with activity, 0/10 at rest
  - Pain-free ROM: Full opposition to all digits
  - Wrist ROM: Equal to uninvolved extremity
  - Edema: Comparative measurement within 20% or less

Subacute Phase: 3–6 Visits
- Therapeutic exercise and home program
  - Manual resistive exercise
    - Wrist, finger, and thumb extensors
  - ROM and stretching techniques
  - Wrist progressive resistive exercises in all planes
    - Start with 6 oz weight
    - Progress over 1 month to 5 lbs minimum
    - Progress dependent upon grip measurement and motor performance testing before and after exercise
  - Hand progressive resistive exercises in all planes
    - Initiated after achieving 1 lb wrist progressive resistive exercise
    - Graded therapy putty, Hand Helper®, Digi-Flex®
- Manual therapy techniques
  - Soft-tissue techniques
    - Friction massage
    - Soft-tissue mobilization to dorsal forearm
  - Passive stretches
- Therapeutic devices and equipment
  - Thumb post splint worn intermittently to avoid pain with activity
  - Splint is discontinued after 8 weeks of wear

- Physical agents and mechanical modalities
  - Continue effective modalities as in acute phase with increased emphasis on use as needed at home.
- Goals/outcomes
  - Pain: 0/10 with activity
  - Edema: Comparative measurement within 10%
  - Strength: 5/5 on wrist/hand manual muscle test and grip motor performance equal to uninvolved extremity
  - Functional goal: resume functional activities with progression to full previous work and home activities

Functional Carryover
- Increase activity with avoidance of pain in wrist and hand
- Avoid undesirable static wrist position or repetitive activity
- Encourage proper neutral wrist posture
- Provide resources for ergonomic tools (e.g., Saunders' Ergo-Source: Stirex Ergonomic Hand Tools, 4250 Norex Drive, Chaska, MN 55318, 1-800-969-4374)
- Job-site assessment and modification as indicated

DISCHARGE PLANNING AND PATIENT RESPONSIBILITY

Criteria for Discharge
- All rehabilitation goals/outcomes achieved with exception of ability to perform heavy repetitious tasks

Circumstances Requiring Additional Visits
- Reflex sympathetic dystrophy
- Persistent inflammation
- Job tasks of a forceful or repetitive nature that exacerbate symptoms
- Need for modification or replacement of splints

Home Program
- Motor performance and flexibility exercises to increase tolerance and endurance for repetitive tasks
- Self-friction massage

Monitoring
- Patient is instructed to call for advice should progression halt or a negative trend occur
- Follow up at 4–8 weeks post-discharge to ensure expected return to function and progression toward attaining all rehabilitation goals/outcomes

546 DEQUERVAIN'S TENDINITIS | WRIST/HAND

REFERENCES

1. American Academy of Orthopædic Surgeons. *Joint Motion: Method of Measuring and Recording.* Chicago, IL: AAOS; 1965.

2. American Physical Therapy Association. *Guide to Physical Therapist Practice.* Alexandria, VA: APTA; 1997.

3. Dobyns J, O'Brien E, Linscheid R, et al. Bowler's thumb: diagnosis and treatment. *J Bone Joint Surg.* 1972;54A:751-755.

4. Engelberg AL. *Guides to the Evaluation of Permanent Impairment.* 3rd ed. Chicago, IL: American Medical Association; 1989.

5. Gray H; Williams PL, ed. *Gray's Anatomy.* 38th ed. New York, NY: Churchill Livingstone; 1995.

6. Grundberg AB, Reagan DS. Pathologic anatomy or the forearm: intersection syndrome. *J Hand Surg (Am).* 1985;10:299-302.

7. Hurley R, ed. *Rehabilitation of the Hand.* St Louis, MO: CV Mosby; 1995.

8. Ippolito E, Postacchini F, Scola E, et al. DeQuervain's disease: An ultrastructural study. *Int Orthop.* 1985;9(4):41-47.

9. Mathiowetz V, Kashman N, Volland G, et al. Grip and pinch strength: normative data for adults. *Arch Phys Med Rehabil.* 1985;66:69-74.

10. Moore JS. DeQuervain's tenosynovitis: stenosing tenosynovitis of the first dorsal compartment. *J Occup Environ Med.* 1997;39:990-1002.

11. Muckart R. Stenosing tenovaginitis of abductor pollicis longus and extensor pollicis brevis at the radial styloid (DeQuervain's disease). *Clin Orthop Rel Res.* 1964;33:201-208.

12. Putz-Anderson V. *Cumulative Trauma Disorders: A Manual for Musculoskeletal Diseases of the Upper Limbs.* Philadelphia, PA: Taylor & Francis; 1988.

13. Reinstein L. DeQuervain's stenosing tenosynovitis in a video games player. *Arch Phys Med Rehabil.* 1983;64:434-435.

14. Totten P. Therapist's management of DeQuervain's disease. In: Hunter JM, Macklin EJ, Callahan AD, eds. *Rehabilitation of the Hand: Surgery and Therapy.* 3rd ed. St Louis, MO: CV Mosby; 1990.

15. Witt J, Pess G, Geberman RH. Treatment of DeQuervain's tenosynovitis: a prospective study of the results of injection of steroids and immobilization in a splint. *J Bone Joint Surg (Am).* 1991;73:219-222.

548 DEQUERVAIN'S TENDINITIS | WRIST/HAND

FLEXOR TENDON REPAIR
SUMMARY OVERVIEW

ICD-9

882.2   883.2

APTA Preferred Practice Pattern: **4J, 7E**

EXAMINATION

- History and Systems Review
- Tests and Measures
  Systems review per APTA's *Guide to Physical Therapy Practice*
  - Anthropometric characteristics
  - Integumentary integrity
  - Motor function
  - Pain
  - ROM
- Establish Plan of Care

GOALS/OUTCOMES

- Digit and thumb ROM: 100% of American Academy of Orthopædic Surgeons norms
- Wrist and forearm ROM: 100% of AMA guides
- Pain: 3/10 or less
- Decrease edema to within 10% of uninvolved side
- Prehensile (grip and pinch) strength: Mean for age/gender norms
- Return to prior functional status and activity level for ADLs and vocational, recreational, and sports activities as identified by patient
- Independence in a progressive home exercise program emphasizing function

INTERVENTION
NUMBER OF VISITS: 8–18

- Patient Instruction
  - Basic Anatomy and Biomechanics
  - Patient-Related Instruction
  - Functional Training in Self-Care and Home Management
  - Description of Surgical Procedure
- Direct Interventions
  - Acute Phase I: 3–6 Visits, Weeks 1–3
  - Acute Phase II: 3–6 Visits, Weeks 4–5
  - Phase III: 2–6 Visits, Weeks 6–12
- Functional Carryover

DISCHARGE PLANNING AND PATIENT RESPONSIBILITY

- Criteria for Discharge
  - All rehabilitation goals/outcomes achieved
- Circumstances Requiring Additional Visits
  - Postoperative infection/complications
  - Nerve laceration
  - Fracture/crush injury
  - Persistent edema
  - Two-stage repair
  - Scar adhesion
  - Persistent PROM limitation
  - Poor/limited active distal interphalangeal flexion
  - Contracture development
  - Job tasks of a forceful or repetitive nature that exacerbate symptoms
- Home Program
  - Resistive exercise
  - Scar reduction techniques
  - Flexibility exercises
- Monitoring

SUMMARY OVERVIEW | WRIST/HAND | FLEXOR TENDON REPAIR   549

FLEXOR TENDON REPAIR

Modified Four-Strand Tendon Repair
Modified Duran Repair Program
ICD-9

882.2	Open wound of hand except finger(s) alone, with tendon involvement
883.2	Open wound of finger(s) with tendon involvement

APTA Preferred Practice Pattern: 4J, 7E

EXAMINATION

Surgical techniques will dictate the rehabilitation program. It is recommended that the therapist consult with the surgeon.

History and Systems Review
- History of current condition
  - Mechanism of injury/onset
  - Date of injury/onset
  - Date and type of surgical procedure
    - Presence of stabilizing pins
    - Presence of digital nerve repair
    - Presence of skin grafts
- Past history of current condition
  - Upper extremity or cervical spine injuries
  - Surgeries
    - ZONE I-Area distal to insertion of flexor digitorum superficialis tendon; injury here involves only flexor digitorum profundus.
    - ZONE II-Injury here involves flexor digitorum profundus and two slips of flexor digitorum superficialis. This zone is sub-divided into distal, middle, and proximal areas. A series of fibrous pulleys and tendons/sheaths contribute to unpredictable repairs.
    - ZONE III-Extends from distal edge of transverse carpal ligament to just beyond distal palmar crease. This area is transversed by the finger flexors in the palm and without fibrous pulleys. Recovery is typically good.
    - ZONE IV-Area of carpal tunnel; the transverse carpal ligament acts as a pulley for the finger flexors.
    - ZONE V-Area of forearm and wrist proximal to transverse carpal ligament; injury here may involve up to 12 tendons and may be associated with injury to median and ulnar nerves.
  - Direct intervention

- Functional status and activity level (current/prior)
  - Occupation
- Patient's functional goals/outcomes

Tests and Measures
Systems review per APTA's *Guide to Physical Therapy Practice*
- Anthropometric characteristics
  - Circumferential measurement for edema
    - Middle and proximal phalanx of digit(s)
    - Distal palmar crease (DPC)
    - Wrist flexor crease

Flexor Tendon Zones

Adapted from lecture: Robert Duran MD and Scott Jaeger MD, American Society for Surgery of the Hand, Symposium 1981. Philadelphia.

- Integumentary integrity
  - Observation of laceration or surgical incision
  - Skin condition
    - Hematomas
    - Vascularization
  - Zone of injury (see diagram)
- Motor function
  - Resting posture of upper extremity
  - Movement patterns
- Pain
  - Measured on visual analog scale
- ROM
  - Within parameters of post-op precautions
  - Gross measure of distance from flexed finger tip to DPC, measured in centimeters
    - Index
    - Long
    - Ring
    - Small

Establish Plan of Care
- Based on history, tests, and measures

GOALS/OUTCOMES
- Digit and thumb ROM: 100% of American Academy of Orthopædic Surgeons (AAOS) norms
  - Passive/active digit
    - Metacarpal phalangeal (MCP): 0–90°
    - Proximal interphalangeal (PIP): 0–100°
    - Distal interphalangeal (DIP): 0–70°
  - Thumb
    - MCP: 0–60°
    - Interphalangeal (IP): 0–80°
    - Radial abduction: 50°
    - Adduction: 0 cm
- Wrist and forearm ROM: 100% of AMA guides
  - Wrist
    - Flexion: 60°
    - Extension: 60°
    - Ulnar deviation: 30°
    - Radial deviation: 20°
  - Forearm
    - Pronation: 80°
    - Supination: 80°

- Pain: 3/10 or less
- Decrease edema to within 10% of uninvolved side
- Prehensile (grip and pinch) strength: mean for age/gender norms
- Return to prior functional status and activity level for ADLs and vocational, recreational, and sports activities as identified by patient
- Independence in a progressive home exercise program emphasizing function

INTERVENTION
NUMBER OF VISITS: 8–18

Coordination, Communication, and Documentation
- Provision of services between admission and discharge that facilitate cost-effective and efficient integration or reintegration to home, community, or work
- Documentation of therapeutic intervention is required for each episode of care and serves as the basic foundation for communication
- Coordination and additional communication will depend on the patient's impairment and home/work/community/leisure situation and requirements. Such services may include:
  - Case management
  - Coordination of care and collaboration with those integral to the patient's rehabilitation program
  - Coordination and monitoring of the delivery of available resources
  - Referrals to other health-care professionals
  - Identification of resources, support groups, or advocacy services
  - Provision of educational or training information
  - Technical assistance

Patient Instruction

Basic Anatomy and Biomechanics
- Hand and wrist anatomical chart, focus on area of repair, surgical procedure, and function of sublimus vs. profundus tendons
- Surgical anatomy of the hand (Netter. 1969. 33–34)
- Pertinent Gray's Anatomy (Gray. 1995. 649–654, 847–848, 857)

WRIST/HAND | FLEXOR TENDON REPAIR 551

Patient-Related Instruction

- Specific exercise instructions
  - Self-PROM
  - Massage techniques to minimize adhesion
  - Edema reduction techniques
- Postoperative precautions
- Splint wear and care

Functional Training in Self-Care and Home Management

- Postoperative precautions
  - Avoid active flexion of all digits to prevent tendon rupture. Any active use of the involved hand is not allowed, such as for holding, grasping.
  - Avoid extension of the digit and wrists beyond the limits of the dorsal block splint
- Skin care
  - On postoperative day 5, the splint is removed 1 time per day for skin care. The patient is cautioned to keep hand and wrist positioned in protective, passive flexion posture. The hand is cleansed with alcohol once a day while sutures remain.
  - In postoperative week 2, begin scar/desensitization massage after suture removal
- Edema control
  - Instruct patient to maintain hand in elevated position at all times
  - Elevation with retrograde massage may be initiated
  - Review low-sodium diet
  - Compression wrapping

Description of Surgical Procedure

- Review operative report

Direct Interventions

Acute Phase: 3–6 Visits, Weeks 1–3

- Status of hand
  - At the time of surgery the patient is fit with a postoperative plaster splint and bulky dressing
  - The patient's wrist and digits are positioned in a protective flexion posture
  - By postoperative day 5 the patient's cast and dressings are removed and the patient is referred for hand therapy
  - Sutures are present until postoperative day 10–14

- Therapeutic exercise and home program
  - Modified Duran Exercise Program
    Exercises should not cause an increase in pain, edema, or stiffness. Perform 10 repetitions each hour while wearing the dorsal block splint.
    - Passive MCP flexion to 90° followed by active extension of MCP and IP joints to within limits of dorsal splint
    - Passive IP flexion followed by active extension of IP joints within the splint
    - Passive fisting followed by active digit extension
      NOTE: Extension exercises may be done passively instead of actively, per physician order
  - Modified four-strand tendon repair program
    Postoperative week 1–3
    - Controlled passive flexion and active extension of the digit
    - Initiate use of the Strickland hinged wrist splint
      a. Exercise sequence is performed 25 repetitions each hour while wearing splint
      b. Passive fisting with active wrist extension, patient holds position gently (comparable to less than 10 microvolts) for 5 seconds; patient allows the wrist to drop into flexion
      c. Digits follow this tenodesis pattern and will straighten
- Manual therapy techniques
  - Initiated following suture removal at approximately 2 weeks postoperative
  - Soft-tissue techniques
    - Retrograde massage for edema reduction
    - Soft-tissue mobilization
    - Scar massage
- Fabrication of devices and equipment
  - Splinting
  - Postoperative day 5 the patient is fitted with a dorsal-based extension block splint (DBS)
    - The wrist is held in 20–30° flexion, MCP joint in 50–70° flexion, and IPs in a neutral position
    - The splint is to be worn at all times except for hand hygiene
  - Kleinert traction option if additional protection required
    - The patient is fitted with a dorsal-based extension block splint as above
    - The digit(s) is held in flexion with dynamic traction using a resistive spring/rubber and nylon thread

552   FLEXOR TENDON REPAIR | WRIST/HAND

- NOTE: The direction of pull should be along the axis of normal flexion of the involved digit
- Tension should be adjusted to allow extension of the digit to the limit of the splint
- Continue intermittent splinting until postoperative week 5
  - For exercise program with modified four-strand repair, Strickland tenodesis splint is fabricated
    - This splint allows full active wrist flexion and 30° wrist dorsiflexion, MCPs extend to 60° and IP's full motion
    - The splint is applied during hourly exercise sessions beginning postoperative week 1
- Wound management
  - Dressing
  - Debridement—selective
  - Topical agents
- Physical agents and mechanical modalities
  - Superficial thermal modalities in an elevated position, after suture removal (optional)
- Goals/outcomes
  - Stabilize/protect surgical site with proper use of splints
  - Decrease edema to within 50% of uninvolved side
  - ROM of all digits to 80% of AAOS norms
    - MCP: 0–75°
    - PIP: 10–90°
    - DIP: 0–55° (unless Zone 1 repair)
  - Decrease scar density
  - Independent self-care within limits of postoperative precautions

Acute Phase II: 3–6 Visits, Weeks 4–5
- Status of the hand:
  - The patient's wrist and digits may have some extension limitations
  - Edema may still be apparent in the hand
  - Patients with early full ROM of the digits may need longer time in protective splint to avoid tendon rupture
- Therapeutic exercise and home program
  Exercises are performed out of the splints. Perform 25 repetitions every 2 hours beginning week 4.
  - Continue passive flexion exercises of the digits
  - Wrist flexion with finger extension to neutral
  - For modified four-strand

- Gentle passive PIP extension with MCPs and wrist flexed
- Progress to PIP extension with the wrist in neutral and only the MCPs flexed
- The shelf position allows increased tendon excursion into the palm
- Beginning week 5, perform 50 repetitions every 2 hours
  - Isolated tendon excursion exercises are begun
    - Flex the IPs while actively extending the MCPs and then extend the digits
  - Active wrist flexion and gradually increase extension beyond neutral with digits held in flexion
  - Light passive IP stretching exercise may be started for Duran repair
- Manual therapy techniques
  - Soft-tissue techniques
    - Soft-tissue mobilization
    - Friction massage
  - Joint mobilization
    - Grades III–V for hypermobility in carpal and MCP joint
- Therapeutic devices and equipment
  - Splinting
    - Modify degree of wrist flexion of dorsal block splint per physician's orders
    - Kleinert traction should be removed at 5 weeks or earlier, dependent upon physician preference. The patient continues to wear the dorsal block splint without flexion traction.
    - Use a dynamic digit extension splint if passive extension is limited. This splint can be worn intermittently as tolerated.
- Physical agents and mechanical modalities
  - Superficial thermal modalities in elevated position
  - Contrast baths
- Goals/outcomes
  - Wrist and hand PROM: 100% of AMA guides or AAOS norms
  - Decrease edema to within 25% of uninvolved side
  - Decrease scar density
  - Pain: 3/10 or less with activity, 0/10 at rest

Phase III: 2–6 Visits, Weeks 6–12
- Therapeutic exercise and home program
  - Resume use of involved hand for light ADLs
  - MCP blocking during IP joint flexion

- The patient can be given a wood block or Swanson Finger Crutch™ for home use
- No blocking is performed to small finger flexor digitorum profunds due to the diameter and vascular supply of the tendon
  - Passive IP extension with the more proximal joints in increasing degrees of extension
  - Active IP and MCP flexion with increasing intensity of contraction
  - Taper active wrist flexion/extension exercises as ROM approaches full range
  - Prehension
    - Introduce active prehensile tasks with light resistance, such as peg boards or foam cubes
  - Week 7
    - Light resistance for prehensile activity with gradual progression: Foam gripping, therapy putty
  - Week 8
    - ROM should now be within normal limits in the involved hand and wrist
    - The patient should continue to avoid heavy resistance activities
    - Progress strengthening exercises
  - Week 12
    - Heavy resistive exercises and use of hand in all ADLs
- Manual therapy techniques
  - Soft-tissue techniques
    - Soft-tissue mobilization
    - Scar massage/desensitization
  - Joint mobilization
- Therapeutic devices and equipment
  - Splinting
    - Discontinue the dorsal block splint unless the patient is in an environment where they may fall or their hand may be "bumped"
    - Scar conformer, elastomer sheeting may be used daytime or nocturnally as needed
- Electrotherapeutic modalities
- Physical agents and mechanical modalities
  - Ultrasound

- Goals/outcomes
  - Digit and thumb AROM: achieve 80% of AAOS norms
    - Digit
      a. MP: 0–75°
      b. IP: 0–80°
      c. DIP: 0–55° (unless Zone 1 repair)
    - Thumb
      a. MP: 0–50°
      b. IP: 0–65°
      c. Radial abduction: 40°
      d. Adduction: -2 cm
  - Independent ADLs and vocational function
  - Strength: Tensile force 5,000 g mean for age/gender norms
  - Return to preoperative, unresisted activity level

Functional Carryover
- Compliance with early postoperative precautions and maintaining protective flexion posture in spite of patient performing adapted ADLs
- Week 6: The patient is allowed use of the involved hand for ADLs, including using utensil for eating and performing self care
- Week 8–10: The patient should be encouraged to progress with hand use for housekeeping and meal preparation
- Week 12: Heavy resistive exercise and functional activity, including simulation of work activity is encouraged
- Ergonomic modifications to the work site as necessary

DISCHARGE PLANNING AND PATIENT RESPONSIBILITY

Criteria for Discharge
- All rehabilitation goals/outcomes achieved

Circumstances Requiring Additional Visits
- Postoperative infection/complications
- Nerve laceration
- Fracture/crush injury
- Persistent edema
- Two-stage repair
- Scar adhesion
- Persistent PROM limitation

554   FLEXOR TENDON REPAIR | WRIST/HAND

- Poor/limited active DIP flexion
- Contracture development
- Job tasks of a forceful or repetitive nature that exacerbate symptoms

Home Program
- Resistive exercise
- Scar reduction techniques
- Flexibility exercises

Monitoring
- Patient is instructed to call for advice should progression halt or a negative trend occur
- Follow up at 4–8 weeks post-discharge to ensure expected return to function and progression toward attaining all rehabilitation goals/outcomes

REFERENCES

1. American Academy of Orthopædic Surgeons. *Joint Motion: Method of Measuring and Recording.* Chicago, IL: AAOS; 1965.

2. American Physical Therapy Association. *Guide to Physical Therapist Practice.* Alexandria, VA: APTA; 1997.

3. Chow J, Thomas L, Dorelle S, et al. A combined regimen of controlled motion following flexor tendon repair in "No Man's Land." *Plast Reconstr Surg.* 1987;79:447-455.

4. Engelberg AL. *Guides to the Evaluation of Permanent Impairment.* 3ʳᵈ ed. Chicago, IL: American Medical Association; 1989.

5. Gray H; Williams PL, ed. *Gray's Anatomy.* 38ᵗʰ ed. New York, NY: Churchill Livingstone; 1995.

6. Hurley R, ed. *Rehabilitation of the Hand.* St Louis, MO: CV Mosby; 1995.

7. Kleinert H, McGoldrick F, Papas N. Concepts that changed flexor tendon surgery. In: Hunter JM, Schneider LH, Mackin EJ, eds. *Nerve Surgery in the Hand: A Third Decade.* St. Louis, MO: CV Mosby; 1997.

8. Lister GD, Kleinert HE, Kutz JE, Atasoy E. Primary flexor tendon repair followed by immediate controlled mobilization. *J Hand Surg.* 1997;2:441-445.

9. Madan E, Hunter J. *Hand Therapy Program for Patients With Staged Gliding Tendon Prosthesis.* 5ᵗʰ ed. Philadelphia, PA: Hand Rehabilitation Foundation; 1986.

10. Mathiowetz V, Kashman N, Volland G, et al. Grip and pinch strength: normative data for adults. *Arch Phys Med Rehabil.* 1985;66:69-74.

11. Netter F. Surgical anatomy of the hand. *Clin Symp.* 1969;21(3):1-46.

12. Silfverskiold K, May E. Flexor tendon repair zone II with a new suture technique and an early mobilization program combining passive and active flexion. *J Hand Surg.* 1994;19A:153.

13. Silfverskiold K, May E. Flexor tendon repair with active mobilisation: the Gothenburg experience. In: Hunter JM, Schneider LH, Mackin EJ, eds. *Tendon and Nerve Surgery in the Hand: A Third Decade.* St. Louis, MO: CV Mosby; 1997.

14. Small J, Brennan M, Colville J. Early active Mobilisation following flexor tendon repair in zone II. *J Hand Surg.* 1989;14B:383-391.

15. Stewart K, van Strien G. Postoperative management of flexor tendon injuries. In: Hunter JM, Macklin EJ, Callahan AD, eds. *Rehabilitation of the Hand.* St. Louis, MO: CV Mosby; 1996.

16. Stewart Pettengill K. Postoperative therapy concepts I: management of flexor tendon injuries: early mobilization. In: Hunter JM, Schneider LH, Macklin EJ eds. *Tendon and Nerve Surgery in the Hand: A Third Decade.* St. Louis, MO: CV Mosby; 1997.

17. Strickland J, Gettle K. Flexor tendon repair: the Indianapolis method. In: Hunter JM, Schneider LH, Macklin EJ, eds. *Tendon and Nerve Surgery in the Hand: A Third Decade.* St. Louis, MO: CV Mosby; 1997.

18. Van Strien G. Postoperative management of flexor tendon injuries. In: Hunter JM, Mackin EJ, Callahan AD, eds. *Rehabilitation of the Hand.* 3ʳᵈ ed. St. Louis, MO: CV Mosby; 1990.

556   FLEXOR TENDON REPAIR | WRIST/HAND

HAND ARTHROPATHY
SUMMARY OVERVIEW

ICD-9

716.94   719.44

APTA Preferred Practice Pattern: **4D, 4E, 4F**

EXAMINATION

- History and Systems Review
- Tests and Measures
  Systems review per APTA's *Guide to Physical Therapy Practice*
  - Anthropometric characteristics
  - Ergonomics and body mechanics
  - Integumentary integrity
  - Joint integrity and mobility
  - Motor function
  - Muscle performance
  - Orthotics, protective and supportive devices
  - Pain
  - Posture
  - ROM
  - Reflex integrity
  - Self-care and home management
  - Sensory integrity
  - Work (job/school/play), community, and leisure integration or reintegration (including instrumental ADLs)
- Establish Plan of Care

GOALS/OUTCOMES

- Functional mobility for metacarpal phalangeal (MCP) and interphalangeal (IP) joints: MCP 0–60°, proximal IP 0–80°, distal IP 0–60°
- Stability and joint protection for carpo-metacarpal joints: Functional splint for ADLs/night splint
- Joint conservation education: Patient to show understanding of joint protection and ability to adjust activities to reduce joint stress
- Functional strength appropriate to age, gender, and occupation. May be tested with splint.
- Pain control: 3/10 for ADLs—may be with use of splints
- Edema control: Home techniques

INTERVENTION
NUMBER OF VISITS: 5–10

- Patient Instruction
  - Handouts
  - Functional considerations
- Direct Interventions
  - Acute Phase: 2–5 Visits
  - Subacute Phase: 3–5 Visits
- Functional Carryover

DISCHARGE PLANNING AND PATIENT RESPONSIBILITY

- Criteria for Discharge
  - Independence in performance of home program
  - Ability to modify tasks to decrease joint stress
  - Pain and inflammation reduced to functional tolerance (3/10 pain or less)
  - Functional grip and pinch strength (may be tested with splints if appropriate) and should be within 10% of unaffected hand or functional for age/gender normative values (Mankowitz)
- Circumstances Requiring Additional Visits
  - Severe degenerative changes
  - History of other pathology
  - Previous surgeries
  - Cognitive limitations
  - Excessive environmental barriers to discharge
  - Additional joint pathology/bilateral symptoms
- Home Program
  - Ongoing use of resting splints for joint protection in ADLs and for night positioning
  - Stretching to maintain hand functional mobility
  - Strengthening within limits of joint protection to maintain functional use of hand
  - Understanding by patient of assistive devices available for minimizing joint stress in ADLs and work activities
- Monitoring

SUMMARY OVERVIEW | WRIST/HAND | HAND ARTHROPATHY   557

HAND ARTHROPATHY

ICD-9

716.94   Arthropathy, unspecified, hand
719.44   Pain in joint, hand
APTA Preferred Practice Pattern: 4D, 4E, 4F

EXAMINATION

History and Systems Review

- History of current condition
  - Location, nature, and behavior of symptoms, relieving/aggravating factors
  - Date of onset/previous treatment
- Past history of current condition
  - Splinting, surgeries, injections
- Other tests and measures
  - Hand dominance
  - ROM, grip/pinch strength
  - Skin condition
- Medications
- Past medical/surgical history
  - Any continuing need of assistive devices for gait affecting upper-extremity use
- Functional status and activity level (current/prior)
- Patient's functional goals
- Surgical reports if applicable

Tests and Measures

Systems review per APTA's *Guide to Physical Therapy Practice*

- Anthropometric Characteristics
  - Hand joint deformities and posture (Heberden's Nodes, Bouchard's Nodes, boutonnière deformity, swan neck deformity, ulnar drift, metacarpal phalangeal (MCP) joint deformity, MCP joint synovitis, intrinsic muscle imbalance, wrist deformity, extensor tendon/flexor tendon subluxation
  - Circulation (arterial, venous, lymphatic): Raynaud's phenomenon
- Ergonomics and body mechanics
- Integumentary integrity
- Joint integrity and mobility: Joint size, inflammation
- Motor function (motor control and motor learning)
- Muscle performance (including strength, power, and endurance)
- Orthotics, protective and supportive devices

- Pain
- Posture
- ROM (including muscle length)
- Reflex integrity
- Self-care and home management (including ADLs and instrumental ADLs)
- Sensory integrity
- Work (job/school/play), community, and leisure integration or reintegration (including instrumental ADLs)

Establish Plan of Care

- Based on history, tests, and measures

GOALS/OUTCOMES

- Functional mobility for MCP and interphalangeal joints: MCP 0–60°, proximal interphalangeal: 0–80°, distal interphalangeal: 0–60°
- Stability and joint protection for carpo-metacarpal (CMC) joints: Functional splint for ADLs/night splint
- Joint conservation education: Patient to show understanding of joint protection and ability to adjust activities to reduce joint stress
- Functional strength appropriate to age, gender, and occupation. May be tested with splint.
- Pain control: 3/10 for ADLs—may be with use of splints
- Edema control: Home techniques

INTERVENTION

NUMBER OF VISITS: 5–10

Coordination, Communication, and Documentation

- Provision of services between admission and discharge that facilitate cost-effective and efficient integration or reintegration to home, community, or work
- Documentation of therapeutic intervention is required for each episode of care and serves as the basic foundation for communication

- Coordination and additional communication will depend on the patient's impairment and home/work/community/leisure situation and requirements. Such services may include:
  - Case management
  - Coordination of care and collaboration with those integral to the patient's rehabilitation program
  - Coordination and monitoring of the delivery of available resources
  - Referrals to other health-care professionals
  - Identification of resources, support groups, or advocacy services
  - Provision of educational or training information
  - Technical assistance
- Specific coordination and communication provisions

Patient Instruction
- Green's Operative Hand Surgery, Netter's Orthopædics (online program), Rehabilitation of the Hand and Upper Extremity (pg 1560, 1576, 1579, 1649, 1653, 1654), Orthopædic Examination, Evaluation, and Intervention (pg 584, 586, 607), Clinical Orthopædic Rehabilitation (pg 52, 53).

Handouts
- Krames Communications (1100 Grundy Lane, San Bruno, CA 94066):
  - *Joint Conservation*
  - *Ergonomics*
  - *Arthritis*
- Sammons-Preston home catalog of ADLs assistive devices
- Home program to cover joint protection considerations, ergonomic changes, and exercises to maintain hand strength/mobility while minimizing joint stress

Functional considerations
- Posture (sitting, standing, sleeping, driving)
- Assistive devices: Splints for carpal tunnel, CMC arthritis, ulnar deviation of digits
- Precautions: Avoidance of stress postures, excessive grip, excessive pinch, especially to avoid thumb CMC and MCP hyperextension, overuse of joints when inflamed
- Alteration of ADLs: Avoid positions of wrist flexion, ulnar deviation, thumb MCP and CMC hyperextension in ADLs. Do not lean on palms, push up from chair with wrists hyperextended, pick up items with pinch grip
- Avoidance of prolonged postures
- Positioning for relief of symptoms
- Body mechanic instruction for lifting, pushing, pulling
- Alternative exercise options (i.e. swimming, sitting ergometer)

Direct Interventions

Acute Phase: 2–5 Visits
- Splinting for joint protection and rest
- Therapeutic exercise for mobility
- Modalities for edema and inflammatory control
- Home exercise program

Subacute Phase: 3–5 Visits
- Therapeutic activities and ADL retraining, concentrating on joint stabilization (no exercise except AROM)
- Night splinting and review of assistive devices for home and work
- Functional activity training for joint protection
- Silver Ring Splinting™ for finger and thumb deformities

Functional Carryover
- Integration of home exercise program into vocational environment
- Completion of ergonomic adjustments to home, automobile, and vocational areas
- Incorporation of proper posture and body mechanics to avoid exacerbation of symptoms
- Recognition/avoidance of activities that increase or exacerbate symptoms
- Incorporation of pain/edema control techniques as part of home program

DISCHARGE PLANNING AND PATIENT RESPONSIBILITY

Criteria for discharge
- Independence in performance of home program
- Ability to modify tasks to decrease joint stress
- Pain and inflammation reduced to functional tolerance (3/10 pain or less)
- Functional grip and pinch strength (may be tested with splints if appropriate) should be within 10% of unaffected hand or functional for age/gender normative values (Mankowitz)

Circumstances Requiring Additional Visits
- Severe degenerative changes
- History of other pathology
- Previous surgeries
- Cognitive limitations
- Excessive environmental barriers to discharge
- Additional joint pathology/bilateral symptoms

Home Program
- Ongoing use of resting splints for joint protection in ADLs and for night positioning
- Stretching to maintain hand functional mobility
- Strengthening within limits of joint protection to maintain functional use of hand
- Understanding by patient of assistive devices available for minimizing joint stress in ADLs and work activities

Monitoring
- Patient may need replacement or revision of splints over time
- Reassessment at 6 months by physician, with possible further treatment as joint degeneration may progress

REFERENCES

1. American Physical Therapy Association. *Guide to Physical Therapist Practice*. Alexandria, VA: APTA; revised 2003.
2. Brotzman SB, Wilk KE. *Clinical Orthopaedic Rehabilitation*. 2nd ed. Mosby Inc; 2003.
3. Dutton M. *Orthopaedic Examination, Evaluation and Intervention*. McGraw-Hill; 2004.
4. Jacobs M, Austin N. *Splinting of the Hand and Upper Extremity*. Lippincott Williams & Wilkins; 2003.
5. Green D, Hotchkiss R, Peterson WC. *Green's Operative Hand Surgery*. Elsevier Inc.; 2005.
6. Mackin EJ, Callahan AD, Osterman AL, et al. *Hunter, Makin, & Callahan's Rehabilitation of the Hand and Upper Extremity*. 5th ed. Mosby Inc; 2002.

HAND FRACTURE
SUMMARY OVERVIEW

ICD-9

    815.00   816.00   816.01

APTA Preferred Practice Pattern: **4G, 4H, 4I**

EXAMINATION

- History and Systems Review
- Tests and Measures

  Systems review per APTA's *Guide to Physical Therapy Practice*
  - Anthropometric characteristics
  - Environmental, home, and work (job/school/play) barriers
  - Ergonomics and body mechanics
  - Integumentary integrity
  - Joint integrity and mobility
  - Muscle performance
  - Orthotics, protective and supportive devices
  - Pain
  - Posture
  - ROM
  - Reflex integrity
  - Self-care and home management
  - Sensory integrity
  - Work (job/school/play), community, and leisure integration or reintegration (including instrumental ADLs)
- Establish Plan of Care

GOALS/OUTCOMES

- Hand, wrist, and forearm ROM: 80–100% of AMA guidelines
- Prehensile strength (grip and pinch): Mean for age/gender norms or equal to uninvolved side if injury is to dominant side, 80% of uninvolved side if non-dominant. Functional needs of work or home ADLs must be met by grip/pinch values.
- Pain: 2/10 or less with activity, 1/10 at rest
- Return to prior functional status for home or work activities
- Return to previous sports or recreational activities
- Ability to maintain home exercise activities if goals not fully met

INTERVENTION
NUMBER OF VISITS: 4–12

- Patient Instruction
  - References
  - Home Program
  - Functional considerations
- Direct Interventions
  - Acute Phase: 2–6 Visits
  - Subacute Phase: 2–6 Visits
- Functional Carryover

DISCHARGE PLANNING AND PATIENT RESPONSIBILITY

- Criteria for Discharge
  - Patient has achieved goals for ROM
  - Pain at 1–2/10 or less
  - Functional pinch or grip related to norms for gender and age
  - Independent performance of home exercises and understanding of any further precautions
  - Patient able to return to previous work or home activities
  - Patient understands goals/precautions for return to sports/recreational activities
- Circumstances Requiring Additional Visits
  - Delay in wound healing
  - Infection
  - Excessive environmental barriers to discharge
  - Chronic reflexive pain syndrome
  - Contractures
- Home Program
  - Home program is to provide frequent, low-level stretching to involved joints, stimulation of circulatory system to reduce swelling and prevent infection. Patient must be able to follow exercise directions, don and doff any assistive devices, and be aware of precautions for fracture and infection potential.
- Monitoring

SUMMARY OVERVIEW | WRIST/HAND | HAND FRACTURE   561

HAND FRACTURE

ICD-9

815.00	Closed fracture of metacarpal bone(s), site unspecified
816.00	Closed fracture of phalanx or phalanges of hand, unspecified
816.01	Closed fracture of middle or proximal phalanx or phalanges of hand

APTA Preferred Practice Pattern: **4G, 4H, 4I**

EXAMINATION

History and Systems Review

- History of current condition
  - Onset of injury, surgical intervention, casting
  - Mechanism of injury/fall risk
- Previous upper extremity fractures
- Other tests and measures
  - ROM
  - Comparative measure of edema
  - Grip/pinch if appropriate to length of time from injury
  - Pain and what aggravates/alleviates
  - Sensory status
  - Hand dominance
- Medications
- Past medical/surgical history
- Functional status and activity level (current/prior)
- Work status/home environment
- Patient's functional goals

Tests and Measures

Systems review per APTA's *Guide to Physical Therapy Practice*

- Anthropometric characteristics
  - Assistive and adaptive devices
  - Circulation (arterial, venous, lymphatic)
- Environmental, home, and work (job/school/play) barriers
- Ergonomics and body mechanics
- Integumentary integrity: Assess scar mobility if open reduction, internal fixation
- Joint integrity and mobility
- Muscle performance (including strength, power, and endurance)
- Orthotics, protective and supportive devices
- Pain
- Posture
- ROM (including muscle length)
- Reflex integrity
- Self-care and home management (including ADLs and instrumental ADLs)
- Sensory integrity
- Work (job/school/play), community, and leisure integration or reintegration (including instrumental ADLs)

Establish Plan of Care

- Based on history, tests, and measures

GOALS/OUTCOMES

- Hand, wrist, and forearm ROM: 80–100% of AMA guidelines
  - Wrist
    - Flexion: 60°
    - Extension: 60°
    - Ulnar deviation: 0–30°
    - Radial deviation: 0–20°
  - Metacarpal phalangeal (MCP) joint: 0–90°
  - Interphalangeal (IP) joints: 0–100°
  - Thumb MCP joint: 0–50°
  - Thumb IP joint: 0–60°
  - Forearm pronation/supination: 80° each
- Prehensile strength (grip and pinch): Mean for age/gender norms or equal to uninvolved side if injury is to dominant side, 80% of uninvolved side if non-dominant. Functional needs of work or home ADLs must be met by grip/pinch values
- Pain: 2/10 or less with activity, 1/10 at rest
- Return to prior functional status for home or work activities
- Return to previous sports or recreational activities
- Ability to maintain home exercise activities if goals not fully met

INTERVENTION
NUMBER OF VISITS: 4–12

Coordination, Communication, and Documentation

- Provision of services between admission and discharge that facilitate cost-effective and efficient integration or reintegration to home, community, or work
- Documentation of therapeutic intervention is required for each episode of care and serves as the basic foundation for communication
- Coordination and additional communication will depend on the patient's impairment and home/work/community/leisure situation and requirements. Such services may include:
  - Case management
  - Coordination of care and collaboration with those integral to the patient's rehabilitation program
  - Coordination and monitoring of the delivery of available resources
  - Referrals to other health-care professionals
  - Identification of resources, support groups, or advocacy services
  - Provision of educational or training information
  - Technical assistance
- Specific coordination and communication provisions

Patient Instruction

- Edema control with contrast baths, cold packs, retrograde massage, elevation
- Mobility exercises for both involved and uninvolved joints
- Home interferential or TENS unit for edema control and pain control

References

- *Rehabilitation of the Hand and Upper Extremity* (Mackin EJ, Callahan AD, Osterman AL, et al. 371–395)
- *Green's Operative Hand Surgery* (Green D, Hotchkiss R, Peterson WC. Chapters 8, 17)
- *Splinting the Hand and Upper Extremity* (Jacobs M, Austin N. 100–113)

Home Program

Should include exercises for mobility appropriate to fracture maturity and healing, edema control measures, instruction in protection of fracture with use of cast, splints, and appropriate wound care if needed. Patient should be able to don and doff any splint independently, or a family member will need to be instructed in this activity. Instruction should include skin care and attention to signs of infection.

Functional considerations

- Posture (sitting, standing, sleeping, driving)
  - Avoid dependent positioning
  - Sleep instructions to protect fracture
- Assistive devices: Splints, cast care, wear instructions
- Precautions
  - Review the time required for fracture healing with patient
  - Review the signs of infection and wound care with patient
- Alteration of ADLs
- Avoidance of prolonged postures
- Positioning for relief of symptoms
- Body mechanic instruction for lifting, pushing, pulling
- Training recommendations: Cross training, importance of aerobic activity for healing

Direct Interventions

Acute Phase: 2–6 Visits

- Heat or cold
- Ultrasound at 20–50% to assist fracture healing
- Wound care for pins or incisions with surgical repairs
- Active exercises for uninvolved joints of injured arm
- Active or active-assisted exercises as appropriate to fracture healing
- Retrograde massage/interferential for edema control

Subacute Phase: 2–6 Visits

- Light strengthening activities as able, with fracture healing to include sensory bins, therapy putty, table top wipe, soft ball squeeze, Baltimore Therapeutic Equipment if available
- Continue edema control as needed
- TENS for pain as needed

WRIST/HAND | HAND FRACTURE   563

Functional Carryover

- Integration of home exercise program into vocational environment
- Completion of ergonomic adjustments to home, automobile, and vocational areas
- Incorporation of proper posture and body mechanics to avoid exacerbation of symptoms
- Recognition/avoidance of activities that increase or exacerbate symptoms

DISCHARGE PLANNING AND PATIENT RESPONSIBILITY

Criteria for Discharge

- Patient has achieved goals for ROM (see goals)
- Pain at 1–2/10 or less
- Functional pinch or grip related to norms for gender and age
- Independent performance of home exercises and understanding of any further precautions
- Patient able to return to previous work or home activities
- Patient understands goals/precautions for return to sports/recreational activities

Circumstances Requiring Additional Visits

- Delay in wound healing
- Infection
- Excessive environmental barriers to discharge
- Chronic reflexive pain syndrome
- Contractures

Home Program

- Home program is to provide frequent, low level stretching to involved joints, stimulation of circulatory system to reduce swelling and prevent infection. Patient must be able to follow exercise directions, don and doff any assistive devices, be aware of precautions for fracture and infection potential.
  - Active and active-assisted exercises for tendon gliding, digit mobility, wrist mobility, forearm mobility
  - Edema control with contrast baths, retrograde massage, positioning, TENS, and cold
  - Strengthening when appropriate using resistive bands, therapy putty, bin exercises, and light weights

Monitoring

- Patient will need to return to physician for follow-up if fracture healing is significantly delayed, and may need specific activity strengthening or work conditioning to return to full activities

REFERENCES

1. American Physical Therapy Association. *Guide to Physical Therapist Practice*. Alexandria, VA: APTA; revised 2003.
2. Gogia PP. *Clinical Wound Management*. Thorofare, NJ: Slack Inc; 1995.
3. Green D, Hotchkiss R, Peterson WC. *Green's Operative Hand Surgery*. Elsevier Inc; 2005.
4. Jacobs M, Austin N. *Splinting of the Hand and Upper Extremity*. Lippincott Williams & Wilkins; 2003.
5. Mackin EJ, Callahan AD, Osterman AL, et al. *Hunter, Makin, & Callahan's Rehabilitation of the Hand and Upper Extremity*. 5th ed. Mosby Inc; 2002.

POSTOPERATIVE CARPAL TUNNEL RELEASE
SUMMARY OVERVIEW

ICD-9
    354.0
APTA Preferred Practice Pattern: **4F**

EXAMINATION
- History and Systems Review
- Tests and Measures
  Systems review per APTA's *Guide to Physical Therapy Practice*
  - Anthropometric characteristics
  - Integumentary integrity
  - Muscle performance
  - Pain
  - ROM and motor performance
  - Sensory integrity
  - Special tests
- Establish Plan of Care

GOALS/OUTCOMES
- Pain-free wrist and forearm AROM: 100% of AMA guides
- Pain-free thumb AROM: 100% of American Academy of Orthopædic Surgeons norms
- Pain: 3/10 or less with activity, 0/10 at rest
- Prehensile (grip and pinch) motor performance: 90% of uninvolved hand or mean for age/gender norms
- Strength: 5/5 on manual muscle test for wrist and forearm
- Sensory integrity: At 6 mm or less on two-point discrimination test
- Return to prior functional status and activity level (current/prior) for ADLs and vocational, recreational, and sports activities as identified by patient
- Independence in a progressive home exercise program emphasizing function

INTERVENTION
NUMBER OF VISITS: 5–12

- Patient Instruction
  - Basic Anatomy and Biomechanics
  - Handouts
  - Functional Considerations
  - Description of Surgical Procedure
- Direct Interventions
  - Acute Phase: 2–6 Visits; Weeks 1–2
  - Subacute Phase: 3–6 Visits, Weeks 3–8
- Functional Carryover

DISCHARGE PLANNING AND PATIENT RESPONSIBILITY
- Criteria for Discharge
  - All rehabilitation goals/outcomes achieved except may experience intermittent recurrence of symptoms
- Circumstances Requiring Additional Visits
  - Postoperative infection/complications
  - Reflex sympathetic dystrophy
  - Scar hypersensitivity
  - Persistent edema altering functional use
  - Slow recovery of prehensile motor performance
  - Job tasks of a forceful or repetitive nature that exacerbate symptoms
  - Wound dehiscence
  - Pillar pain
  - Triggering
- Home Program
  - Stretching exercises
  - Tendon gliding exercise
  - Nerve gliding
  - Use of splint if symptoms recur
- Monitoring

SUMMARY OVERVIEW | WRIST/HAND | POSTOPERATIVE CARPAL TUNNEL RELEASE   565

POSTOPERATIVE CARPAL TUNNEL RELEASE

ICD-9
>   354.0   Carpal tunnel syndrome

APTA Preferred Practice Pattern: 4F

EXAMINATION

History and Systems Review

- History of current condition
  - Date and mechanism of injury/onset
  - Date and type of surgical procedure
  - Location, nature, and behavior of symptoms
    - Aggravating/relieving factors
- Past history of current condition
  - Upper extremity or cervical injury
  - Surgery
    - Ganglion cysts
  - Therapeutic intervention
- Past medical/surgical history
  - Inquire regarding systemic pathology
- Functional status and activity level (current/prior)
  - Current functional limitations
  - Occupational activities and work status
  - Leisure/recreational activities
- Growth and development
  - Hand dominance
- Patient's functional goals/outcomes

Tests and Measures

Systems review per APTA's *Guide to Physical Therapy Practice*

- Anthropometric characteristics
  - Atrophy of thenar eminence
  - Deformity
- Integumentary integrity
  - Scars
- Muscle performance
  - Strength
    - Elbow, wrist, digits, and thumb
    - Grip and pinch
- Pain
  - Measured on visual analog scale
- ROM and motor performance
  - Upper extremity functional ROM
  - Active ROM and strength
    - Forearm
    - Wrist
    - Digits

- Sensory integrity
  - Two-point discrimination
  - Dermatomal patterns
- Special tests
  - Semmes-Weinstein Monofilament
    - Sensory discrimination test
  - To monitor surgical recovery of median nerve
    - Reverse Phalen's
      a. Replication of symptoms by wrist hyperextension
      b. Hold 30–60 seconds
    - Phalen's
      a. Palmar pinch with maximal active wrist flexion
      b. Hold 60 seconds
    - Tinel's
      a. Tap along nerve at wrist flexion creases
      b. Symptoms will occur along distribution of nerve distally

Establish Plan of Care

- Based on history, tests, and measures

GOALS/OUTCOMES

- Pain-free wrist and forearm AROM: 100% of AMA guides
  - Wrist
    - Flexion: 60°
    - Extension: 60°
    - Ulnar deviation: 30°
    - Radial deviation: 20°
  - Forearm
    - Pronation: 80°
    - Supination: 80°
- Pain-free thumb AROM: 100% of American Academy of Orthopædic Surgeons (AAOS) norms
  - Metacarpal phalangeal (MCP): 0–60°
  - Interphalangeal (IP): 0–80°
  - Radial abduction: 50°
  - Adduction: 0 cm
  - Opposition: 8 cm

566   PostOp Carpal Tunnel Release | Wrist/Hand

- Pain: 3/10 or less with activity, 0/10 at rest
- Prehensile (grip and pinch) motor performance: 90% of uninvolved hand or mean for age/gender norms
- Strength: 5/5 on manual muscle test for wrist and forearm
- Sensory integrity: at 6 mm or less on two-point discrimination test
- Return to prior functional status and activity level (current/prior) for ADLs and vocational, recreational, and sports activities as identified by patient
- Independence in a progressive home exercise program emphasizing function

INTERVENTION
NUMBER OF VISITS: 5–12

Coordination, Communication, and Documentation
- Provision of services between admission and discharge that facilitate cost-effective and efficient integration or reintegration to home, community, or work
- Documentation of therapeutic intervention is required for each episode of care and serves as the basic foundation for communication
- Coordination and additional communication will depend on the patient's impairment and home/work/community/leisure situation and requirements. Such services may include:
  ○ Case management
  ○ Coordination of care and collaboration with those integral to the patient's rehabilitation program
  ○ Coordination and monitoring of the delivery of available resources
  ○ Referrals to other health-care professionals
  ○ Identification of resources, support groups, or advocacy services
  ○ Provision of educational or training information
  ○ Technical assistance

Patient Instruction

Basic Anatomy and Biomechanics
- Refer to anatomical charts for relation of surgical procedure to nerves and tendons
- Pertinent Gray's Anatomy (Gray. 1995. 649–654, 852, 1272)
- *Surgical Anatomy Of The Hand* (Netter. 1969)

Handouts
- Home exercise program for stretching
- Skin and surgical wound care
  ○ Scar mobilization/management
- Postoperative edema control
- Splint utilization
- Commercially available products, such as:
  ○ Krames Communications (1100 Grundy Lane, San Bruno, CA 94066):
    - *Carpal Tunnel Syndrome: Relieving the Pressure in Your Wrist*

Functional Considerations
- Avoidance of activities placing force on wrist extension/flexion

Description of Surgical Procedure
- Review of operative procedure and relation to joint biomechanics, rehabilitation, and function

Direct Interventions

Acute Phase: 2–6 Visits; Weeks 1–2
- Therapeutic exercise and home program 3 times per day; 10 repetitions each
  ○ Tendon gliding exercises
    - IP flexion or "claw"
    - MCP flexion, followed by proximal interphalangeal flexion "straight fist"
    - Full fisting: Active-assisted/gentle
  ○ Thumb flexion/extension
  ○ Opposition
  ○ Digit abduction/adduction
  ○ Sensory training or retraining
- Manual therapy techniques
  ○ Soft-tissue techniques
    - Soft-tissue mobilization of thenar eminence

WRIST/HAND | POSTOP CARPAL TUNNEL RELEASE   567

- Friction massage to reduce scar adhesion following suture removal
- Manual lymphatic drainage
- Silicone gel/elastomer
  - Joint mobilization
- Therapeutic devices and equipment
  - Wrist splint, maintaining neutral position
  - Custom or prefabricated
  - Worn nocturnally and during strenuous activity
- Physical agents and mechanical modalities
  - Thermal modalities in elevated position
  - Contact particles for desensitization, Fluidotherapy®
- Goals/outcomes
  - Pain: 3/10 with activity, 0/10 at rest
  - Wrist ROM: 80% of AMA guides
    - Flexion: 50°
    - Extension: 50°
    - Ulnar deviation: 25°
    - Radial deviation: 15°

Subacute Phase: 3–6 Visits, Weeks 3–8
- Therapeutic exercise and home program
  3 times per day; 10 repetitions each as tolerated
  - Week 3: Endoscopic release
    - Full fisting
    - Resistive exercise: therapy putty (grade determined by motor performance and pinch assessment)
    - Isometric and isotonic resistance for wrist and hand
    - Resume use of involved hand for light ADLs and hand crafts
    - Sensory training/retraining
  - Weeks 4–5
    - Open-palm release will begin graded isometric and isotonic strengthening
    - Wrist progressive resistance exercise
      a. Begin with 1 lb and progress to minimum of 5 lbs
  - Weeks 6–8
    - Functional training
      a. Motor performance, work simulation
      b. Work tolerance program
- Manual therapy techniques
  - Joint mobilization
    - Anterior/posterior glide of the distal radius and proximal row of carpals
    - Distal radio-ulnar joint
    - Scaphoid distraction

- Soft-tissue techniques
  - Friction massage for reduction of scar adhesion
- Passive stretches
  - Thumb abduction
  - Median nerve glide
    a. Shoulder abduction to 110°, forearm supination and extension of the elbow, wrist, and fingers
  - Wrist extension
- Therapeutic devices and equipment
  - Worn during strenuous activity and as needed nocturnally
  - Utilization decreases with adequate motor performance for activity
- Wound management
- Electrotherapeutic modalities
  - Iontophoresis
  - TENS
- Physical agents and mechanical modalities
  Continue effective modalities as in acute phase, with increased emphasis on use as needed at home.
  - Deep thermal modalities
    - Ultrasound
    - Phonophoresis
  - Superficial thermal modalities
    - Paraffin baths
    - Hot packs
  - Hydrotherapy
    - Contrast baths
  - Mini-vibrator for desensitization
  - Silicone gel/elastomer for scar management
- Goals/outcomes
  - ROM: 100% of AMA guides for wrist and 100% of AAOS norms for thumb
  - Pain: 3/10 or less
  - Strength: Gain 15 lbs in grip motor performance by postoperative week 6
  - Prehensile (grip and pinch) motor performance: 90% of uninvolved hand or mean for age/gender norms
  - Absence of scar adhesion

Functional Carryover
- Use of hand for ADLs and leisure activities that do not promote symptoms
- Consideration of referral to work tolerance program
- Ergonomic modifications to work site as necessary

DISCHARGE PLANNING AND PATIENT RESPONSIBILITY

Criteria for Discharge
- All rehabilitation goals/outcomes achieved except may experience intermittent recurrence of symptoms

Circumstances Requiring Additional Visits
- Postoperative infection/complications
- Reflex sympathetic dystrophy
- Scar hypersensitivity
- Persistent edema altering functional use
- Slow recovery of prehensile motor performance
- Job tasks of a forceful or repetitive nature that exacerbate symptoms
- Wound dehiscence
- Pillar pain
- Triggering

Home Program
- Stretching exercises
- Tendon gliding exercise
- Nerve gliding
- Use of splint if symptoms recur

Monitoring
- Patient is instructed to call for advice should progression halt or a negative trend occur
- Follow up at 4–8 weeks post-discharge to ensure expected return to function and progression toward attaining all rehabilitation goals/outcomes

REFERENCES

1. American Academy of Orthopedic Surgeons. *Joint Motion: Method of Measuring and Recording.* Chicago, IL: AAOS; 1965.
2. American Physical Therapy Association. *Guide to Physical Therapist Practice.* Alexandria, VA: APTA; 1997.
3. Banta CA. A prospective, nonrandomized study of iontophoresis wrist splinting and anti-inflammatory medication in the treatment of early-mild carpal tunnel syndrome. *J Occup Med.* 1994;36:166-168.
4. Gellman H, Kan D, Gee V, Kushner SH, Botte MJ. Analysis of pinch and grip strength after carpal tunnel release. *J Hand Surg (Am).* 1989;14(5):863-864.
5. Ghavanini MR. Carpal tunnel syndrome: reappraisal of five clinical tests. *Electromyogr Clin Neurophysiol.* 1998;38:437-441.
6. Gray H; Williams PL, ed. *Gray's Anatomy.* 38th ed. New York, NY: Churchill Livingstone; 1995.
7. Hurley R, ed. *Rehabilitation of the Hand.* St Louis, MO: CV Mosby; 1995.
8. Mathiowetz V, Kashman N, Volland G, et al. Grip and pinch strength: normative data for adults. *Arch Phys Med Rehabil.* 1985;66:69-74.
9. Menon J, Etter C. Endoscopic carpal tunnel release. *J Hand Ther.* 1993;6(2):139-144.
10. Netter F. Surgical anatomy of the hand. *CIBA Clin Symp.* 1969;21(3):1-46.
11. Ozatas O, Turan B, Bora I, et. al. Ultrasound therapy effect on carpal tunnel syndrome. *Arch Phys Med Rehabil.* 1998;79:1540-1544.
12. Rozymaryn LM, Dovelle S, Rothman ER, et al. Nerve and tendon gliding exercises and the conservative management of carpal tunnel syndrome. *J Hand Ther.* 1998;11(3):171-179.

570   PostOp Carpal Tunnel Release | Wrist/Hand

POSTOPERATIVE DEQUERVAIN'S SYNDROME
SUMMARY OVERVIEW

ICD-9

727.04

APTA Preferred Practice Pattern: **4F**

EXAMINATION

- History and Systems Review
- Tests and Measures
  Systems review per APTA's *Guide to Physical Therapy Practice*
  - Anthropometric characteristics
  - Pain
  - ROM
- Establish Plan of Care

GOALS/OUTCOMES

- Pain-free wrist ROM: 100% of AMA guides
- Pain-free thumb ROM: 100% of American Academy of Orthopædic Surgeons norms
- Pain: 0/10
- Strength: 4/5 on manual muscle tests for thumb and wrist musculature
- Prehensile (grip and pinch) motor performance: Mean for age/gender norms
- Return to prior functional status and activity level (current/prior) for ADLs and vocational, recreational, and sports activities as identified by patient
- Independence in a progressive home exercise program emphasizing function

INTERVENTION
NUMBER OF VISITS: 6–12

- Patient Instruction
  - Basic Anatomy and Biomechanics
  - Handouts
  - Functional Considerations
  - Description of Surgical Procedure
- Direct Interventions
  - Acute Phase: 3–6 Visits, Weeks 1–6
  - Subacute Phase: 3–6 Visits, Weeks 7–12
- Functional Carryover

DISCHARGE PLANNING AND PATIENT RESPONSIBILITY

- Criteria for Discharge
  - All rehabilitation goals/outcomes achieved, but may discharge at 90% ROM if all other goals/outcomes attained
- Circumstances Requiring Additional Visits
  - Postoperative infection/complications
  - Scar hypersensitivity
  - Reflex sympathetic dystrophy
  - Job tasks of a forceful or repetitive nature that exacerbate symptoms
  - Scar adhesion causing pain
  - Limited ROM
- Home Program
  - Discontinue use of splint at discharge
  - Scar reduction techniques as needed
  - Exercise
- Monitoring

SUMMARY OVERVIEW | WRIST/HAND | POSTOPERATIVE DEQUERVAIN'S SYNDROME 571

POSTOPERATIVE DEQUERVAIN'S SYNDROME

ICD-9
> 727.04   Radial styloid tenosynovitis

APTA Preferred Practice Pattern: **4F**

EXAMINATION

DeQuervain's is inflammation of a tendon sheath (tenosynovitis) that commonly involves the tendons that straighten or span the thumb away from the hand (abductor longus and extensor pollicis brevis tendons), producing a constricture of their sheaths in their common osteofibrous canal.

History and Systems Review

- History of current condition
  - Date and mechanism of surgical procedures
    - Postoperative precautions
    - Splinting/casting
  - Location, nature, and behavior of symptoms
    - Aggravating/relieving factors
- Past history of current condition
  - Upper extremity or cervical injury
  - Surgery
    - Ganglion cysts
  - Therapeutic intervention
- Functional status and activity level (current/prior)
- Growth and development
  - Hand dominance
- Patient's functional goals/outcomes

Tests and Measures

Systems review per APTA's *Guide to Physical Therapy Practice*

- Anthropometric characteristics
  - Observation
    - Extremity position
  - Comparative circumferential measurements for edema
    - Distal palmar crease
    - Wrist flexion crease
- Pain
  - Measured on visual analog scale
- ROM
  - Active ROM of thumb and wrist

Establish Plan of Care

- Based on history, tests, and measures

GOALS/OUTCOMES

- Pain-free wrist ROM: 100% of AMA guides
  - Flexion: 60°
  - Extension: 60°
  - Ulnar deviation: 30°
  - Radial deviation: 20°
- Pain-free thumb ROM: 100% of American Academy of Orthopædic Surgeons (AAOS) norms
  - Metacarpal phalangeal (MCP): 0–60°
  - Interphalangeal (IP): 0–80°
  - Radial abduction: 50°
  - Adduction: 0 cm
  - Opposition: 8 cm
- Pain: 0/10
- Strength: 4/5 on manual muscle tests for thumb and wrist musculature
- Prehensile (grip and pinch) motor performance: Mean for age/gender norms
- Return to prior functional status and activity level (current/prior) for ADLs and vocational, recreational, and sports activities as identified by patient
- Independence in a progressive home exercise program emphasizing function

INTERVENTION
NUMBER OF VISITS: 6–12

Coordination, Communication, and Documentation

- Provision of services between admission and discharge that facilitate cost-effective and efficient integration or reintegration to home, community, or work
- Documentation of therapeutic intervention is required for each episode of care and serves as the basic foundation for communication
- Coordination and additional communication will depend on the patient's impairment and home/work/

community/leisure situation and requirements. Such services may include:

- Case management
- Coordination of care and collaboration with those integral to the patient's rehabilitation program
- Coordination and monitoring of the delivery of available resources
- Referrals to other health-care professionals
- Identification of resources, support groups, or advocacy services
- Provision of educational or training information
- Technical assistance

Patient Instruction

Basic Anatomy and Biomechanics
- Refer to anatomical chart with focus on mechanism of surgical release
- Pertinent Gray's Anatomy (Gray. 1995. 649–654. 851–852, 1927)
- Therapist's management of DeQuervain's disease (Totten. 1990. 308–320)

Handouts
- Home exercise program
- Cryotherapy or thermal modalities in elevated positions
- Edema reduction techniques
- Scar reduction/desensitization techniques
  - Silicone gel/elastomer for scar management

Functional Considerations
- Use of splint for all activity
- Use of assistive devices to maintain independence in ADLs
- Edema control
  - Retrograde massage
  - Compression glove
  - Coban™ wrap
- Following suture removal, begin scar desensitization

Description of Surgical Procedure
- Review of operative procedure and relation to joint biomechanics, rehabilitation, and function

Direct Interventions

Acute Phase: 3–6 Visits, Weeks 1–6
- Therapeutic exercise and home program
  Perform 4–6 times per day, 10 repetitions, avoiding pain, stiffness, or increase in edema
  - Digit abduction/adduction
  - Intrinsic-plus position
    - MCP flexion, proximal interphalangeal, and distal interphalangeal extension
  - Fisting
  - Thumb flexion
  - Thumb radial abduction
  - Thumb palmar abduction
  - Opposition
  - Wrist flexion/extension
  - Wrist radial deviation and ulnar deviation
  - Pronation/supination
- Manual therapy techniques
  - Soft-tissue techniques
    - Soft-tissue mobilization
    - Friction massage to scar following suture removal
- Therapeutic devices and equipment
  - Thumb post spica splint
    - Wrist in 10–20° extension
    - Thumb in mid-position with IP free, allowing for thumb to index opposition
  - Continuous utilization except during exercise and hygiene
- Electrotherapeutic modalities
  - Iontophoresis
  - TENS
- Physical agents and mechanical modalities
  - Thermal agents in elevated position
- Goals/outcomes
  - Pain: 3/10 or less
  - Pain-free ROM: 75% of AMA guides for wrist and AAOS norms for thumb
    - Wrist
      a. Ulnar deviation: 25°
      b. Radial deviation: 15°
    - Thumb
      a. MCP: 45°
      b. IP: 60°
      c. Radial abduction: 40°
      d. Adduction: -2 cm
      e. Opposition: 6 cm

- Stabilize/protect surgical site with use of splint
- Edema: reduce to within 10% of uninvolved limb

Subacute Phase: 3–6 Visits, Weeks 7–12

- Therapeutic exercise and home program
  - Stretching pre- and post-exercise
  - Wrist and hand progressive resistive exercise
    - Start with 6 oz weight
    - Progress during subacute phase to 5 lbs
    - Progress dependent upon grip measurement and motor performance testing
    - Use graded therapy putty or grip exercisers
    - Week 8, initiate grip isometrics
    - Baltimore Therapeutic Equipment, work simulation with gentle, progressive resistance/endurance
  - Upper extremity endurance activity
    - Simulation of work activities or sports participation
- Manual therapy techniques
  - Soft-tissue techniques
    - Soft-tissue mobilization for dorsal forearm
    - Friction massage at surgical site
  - Passive stretches
- Therapeutic devices and equipment
  Per physician orders
  - Use only for resistive daily activities, such as driving, laundry, raking leaves, vacuuming
    - Gradual reduction of splint wear as indicated by decreased edema and increased pain-free activity
  - Nocturnal wear only if sleep is disrupted due to pain
- Physical agents and mechanical modalities
  Continue effective modalities as in acute phase with increased emphasis on use as needed at home.
  - Scar desensitization techniques
    - Contact particles, Fluidotherapy®
    - Friction massage
    - Vibration
- Goals/outcomes
  - Pain: 0/10 or less
  - AROM: 100% of AMA guides for wrist and 100% of AAOS norms for thumb
  - Strength: 4/5 on manual muscle test for wrist and thumb
  - Prehensile (grip and pinch) motor performance: Mean for age/gender norms

Functional Carryover

- Modification of daily activity to avoid repetitive thumb extension
- Job-site assessment or modification as appropriate

DISCHARGE PLANNING AND PATIENT RESPONSIBILITY

Criteria for Discharge

- All rehabilitation goals/outcomes achieved, but may discharge at 90% ROM if all other goals/outcomes attained

Circumstances Requiring Additional Visits

- Postoperative infection/complications
- Scar hypersensitivity
- Reflex sympathetic dystrophy
- Job tasks of a forceful or repetitive nature that exacerbate symptoms
- Scar adhesion causing pain
- Limited ROM

Home Program

- Discontinue use of splint at discharge
- Scar reduction techniques as needed
- Exercise
  - Flexibility
  - Motor performance
  - Functional progression of activities to enable patient to return to previous recreational and sport status

Monitoring

- Patient is instructed to call for advice should progression halt or a negative trend occur
- Follow up at 4–8 weeks post-discharge to ensure expected return to function and progression toward attaining all rehabilitation goals/outcomes

REFERENCES

1. American Academy of Orthopædic Surgeons. *Joint Motion: Method of Measuring and Recording.* Chicago, IL: AAOS; 1965.

2. American Physical Therapy Association. *Guide to Physical Therapist Practice.* Alexandria, VA: APTA; 1997.

3. Armstrong TJ, Fine LJ, Goldstein SA, Lifshitz YR, Silverstein BA. Ergonomics considerations in hand and wrist tendinitis. *J Hand Surg [Am].* September 1987;12(5 Pt 2):830-7.

4. Arons MS. DeQuervain's release in working women. *J Hand Surg.* 1987;12A(4):540.

5. Engelberg AL. *Guides to the Evaluation of Permanent Impairment.* 3rd ed. Chicago: American Medical Association; 1989.

6. Gray H; Williams PL, ed. *Gray's Anatomy.* 38th ed. New York, NY: Churchill Livingstone; 1995.

7. Grundberg AB, Reagan DS. Pathologic anatomy of the forearm: intersection syndrome. *J Hand Surg [Am].* 1985;10(2):299-302.

8. Hurley R, ed. *Rehabilitation of the Hand.* St Louis, MO: Mosby; 1995.

9. Ippolito E, Postacchini F, Scola E, et al. DeQuervain's disease: An ultrastructural study. *Int Orthop.* 1985:9(4):41-47.

10. Jackson WT, et al. Anatomical variations in the first extensor compartment of the wrist. *J Bone Joint Surg.* 1986;68A(6):923.

11. Mathiowetz V, Kashman N, Volland G, et al. Grip and pinch strength: normative data for adults. *Arch Phys Med Rehabil.* 1985;66:69-73.

12. Moore JS. DeQuervain's tenosynovitis: stenosing tenosynovitis of the first dorsal compartment. *J Occup Environ Med.* 1997;39(1):990-1002.

13. Reinstein L. DeQuervain's stenosing tenosynovitis in a video games player. *Arch Phys Med Rehabil.* 1983:64(9):434-435.

14. Totten P. Therapist's management of DeQuervain's disease. In: Hunter JM, Mackin EJ, Callahan, eds. *Rehabilitation of the Hand.* 3rd ed. St. Louis, MO: CV Mosby; 1990:308-320.

15. Viegas SF. Trigger Thumb of DeQuervain's disease. *J Hand Surg.* 1986;11A(2):235.

16. Witt J, Pess G, Geberman RH. Treatment of DeQuervain's tenosynovitis: a prospective study of the results of injection of steroids and immobilization in a splint. *J Bone Joint Surg (Am).* 1991;73(2):219-222.

576   POSTOPERATIVE DEQUERVAIN'S SYNDROME | WRIST/HAND

POSTOPERATIVE DUPUYTREN'S FASCIECTOMY
SUMMARY OVERVIEW

ICD-9

728.6

APTA Preferred Practice Pattern: **4D, 4J**

EXAMINATION

- History and systems review
- Tests and Measures
  Systems review per APTA's *Guide to Physical Therapy Practice*
  - Anthropometric characteristics
  - Integumentary integrity
  - Joint integrity and mobility
  - Motor function
  - Pain
  - ROM
  - Sensory integrity
- Establish Plan of Care

GOALS/OUTCOMES

- ROM: 100% of AMA guides or American Academy of Orthopædic Surgeons (AAOS) norms for uninvolved joints of the wrist, thumb, and digits
- Achieve 80% of AAOS norms for proximal interphalangeal of involved joint, minimizing joint contracture
- Pain: 0/10
- Prehensile (grip and pinch) strength: Mean for age/gender norms
- Strength: 5/5 on manual muscle test for extensors of involved digits
- Return to prior functional status and activity level for ADLs and vocational, recreational, and sports activities as identified by patient
- Independence in a progressive home exercise program emphasizing function
- Prevent scar adhesion and minimize scar density

INTERVENTION
NUMBER OF VISITS: 6–11

- Patient Instruction
  - Basic Anatomy and Biomechanics
  - Patient-Related Instruction
  - Functional Considerations
  - Description of Surgical Procedure
- Direct Interventions
  - Acute Phase: 3–5 Visits, Days 10–21 Postoperative
  - Subacute Phase: 3–6 Visits, Weeks 4–8
- Functional Carryover

DISCHARGE PLANNING AND PATIENT RESPONSIBILITY

- Criteria for Discharge
  - All rehabilitation goals/outcomes achieved with the exception of return to prior functional status and activity level for recreational and sports activities
- Circumstances Requiring Additional Visits
  - Underlying medical complications, such as diabetes or arthritis
  - Scar hypersensitivity
  - Presence of reflex sympathetic dystrophy
  - Postoperative infection/complications
  - Need for ongoing modification of splints
- Home Program
  - Progressive strengthening and conditioning of upper extremity as patient resumes/expands activities
  - Long-term splinting
  - Scar reduction techniques
- Monitoring

SUMMARY OVERVIEW | WRIST/HAND | POSTOPERATIVE DUPUYTREN'S FASCIECTOMY   577

POSTOPERATIVE DUPUYTREN'S FASCIECTOMY

ICD-9
728.6   Contracture of palmar fascia
APTA Preferred Practice Pattern: 4D, 4J

EXAMINATION

Dupuytren's contracture is a contracture of the proliferated longitudinal bands of the palmar aponeurosis lying between the skin and flexor tendons in the distal palm and fingers. It begins as a nodule and progresses to fibrous bands with contracture of the fingers. It occurs most often in the ring and little fingers.

History and systems review
- History of current condition
  - Mechanism of injury
  - Date of injury/onset
  - Surgical procedures and postoperative limitations
  - Location, nature, and behavior of symptoms
    - Aggravating/relieving factors
- Growth and development
  - Hand dominance
- Functional status and activity level (current/prior)
  - Occupational activities
  - Recreational activities
- Patient's functional goals

Tests and Measures
Systems review per APTA's *Guide to Physical Therapy Practice*
- Anthropometric characteristics
  - Circumferential measurement for edema
    - Distal palmar crease
    - Middle and proximal phalanx of involved digit
- Integumentary integrity
  - Observation
    - Appearance of wound
    - Integument (capillary refill)
    - Obvious deformities
- Joint integrity and mobility
- Motor function
  - Assessed as appropriate to postoperative healing status
- Pain
  - Measured on visual analog scale

- ROM
  - Wrist
  - Thumb
  - Digits
- Sensory integrity
  - Protective sensibility
    - Semmes-Weinstein monofilament
  - Discrimination sensibility
    - Two-point discrimination, static

Establish Plan of Care
- Based on history, tests, and measures

GOALS/OUTCOMES
- ROM: 100% of AMA guides or American Academy of Orthopædic Surgeons (AAOS) norms for uninvolved joints of the wrist, thumb, and digits
  - Wrist
    - Flexion: 60°
    - Extension: 60°
    - Ulnar deviation: 30°
    - Radial deviation: 20°
  - Thumb
    - Metacarpal phalangeal (MCP): 0–60°
    - Interphalangeal (IP): 0–80°
    - Radial abduction: 50°
    - Adduction: 0 cm
    - Opposition: 8 cm
  - Digit
    - MCP: 0–90°
    - Proximal interphalangeal (PIP): 0–100°
    - Distal interphalangeal (DIP): 0–70°
- Achieve 80% of AAOS norms for PIP of involved joint, minimizing joint contracture
  - PIP: 10–90°

578   PostOp Dupuytren's Fasciectomy | Wrist/Hand

- Pain: 0/10
- Prehensile (grip and pinch) strength: Mean for age/gender norms
- Strength: 5/5 on manual muscle test for extensors of involved digits
- Return to prior functional status and activity level for ADLs and vocational, recreational, and sports activities as identified by patient
- Independence in a progressive home exercise program emphasizing function
- Prevent scar adhesion and minimize scar density

INTERVENTION
NUMBER OF VISITS: 6–11

Coordination, Communication, and Documentation
- Provision of services between admission and discharge that facilitate cost-effective and efficient integration or reintegration to home, community, or work
- Documentation of therapeutic intervention is required for each episode of care and serves as the basic foundation for communication
- Coordination and additional communication will depend on the patient's impairment and home/work/community/leisure situation and requirements. Such services may include:
  - Case management
  - Coordination of care and collaboration with those integral to the patient's rehabilitation program
  - Coordination and monitoring of the delivery of available resources
  - Referrals to other health-care professionals
  - Identification of resources, support groups, or advocacy services
  - Provision of educational or training information
  - Technical assistance

Patient Instruction

Basic Anatomy and Biomechanics
- Anatomy of hand and wrist structure
- Pertinent Gray's Anatomy (Gray. 1995. 649–654, 854, 857)

Patient-Related Instruction
- Home exercise program
- Wound care and dressing change
  - Saline soaks
    - 9 g (1 heaping tsp) table salt to 1 qt lukewarm water
    - 2–3 times per day
    - Squeeze soft foam ball in water (closed wound only)
- Edema control by elevation, retrograde massage, compression wrap, compression glove, or low sodium diet

Functional Considerations
- Adaptive equipment or one-handed techniques for daily activities

Description of Surgical Procedure
- Review of operative report
- Review of operative procedures in relation to joint biomechanics, rehabilitation, function, scar formation, and postoperative limitations

Direct Interventions

Acute Phase: 3–5 Visits, Days 10–21 Postoperative
- Therapeutic exercise and home program
  Exercise within postoperative limitations per physician should not cause increased pain, edema, or stiffness (3–6 times per day, 10 repetitions each)
  - Flexibility exercises
    - Active wrist and digit flexion/extension in whirlpool
    - Abduction/adduction digits
    - Thumb circumduction, opposition to all digits
    - IP blocking: Full flexion and extension of the PIP and DIP with support at each more proximal joint
    - Fisting
    - Digit extension
    - Cross digits for MCP rotation
    - Intrinsic-plus position
      a. MCP flexion with PIP and DIP extension
- Manual therapy techniques
  - Soft-tissue techniques
    - Elevation with retrograde massage

WRIST/HAND | POSTOP DUPUYTREN'S FASCIECTOMY   579

- Joint mobilization
  - PIP and MCP joints
    a. Particularly of involved digits
- Therapeutic devices and equipment
  - Splinting
    - Custom fabrication of hand-based resting pan or modified ulnar gutter splint
    - Maintain postoperative positioning in full MCP and IP extension
- Wound management
  - Cleansing whirlpool (92–96° F), followed by rinse with saline or water and elevation
  - Debridement (selective)
  - Topical agents
  - Dressings
    - Dry, sterile dressing applied after soak
    - Reapply following whirlpool and debridement
    - Support tissues to prevent hematoma
      a. Gauze dressing and Coban™ or Bandnet®
- Goals/outcomes
  - Pain-free wrist ROM: 100% of AMA guides or AAOS norms for the wrist, thumb, and uninvolved digits
  - Promote wound healing
  - Reduction of edema to within 25% of contralateral side
  - Maintain/gain extension posture through proper splinting

Subacute Phase: 3–6 Visits, Weeks 4–8
- Therapeutic exercise and home program
  - Passive stretches
  - Prehensile, graded activity
    - Foam cubes
    - Chinese chime balls
    - Scarf-walking
  - Progression of flexibility exercises
    - Contract-relax
    - ROM
  - Therapy putty
    10 repetitions 3–6 times per day
    - Rolling out the putty
    - Press/flatten the putty
    - Three-jaw chuck pinch
    - Palmar pinch to individual digits
    - Squeeze

  - Individual digit/thumb extension loops
  - Individual digit pokes
- Manual therapy techniques
  - Joint mobilization
    - PIP, MCP joints
  - Manual resistive exercise
  - Soft-tissue techniques
    - Techniques for reduction of adhesion formation
    - Deep tissue massage (delay to areas of skin grafting)
- Therapeutic devices and equipment
  - Scar conformer (Otoform K™) is fabricated once sutures are removed
  - Silicone gel sheet and Coban™, nocturnal wear, as needed
  - Continue resting pan splint nocturnally, up to 6 months postoperatively
  - Postoperative week 6 (option) dynamic PIP extension splint (such as splint #501 made by LMB)
  - During wound maturation phase (postoperative week 6+) optional PIP serial extension casts may be considered
- Physical agents and mechanical modalities
  - Elevated thermal modalities prior to mobilization or exercise
  - Ultrasound
- Goals/outcomes
  - Reduce scar density
  - Rebalance the muscle-tendon structure
    - 5/5 strength for extensors of involved digits
    - Maximize flexor tendon excursion
    - Prehensile (grip and pinch) motor performance: mean for age/gender norms
  - Return to resistive grasp with leisure/work activity (such as golf club, tennis racquet)

Functional Carryover
- Scar conformer and splinting may continue up to 6 months postoperative
- Taper structured exercise, as work/leisure activities are resumed (generally during the third month postoperative)

DISCHARGE PLANNING AND PATIENT RESPONSIBILITY

Criteria for Discharge
- All rehabilitation goals/outcomes achieved with the exception of return to prior functional status and activity level for recreational and sports activities

Circumstances Requiring Additional Visits
- Underlying medical complications, such as diabetes or arthritis
- Scar hypersensitivity
- Presence of reflex sympathetic dystrophy
- Postoperative infection/complications
- Need for ongoing modification of splints

Home Program
- Progressive strengthening and conditioning of upper extremity as patient resumes/expands activities
- Long-term splinting
- Scar reduction techniques

Monitoring
- Patient will call for splint adjustment as needed
- Patient is instructed to call for advice should progression halt or a negative trend occur

REFERENCES

1. American Physical Therapy Association. *Guide to Physical Therapist Practice*. Alexandria, VA: APTA; 1997.
2. Boyer M, Gelberman R. Complications of the operative treatment of Dupuytren's disease. *Hand Clin.* 1999;15(1):161-166.
3. Crowley B, Tonkin M. The proximal interphalangeal joint in Dupuytren's disease. *Hand Clin.* 1999;15(1):137-146.
4. Engelberg AL. *Guides to the Evaluation of Permanent Impairment.* 3rd ed. Chicago, IL: American Medical Association; 1989.
5. Gray H; Williams PL, ed. *Gray's Anatomy.* 38th ed. New York, NY: Churchill Livingstone; 1995.
6. Hurley R, ed. *Rehabilitation of the Hand.* St. Louis, MO: CV Mosby; 1995.
7. Lubahn J. Open-palm techniques and soft-tissue coverage in Dupuytren's disease. *Hand Clin.* 1999;15(1):127-136.
8. Lubahn JD, Lister GD, Wolfe T. Fasciectomy and Dupuytren's disease: a comparison between the open-palm technique and wound closure. *J Hand Surg.* 1984;9A:53-58.
9. Mullins P. Postsurgical rehabilitation of Dupuytren's disease. *Hand Clin.* 1999;15(1):167-174.
10. Tubiana R. Dupuytren's disease of the radial side of the hand. *Hand Clin.* 1999;15(1):149-159.

582   PostOp Dupuytren's Fasciectomy | Wrist/Hand

PROXIMAL INTERPHALANGEAL JOINT INJURIES COLLATERAL LIGAMENT SPRAIN

SUMMARY OVERVIEW

ICD-9

842.1

APTA Preferred Practice Pattern: 4E, 4J

EXAMINATION

- History and Systems Review
- Tests and Measures
  Systems review per APTA's *Guide to Physical Therapy Practice*
  - Anthropometric characteristics
  - Integumentary integrity
  - Joint integrity and mobility
  - Muscle performance
  - Pain
  - ROM
- Establish Plan of Care

GOALS/OUTCOMES

- ROM: 70% of American Academy of Orthopædic Surgeons norms for interphalangeal joints and 100% for metacarpal phalangeal joints
- Prevention of proximal interphalangeal (PIP) flexion contracture
- Edema: Within 5 mm or less, as compared to contralateral digit
- Prehensile (grip and pinch) strength: 90% of uninvolved hand or mean for age/gender norms
- Return to previous functional status and activity level; without recurrent injury
- Independence in a progressive home exercise program emphasizing function

INTERVENTION
NUMBER OF VISITS: 8–14

- Patient Instruction
  - Basic Anatomy and Biomechanics
  - Handouts
  - Functional Considerations
- Direct Interventions
  - Acute Phase: 4–7 Visits
  - Subacute Phase: 4–7 Visits
- Functional Carryover

DISCHARGE PLANNING AND PATIENT RESPONSIBILITY

- Criteria for Discharge
  - All rehabilitation goals/outcomes achieved with possible exceptions listed in guideline
- Circumstances Requiring Additional Visits
  - Need for modification or replacement of splints
  - Negative trend with PIP flexion contracture
- Home Program
  - Therapeutic devices and equipment
  - Progressive strengthening program with various therapy putty or resistive grip exercises
- Monitoring

PROXIMAL INTERPHALANGEAL JOINT INJURIES COLLATERAL LIGAMENT SPRAIN

ICD-9

842.1   Hand sprain

APTA Preferred Practice Pattern: 4E, 4J

EXAMINATION

History and Systems Review

- History of current condition
  - Mechanism of injury/onset
  - Date of injury/onset
  - Location, nature, and behavior of symptoms
    - Radiating symptoms
    - Aggravating/relieving factors
  - Current medical interventions
- Past history of current condition
  - Upper extremity injuries
  - Surgery
  - Direct intervention
- Other tests and measures
- Functional status and activity level (current/prior)
  - ADLs
  - Occupational activities
  - Recreational activities
- Growth and development
  - Hand dominance
- Patient's functional goals/outcomes

Tests and Measures

Systems review per APTA's *Guide to Physical Therapy Practice*

- Anthropometric characteristics
  - Edema
  - Comparative circumferential measurements
- Integumentary integrity
  - Scars
  - Discoloration or bruising
- Joint integrity and mobility
  - Deformities
  - Triggering
    - Patient actively flexes and extends fingers
    - A sudden palpable and audible snapping indicates a trigger finger
- Muscle performance
  - Grip and pinch strength

- Pain
  - Measured on visual analog scale
  - Location
  - Palpable, resisting, with motion
  - Intensity and duration
- ROM
  - Nature and quality of movement

Establish Plan of Care

- Based on history, tests, and measures

GOALS/OUTCOMES

- ROM: 70% of American Academy of Orthopædic Surgeons (AAOS) norms for interphalangeal (IP) joints and 100% for metacarpal phalangeal (MCP) joints

	Normal	70%
MCP	0–90°	NA
Proximal IP (PIP)	0–100°	10–80°
Distal IP (DIP)	0–70°	0–50°

- Prevention of PIP flexion contracture
- Edema: Within 5 mm or less, as compared to contralateral digit
- Prehensile (grip and pinch) strength: 90% of uninvolved hand or mean for age/gender norms
- Return to previous functional status and activity level without recurrent injury
- Independence in a progressive home exercise program emphasizing function

INTERVENTION
NUMBER OF VISITS: 8–14

Coordination, Communication, and Documentation

- Provision of services between admission and discharge that facilitate cost-effective and efficient integration or reintegration to home, community, or work
- Documentation of therapeutic intervention is required for each episode of care and serves as the basic foundation for communication
- Coordination and additional communication will depend on the patient's impairment and home/work/community/leisure situation and requirements. Such services may include:
  - Case management
  - Coordination of care and collaboration with those integral to the patient's rehabilitation program
  - Coordination and monitoring of the delivery of available resources
  - Referrals to other health-care professionals
  - Identification of resources, support groups, or advocacy services
  - Provision of educational or training information
  - Technical assistance

Patient Instruction

Basic Anatomy and Biomechanics

- Refer to hand anatomical chart to help patient understand area of injury, ligamentous structure, and PIP joint biomechanics
- Surgical anatomy of the hand (Netter. 1969)
- Length of time required for ligament healing
- Pertinent Gray's Anatomy (Gray. 1995. 658–659, 858)

Handouts

- Home exercise program
  - Specific ROM exercises
  - Edema reduction techniques
- Splint wear and care instructions

Functional Considerations

- Joint protection techniques and advice regarding appropriate hand use/activity
- Utilization of adaptive aides, such as compression wrap, finger sleeve

Direct Interventions

Acute Phase: 4–7 Visits

- The most important small hand joints are the PIP joints. These have the greatest joint motion of the individual finger joints; if motion is lost at this level, significant restriction in hand function often occurs.
  - Stiffness of the PIP joint occurs rapidly, but healing of the injured ligaments surrounding the joint is notoriously slow, and symptoms may persist for many months
  - Ligaments that are stable to stress and active motion testing are immobilized until the acute discomfort subsides (usually 3–10 days)
  - Partial or near complete ligament tears may require immobilization up to 3 weeks, before gradual mobilization begins
- Therapeutic exercise and home program
  - ROM exercises, in elevated position
    - Pay particular attention to intrinsic stretch and direction of pull of lateral bands
    - Intrinsic plus position
      a. MCP flexion, PIP, and DIP extension
    - MCP flexion, PIP extension, DIP flexion
    - MCP flexion, PIP flexion, DIP extension
  - Reinforce exercise technique/position for mobilization of lateral bands and intrinsic myotendon unit
  - Repeated every hour for 3–5 minutes to prevent further joint edema
- Manual therapy techniques
  - Soft-tissue techniques
    - Friction massage
    - Soft-tissue mobilization and stretching
  - Joint mobilization
    - Grades I–II to areas of hypomobility in the wrist, thumb, and digits
- Therapeutic devices and equipment
  - Fabrication of devices and equipment
  - Dynamic PIP joint splints to facilitate motion in flexion/extension
  - Adjacent digit taping with Velcro® finger loops, worn daytime
  - Static night splinting, if flexion contractures appear likely
  - Splint size needs to accommodate compression wraps (worn in conjunction for edema)

WRIST/HAND | PROXIMAL INTERPHALANGEAL JOINT INJURIES COLLATERAL LIGAMENT SPRAIN   585

- Physical agents and mechanical modalities
  - Cryotherapy for edema
  - Ultrasound, nonthermal
  - Contrast bath
- Goals/outcomes
  - ROM: 20° or less PIP joint lag in extension
  - Strength: 3 lbs palmar pinch and lateral pinch
  - Edema
    - Has not increased with exercise or activity
    - Controlled to within 7 mm difference of contralateral digit, when wearing compression wrap

Subacute Phase: 4–7 Visits

- Therapeutic exercise and home program
  - Progression of flexibility exercises
  - Resistive exercises, such as:
    - Graded pinch pins
    - Graded therapy putty
    - Digi-flex® gripper
- Manual therapy techniques
  - Retrograde massage
  - Joint mobilization
    - Grades III–IV to persistent hypomobilities in the digit
  - Soft-tissue techniques
    - Soft-tissue mobilization and stretching
- Therapeutic devices and equipment
  - Long-term use of dynamic PIP joint extension splint to prevent flexion contracture
- Physical agents and mechanical modalities
  - Continue effective modalities as in acute phase with increased emphasis on use as needed at home
- Goals/outcomes
  - ROM: 70% of AAOS norms for IP motion in digits
    - PIP: 10–70°
    - DIP: 0–50°
  - Edema: within 5 mm or less as compared to contralateral digit
  - Prehensile (grip and pinch) strength: 75–100% of mean for age/gender norms
  - Resume functional activities with progression into work and leisure activities

Functional Carryover

- Instruction in prolonged use of and tapering from compression wrap and splints
- Instruction in "handle" adaptations for work and home (e.g., golf club, racquet, screwdriver, or gardening implements)

DISCHARGE PLANNING AND PATIENT RESPONSIBILITY

Criteria for Discharge

- All rehabilitation goals/outcomes achieved except:
  - Stabilized edema, without compression wrap
  - Maximal gain of grip and pinch motor performance

Circumstances Requiring Additional Visits

- Need for modification or replacement of splints
- Negative trend with PIP flexion contracture

Home Program

- Therapeutic devices and equipment
- Progressive strengthening program with various therapy putty or resistive grip exercises

Monitoring

- Patient is instructed to call for advice should progression halt or a negative trend occur
- Patient to recheck/call at 2 weeks post-discharge to ensure return to function and achieve all rehabilitation goals/outcomes

REFERENCES

1. American Academy of Orthopædic Surgeons. *Joint Motion: Method of Measuring and Recording.* Chicago, IL: AAOS; 1965.
2. American Physical Therapy Association. *Guide to Physical Therapist Practice.* Alexandria, VA: APTA; 1997.
3. Engelberg AL. *Guides to the Evaluation of Permanent Impairment.* 3rd ed. Chicago, IL: American Medical Association; 1989.
4. Gray H; Williams PL, ed. *Gray's Anatomy.* 38th ed. New York, NY: Churchill Livingstone; 1995.
5. Hunter JM, Mackin EJ, Callahan AD. Joint injuries in the hand: preservation of proximal interphalangeal joint function. *Rehabilitation of the Hand.* 3rd ed. St. Louis, MO: CV Mosby; 1990:295-303.

6. Hurley R, ed. *Rehabilitation of the Hand.* St Louis, MO: CV Mosby; 1995.

7. Mathiowitz V, Kashman N, Volland G, et al. Grip and pinch strength: normative data for adults. *Arch Phys Med Rehabil.* 1985;66:69-74.

8. Netter F. Surgical anatomy of the hand. *CIBA Clin Symp.* 1969;21(3):34-35.

PROXIMAL INTERPHALANGEAL JOINT INJURIES DORSAL DISLOCATION

SUMMARY OVERVIEW

ICD-9

834.0

APTA Preferred Practice Pattern: 4J

EXAMINATION

- History and Systems Review
- Tests and Measures
  Systems review per APTA's *Guide to Physical Therapy Practice*
  - Anthropometric characteristics
  - Integumentary integrity
  - Joint integrity and mobility
  - Muscle performance
  - Pain
  - ROM
- Establish Plan of Care

GOALS/OUTCOMES

- ROM: restore a minimum of 70% of American Academy of Orthopædic Surgeons norms for interphalangeal motion in digits and 100% for metacarpal phalangeal joints
- Prevention of proximal interphalangeal flexion contracture
- Edema: Within 5 mm or less, as compared to contralateral digit
- Prehension (grip and pinch) strength: 90% of uninvolved hand or mean for age/gender norms
- 5/5 on manual muscle test for wrist, forearm, and elbow
- Return to prior functional status and activity level (current/prior) for ADLs and vocational, recreational, and sports activities as identified by patient
- Independence in a progressive home exercise program

INTERVENTION

NUMBER OF VISITS: 12–20

- Patient Instruction
  - Basic Anatomy and Biomechanics
  - Handouts
  - Functional Considerations
- Direct Interventions
  - Acute Phase: 2–4 Visits
  - Subacute Phase: 10–16 Visits
- Functional Carryover

DISCHARGE PLANNING AND PATIENT RESPONSIBILITY

- Criteria for Discharge
  - All rehabilitation goals/outcomes achieved except may discharge prior to attaining maximal recovery of prehensile strength
- Circumstances Requiring Additional Visits
  - Postoperative infection/complications
  - Need for modification or replacement of splints
  - Job tasks of a forceful or repetitive nature that exacerbate symptoms
- Home Program
  - Splinting, up to 3 months post-injury or longer
  - Motor performance exercises and activities
- Monitoring

PROXIMAL INTERPHALANGEAL JOINT INJURIES DORSAL DISLOCATION

ICD-9

> 834.0   Closed dislocation of finger

APTA Preferred Practice Pattern: 4J

EXAMINATION

History and Systems Review

- History of current conditions
  - Mechanism of injury/onset
  - Date of injury/onset
  - Onset and pattern of symptoms
  - Current therapeutic interventions
- Past history of current condition
  - Previous upper extremity injuries
  - Surgery
  - Direct intervention
  - Prior therapeutic interventions
  - Surgical intervention
    - Pin fixation
  - Bracing, injections, etc.
- Functional status and activity level (current/prior)
  - ADLs
  - Occupational activities
  - Recreational activities
- Social habits
- Growth and development
  - Hand dominance
- Patient's functional goals/outcomes

Tests and Measures

Systems review per APTA's *Guide to Physical Therapy Practice*

- Anthropometric characteristics
  - Circumferential measurement for edema
- Integumentary integrity
  - Skin color
  - Scar tissue
- Joint integrity and mobility
  - Deformities
  - Nature and quality of movement
  - Capsular tightness

- Muscle performance
  - Grip strength
  - Pinch strength
  - Intrinsic strength
- Pain
  - Measured on visual analog scale
  - Location
  - Palpable, resting, motion
  - Intensity and duration
- ROM
  - Flexor digitorum profundus and flexor digitorum superficialis individual tendon gliding
  - Nature and quality of movement

Establish Plan of Care

- Based on history, tests, and measures

GOALS/OUTCOMES

- ROM: Restore a minimum of 70% of American Academy of Orthopædic Surgeons (AAOS) norms for interphalangeal (IP) motion in digits and 100% for metacarpal phalangeal (MCP) joints

	Normal	*70%*
MCP	0–90°	
Proximal IP (PIP)	0–100°	10–80°
Distal IP (DIP)	0–70°	0–50°

- Prevention of PIP flexion contracture
- Edema: Within 5 mm or less, as compared to contralateral digit
- Prehension (grip and pinch) strength: 90% of uninvolved hand or mean for age/gender norms
- 5/5 on manual muscle test for wrist, forearm, and elbow
- Return to prior functional status and activity level (current/prior) for ADLs and vocational, recreational, and sports activities as identified by patient
- Independence in a progressive home exercise program

INTERVENTION
NUMBER OF VISITS: 12–20

Coordination, Communication, and Documentation
- Provision of services between admission and discharge that facilitate cost-effective and efficient integration or reintegration to home, community, or work
- Documentation of therapeutic intervention is required for each episode of care and serves as the basic foundation for communication
- Coordination and additional communication will depend on the patient's impairment and home/work/community/leisure situation and requirements. Such services may include:
  - Case management
  - Coordination of care and collaboration with those integral to the patient's rehabilitation program
  - Coordination and monitoring of the delivery of available resources
  - Referrals to other health-care professionals
  - Identification of resources, support groups, or advocacy services
  - Provision of educational or training information
  - Technical assistance

Patient Instruction

Basic Anatomy and Biomechanics
- Refer to hand anatomical chart to help patient understand mechanics of injury, involved structures, and PIP joint biomechanics
- Length of time required for ligament healing
- Pertinent Gray's Anatomy (Gray. 1995. 658–659, 858)

Handouts
- Specific home program
  - Specific ROM exercises
  - Edema reduction techniques
- Splint wear and care instructions

Functional Considerations
- Joint protection techniques and advice regarding appropriate hand use/activity
- Utilization of adaptive aids, compression wrap, finger sleeve, etc.

Direct Interventions

Acute Phase: 2–4 Visits
- Status of hand
  - Dorsal dislocations of the PIP joint are common and may be associated with a fracture or injury of tendon/ligament
  - If reduction is stable and there is no fracture, the PIP joint is splinted in 25° flexion for 3 weeks to allow soft-tissue healing
  - Unstable PIP joint (after reduction) will require 5 weeks of cast immobilization limiting 25° of full PIP joint extension. The patient should receive home exercise program during the interim to maintain range of uninvolved joint.
- Therapeutic exercise and home program
  - ROM exercises, in elevated position
    - Differential tendon gliding
      a. Intrinsic plus position: MCP flexion, PIP and DIP extension
      b. MCP flexion, PIP extension, DIP flexion
      c. MCP flexion, PIP flexion, DIP extension
    - Intrinsic stretching
- Manual therapy techniques
  - Soft-tissue techniques
    - Soft-tissue mobilization
    - Retrograde massage for edema reduction
  - Joint mobilization
    - Grades I–II for pain relief
    - Grades III–IV to specific areas of hypomobility in surrounding joints
- Therapeutic devices and equipment
  - Fabrication of devices and equipment
    - Protective splint
- Goals/outcomes
  - ROM within limits of cast/splint; PIP 25–80°
  - Edema
    - Has not increased with exercise or activity
    - Controlled to within 7 mm difference of contralateral digit

Subacute Phase: 10–16 Visits
- Status of the hand
  - Period of immobilization ends. Uninvolved joints will be stiff.
- Therapeutic exercise and home program
  - Progression of flexibility exercises

WRIST/HAND | PROXIMAL INTERPHALANGEAL JOINT INJURIES DORSAL DISLOCATION 591

- Wrist and forearm as needed
  - Contract/relax techniques to pain tolerance
  - Progressive resistive exercise
    - Wrist
    - Fingers
    - Thumb
  - Progressive activities
    - Gripping activities
    - Baltimore Therapeutic Equipment work simulator
- Manual therapy techniques
  - Retrograde massage
  - Joint mobilization
    - Carpal mobilization following cast removal
  - Soft-tissue techniques
    - Attention to volar plate and lateral structures
  - Passive stretches
    - Gradual PIP extension with MCP held in flexion
- Therapeutic devices and equipment
  - Removable, protective splinting for daytime activities
  - May continue until 3 months post-injury, or longer if needed
- Physical agents and mechanical modalities
  - Ultrasound
  - Contrast bath for edema and pain management
  - Cryotherapy for edema
- Goals/outcomes
  - ROM: Stable PIP joint with 70% of AAOS norms
    - PIP: 10–80°
    - DIP: 0–50°
  - Edema: within 5 mm or less as compared to contralateral digit
  - Prehensile (grip and pinch) strength: 75–100% of mean for age/gender norms

Functional Carryover
- Instruction in prolonged use of and tapering off of compression wrap and splints
- Adapt prehensile patterns and/or "handle" adaptations for writing and leisure/sports (e.g., racquet-grip or golf club handles)

DISCHARGE PLANNING AND PATIENT RESPONSIBILITY

Criteria for Discharge
- All rehabilitation goals/outcomes achieved except may discharge prior to attaining maximal recovery of prehensile strength

Circumstances Requiring Additional Visits
- Postoperative infection/complications
- Need for modification or replacement of splints
- Job tasks of a forceful or repetitive nature that exacerbate symptoms

Home Program
- Splinting, up to 3 months post-injury or longer
- Motor performance exercises and activities

Monitoring
- Taper therapeutic sessions after 8–10 weeks following injury
- Patient to be seen for reconditioning and building tolerance to repetitive materials handling, if needed, prior to return to work
- Patient is instructed to call for advice should progression halt or a negative trend occur

REFERENCE
1. American Physical Therapy Association. *Guide to Physical Therapist Practice.* Alexandria, VA: APTA; 1997.
2. Engelberg AL. *Guides to the Evaluation of Permanent Impairment.* 3rd ed. Chicago, IL: American Medical Association; 1989.
3. Gray H; Williams PL, ed. *Gray's Anatomy.* 38th ed. New York, NY: Churchill Livingstone; 1995.
4. Hunter JM, Mackin EJ, Callahan AD. Joint injuries in the hand: preservation of proximal interphalangeal joint function. In: *Rehabilitation of the Hand.* 3rd ed. St. Louis, MO: CV Mosby; 1990:295-303.
5. Hurley R, ed. *Rehabilitation of the Hand.* St Louis, MO: CV Mosby; 1995.
6. Mathiowetz V, Kashman N, Volland G, et al. Grip and pinch strength: normative data for adults. *Arch Phys Med Rehabil.* 1985;66:69-74.
7. Netter F. Surgical anatomy of the hand. *CIBA Clin Symp.* 1969;21(3):34-35.

REFLEX SYMPATHETIC DYSTROPHY OF THE UPPER EXTREMITY

SUMMARY OVERVIEW

ICD-9

337.20   337.21   337.29

APTA Preferred Practice Pattern: **4D**

EXAMINATION

- History and Systems Review
- Tests and Measures
  Systems review per APTA's *Guide to Physical Therapy Practice*
  - Anthropometric characteristics
  - Integumentary integrity
  - Joint integrity and mobility
  - Muscle performance
  - Pain
  - Posture
  - ROM
  - Reflex integrity
  - Sensory integrity
- Establish Plan of Care

GOALS/OUTCOMES

- Prognosis: Patient will return to pre-morbid status or achieve highest level of function
- Wrist and elbow ROM: 80% of AMA guides
- Hand ROM: 100% of American Academy of Orthopædic Surgeons norms for metacarpal phalangeal and interphalangeal joints
- Functional shoulder ROM
- Pain: 2/10 or less
- Prehensile (grip and pinch) strength: 90% of mean for age/gender norms
- Increase patient's ability to interpret tactile stimuli, understanding of the need for protection, and ability to compensate for sensory loss
- Edema: Reduce to within 10% of uninvolved limb
- Return to prior functional status and activity level (current/prior) for ADLs and vocational, recreational, and sports activities as identified by patient
- Independence in a progressive home exercise program emphasizing function

INTERVENTION

NUMBER OF VISITS: 16–32

- Patient Instruction
  - Basic Anatomy and Biomechanics
  - Handouts
  - Functional Considerations
- Direct Interventions
  - Acute Phase: 8–16 Visits
  - Progressive Phase: 8–16 Visits
- Functional Carryover

DISCHARGE PLANNING AND PATIENT RESPONSIBILITY

- Criteria for Discharge
  - All rehabilitation goals/outcomes achieved with possible exceptions listed in guideline
- Circumstances Requiring Additional Visits
  - Series of nerve blocks requiring immediate PROM
  - Persistent edema altering functional use
  - Contracture development
  - Psychosocial complicating factors
  - Special occupational needs requiring extensive conditioning
- Home Program
  - Motor performance
  - Flexibility
  - Desensitization techniques
- Monitoring

SUMMARY OVERVIEW | WRIST/HAND | REFLEX SYMPATHETIC DYSTROPHY OF THE UPPER EXTREMITY   593

REFLEX SYMPATHETIC DYSTROPHY OF THE UPPER EXTREMITY

ICD-9

337.20　Reflex sympathetic dystrophy, unspecified

337.21　Reflex sympathetic dystrophy of the upper limb

337.29　Reflex sympathetic dystrophy of other specified site

APTA Preferred Practice Pattern: **4D**

EXAMINATION

History and Systems Review

- History of current condition
  - Current therapeutic interventions
  - Onset and course of events
  - Location, nature, and behavior of symptoms
    - Aggravating/relieving factors
- Past history of current condition
  - Upper extremity or cervical spine injury
  - Surgery
  - Direct intervention
  - Psychological intervention
- Other tests and measures
  - Stage of reflex sympathetic dystrophy (RSD)
  - Lab diagnostic tests (EMG, MRI)
- Medications
- Growth and development
  - Hand dominance
- Functional status and activity level (current/prior)
  - Self-care activities
  - Assistive devices/splints
  - Occupational activities
  - Recreational activities
- Social habits
  - Behavioral health risks/physical fitness
- Social history
  - Language/culture
  - Care giver status
  - Family/significant other resources
- Living environment
- Growth and development
- Occupation/employment
- General demographics
  - Age
- Patient's functional goals/outcomes

Tests and Measures

Systems review per APTA's *Guide to Physical Therapy Practice*

- Anthropometric characteristics
  - Comparative circumferential or volumetric measurement for edema
- Integumentary integrity
  - Skin color
  - Skin moisture and temperature
  - Tone and trophic changes
  - Nail changes
  - Hair growth
- Joint integrity and mobility
  - Deformities
- Muscle performance
  - Grip and pinch measurement
  - Manual muscle test for upper extremity as tolerated
- Pain
  - Measured on visual analog scale/numerical
- Posture
  - Cervical/thoracic/hand posturing
  - Resting postures/attitude of the hand
- ROM
  - Active/passive ROM and functional ROM
    - Cervical spine
    - Shoulder
    - Elbow
    - Wrist
    - Hand
- Reflex integrity
- Sensory integrity
  - Vibration (256 cps, 30 cps tuning fork)
  - Sensory evaluation
    - Proprioception and kinesthesia (sharp-dull, temperature, touch, pressure)

Establish Plan of Care

- Based on history, tests, and measures

GOALS/OUTCOMES

- Prognosis: Patient will return to pre-morbid status or achieve highest level of function
  - Expected length of care: 2–4 months
  - Visits: 16–32
- Wrist and elbow ROM: 80% of AMA guides

Wrist	Normal	80%
Flexion	60°	50°
Extension	60°	50°
Ulnar deviation	30°	25°
Radial deviation	20°	15°

Elbow	Normal	80%
Flexion	140°	115°
Extension	0°	0°
Pronation	80°	65°
Supination	80°	65°

- Hand ROM: 100% of American Academy of Orthopædic Surgeons (AAOS) norms for metacarpal phalangeal (MCP) and interphalangeal (IP) joints
  - Digit
    - MCP: 0–90°
    - Proximal IP (PIP): 0–100°
    - Distal IP (DIP): 0–70°
  - Thumb
    - MCP: 0–60°
    - IP: 0–80°
    - Radial abduction: 50°
    - Adduction: 0 cm
    - Opposition: 8 cm
- Functional shoulder ROM
  - Flexion: 162°
  - External rotation: 60°
- Pain: 2/10 or less
- Prehensile (grip and pinch) strength: 90% of mean for age/gender norms
- Increase patient's:
  - Ability to interpret tactile stimuli
  - Understanding of the need for protection
  - Ability to compensate for sensory loss
- Edema: Reduce to within 10% of uninvolved limb
- Return to prior functional status and activity level (current/prior) for ADLs and vocational, recreational, and sports activities as identified by patient
- Independence in a progressive home exercise program emphasizing function

INTERVENTION
NUMBER OF VISITS: 16–32

Coordination, Communication, and Documentation

- Provision of services between admission and discharge that facilitate cost-effective and efficient integration or reintegration to home, community, or work
- Documentation of therapeutic intervention is required for each episode of care and serves as the basic foundation for communication
- Coordination and additional communication will depend on the patient's impairment and home/work/community/leisure situation and requirements. Such services may include:
  - Case management
  - Coordination of care and collaboration with those integral to the patient's rehabilitation program
  - Coordination and monitoring of the delivery of available resources
  - Referrals to other health-care professionals
  - Identification of resources, support groups, or advocacy services
  - Provision of educational or training information
  - Technical assistance

Patient Instruction

Basic Anatomy and Biomechanics
- Autonomic nervous system vs. central nervous system

Handouts
- Home exercise program including graded activities
- Edema reduction techniques
- Desensitization program
  - Texture desensitization
  - Particle immersion
  - Vibration desensitization
  - Active traction and compression exercises; stress loading techniques
- Orthotic wear, care, and precautions
- Home application of modalities

Functional Considerations
- Review treatment and functional precautions
  - Activity should not cause an increase in pain, edema, or stiffness

- Extremes of temperature should be avoided as this may increase afferent transmission and exacerbate condition
- ROM performed in pain-free range
- Edema control techniques
  - Elevation
  - Intermittent compression pump
  - Retrograde massage
  - External pressure wraps
  - Active exercise
  - Compression glove for nocturnal wear
- Pain control techniques and sensory precautions
  - Awareness of RSD cycle: Disuse, edema, immobility contribute to a stiff, swollen, painful extremity
- The patient should perform his or her own ADL tasks. The hand must be exercised or used in active tasks a few minutes out of each half hour.

Direct Interventions

Acute Phase: 8–16 Visits

- Natural progression of the RSD process (Lankford L, Thompson J. 1977.)
  - Stage I: A hot erythematous swollen extremity
  - Stage II: A cold, cyanotic limb with progressive trophic changes
  - Stage III: Extremity with fixed fibrotic change and atrophy
- Therapeutic exercise and home program
  - Alternating dynamic flexion and extension of digits
  - Active and active-assistive exercise of the entire extremity
    - Performed sequentially from distal to proximal joints
    - Sustained effort exercise for 5–10 seconds in each direction is encouraged
    - Reciprocal pulleys
    - Towel or dowel exercises
  - Stress loading techniques
    - "Scrubbing": Holding a course bristle brush, applying as much pressure as possible
    - Continue for 3 minutes, 5 times a day initially
    - Progress exercise time to 5–10 minutes, 3 times a day
    - Dystrophile®
  - Proprioceptive activities
    - Shoulder-elbow-hand loading axis

- Quadriped progression
  - Activities in clinic, such as:
    - Valpar whole-body ROM
    - Elevated washers
    - Peg board work
    - Upper extremity wall ladder
    - Removal of objects from rice
    - Activities should be elevated whenever possible to control edema and promote active shoulder ROM
- Manual therapy techniques
  - Soft-tissue techniques
    - Pain-free, elevated retrograde massage for desensitization, progressing to 10–15 minutes
  - ROM
    - If a stellate ganglion block is used, maintain ROM immediately after the vasodilation
    - Range by the therapist is always within pain tolerance
    - Heat application with gentle Coban™ wrapping for flexion
- Therapeutic devices and equipment
  - Static splints
    - Resting or cock-up splint to support wrist or digits
    - Splint wear will be intermittent to allow the patient intermittent use of the involved extremity
    - Splints must be comfortable and easy to apply and accommodate for edema
- Electrotherapeutic modalities
  - TENS applied for relief of vasomotor instability and pain
    - Conventional TENS high rate (80 pps) and low width (50 microseconds), amplitude controlled by the patient
    - Greatest relief may be achieved with electrode placement over the lower trunk of the brachial plexus
  - H-Wave®: Applied for edema/pain
  - Interferential: Applied for edema/pain
  - MENS: For example, use of the Myomatic I
    - Probes for pain relief
      a. 30 Hz and maximal subsensory microamperage (try 100 mA)
      b. Adjust downward if needed to keep the treatment subsensory
      c. Wave slope setting of 10

- Follow with probe/electrode treatment of same areas with settings of 0.3 Hz and 40 mA, wave slope 1–3
  a. The unattended treatment is set up by placing electrodes on or around the periphery of the effected area
  b. Set at 30 Hz, 100 mA or subsensory for the initial 10 minutes of treatment, follow with 10 minutes of 0.3 Hz and 40 mA for an additional 20 minutes
- Physical agents and mechanical modalities
  o Sensory stimulation
    ▪ Graded sensory mediums
    ▪ Functional activities involving tactile stimulation
  o Contrast baths at moderate temperature only, to avoid exacerbation of symptoms
  o Jobst Intermittent Compression Pump
    ▪ 60–90 mm Hg
    ▪ 45–60 minutes
- Goals/outcomes
  o Pain: 5/10 or less
  o Edema: Reduce to within 30% of uninvolved limb
  o ROM: Ability to make a loose fist and oppose thumb to index and long finger
  o Independence in self-care activities
  o Resume home/leisure activity with tolerance of uninterrupted, bilateral hand use for 15–30 minutes

Progressive Phase: 8–16 Visits
- Therapeutic exercise and home program
  o Motor performance exercise and graded activities are initiated as pain is controlled and active ROM is 80% of AMA guides
  o Baltimore Therapeutic Equipment work simulator
    ▪ Light work with emphasis on pain-free use
    ▪ Allows for goal directed exercise with patient controlling resistance and time worked
    ▪ Include shoulder wheel, gross grasp, wrist flexion/extension, supination/pronation, and elbow flexion/extension
  o Therapeutic activities
    ▪ Squeeze water from sponge during contrast bath
    ▪ Pinch pins, Velcro exercise boards
    ▪ Graded hand exercise with light resistance therapy putty
  o Weight well
    ▪ Graded exercise program

- ▪ Positions upper extremity in elevation
- Manual therapy techniques
  o Joint mobilization
    ▪ Grades II–III mobilization and oscillation
  o Soft-tissue techniques
- Therapeutic devices and equipment
  o Monitor contracture formation
  o Use dynamic splints accordingly
- Physical agents and mechanical modalities Continue effective modalities as in acute phase with increased emphasis on use as needed at home.
  o Superficial thermal modalities with extremity in elevated position
    ▪ Moist hot pack, paraffin, Fluidotherapy®, ultrasound
- Goals/outcomes
  o Edema: Reduce to within 20% of uninvolved limb
  o Pain: 2/10 or less
  o Uninterrupted use of hand for a minimum of 1 hour
  o Independence in ADLs and leisure/sport activity
  o Prehensile (grip and pinch) strength: 75% of mean age/gender norms
  o Independence in a progressive home exercise program with focus on strengthening and function

Functional Carryover
- Appropriate referral for prevocational/vocational assessment, determined by patient's age and functional status
- Therapist may perform a job site analysis and provide information regarding work station, adaptive equipment, and techniques to promote safety
- Recommendations for job training or pre-work conditioning
- A successful course of treatment may require treatment for 6 months or longer
- The patient should be encouraged to perform their own ADLs tasks
- Assist the patient and family in understanding and coping with the nature of RSD
- Encourage the patient to gradually resume functional roles as progress occurs

DISCHARGE PLANNING AND PATIENT RESPONSIBILITY

Criteria for Discharge
- All rehabilitation goals/outcomes achieved except:
  - May not return to functional status and activity level (current/prior) for ADLs and vocational activities
  - May discharge with grip motor performance of 80% of mean for age/gender norms if all other goals/outcomes achieved

Circumstances Requiring Additional Visits
- Series of nerve blocks requiring immediate PROM
- Persistent edema altering functional use
- Contracture development
- Psychosocial complicating factors
- Special occupational needs that require extensive conditioning

Home Program
- Motor performance
- Flexibility
- Desensitization techniques

Monitoring
- Patient is instructed to call for advice should progression halt or a negative trend occur
- Patient to recheck at monthly intervals post-discharge to monitor functional gains and recovery of motor performance. Periodic follow-up visits can be made up to 1 year after involvement.

REFERENCE

1. American Academy of Orthopædic Surgeons. *Joint Motion: Method of Measuring and Recording.* Chicago, IL: AAOS; 1965.
2. American Physical Therapy Association. *Guide to Physical Therapist Practice.* Alexandria, VA: APTA; 1997.
3. Aronoff GM, Harden N, Stanton-Hicks M, et al. American Academy of Disability Evaluating Physicians (AADEP) position paper: complex regional pain syndrome I (RSD): impairment and disability issues. *Pain Med.* September 2002;3(3):274-88.
4. Bandyk DF, Johnson BL, Kirkpatrick AF, et al. Surgical sympathectomy for reflex sympathetic dystrophy syndromes. *J Vasc Surg.* February 2002;35(2):269-77.

5. Barber LM. Desensitization of the traumatized hand. In: Hunter JM, Mackin EJ, Callahan AD, et al, eds. *Rehabilitation of the Hand: Surgery and Therapy.* 3rd ed St. Louis, MO: CV Mosby; 1990:721-730.
6. Carlsen LK, Watson. Treatment of reflex sympathetic dystrophy using the stress-loading program. *J Hand Ther.* 1983;1(4):149-153.
7. Daniel M, Strickland LR. *Occupational Therapy Protocol Management in Adult Physical Dysfunction.* Gaithersburg, MD: Aspen Publishers; 1992.
8. Engelberg AL. *Guides to the Evaluation of Permanent Impairment.* 3rd ed. Chicago, IL: American Medical Association; 1989.
9. Gray H; Williams PL, ed. *Gray's Anatomy.* 38th ed. New York, NY: Churchill Livingstone; 1995.
10. Hurley R, ed. *Rehabilitation of the Hand.* St Louis, MO: CV Mosby; 1995.
11. Kemler MA, Rijks CP, de Vet HC. Which patients with chronic reflex sympathetic dystrophy are most likely to benefit from physical therapy? *J Manipulative Physiol Ther.* May 2001;24(4):272-8.
12. Lankford L, Thompson J. Reflex sympathetic dystrophy, upper and lower extremity: diagnosis and management. *American Academy of Orthopædic Surgeons (Course Lectures).* St. Louis, MO: CV Mosby; 1977;26:163-178.
13. Mathiowetz V, Kashman N, Volland G, et al. Grip and pinch strength: normative data for adults. *Arch Phys Med Rehabil.* 1985;66:69-74.
14. Okudan B, Celik C, Serttas S, Ozgirgin N. The predictive value of additional late blood pool imaging to the three-phase bone scan in the diagnosis of reflex sympathetic dystrophy in hemiplegic patients. *Rheumatol Int.* December 2005;26(2):126-31.
15. Schutzer SF, Gossling HR. Current concepts review: the treatment of reflex sympathetic systrophy syndrome. *J Bone Joint Surg.* 1984;66A:625-629.
16. Waylett-Randall J. Therapist's management of reflex sympathetic dystrophy. In: Hunter JM, Mackin EJ, Callahan AD, eds. *Rehabilitation of the Hand: Surgery and Therapy.* 3rd ed. St. Louis, MO: CV Mosby; 1990:787-792.
17. Zyluk A. A new clinical severity scoring system for reflex sympathetic dystrophy of the upper limb. *J Hand Surg [Br].* June 2003;28(3):238-41.

WRIST FRACTURE
SUMMARY OVERVIEW

ICD-9

   813.4   813.8   814.00

APTA Preferred Practice Pattern: **4D, 4H, 4J**

EXAMINATION

- History and Systems Review
- Tests and Measures
  Systems review per APTA's *Guide to Physical Therapy Practice*
  - Anthropometric characteristics
  - Ergonomics/body mechanics
  - Joint integrity and mobility
  - Motor function
  - Muscle performance
  - Pain
  - ROM
  - Sensory integrity
- Establish Plan of Care

GOALS/OUTCOMES

- Wrist and forearm ROM: 100% of AMA guides
- Metacarpal phalangeal ROM: 100% of American Academy of Orthopædic Surgeons norms
- Pain: 2/10 with activity, 0/10 at rest
- Prehensile (grip and pinch) strength: Mean for age/gender norms or equal to uninvolved side, or adequate for work/home tasks performance
- Return to prior functional status and activity level for ADLs and vocational, recreational, and sports activities as identified by patient
- Independence in a progressive home exercise program emphasizing function

INTERVENTION
NUMBER OF VISITS: 8–16

- Patient Instruction
  - Basic Anatomy and Biomechanics
  - Handouts
  - Functional Considerations
- Direct Interventions
  - Acute Phase: 4–8 Visits, Weeks 1–4 After Cast Removal
  - Subacute Phase: 4–8 Visits, Weeks 5–8 After Cast Removal
- Functional Carryover

DISCHARGE PLANNING AND PATIENT RESPONSIBILITY

- Criteria for Discharge
  - All rehabilitation goals/outcomes achieved with the exception of the final 10% of wrist and forearm range
- Circumstances Requiring Additional Visits
  - Presence of reflex sympathetic dystrophy of the upper extremity
  - Presence of stiff hand syndrome
  - Carpal tunnel syndrome
  - Open reduction or surgical fixation
  - Postoperative infection/complications
  - Underlying medical conditions, e.g., arthritis
  - Persistent or worsening edema
  - Special occupational needs that require extensive strengthening
- Home Program
  - Edema reduction techniques
  - Self-mobilization
  - Motor performance exercise
- Monitoring

SUMMARY OVERVIEW | WRIST/HAND | WRIST FRACTURE   599

WRIST FRACTURE

ICD-9

813.4	Closed fracture of lower end of radius and ulna
813.8	Closed fracture of unspecified part of radius and ulna
814.00	Closed fracture of carpal bone, unspecified

APTA Preferred Practice Pattern: 4D, 4H, 4J

EXAMINATION

History and Systems Review

- History of current condition
  - Mechanism of injury/onset
  - Date of injury/onset
  - Patient/family/caregiver
    - Concerns leading patient to seek therapeutic intervention
  - Current therapeutic intervention
  - Post-injury progression
    - Casting
    - Surgical procedure and postoperative precautions
    - Dressings and splints applied by physician
  - Location, nature, and behavior of symptoms
    - Radiating symptoms
    - Aggravating/relieving factors
- Past history of current condition
  - Prior medications
  - Surgical intervention
  - Upper extremity injury
  - Prior therapeutic interventions
- Growth and development
  - Hand dominance
- Functional status and activity level (current/prior)
  - Ambulatory aids/splints
  - Occupational activities
  - Recreational activities
- Social habits
  - Behavioral health risks (i.e., substance abuse)
  - General level of fitness
- Occupation/employment
- Patient's functional goals/outcomes

Tests and Measures

Systems review per APTA's *Guide to Physical Therapy Practice*

- Anthropometric characteristics
  - Circumferential measurements for edema

- Distal palmar crease
- Wrist flexion crease
- 10 cm proximal to wrist
- Ergonomics/body mechanics
- Joint integrity and mobility
  - Capsular tightness
  - Deformities
  - Nature and quality of movement
- Motor function
  - Autonomic function
  - Dexterity
  - Coordination
- Muscle performance
  - Grip: Include functional measures (i.e., palmar flexion)
  - Pinch
- Pain
  - Measured on visual analog scale
- ROM
  - Elbow
  - Wrist
  - Hand
- Sensory integrity
  - Superficial

Establish Plan of Care

- Based on history, tests, and measures

GOALS/OUTCOMES

- Wrist and forearm ROM: 100% of AMA guides
  - Wrist
    - Flexion: 60°
    - Extension: 60°
    - Ulnar deviation: 30°
    - Radial deviation: 20°
  - Forearm
    - Pronation: 80°
    - Supination: 80°

- Metacarpal phalangeal (MCP) ROM: 100% of American Academy of Orthopædic Surgeons norms
  - Flexion: 90°
  - Extension: 0°
- Pain: 2/10 with activity, 0/10 at rest
- Prehensile (grip and pinch) strength: Mean for age/gender norms or equal to uninvolved side, or adequate for work/home tasks performance
- Return to prior functional status and activity level for ADLs and vocational, recreational, and sports activities as identified by patient
- Independence in a progressive home exercise program emphasizing function

INTERVENTION
NUMBER OF VISITS: 8–16

Coordination, Communication, and Documentation
- Provision of services between admission and discharge that facilitate cost-effective and efficient integration or reintegration to home, community, or work
- Documentation of therapeutic intervention is required for each episode of care and serves as the basic foundation for communication
- Coordination and additional communication will depend on the patient's impairment and home/work/community/leisure situation and requirements. Such services may include:
  - Case management
  - Coordination of care and collaboration with those integral to the patient's rehabilitation program
  - Coordination and monitoring of the delivery of available resources
  - Referrals to other health-care professionals
  - Identification of resources, support groups, or advocacy services
  - Provision of educational or training information
  - Technical assistance

Patient Instruction

Basic Anatomy and Biomechanics
- Review of bony, musculature, and ligamentous structures of the forearm, wrist, and hand
- Relation of radius and ulna during forearm rotation
- Pertinent Gray's Anatomy (Gray. 1995. 645–654)

Handouts
- Home exercise program
- Application of superficial thermal modalities/cryotherapy
- Edema control techniques
- Self-mobilization, massage, and stretching techniques

Functional Considerations
- Assistive devices to avoid stress on fracture site/splinting
- Modification/accommodation for one-handed daily activities

Direct Interventions

Acute Phase: 4–8 Visits, Weeks 1–4
After Cast Removal
- Therapeutic exercise and home program
  - Flexibility exercises
    - Digit flexion with wrist extension to reestablish normal tenodesis pattern and to avoid substitution of digit extensors for wrist extensors
  - ROM following cast removal
    - Passive ROM
    - Active-assisted ROM
    - Exercise should not cause increase in pain, edema, or stiffness. Perform 4–6 times per day, 10 repetitions each.
    - Digit abduction/adduction
    - Intrinsic-plus position: "Shelf"
      a. MCP flexion, distal interphalangeal and proximal interphalangeal extension
    - Thumb radial abduction, palmar abduction
    - Opposition
    - Fisting sequence
    - Wrist flexion/extension
    - Wrist extension with digit flexion
    - Forearm pronation/supination
    - Wrist ulnar/radial deviation
- Manual therapy techniques
  - Soft-tissue techniques
    - Soft-tissue mobilization for edema reduction
      a. Performed with upper extremity elevated, elbow extended
  - Joint mobilization
    - Gliding of individual carpals
- Therapeutic devices and equipment
  - Splinting

WRIST/HAND | WRIST FRACTURE   601

- Elastic wrist splint or wrist cock-up splint following cast removal
- With increased ROM, wean from splint wear except for vigorous activities, such as lifting, driving
  - Compression glove for edema
- Electrotherapeutic modalities
- Physical agents and mechanical modalities
  - Contrast bath
  - Cryotherapy/thermal modalities
  - Ultrasound
- Goals/outcomes
  - Edema: Reduction to within 25% of uninvolved hand/wrist
  - Independence with self-care
  - Forearm rotation to 75% of AMA guides and ability to make complete fist
    - Wrist
      a. Flexion: 45°
      b. Extension: 45°
      c. Ulnar deviation: 25°
      d. Radial deviation: 15°
    - Forearm
      a. Pronation: 60°
      b. Supination: 60°

Subacute Phase: 4–8 Visits, Weeks 5–8 After Cast Removal
- Therapeutic exercise and home program
  - Passive ROM
  - Motor performance
    Initiated when wrist ROM is 75% of anticipated goal
    - Therapy putty
    - Foam and grippers
    - Exerstick™
    - Resisted exerciser
    - Baltimore Therapeutic Equipment
    - Free weights
    - Contract-relax
    - Over-pressure
    - Pronation/supination without substituted wrist rotation, ulnar deviation, or palmar flexion
- Manual therapy techniques
  - Joint mobilization
  - Manual resistive exercise
  - Soft-tissue techniques

- Therapeutic devices and equipment
  - Splinting
    - Worn for heavy activities that cause pain without splint
  - Compression glove worn nocturnally
    - Taper off as edema stabilizes
- Physical agents and mechanical modalities
  - Continue effective modalities as in acute phase with increased emphasis on use as needed at home
- Goals/outcomes
  - ROM: 90% of AMA guides for wrist and forearm
    - Wrist
      a. Flexion: 55°
      b. Extension: 55°
      c. Ulnar deviation: 30°
      d. Radial deviation: 20°
    - Forearm
      a. Pronation: 70°
      b. Supination: 70°
  - Prehensile (grip and pinch) strength: Mean for age/gender norms
  - Resume functional activities
  - Pain: 0/10

Functional Carryover
- Ergonomic assessment and modifications as needed
- Orientation of exercise program toward individualized work simulation

DISCHARGE PLANNING AND PATIENT RESPONSIBILITY

Criteria for Discharge
- All rehabilitation goals/outcomes achieved with the exception of the final 10% of wrist and forearm range

Circumstances Requiring Additional Visits
- Presence of reflex sympathetic dystrophy of the upper extremity
- Presence of stiff hand syndrome
- Carpal tunnel syndrome
- Open reduction or surgical fixation
- Postoperative infection/complications
- Underlying medical conditions, e.g., arthritis
- Persistent or worsening edema
- Special occupational needs that require extensive strengthening

Home Program

- Edema reduction techniques
- Self-mobilization
- Motor performance exercise

Monitoring

- Patient is instructed to call for advice should progression halt or a negative trend occur
- Follow up at 4–8 weeks post-discharge to ensure expected return to function and progression toward attaining all rehabilitation goals/outcomes
- If symptoms consistently recur, consideration of reassessment for direct intervention or potential as surgical candidate
- Awareness of complications
  - Volkman's ischemic contracture
  - Nerve compression syndrome
  - Reflex sympathetic dystrophy
  - Traumatic arthritis
  - Cosmetic deformity

REFERENCES

1. American Physical Therapy Association. *Guide to Physical Therapist Practice*. Alexandria, VA: APTA; 1997.
2. Clyburn TA. Dynamic external fixation for comminuted intra-articular fractures of the distal end of the radius. *J Bone Surg.* 1987;69A:248.
3. Engelberg AL. *Guides to the Evaluation of Permanent Impairment.* 3rd ed. Chicago, IL: American Medical Association; 1989.
4. Gray H; Williams PL, ed. *Gray's Anatomy.* 38th ed. New York, NY: Churchill Livingstone; 1995.
5. Hunter JM, Mackin EJ, Callahan AD. Fractures and traumatic conditions of the wrist. *Rehabilitation of the Hand.* 3rd ed. St. Louis, MO: CV Mosby; 1990:267-283.
6. Hurley R, ed. *Rehabilitation of the Hand.* St Louis, MO: CV Mosby; 1995.
7. Lyngcoln A, Taylor N, Pizzari T, Baskus K. The relationship between adherence to hand therapy and short-term outcome after distal radius fracture. *J Hand Ther.* 2005;18:2-8.
8. Mathiowetz V, Kashman N, Volland G, et al. Grip and pinch strength: normative data for adults. *Arch Phys Med Rehabil.* 1985;66:69-74.
9. Wakefield AE, McQueen MM. The role of physiotherapy and clinical predictors of outcome after fracture of the distal radius. *J Bone Joint Surg (Br).* 2000;82-B:972-6.

604   WRIST FRACTURE | WRIST/HAND

WRIST SPRAIN/STRAIN
SUMMARY OVERVIEW

ICD-9

842.0   842.1

APTA Preferred Practice Pattern: 4D, 4I

EXAMINATION

- History and Systems Review
- Tests and Measures
  Systems review per APTA's *Guide to Physical Therapy Practice*
  - Circulation
  - Ergonomics and body mechanics
  - Integumentary integrity
  - Joint integrity and mobility
  - Muscle performance
  - Neuromotor development and sensory integration
  - Pain
  - Posture
  - ROM
  - Reflex integrity
  - Self-care and home management
  - Sensory integrity
  - Work (job/school/play), community, and leisure integration or reintegration (including instrumental ADLs)
- Establish Plan of Care

GOALS/OUTCOMES

- Pain reduced to 1/10 with activity, 0/10 at rest
- Full wrist and hand mobility (wrist flexion/extension 60°/60° or equal to uninvolved extremity): Digits able to complete full hook, fist positioning, thumb to base of small finger
- Functional strength of grip and pinch to meet norms for age and gender, work, or home activity level, or comparative to uninvolved extremity
- Return of patient to home, work, and sports/recreational activities

INTERVENTION
NUMBER OF VISITS: 5–10

- Patient Instruction
  - Basic Anatomy and Biomechanics
  - Handouts
  - Functional Considerations
- Direct Interventions
  - Acute Phase: 3–5 Visits
  - Subacute Phase: 2–5 Visits
- Functional Carryover

DISCHARGE PLANNING AND PATIENT RESPONSIBILITY

- Criteria for Discharge
  - Independence in strengthening exercise program
  - Full active mobility in all involved joints
  - Functional grip and pinch to meet norms for age/gender or equal to uninvolved extremity and work/home activities
  - Pain: 0/10 at rest, 1/10 with use
  - Client able to return to full work or recreational activities
- Circumstances Requiring Additional Visits
  - History of other pathology
  - Osteoarthritis
  - Unstable ligamentous support
  - Surgery to repair injury
  - Significant return to work or sport requirements
- Home Program
  - Home program should include activities for controlling edema, reducing pain, increasing mobility of hand, wrist, and forearm, gradual progression of activity to return strength, and instruction in precautions for healing and correct use of protective support
- Monitoring

SUMMARY OVERVIEW | WRIST/HAND | WRIST SPRAIN/STRAIN   605

WRIST SPRAIN/STRAIN

ICD-9

    842.0   Wrist sprain

    842.1   Hand sprain

APTA Preferred Practice Pattern: 4D, 4I

EXAMINATION

History and Systems Review

- History of current condition
  - Mechanism of injury, onset date
  - Pain and movements/activities that aggravate/alleviate pain
  - Mobility of wrist and associated joints, with notes on active vs. passive response
- Past history of current condition
- Other tests and measures
  - Appropriate testing of ligamentous stability, in particular the TFCC and carpal joints
- Medications
- Past medical/surgical history
- Functional status and activity level (current/prior)
- Patient's functional goals

Tests and Measures

Systems review per APTA's *Guide to Physical Therapy Practice*

- Circulation (arterial, venous, lymphatic)
- Ergonomics and body mechanics
- Integumentary integrity
- Joint integrity and mobility
- Muscle performance (including strength, power, and endurance)
- Neuromotor development and sensory integration
- Pain
- Posture
- ROM (including muscle length)
- Reflex integrity
- Self-care and home management (including ADLs and instrumental ADLs)
- Sensory integrity
- Work (job/school/play), community, and leisure integration or reintegration (including instrumental ADLs)

Establish Plan of Care

- Based on history, tests, and measures

GOALS/OUTCOMES

- Pain: reduced to 1/10 with activity, 0/10 at rest
- Full wrist and hand mobility (wrist flexion/extension 60°/60° or equal to uninvolved extremity): Digits able to complete full hook, fist positioning, thumb to base of small finger
- Functional strength of grip and pinch to meet norms for age and gender, work or home activity level, or comparative to uninvolved extremity
- Return to home, work, and sports/recreational activities

INTERVENTION

NUMBER OF VISITS: 5–10

Coordination, Communication, and Documentation

- Provision of services between admission and discharge that facilitate cost-effective and efficient integration or reintegration to home, community, or work
- Documentation of therapeutic intervention is required for each episode of care and serves as the basic foundation for communication
- Coordination and additional communication will depend on the patient's impairment and home/work/community/leisure situation and requirements. Such services may include:
  - Case management
  - Coordination of care and collaboration with those integral to the patient's rehabilitation program
  - Coordination and monitoring of the delivery of available resources
  - Referrals to other health-care professionals
  - Identification of resources, support groups, or advocacy services
  - Provision of educational or training information
  - Technical assistance
- Specific coordination and communication provisions

Patient Instruction

Basic Anatomy and Biomechanics
- Review with patient the hand and wrist anatomy and ligamentous structures
- Krames has a handout for Wrist Sprain and Clinical Orthopædic Rehabilitation by S. Brent Brotzman has very good drawings of the hand.

Handouts
- Home program
  - Edema control with contrast baths, retrograde massage, elevation or TENS
  - Tendon glide exercises to maintain length of hand musculature and active/assisted exercises as appropriate to pain level and length of time post injury
  - Appropriate donning/doffing and wear of splints as needed
  - Gradual, progressive strengthening as allowed by stage of sprain

Functional Considerations
- Posture (avoid dependent postures, elevate for swelling)
- Assistive devices (splints for resting of joints to improve function of hand)
- Precautions (pain as initial guideline to minimize trauma to sprain)
- Alteration of ADLs
- Avoidance of prolonged postures
- Positioning for relief of symptoms
- Body mechanic instruction for lifting, pushing, pulling, etc.
- Training recommendations (graded exercises with weights as sprain improves and tolerates increased resistance)

Direct Interventions

Acute Phase: 3–5 Visits
- Edema control
- Active exercises for tendon gliding
- Isometric exercises for stability of wrist
- Modalities for pain and swelling
- Splinting to rest affected joints and improve total hand function
- Home exercise program
- Joint protection and splinting

Subacute Phase: 2–5 Visits
- Isometric strengthening
- Active exercises
- Baltimore Therapeutic Equipment program
- Light progressive weight exercises for strengthening
- Home exercise program progression
- Work conditioning

Functional Carryover
- Integration of home exercise program into vocational environment
- Completion of ergonomic adjustments to home, automobile, and vocational areas
- Incorporation of proper posture and body mechanics to avoid exacerbation of symptoms
- Recognition/avoidance of activities that increase or exacerbate radiating symptoms

DISCHARGE PLANNING AND PATIENT RESPONSIBILITY

Criteria for Discharge
- Independence in strengthening exercise program
- Full active mobility in all involved joints
- Functional grip and pinch to meet norms for age/gender or equal to uninvolved extremity and work/home activities
- Pain: 0/10 at rest, 1/10 with use
- Client able to return to full work or recreational activities

Circumstances Requiring Additional Visits
- History of other pathology
- Osteoarthritis
- Unstable ligamentous support
- Surgery to repair injury
- Significant return to work or sport requirements

Home Program
- Home program should include activities for controlling edema, reducing pain, increasing mobility of hand, wrist, and forearm, gradual progression of activity to return strength, and instruction in precautions for healing and correct use of protective supports

Monitoring
- Needed only if client is to have further surgical address to injury

REFERENCES

1. American Physical Therapy Association. *Guide to Physical Therapist Practice*. Alexandria, VA: APTA; revised 2003.
2. Berger R, et al. Physical examination and provocative maneuvers of the wrist. In: Gilula LA, Yin Y. *Imaging of the Wrist and Hand*. Philadelphia: W.B. Saunders, 1996.
3. Brotzman SB, Wilk KE. *Clinical Orthopaedic Rehabilitation*. 2nd ed. Mosby Inc; 2003.
4. Jacobs M, Austin N. *Splinting of the Hand and Upper Extremity*. Lippincott Williams & Wilkins; 2003.
5. Larsen CF, Amadio PC, Gilula LA, Hodge JC. Analysis of carpal instability: description of the scheme. *J Hand Surg [Am]*. Sept. 1995;20(5):757-64.
6. LaStayo P, Howell J. Clinical provocative tests used in evaluating wrist pain. *J Hand Ther*. 1995;8(1):10-7.
7. Levine WR. Rehabilitation techniques for ligament injuries of the wrist. *Hand Clinics*. November 1992;8(4):669-81.
8. Mackin EJ, Callahan AD, Osterman AL, et al. *Hunter, Makin, & Callahan's Rehabilitation of the Hand and Upper Extremity*. 5th ed. Mosby Inc; 2002.

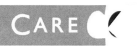

RETURN TO SPORT

Ankle Sprain/Instability—Return To Sport	611
Anterior Cruciate Ligament Reconstruction—Return To Sport	613
Elbow/Shoulder Injury—Return To Tennis	615
Exercise Sequence: Elbow/Shoulder Injury—Return To Tennis	617
Hamstring Injury—Return To Sport	621
Hip Pain In Runners—Return To Sport	623
Exercise Sequence: Hip Pain In Runners—Return To Sport	625
Upper Extremity Injury—Return To Throwing	627
Exercise Sequence: Upper Extremity Injury—Return To Throwing	629
Walking Program—Walking For The Health Of It	635
Patient Information Sheet: Walking For The Health Of It	637
Activity Questionnaire for Runners/Walkers	639

610   RETURN TO SPORT

ANKLE SPRAIN/INSTABILITY—RETURN TO SPORT

ICD-9
837   Dislocation of ankle
845   Sprains and strains of ankle and foot

APTA Preferred Practice Pattern: 4E, 4J

This guideline is for returning to active sports participation and is appropriate after the subacute phase of rehabilitation has been completed. Following initial assessment and instruction by the physical therapist, the program outlined will be primarily performed independently (at home or in a health club). Periodic assessment by the physical therapist, with incorporation of physician recommendations, will allow progression toward goals. The phases within the guideline have been formatted so that they can be copied and distributed to the patient as a home program.

CONDITIONS

Individuals not meeting the following conditions should follow the *Ankle Sprain/Instability* guideline.
- Ankle pain: 2/10 or less as measured on visual analog scale
- Pain-free AROM:
  ○ Plantarflexion: 40°
  ○ Dorsiflexion: 8° in subtalar neutral with knee flexed
- Foot and ankle strength: 4+/5 on manual muscle tests
- Minimal edema (less than 1 cm difference as measured in figure eight compared to uninvolved leg)
- Normal gait pattern

HISTORY

It is assumed that the patient was thoroughly evaluated in the earlier stages of his or her rehabilitation process. However, if this is the patient's initial presentation, conduct a full evaluation in addition to gathering the sport-specific information below.
- History of sports activity
- Sports of choice
  ○ Team
    ▪ Position played
  ○ Individual
- Competitive level
- Specific sport goals/timeline
- Orthotics, protective and supportive devices
  ○ Shoe style
  ○ Orthotics
  ○ Braces
  ○ Taping
  ○ Other

PROGRESSION

This guideline has been divided into three phases. Within each phase, a number of exercise options are presented. It is not intended that each individual will do every exercise; rather, the physical therapist will determine the appropriate combination of exercises based on the individual's sport-specific needs and availability of equipment. It is assumed that the physical therapist possesses the kinesiological and sports knowledge base to correlate the appropriate exercises with the sport-specific demands.

Progression from one phase to the next will be determined by the physical therapist on the basis of the individual's mastery of and tolerance for the exercises and skills within the previous phase.

Based upon the home program model, the following visits are suggested per phase:
- Phase I: 1–2 visits
- Phase II: 1–2 visits
- Phase III: 1–2 visits

However, the guideline can be adapted to the clinical setting (for inclusion of manual therapy techniques and taping techniques) and the visits adjusted according to the physician/physical therapist recommendations.

PATIENT EDUCATION
- Instruct patient in self-monitoring of heart rate and perceived exertion
- Educate patient as to the influence of proper biomechanical alignment and adequate flexibility on

the kinematics of the lower quarter, as well as the influence of ankle pathology on the entire lower quarter

- Instruct patient in proper training progression per the patient's individual fitness level
- Instruct patient in monitoring the signs of overtraining:
  - Elevated resting morning heart rate
  - General sense of listlessness or fatigue
  - Soreness/aching/effusion
- Advise patient regarding the importance of each segment of training, including aerobic conditioning, flexibility, strengthening, and neuromuscular/balance/proprioceptive reeducation in the overall scheme of returning to full fitness

GOALS/OUTCOMES

- Patient will be able to pursue his or her sports activity without exacerbation of symptoms
- Patient displays a good understanding of the return to sport progression and the risks of overtraining

REFERENCES

1. Borg G. Perceived exertion: a note on history and methods. *Med Sci Sports Exerc.* 1973;2:90-93.
2. Cyriax JH, Cyriax PJ. *Illustrated Manual of Orthopedic Medicine.* London, England: Butterworths; 1983.
3. Gray G. *Lower Extremity Functional Profile.* Adrian, MI: Wynn Marketing; 1995.
4. Hart A, Hopkins C, Ford B. *ICD-9-CM Expert for Physicians, Volume 1&2.* 7th ed. USA: Ingenix; 2005.
5. Kendall F. *Muscles, Testing and Function.* 3rd ed. Baltimore, MD: Williams & Wilkins; 1983.
6. Lantell G, Baas B, Lopez D, et al. The contributions of proprioceptive defects, muscle function, and anatomic laxity to functional instability of the ankle. *J Orthop Sports Phys Ther.* 1995;4(8):206-213.
7. Malone TR, Hardacker MT. Rehabilitation of foot and ankle injuries in ballet dancers. *J Orthop Sports Phys Ther.* 1990;11:355-361.
8. Roy S, Irvine R. *Sports Medicine, Prevention, Evaluation, Management, and Rehabilitation.* Englewood Cliffs, NJ: Prentice Hall; 1983.
9. Wilkerson GB. Treatment of ankle sprains with external compression and early immobilization. *Phys Sports Med.* 1985;13:83-90.

ANTERIOR CRUCIATE LIGAMENT RECONSTRUCTION
RETURN TO SPORT

ICD-9

844.2   Sprain of cruciate ligament of knee

APTA Preferred Practice Pattern: **4E, 4J**

This guideline is for returning to active sports participation and is appropriate after the subacute phase of rehabilitation has been completed. Following initial assessment and instruction by the physical therapist, the program outlined will be primarily performed independently (at home or in a health club). Periodic assessment by the physical therapist, with incorporation of physician recommendations, will allow progression toward goals. The phases within the guideline have been formatted so that they can be copied and distributed to the patient as a home program.

CONDITIONS

Individuals not meeting the criteria below should be referred to the *Accelerated Anterior Cruciate Ligament Reconstruction* guideline.

- No pain during subacute phase exercise
- No joint edema
- Confirmation of 0–135° active ROM of involved knee
- Full functional performance of ADLs and vocational activity
- Patellar range of motion within 80% relative to uninvolved leg
- Functional strength testing: 60% of uninvolved leg (i.e., single-leg quarter squat, single-leg press)

HISTORY

It is assumed that the patient was thoroughly evaluated in the earlier stages of his or her rehabilitation process. However, if this is the patient's initial presentation, conduct a full evaluation in addition to gathering the sport-specific information below.

- History of sports activity
- Sports of choice
  - Team
    - Position played
  - Individual
- Competitive level
- Specific sport goals/timeline
- Orthotics, protective and supportive devices
  - Shoe style
  - Orthotics
  - Braces
  - Other

PROGRESSION

This guideline has been divided into three phases. Within each phase, a number of exercise options are presented. It is not intended that each individual will do every exercise; rather, the physical therapist will determine the appropriate combination of exercises on the basis of the individual's sport-specific needs and the availability of equipment. It is assumed that the physical therapist possesses the kinesiological and sports knowledge base to correlate the appropriate exercises with the sport-specific demands.

Progression from one phase to the next will be determined by the physical therapist based on the individual's mastery of and tolerance for the exercises and skills within the previous phase.

Based on the home program model, the following visits are suggested per phase:

- Phase I: 4–6 visits, Weeks 6–12 postoperative
- Phase II: 3–4 visits, Weeks 12–20 postoperative
- Phase III: 8–10 visits, Weeks 20–52 postoperative

However, the guideline can be adapted to the clinical setting and the visits adjusted according to the physician/physical therapist recommendations.

The average patient will end formal progression after Phase II. Phase III is for those individuals requiring greater muscle performance, endurance, or agility to meet sport-specific demands.

PATIENT INSTRUCTION

- The influence of proper biomechanical alignment, adequate flexibility, and muscle performance on the

RETURN TO SPORT | ANTERIOR CRUCIATE LIGAMENT RECONSTRUCTION   613

kinematics of the knee as well as the influence of knee pathology on the other joints of the lower quarter
- Self-monitoring of heart rate
- Self-monitoring of perceived exertion
- Monitoring the signs of overtraining
  - Attention to soreness/aching/effusion
  - Elevated resting morning heart rate
  - General sense of listlessness or fatigue

GOALS/OUTCOMES
- Patient will be able to monitor his or her own heart rate
- Patient will be able to pursue his or her sports of choice without exacerbation of symptoms as noted on the visual analog scale
- Patient will display good understanding of the sport-specific progression and the risks of overtraining

REFERENCE
1. Bak K, Jorgensen U, Ekstrand J, Scavenius M. Results of reconstruction of acute ruptures of the anterior cruciate ligament with an iliotibial band autograft. *Knee Surg Sports Tramatol Arthrosc.* 1999;7(2);111-117.
2. Borg G. Perceived exertion: a note on history and methods. *Med Sci Sports Exer.* 1973;2:90-93.
3. Chen CH, Chen WJ, Shih CH. Arthroscopic anterior cruciate ligament reconstruction with quadriceps tendon-pattar bone autograft. *J Trauma.* 1999;46:678-682.
4. Cyriax JH, Cyriax, PJ. *Illustrated Manual of Orthopedic Medicine.* London, England: Butterworths; 1983.
5. Fleming BC, Beynnon BD, Renstrom PA, et al. The strain behavior of the anterior cruciate ligament during stair climbing: an in vivo study. *Arthroscopy.* 1999;15:185-191.
6. Gray G. *Lower Extremity Functional Profile.* Adrian, MI: Wynn Marketing; 1995.
7. Gray H; Williams PL, ed. *Gray's Anatomy.* 38th ed. New York, NY: Churchill Livingstone; 1995.
8. Hart A, Hopkins C, Ford B. *ICD-9-CM Expert for Physicians, Volume 1&2.* 7th ed. USA: Ingenix. 2005.
9. Muneta T, Sekiya I, Ogiuchi T, et al. Effects of aggressive early rehabilitation on the outcome of anterior cruciate ligament reconstruction with multi-stand semitendinosus tendon. *Int Orthop.* 1998;22:352-356.
10. Petersen W, Laprell H. Combined injuries of the medial collateral ligament and the anterior cruciate ligament: early ACL reconstruction versus late ACL reconstruction. *Arch Orthop Trauma Surg.* 1999;119:258-262.
11. Petshe TS, Hutchinson MR. Loss of extension after reconstruction of the anterior cruciate ligament. *J Am Acad Orthop Surg.* 1999:7(2);119-127.
12. Roy S, Irvine R. *Sports Medicine: Prevention, Evaluation, Management and Rehabilitation.* Englewood Cliffs, NJ: Prentice-Hall; 1983.
13. Shelbourne KD, Davis TJ. Evaluation of knee stability before and after participation in a functional sports agility program during rehabilitation after anterior cruciate ligament reconstruction. *Am J Sports Med.* 1999;27:156-161.
14. Shelbourne KD, Knitz PA. Accelerated rehabilitation after anterior cruciate ligament reconstruction. *Am J Sports Med.* 1990;18:389-417.
15. Shelbourne KD, Patel DV. Treatment of limited motion after anterior cruciate ligament reconstruction. *Knee Surg Sports Traumatol Arthrosc.* 1999;7(2):85-92.
16. Shelbourne KD, Klootwyk TE, DeCarlo MS. Update on accelerated rehabilitation after ACL reconstruction. *J Orthop Sports Phys Ther.* 1992;15:303-308.
17. Wile KE, Arrigo C, Andrews JR, Clancy WG Jr. Rehabilitation after all reconstruction in the female athlete. *J Athletic Training.* 1999;34:177-193.

ELBOW/SHOULDER INJURY RETURN TO TENNIS
RETURN TO SPORT

ICD-9

716.91	Arthropathy, unspecified, shoulder region
718.21	Pathological dislocation, shoulder region
718.31	Recurrent dislocation of joint, shoulder region
718.81	Other joint derangement, not elsewhere classified, shoulder region
718.91	Unspecified derangement of joint, shoulder region
719.41	Pain in joint, shoulder region
719.42	Pain in joint, upper arm
719.43	Pain in joint, forearm
719.51	Stiffness of joint, not elsewhere classified, shoulder region
719.52	Stiffness of joint, not elsewhere classified, upper arm
719.91	Unspecified disorder of joint, shoulder region
726.0	Adhesive capsulitis of shoulder
726.1	Rotator cuff syndrome of shoulder and allied disorders
726.2	Other affections of shoulder region, not elsewhere classified
726.3	Enthesopathy of elbow region
726.91	Exostosis of unspecified site
727.3	Other bursitis
727.61	Complete rupture of rotator cuff
727.62	Nontraumatic rupture of tendons of biceps (long head)
810	Fracture of clavicle
812	Fracture of humerus
813.0	Closed fracture of upper end of radius and ulna
831.0	Closed dislocation of shoulder
831.1	Open dislocation of shoulder
840	Sprains and strains of shoulder and upper arm
841	Sprains and strains of elbow and forearm
959.2	Other and unspecified injury to shoulder and upper arm

APTA Preferred Practice Pattern: 4B,4C, 4D, 4E, 4F, 4G, 4I, 5D, 5H

This is intended to be a progression for return to tennis, to be initiated after the subacute phase of rehabilitation has been completed. Following initial assessment and instruction by the physical therapist, the program outlined will be primarily performed independently (at home or in a health club). Periodic assessment by the physical therapist, with incorporation of physician recommendations, will allow progression toward goals. The phases within the guideline have been formatted so that they can be copied and distributed to the patient as a home program.

CONDITIONS

Individuals not meeting the criteria below should be referred to the appropriate guideline.

- No pain during subacute phase exercise
- No joint swelling
- Full active ROM of the involved extremity
- Motor performance: 75% of uninvolved extremity
  - Shoulder flexion/extension
  - Shoulder internal/external rotation
  - Elbow flexion/extension
  - Forearm supination/pronation
  - Normal scapular strength to provide a stable base for elbow function
- Grip motor performance: 90% of uninvolved extremity

HISTORY

It is assumed that the patient was thoroughly evaluated in the earlier stages of his or her rehabilitation process.

RETURN TO SPORT | ELBOW/SHOULDER INJURY—RETURN TO TENNIS **615**

However, if this is the patient's initial presentation, conduct a full evaluation in addition to gathering the sport-specific information below.
- History of sports activity
- Competitive level and frequency of participation
- Specific sports goals and timeline
- Adaptive equipment
  - Braces
  - Racquet style and size
  - Other

PROGRESSION

This guideline has been divided into four phases. Progression from one phase to the next will be determined by the physical therapist on the basis of the individual's mastery of and tolerance for the exercises and skills within the previous phase.

Based on the home program model, the following visits are suggested per phase:
- Phase I: 2 visits
- Phase II: 1–2 visits
- Phase III: 1 visit
- Phase IV: 1 visit

PATIENT INSTRUCTION

- The influence of proper biomechanical alignment, adequate flexibility, strength, and motor performance of both the upper and lower extremities on the kinematics of the shoulder and elbow joints
- Monitoring the signs of overtraining
  - Attention to soreness/aching/effusion
  - Elevated resting morning heart rate
  - Generalized sense of listlessness or fatigue
- The importance of adequate warm-up prior to and cool-down following exercise
- May use tennis elbow strap as needed though current research challenges this approach. See referenced articles.
- Use of ice after exercise as well as proper hydration to reduce risk of exacerbating inflammatory processes
- Use of a mid- to large-size racquet head to reduce stress on the upper extremity, and the importance of proper grip size and racquet weight in minimizing stress on the involved extremity
- Utilization of a tennis professional for instruction in proper stroke dynamics

GOALS/OUTCOMES

- Patient will be able to resume tennis without exacerbation of symptoms as noted on the visual analog scale
- Patient displays understanding of the sport-specific progression and the risks of overtraining

REFERENCES

1. Elliot BC. Biomechanics of the serve in tennis: a biomechanical perspective. *Sports Med.* 1988;6:285-302.
2. Hart A, Hopkins C, Ford B. *ICD-9-CM Expert for Physicians, Volume 1&2.* 7th ed. USA: Ingenix; 2005.
3. Litchfield R, Hawkins R, Dillman CJ, Atkins J, Hagerman G. Rehabilitation for the overhead athlete. *J Orthop Sports Phys Ther.* 1993;18(2):433-441.
4. Ng GYF, Chan, H. The immediate effects of tension on counterforce of counterforce forearm brace on neuromuscular performance of wrist extensor muscles in subjects with lateral humeral epicondylitis. *J Orthop Sports Phys Ther.* 2004;2:72-78.
5. Nirschl RP. Prevention and treatment of elbow and shoulder injuries in the tennis player. *Clin Sports Med.* 1988;7:289-308.
6. Perry J. Anatomy and biomechanics of the shoulder in throwing, swimming, gymnastics and tennis. *Clin Sports Med.* 1983;2:379-390.
7. Rhy KN, McCormick J, Jobe FW, et al. An electromyographic analysis of shoulder function in tennis players. *Am J Sports Med.* 1988;16:481-488.
8. Van Gheluwe B, Hebbelinch M. Muscle actions and ground reaction forces in tennis. *Int J Sports Biomech.* 1986;2:88-93.
9. Wilk KE, Arrigo CA. Current concepts in the rehabilitation of the athletic shoulder. *J Orthop Sports Phys Ther.* 1993;18(1):386-391.
10. Wilk KE, Voight ML, Keirns MA, et al. Stretch-shortening drills for the upper extremities: theory and clinical application. *J Orthop Sports Phys Ther.* 1993;17(5):225-239.

EXERCISE SEQUENCE
ELBOW/SHOULDER INJURY RETURN TO TENNIS—RETURN TO SPORT

PHASE I: HOME PROGRAM

Weeks 1 and 2: To be performed 3 times per week. Begin each session with proper stretching to both upper and lower extremities. Proceed to the next day if you are pain-free and have no swelling.

Aerobic Conditioning

Due to the intermittent nature of tennis at the amateur level, regular aerobic conditioning is recommended as a supplement to court time to enhance cardiovascular conditioning and exercise endurance. Perform for 15–20 minutes duration at 60–75% of age-predicted maximum heart rate.

- Walking or intermittent walk/jog on treadmill or outdoors
- Stair machine
- Ski machine
- Upper or lower body cycling

Flexibility

Static stretching of the following muscles should be performed following a warm-up period. Emphasis should be placed on long-duration, low-intensity techniques with use of contract/relax techniques as appropriate.

- Hamstring
- Gastrocnemius/soleus
- Quadriceps
- Hip internal and external rotators
- Psoas
- Pectorals
- Latissimus
- Wrist flexors and extensors

Sport-Specific Agility Drills

- Shuttle drills
  - Lateral shuffle steps, center court to side court line
  - Forward/backward shuttle, base line to net
- Cariocas, right leading and left leading
- Cut and run to the right and to the left
- Diagonal forward/backward running

Strengthening

As with any racquet sport, the element of power in tennis comes not only from the upper body, but is generated in the gluteals, hip abductors, and abdominals. For this reason, lower extremity and abdominal exercises are presented in Phase I and should be continued as needed through the remaining phases.

- Squats progression
  - With body weight only, may be used as a warm-up
  - Light weight
    - 40–55% of one-repetition maximum
    - 15–25 repetitions per set may be used to regain motor performance and endurance
  - Plyometric (jump squats)
    - Very light weights (20% of one-repetition maximum)
    - Used to regain explosive power
- Lunge progression
  - With body weight only, may be used as a warm-up
  - Multidirectional lunges target specific muscles
    - Anterior lunge: Targets gluteals, hamstrings, and quadriceps
    - Lateral lunge: Targets hip abductors, adductors as well as gluteals and hamstrings
    - Rotational lunges: Targets hip rotators as well as abductors, adductors, gluteals, hamstrings, and quadriceps
- Abdominal progression
  - Open-kinetic chain
    - Supine crunches
    - Abdominal bracing with alternate arm and leg lift
  - Closed-kinetic chain functional strengthening. Avoid using nonweight-bearing leg for counterbalance during any of these exercises.
    - Single-leg stand posterior overhead reach
      a. Use one or both arms, reaching to maximum distance directly posteriorly overhead
      b. Progress to holding a racquet for additional weight

RETURN TO SPORT | EXERCISE SEQUENCE—ELBOW/SHOULDER INJURY—RETURN TO TENNIS 617

- Single-leg stand rotational overhead reach
  a. Use one or both arms, reaching diagonally posteriorly overhead
  b. Progress to holding a racquet for additional weight
- Single-leg stand overhead pull using resistive tubing
  a. Attach tubing to top of door frame
  b. Stand with your back to the door and grasp the tubing overhead
  c. Pull down and forward as if swinging an ax, while balancing on one leg
  d. Repeat weight bearing on other leg

Sport-Specific Strengthening

- Day 1
  ○ 10 shadow forehand strokes (without tennis ball)
  ○ 10 shadow backhand strokes (without tennis ball)
  ○ 25 forehand strokes (drop ball and hit to backboard)
  ○ 25 backhand strokes (drop ball and hit to backboard)
- Day 2
  ○ 10 shadow forehand strokes (without tennis ball)
  ○ 10 shadow backhand strokes (without tennis ball)
  ○ 35 forehand strokes (drop ball and hit to backboard)
  ○ 35 backhand strokes (drop ball and hit to backboard)
- Day 3
  ○ 10 shadow forehand strokes (without tennis ball)
  ○ 10 shadow backhand strokes (without tennis ball)
  ○ 35 forehand strokes (drop ball and hit to backboard)
  ○ 35 backhand strokes (drop ball and hit to backboard)
  ○ 10 consecutive forehand strokes against backboard
- Days 4–6
  ○ 10 shadow forehand strokes (without tennis ball)
  ○ 10 shadow backhand strokes (without tennis ball)
  ○ 35 forehand strokes (drop ball and hit to backboard)
  ○ 35 backhand strokes (drop ball and hit to backboard)
  ○ 10 consecutive forehand strokes against backboard
  ○ 10 consecutive backhand strokes against backboard

PHASE II: HOME PROGRAM

Weeks 3 and 4: You may begin to have someone hit balls to you. Continue 3 times per week. Begin each session with proper stretching and warm-up. Aerobic conditioning, strengthening, and flexibility should be continued as in Phase I.

Sport-Specific Agility Drills

- Shuttle drills
  ○ Lateral shuffle steps, center court to side court line, with direction changes on command
  ○ Forward/backward shuttle, base line to net, with direction changes on command
- Cariocas, right leading and left leading
- Cut and run varying directions using backward, forward, and side steps

Sport-Specific Strengthening

- Warm-up
  ○ 10 shadow forehand strokes (without tennis ball)
  ○ 10 shadow backhand strokes (without tennis ball)
  ○ 15 consecutive forehand strokes against backboard
  ○ 15 consecutive backhand strokes against backboard
- Activity
  ○ 25 forehand strokes
  ○ 25 backhand strokes
  ○ Each session increase by 10 strokes
    ▪ By last day of Week 4 you should be hitting 75 forehand and 75 backhand strokes

PHASE III: HOME PROGRAM

Weeks 5 and 6: You may begin to rally with a partner. Begin each session with proper stretching and warm-up. Continue 3 times per week. Only move to next phase if you are pain-free and have no swelling. General aerobic conditioning, strengthening, and flexibility exercises should be continued as in Phase I.

Sport-Specific Agility Drills

- Shuttle drills
  ○ Use a ball machine to determine your direction changes
    ▪ Carry your racquet, and position yourself to hit the ball, but do not hit
    ▪ This is intended to be an agility drill, not a stroke drill
    ▪ You should be using forward and backward as well as lateral shuffle steps to position yourself appropriately on the court
- Cariocas, right leading and left leading
  ○ Focus on increasing speed and holding your racquet

- Cut and run varying directions using backward, forward, side shuffle, and carioca steps

Sport-Specific Strengthening
- Warm-up
  - 10 shadow forehand strokes (without tennis ball)
  - 10 shadow backhand strokes (without tennis ball)
  - 25 consecutive forehand strokes against backboard
  - 25 consecutive backhand strokes against backboard
- Activity
  - 25 forehand strokes (rally)
  - 25 backhand strokes (rally)
  - 75 each alternate forehand and backhand strokes (rally)
  - Limit total playing time to 45 minutes

PHASE IV: HOME PROGRAM

Weeks 7 and 8: Begin each session with proper stretching and warm-up. Continue 3 times per week. General aerobic conditioning, strengthening, and flexibility exercises should be continued as in Phase I. Sport-specific agility drill should be continued as in Phase III.

Sport-Specific Strengthening
- Warm-up
  - 10 shadow forehand strokes (without tennis ball)
  - 10 shadow backhand strokes (without tennis ball)
  - 25 consecutive forehand strokes against backboard
  - 25 consecutive backhand strokes against backboard
- Activity
  - 100 strokes alternate forehand and backhand
  - 10 forehand volleys
  - 10 backhand volleys
  - Increase volleys by 10 each session
  - By the end of Week 7 begin with 10 serves. Add 10 serves each session.
  - Serve only 75% effort; go easy and don't try to kill the ball
- Return to sport at Week 8
  - Begin normal drills including down the line, cross court, volleys, and serves as outlined by your coach
  - Remember: Only progress if you are pain-free and have no swelling
  - Use heat before and ice after workout

RETURN TO SPORT | EXERCISE SEQUENCE—ELBOW/SHOULDER INJURY—RETURN TO TENNIS   619

HAMSTRING INJURY—RETURN TO SPORT

ICD-9

843.9	Sprain of unspecified site of hip and thigh
844.9	Sprain of unspecified site of knee and leg
924.0	Contusion of hip and thigh
928.0	Crushing injury of hip and thigh

APTA Preferred Practice Pattern: **4D, 4E, 4J, 7B, 7E**

This guideline is for returning to active sports participation and is appropriate after the subacute phase of rehabilitation has been completed. Following initial assessment and instruction by the physical therapist, the program outlined will be primarily performed independently (at home or in a health club). Periodic assessment by the physical therapist, with incorporation of physician recommendations, will allow progression toward goals. The phases within the guideline have been formatted so that they can be copied and distributed to the patient as a home program.

CONDITIONS

- Pain-free knee ROM: 0–135°
- Pain-free hip ROM: -10–135°
- Absence of active inflammatory process
- No pain during exercise
- Pain-free active straight-leg raise

HISTORY

It is assumed that the patient was thoroughly evaluated in the earlier stages of his or her rehabilitation process. However, if this is the patient's initial presentation, conduct a full evaluation in addition to gathering the sport-specific information below.

- History of sports activity
- Sports of choice
  - Team
    - Position played
  - Individual
- Competitive level
- Specific sport goals/timeline
- Orthotics, protective and supportive devices
  - Shoe style
  - Orthotics
  - Braces
  - Other

PROGRESSION

This guideline has been divided into three phases. Within each phase, a number of exercise options are presented. It is not intended that each individual will do every exercise; rather, the physical therapist will determine the appropriate combination of exercises on the basis of the individual's sport-specific needs and the availability of equipment. It is assumed that the physical therapist possesses the kinesiological and sports knowledge base to correlate the appropriate exercises with the sport-specific demands.

Progression from one phase to the next will be determined by the physical therapist based on the individual's mastery of and tolerance for the exercises and skills within the previous phase.

Based on the home program model, the following visits are suggested per phase:

- Phase I: 2 visits
- Phase II: 1–2 visits
- Phase III: 1–2 visits

However, the guideline can be adapted to the clinical setting and the visits adjusted according to the physician/physical therapist recommendations.

PATIENT INSTRUCTION

- The influence of proper biomechanical alignment, adequate flexibility, and muscle performance on the kinematics of the knee and hip, as well as the influence of hip and knee pathology on the joints of the lower quarter
- Self-monitoring of heart rate
- Self-monitoring of perceived exertion
- Monitoring the signs of overtraining
  - Attention to soreness/aching
  - Elevated resting morning heart rate
  - General sense of listlessness or fatigue

GOALS/OUTCOMES

- Patient will be able to monitor his or her own heart rate
- Patient will be able to pursue his or her sports of choice without exacerbation of symptoms as noted on visual analog scale
- Patient displays good understanding of the sport-specific progression and the risks of overtraining

REFERENCE

1. American Physical Therapy Association. *Guide to Physical Therapist Practice*. Alexandria, VA: APTA; 1997.
2. Borg G. Perceived exertion: a note on history and methods. *Med Sci Sports Exerc*. 1973;2:90-93.
3. Cyriax JH, Cyriax PJ. *Illustrated Manual of Orthopedic Medicine*. London, England: Butterworths; 1983.
4. Gray G. *Lower Extremity Functional Profile*. Adrian, MI: Wynn Marketing; 1995.
5. Hart A, Hopkins C, Ford B. *ICD-9-CM Expert for Physicians, Volume 1&2*. 7th ed. USA: Ingenix; 2005.
6. Kendall F. *Muscles: Testing and Function*. Baltimore, MD: Williams & Wilkins; 1983.
7. Roy S, Irvine R. *Sports Medicine, Prevention, Evaluation, Management and Rehabilitation*. Englewood Cliffs, NJ: Prentice-Hall; 1983.

HIP PAIN IN RUNNERS—RETURN TO SPORT

ICD-9

715.00	Osteoarthrosis, generalized, site unspecified
715.09	Osteoarthrosis, generalized, multiple sites
726.5	Enthesopathy of hip region
733.14	Pathologic fracture of neck of femur
733.15	Pathologic fracture of other specified part of femur
843.9	Sprain of unspecified site of hip and thigh

APTA Preferred Practice Pattern: 4C, 4D, 4E, 4F, 4G, 4H, 4I,4J, 6B

This guideline is for returning to active sports participation and is appropriate after the subacute phase of rehabilitation has been completed. Following initial assessment and instruction by the physical therapist, the program outlined will be primarily performed independently (at home or in a health club). Periodic assessment by the physical therapist, with incorporation of physician recommendations, will allow progression toward goals. The guideline has been formatted so that it can be copied and distributed to the patient as a home program.

CONDITIONS

Individuals not meeting the criteria below should be referred to the *Hip Soft Tissue Pain* guideline.

- Lower extremity functional ROM:
  - Hip: -10–100°
  - Knee: 5–135°
  - Ankle: 8° dorsiflexion, 40° plantarflexion
- Structural biomechanical aspects that may contribute to overuse injuries have been addressed, including the use of orthotics or special footwear as appropriate
- Pain-free, normal gait pattern without assistive devices
- No pain during exercise

HISTORY

It is assumed that the patient was thoroughly evaluated in the earlier stages of the rehabilitation process. However, if this is the patient's initial presentation, conduct a full evaluation in addition to gathering the sport-specific information below. (See *Activity Questionnaire for Runners/Walkers*)

- Previous running history
  - Mileage
  - Pace
  - Shoe style
  - Terrain
  - Recent racing history
- Cross-training preferences
- Past history of current condition
  - Previous lower quarter injuries/surgeries

PROGRESSION

Within this progression, a number of exercise options are presented. It is not intended that each individual will do every exercise; rather, the physical therapist will determine the appropriate combination of exercises on the basis of the individual's running goals and availability of equipment. It is assumed that the physical therapist possesses the kinesiological and sports knowledge base to correlate the appropriate exercises with the sport-specific demands.

Based upon the home program model, 1–2 visits are suggested. However, the guideline can be adapted to the clinical setting and the visits adjusted according to the physician/physical therapist recommendations.

PATIENT INSTRUCTION

- The influence of proper biomechanical alignment and adequate flexibility on the kinematics of the hip, as well as the influence of hip pathology on lumbar dynamics
- Proper training protocol per the patient's individual fitness level
- Monitoring the signs of overtraining
  - Elevated resting morning heart rate
  - General sense of listlessness or fatigue
  - Attention to soreness/aching
- Self-monitoring of heart rate
- Self-monitoring of perceived exertion

RETURN TO SPORT | HIP PAIN IN RUNNERS   623

GOALS/OUTCOMES

- Patient will be able to monitor his or her own heart rate
- Patient will be able to pursue the running program without exacerbation of symptoms
- Patient displays a good understanding of the running program progression and the risks of overtraining as well as the risks of return to a sedentary lifestyle

REFERENCES

1. American Physical Therapy Association. *Guide to Physical Therapist Practice.* Alexandria, VA: APTA; 1997.

2. Boyd KT, Peirce NS, Batt ME. Common hip injuries in sport. *Sports Med.* 1997;24(4):273-288.

3. Gerard J, Kleinfeld SL. *Orthopaedic Testing, A Rational Approach to Diagnosis.* New York, NY: Churchill Livingstone; 1993.

4. Gray G. *Lower Extremity Functional Profile.* Adrian, MI: Wynn Marketing; 1995.

5. Gray H; Williams PL, ed. *Gray's Anatomy.* 38th ed. New York, NY: Churchill Livingstone; 1995.

6. Hart A, Hopkins C, Ford B. *ICD-9-CM Expert for Physicians, Volume 1&2.* 7th ed. USA: Ingenix; 2005.

7. Hertling D, Kessler R. *Management of Common Musculoskeletal Disorders: Physical Therapy Principles and Methods.* 3rd ed. Philadelphia, PA: Lippincott-Raven Publishers; 1996.

8. Hoppenfeld S. *Physical Examination of the Spine and Extremities.* New York, NY: Appleton-Century-Crofts; 1976.

9. Jenkins, DB. *Hollinshead's Functional Anatomy of the Limbs and Back.* 6th ed. Philadelphia, PA: WB Saunders; 1991.

10. Jones DL, Erhard RE. Diagnosis of trochanteric bursitis versus femoral neck stress fracture. *Phys Ther.* 1997;77:58-67.

11. Kendall FP, McCreary EK, Provance PG. *Muscles: Testing and Function.* 4th ed. Baltimore, MD: Williams & Wilkins; 1993.

12. Magee DJ. *Orthopedic Physical Assessment.* 3rd ed. Philadelphia, PA: WB Saunders; 1997.

13. Porter-Hoke A. North American Institute of Orthopædic Manual Therapy Course Notes, Level 1 and 2. NAIOMT, Inc.; 1993.

14. Richardson JK, Iglarsh AZ. *Clinical Orthopedic Physical Therapy.* Philadelphia, PA: WB Saunders; 1994.

EXERCISE SEQUENCE
HIP PAIN IN RUNNERS—RETURN TO SPORT

PROGRESSIVE PHASE: HOME PROGRAM

Aerobic Capacity and Endurance

Cycling

- Incorporating appropriate warm-up and cool-down intervals, cardiovascular conditioning may be performed on stationary or regular bicycle as symptoms permit
- Attention to proper bike fit is important, as hip and back pain may result from improper biking biomechanics
- If biking has not been used as a cross-training method in the past, an appropriate base building period is necessary:
  - 3–5 minute warm-up at 70–90 rpm, at 55–65% of age-estimated maximum heart rate
  - 10–15 minutes at 80–90 rpm, at 70–75% of age-estimated maximum heart rate, building this phase at no more than 3–5 minutes per session as symptoms and cardiovascular condition permit
  - 3–5 minute cool-down at 70 rpm, at 55–65% of age-estimated maximum heart rate

Aqua Jogging

- Deep water jogging has been shown to be an effective mode of cross-training for runners, with good specificity of carryover
- Use of a flotation device (Wet Vest®) will enhance the comfort of beginners. As you improve, you can enhance cardiovascular training by jogging without the vest.
- Appropriate warm-up and cool-down intervals should be incorporated, as well as a base building period if this is an unfamiliar activity

Running

- As soon as symptoms permit, a return to running should be initiated
  - This should consist of level ground or treadmill running at first, at a speed that brings the heart rate no higher than 60% of age-estimated maximum

(warm-up pace), for durations that do not exacerbate symptoms (generally less than 15 minutes)
  - As symptoms permit, duration (mileage) should be increased by no more than 10% per week
  - Once a substantial base of mileage has been built with no return of symptoms, the addition of speed-specific training may be incorporated
    - This may consist of "fartlek" (short bursts of acceleration within a longer run) or "tempo" (runs of longer duration at or near race pace), or it may be more regimented intervals using a track and stopwatch
    - For marathoners, the distance covered on any interval may range from 400 m at 10K-race pace to 3–5 miles at marathon race pace
    - For shorter distance runners, the intervals would be relatively shorter. For example, a 10K racer may do intervals of 100–400 m at 5K-race pace and 400 m up to 2 mi at 10K-race pace.
    - Speed-specific intervals should be performed no more than once per week initially and should be pursued cautiously. Total speed-work distance should comprise no more than 10% of total weekly mileage.
  - Additional strengthening may be obtained with the incorporation of hill repeats
    - Specific hill training should be performed no more than twice per week and pursued cautiously
    - Monitoring of heart rate will assist in avoiding excessive speed on the uphill
    - Maintaining proper form on the downhill will reduce risk of impact injuries
  - To avoid overuse injury, periodization of mileage, terrain, interval training, proper footwear, etc., is crucial. For example, the following beginning marathon training schedule demonstrates good periodization of intensity, duration, and terrain and could be adjusted to match your individual capabilities:
    - Sun: 10 mi at 70% of age-estimated max heart rate on rolling trails
    - Mon: 3 mi at 70% of age-estimated max heart rate on flat pavement

- Tues: 6 mi at 70% of age-estimated max heart rate on rolling hills
- Wed: Off, or alternate form of training (e.g., swimming, biking)
- Thur: 5 mi consisting of 1 mi warm-up, 2–3 mi of interval work at 80–85% of age-estimated max heart rate, and 1 mi cool-down (track)
- Fri: 3 mi at 70% of age-estimated max heart rate on flat pavement
- Sat: Off, or alternate form of training

Neuromuscular/Balance/ Proprioceptive Reeducation

- Balance/reach drills

  All exercises: 3–5 sets of 10–15 reaches, observing closely for deterioration of proper form due to fatigue

  - Unilateral stance balancing, reaching one or both arms in various directions to maximum distance, avoiding use of other leg for counterbalance. You may obtain additional challenges by holding a light weight or medicine ball, or by using resistive tubing.
    - Anterior reach: Stimulates hamstrings, soleus, gastrocnemius, and hip/back extensors (depending on height of reach)
    - Posterior overhead reach: Stimulates abdominals
    - Lateral rotational reach: Stimulates hip abductors and lateral trunk stabilizers
  - Unilateral stance balancing, reaching opposite leg in various directions to maximum distance
    - Anterior reach: Stimulates quadriceps, soleus
    - Posterior reach: Stimulates gluteals, quadriceps, hip/back extensors
    - Rotational reach to side: Stimulates gluteals, quadriceps, trunk stabilizers, hip abductors, abdominals

Strengthening

- Open kinetic chain exercise using weight machines, cuff weights, or resistive tubing

  All exercises: 3–5 sets of 15–18 repetitions
  - Hip flexion
  - Hip extension
  - Hip abduction
  - Hip adduction
- Closed-kinetic chain functional exercise using body weight only or additional weight as appropriate

  All exercises: 3–5 sets of 15–18 repetitions, observing for deterioration of proper form due to fatigue
  - Squats
    - Progression from mini squats to deeper squats as symptoms permit, with additional challenges from additional weight
  - Lunges
    - Progressing from straight anterior/posterior and lateral lunges to rotational lunges as appropriate, increasing distance lunged or using additional weight as appropriate
  - Step up/step down
    - Varying step height and direction of step (lateral, anterior, posterior, or rotational) as appropriate, with additional challenges of increasing distance from step or use of additional weight as appropriate

Flexibility

- Flexibility exercises
  - Performed preferably when you are warm, e.g.:
    - After walking at least 3–5 minutes
    - After a warm shower or bath
  - Emphasis should be on proper technique and form
    - Holding stretches for 15–30 seconds
  - Perform 3–5 repetitions of each stretch on both sides on a regular basis, even on days when you're not running
    - Gastrocnemius/soleus
    - Hamstrings
    - Quadriceps
    - Gluteals
    - Psoas

UPPER EXTREMITY INJURY—RETURN TO THROWING

This is intended to be a progression for return to throwing, to be initiated after the subacute phase of rehabilitation has been completed. Following initial assessment and instruction by the physical therapist, the program outlined will be primarily performed independently (at home or in a health club). Periodic assessment by the physical therapist, with incorporation of physician recommendations, will allow progression toward goals/outcomes. The phases within the guideline have been formatted so they can be copied and distributed to the patient as a home program.

CONDITIONS

Individuals not meeting the criteria below should be referred to the appropriate guideline.
- No pain during subacute phase exercise
- No joint swelling
- Full active ROM of the involved extremity
- Muscle performance: 75% of uninvolved extremity
  - Shoulder flexion/extension
  - Shoulder internal/external rotation
  - Elbow flexion/extension
  - Forearm supination/pronation
  - Scapular stabilizer strength

HISTORY

It is assumed that the patient was thoroughly evaluated in the earlier stages of his or her rehabilitation process. However, if this is the patient's initial presentation, conduct a full evaluation in addition to gathering the sport-specific information below.
- History of sports activity
- Competitive level and frequency of participation
- Position played
  - Infield
  - Outfield
  - Pitcher
  - Catcher
- Adaptive equipment
  - Braces
  - Other
    - Glove style
    - Bat preference and grip

PROGRESSION

This guideline has been divided into three phases. Progression from one phase to the next will be determined by the physical therapist based on the individual's mastery of and tolerance for the exercises and skills within the previous phase.

Based on the home program model, the following visits are suggested per phase:
- Phase I: 2 visits
- Phase II: 1–2 visits
- Phase III: 1 visit

PATIENT INSTRUCTION

- The influence of proper biomechanical alignment, adequate flexibility and motor performance of both the upper and lower extremities on the kinematics of the shoulder and elbow joints
- Monitoring the signs of overtraining
  - Attention to soreness/aching/effusion
  - Elevated resting morning heart rate
  - Generalized sense of listlessness or fatigue
- The importance of adequate warm-up through the use of moist heat and light activity prior to vigorous exercise
- The importance of exercising within pain-free limitations
  - For infielders, the maximum distance thrown will be 120 ft
  - For outfielders, the maximum distance thrown will be 200 ft
  - For pitchers, the maximum distance thrown will be 150 ft
- Use of ice after exercise to reduce risk of exacerbating inflammatory processes
- Unless otherwise instructed, all throws should have an arc
- The importance of a well-rounded exercise regime in the rehabilitation process, including cardiovascular conditioning, general strengthening and flexibility, agility and eye-hand coordination drills, and sport-specific strengthening

RETURN TO SPORT | UPPER EXTREMITY INJURY—RETURN TO THROWING   627

GOALS/OUTCOMES

- Patient will be able to resume previous sports activity without exacerbation of symptoms as noted on the visual analog scale
- Patient displays understanding of the sport-specific progression and the risks of overtraining

REFERENCES

1. Blackburn TA, Baker C. *Shoulder arthroscopy and rehabilitation: the technique of throwing.* The Sports Medicine Team Concept 8th Annual Conference; Kona Surf Resort, Kona, HI; December 1-6, 1987.

2. Donatelli R, Wooden M. *Orthopaedic Physical Therapy.* Melbourne, Australia: Churchill Livingstone; 1989.

3. Jobe FW. Painful athletic injuries of the shoulder. *Clin Orthop Rel Res.* 1983;173:117-124.

4. Jobe FW, Tibone J, Perry J, et al. An EMG analysis of the shoulder in throwing and pitching. *Am J Sports Med.* 1983;11(1):3-5.

5. Moseley JB, Jobe FW, Pink M, et al. EMG analysis of the scapular muscles during a shoulder rehabilitation program. *Am J Sports Med.* 1992;20(2):128-134.

6. Reid DC. *Sports Injury Assessment and Rehabilitation.* New York, NY; Churchill Livingstone; 1992.

7. Roy S, Irvin R. *Sports Medicine Prevention, Evaluation, Management and Rehabilitation.* Englewood Cliffs, NJ: Prentice Hall; 1983.

8. Wilk KE, Meister K, Andrews JR. Current concepts in the rehabilitation of the overhead throwing athlete. *Am J Sports Med.* 2002;30(1):136-151.

EXERCISE SEQUENCE
UPPER EXTREMITY INJURY—RETURN TO THROWING

PHASE I: HOME PROGRAM

To be performed daily. Begin each session with proper warm-up and gentle stretching of both upper and lower extremities. Proceed to the next day only if you are pain-free and have no swelling.

Aerobic Conditioning

Due to the intermittent nature of baseball and softball at the amateur level, regular aerobic conditioning is recommended as a supplement to field time to enhance cardiovascular conditioning and exercise endurance. Perform at 60–75% of age-predicted maximum heart rate:

- Walking or intermittent walk/jog on treadmill or outdoors
  - 20–30 minutes duration
- Stair machine
  - Will promote cardiovascular conditioning and may also be used to enhance gluteal and quadriceps motor performance by alternating positions, step height, and speed
  - 15–20 minutes duration
- Upper or lower body ergometer
  - Will promote cardiovascular conditioning as well as endurance
  - 15–20 minutes duration
- Ski machine
  - 15–20 minutes duration

Flexibility

Static stretching of the following muscles should be performed following a warm-up period. Emphasis should be placed on long-duration, low-intensity techniques with use of contract/relax techniques as appropriate. Due to the full-body nature of proper throwing mechanics, lower extremity as well as upper extremity stretching should be emphasized.

- Hamstring
- Gastrocnemius/soleus
- Quadriceps
- Hip internal and external rotators

- Psoas
- Pectorals
- Latissimus
- Wrist flexors and extensors
- Shoulder/scapular stabilizers
- Cervical musculature

Sport-Specific Agility Drills

- Shuttle drills
  - Lateral shuffle steps
    - Use stance appropriate to fielding grounders
    - Work to the right and to the left
  - Forward/backward shuffle steps
    - Use stance appropriate to fielding grounders when going forward
    - Use stance appropriate for fly balls when going backward
  - Diagonal forward/backward running
- Cariocas, right leading and left leading
- Cut and run to the right and to the left

Strengthening

As with any throwing sport, the element of power comes not only from the upper body but is generated in the gluteals, hip abductors, and abdominals. For this reason, lower extremity and abdominal exercises are presented in Phase I and should be continued as needed through the remaining phases.

- Squats progression
  - With body weight only, may be used as a warm-up
  - Light weight
    - 40–55% of one-repetition maximum
    - 15–25 repetitions per set
    - May be used to regain endurance
  - Moderate weight
    - 60–80% of one-repetition maximum
    - 8–12 repetitions per set
    - May be used to regain motor performance

- ○ Plyometric (jump squats)
  - ▪ Very light weights (20% of one-repetition maximum)
  - ▪ May be used to regain explosive power
- • Lunge progression
  - ○ With body weight only, may be used as a warm-up
  - ○ With light to moderate weight, may be used to target specific muscles for strengthening
  - ○ Multidirectional lunges target specific muscles
    - ▪ Anterior lunge: Targets gluteals, hamstrings, and quadriceps
    - ▪ Lateral lunge: Targets hip abductors, adductors as well as gluteals and hamstrings
    - ▪ Rotational lunges: Targets hip rotators as well as abductors, adductors, gluteals, hamstrings, and quadriceps
- • Abdominal progression
  - ○ Open-kinetic chain
    - ▪ Supine crunches
    - ▪ Abdominal bracing with alternate arm and leg lift
  - ○ Closed-kinetic chain functional strengthening. Avoid using nonweight-bearing leg for counterbalance during any of these exercises
    - ▪ Single-leg stand posterior overhead reach
      - a. Use one or both arms, reaching to maximum distance directly posteriorly overhead
      - b. Progress to holding a bat or other light weight for additional resistance
    - ▪ Single-leg stand rotational overhead reach
      - a. Use one or both arms, reaching diagonally posteriorly overhead
      - b. Progress to holding a bat or other light weight for additional resistance
    - ▪ Single-leg stand overhead pull using resistive tubing
      - a. Attach tubing to top of door frame, stand with your back to the door and grasp the tubing overhead
      - b. Pull down and forward as if swinging an ax, while balancing on one leg
      - c. Repeat weight bearing on other leg
- • Upper body progression
  - ○ Free weight exercises
    - ▪ Seated rowing
    - ▪ Incline bench press
    - ▪ Overhead press (use caution in patients with history of anterior dislocation or shoulder impingement, or postoperatively)

- ▪ Therapeutic ball activities using free weights for resistance
  - a. Prone flys
  - b. Prone overhead press
  - c. Prone latissimus pulldowns using resistive tubing
  - d. Supine pull-over using resistive tubing
- ▪ Plyometrics: Medicine ball toss and catch
  - a. One- and two-hand techniques
  - b. Incorporating overhand, underhand, and chest press throwing techniques
  - c. Progress to heavier ball as symptoms permit
- ○ Neuromuscular/balance/proprioceptive reeducation
  - ▪ Body Blade® activities utilizing all planes and positions
  - ▪ Push ups
    - a. Hands and knees position
    - b. Hands and toes position
    - c. Pushing off of therapeutic ball

Sport-Specific Strengthening

Infielders and Outfielders
- • Days 1–3: Toss the ball with no wind-up. Stand with your feet shoulder width apart and face the player you are throwing to. Concentrate on staying on top of the ball.
  - ○ 10 throws, 20 ft (warm-up)
  - ○ 15 throws, 30 ft
  - ○ 10 throws, 20 ft (cool-down)
- • Days 4–6: Toss the ball with no wind-up. Stand sideways to the person you are throwing towards with feet shoulder width apart. Close up and pivot onto your back foot as you throw.
  - ○ 10 throws, 20 ft (warm-up)
  - ○ 10 throws, 30 ft
  - ○ 10 throws, 40 ft
  - ○ 10 throws, 50 ft
  - ○ 10 throws, 30 ft (cool-down)
- • Days 7–9: Repeat position from days 4–6. Follow through with your pivot leg.
  - ○ 10 throws, 50 ft (warm-up)
  - ○ 20 throws, 70 ft
  - ○ 20 throws, 80 ft
  - ○ 20 throws, 60 ft (cool-down)

Pitchers

- Days 1–3: Toss the ball with no wind-up against a wall on alternate days. Start with 25–30 throws, building up to 70 throws, and gradually increase the throwing distance.
  - 20 throws, 20 ft (warm-up)
  - 25–40 throws, 30–40 ft
  - 10 throws, 20 ft (cool-down)
- Days 4–6: Toss the ball (playing catch with easy wind-up) on alternate days.
  - 10 throws, 20 ft (warm-up)
  - 10 throws, 30–40 ft
  - 30–40 throws, 50 ft
  - 10 throws, 60 ft
  - 10 throws, 20–30 ft (cool-down)
- Days 7–9: Continue increasing the throwing distance while still tossing the ball with an easy wind-up.
  - 10 throws, 20 ft (warm-up)
  - 10 throws, 30–40 ft
  - 30–40 throws, 50–60 ft
  - 10 throws, 30 ft (cool-down)

PHASE II: HOME PROGRAM

To be performed daily. Begin each session with proper warm-up and gentle stretching of both upper and lower extremities. Proceed to the next day only if you are pain-free and have no swelling. Aerobic conditioning, strengthening, sport-specific agility drills, and flexibility should be continued as in Phase I.

Sport-Specific Drills

Infielders and Outfielders

- Days 10–12: Assume the pitcher's stance. Lift and stride with your lead leg. Follow through with your pivot leg.
  - 10 throws, 60 ft (warm-up)
  - 20 throws, 70 ft
  - 30 throws, 80 ft
  - 10 throws, 60 ft (cool-down)
- Days 13–15
  - Outfielders: Lead with your glove side foot forward. Take one step, crow hop, and throw the ball.
  - Infielders: Lead with your glove side foot forward. Take a shuffle step, and throw the ball.
    - 15 throws, 70 ft (warm-up)
    - 15 throws, 90 ft

- 30 throws, 100 ft (throw the last five throws in a straight line)
- 15 throws, 80 ft (cool-down)

- Days 16–18: Repeat the throwing technique as in Days 13–15. Assume your playing position. Infielders and catchers do not throw greater than 120 ft Outfielders do not throw farther than 150 ft (mid-outfield).
  - 15 throws, 80 ft (warm-up)
  - 15 throws
    - Infielders 80–90 ft
    - Outfielders 90–100 ft
  - 15 throws
    - Infielders 90–100 ft
    - Outfielders 110–125 ft
  - 15 throws
    - Infielders 110–120 ft
    - Outfielders 130–150 ft
  - 15 throws, 80 ft (cool-down)

Pitchers

- Days 10–12: Increase throwing distance to a maximum of 60 ft. Continue tossing the ball with an occasional throw at no more than half speed.
  - 10 throws, 30 ft (warm-up)
  - 10 throws, 40–45 ft
  - 30–40 throws, 60 ft
  - 10 throws, 30 ft (cool-down)
- Days 13–16: During this phase, gradually increase the distance to 150 ft maximum
  - Day 13
    - 10 throws, 40 ft (warm-up)
    - 10 throws, 50–60 ft
    - 30 throws, 70–80 ft
    - 10 throws, 50–60 ft
    - 10 throws, 40 ft (cool-down)
  - Day 14
    - 10 throws, 40 ft (warm-up)
    - 10 throws, 50–60 ft
    - 20–30 throws, 80–90 ft
    - 20 throws, 50–60 ft
    - 10 throws, 40 ft (cool-down)
  - Day 15
    - 10 throws, 40 ft (warm-up)
    - 10 throws, 60 ft
    - 15–20 throws, 100–110 ft
    - 20 throws, 60 ft
    - 10 throws, 40 ft (cool-down)

○ Day 16
  ▪ 10 throws, 40 ft (warm-up)
  ▪ 10 throws, 60 ft
  ▪ 15–20 throws, 120–150 ft
  ▪ 20 throws, 60 ft
  ▪ 10 throws, 40 ft (cool-down)
• Days 17–20: Progress to throwing off the mound at half to three-quarters speed. Try to use proper body mechanics, especially when throwing off the mound.
  ▪ Stay on top of the ball
  ▪ Keep the elbow up
  ▪ Throw over the top
  ▪ Follow through with the arm and trunk
  ▪ Use the legs to push
○ Day 17
  ▪ 10 throws, 60 ft (warm-up)
  ▪ 10 throws, 120–150 ft (lobbing)
  ▪ 30 throws, 45 ft (off the mound)
  ▪ 10 throws, 60 ft (off the mound)
  ▪ 10 throws, 40 ft (cool-down)
○ Day 18
  ▪ 10 throws, 50 ft (warm-up)
  ▪ 10 throws, 120–150 ft (lobbing)
  ▪ 20 throws, 45 ft (off the mound)
  ▪ 20 throws, 60 ft (off the mound)
  ▪ 10 throws, 40 ft (cool-down)
○ Day 19
  ▪ 10 throws, 50 ft (warm-up)
  ▪ 10 throws, 60 ft
  ▪ 10 throws, 120–150 ft (lobbing)
  ▪ 10 throws, 45 ft (off the mound)
  ▪ 30 throws, 60 ft (off the mound)
  ▪ 10 throws, 40 ft (cool-down)
○ Day 20
  ▪ 10 throws, 50 ft (warm-up)
  ▪ 10 throws, 120–150 ft (lobbing)
  ▪ 10 throws, 45 ft (off the mound)
  ▪ 40–50 throws, 60 ft (off the mound)
  ▪ 10 throws, 40 ft (cool-down)

PHASE III: HOME PROGRAM

To be performed daily. Begin each session with proper warm-up and gentle stretching of both upper and lower extremities. Proceed to the next day only if pain-free and no swelling. Aerobic conditioning, strengthening, sport-specific agility drills, and flexibility should be continued as in Phase I.

Sport-Specific Strengthening

Infielders and Outfielders

• Days 19–21: Infielders, catchers, and outfielders may all assume their playing position
  ○ 15 throws, 80 ft (warm-up)
  ○ 15 throws
  ○ Infielders 80–90 ft
  ○ Outfielders 90–100 ft
  ○ 15 throws
    ▪ Infielders 90–100 ft
    ▪ Outfielders 110–120 ft
  ○ 15 throws
    ▪ Infielders 110–120 ft
    ▪ Outfielders 130–150 ft
  ○ 15 throws, 80 ft (cool-down)
• Days 22–24: Repeat exercises as in Days 19–21. Use a fungo bat to hit to the infielders and outfielders while in their normal playing position.

Pitchers

At this time, if the pitcher has successfully completed Phase II without pain or discomfort and is throwing approximately three-quarters speed, the pitching coach may allow the pitcher to proceed to Phase III, "Up/Down Bullpens." This drill is used to simulate a game situation. The pitcher rests in between a series of pitches to reproduce the rest period between innings.

• Days 21–25: "Up/Down Bullpens": (half to three-quarters speed)
  ○ Day 21
    ▪ 10 warm-up throws, 120–150 ft (lobbing)
    ▪ 10 warm-up throws, 60 ft (off the mound)
    ▪ 40 pitches, 60 ft (off the mound)
    ▪ Rest 10 minutes
    ▪ 20 pitches, 60 ft (off the mound)
  ○ Day 22
    ▪ Off
  ○ Day 23
    ▪ 10 warm-up throws, 120–150 ft (lobbing)
    ▪ 10 warm-up throws, 60 ft (off the mound)
    ▪ 30 pitches, 60 ft (off the mound)
    ▪ Rest 10 minutes
    ▪ 10 warm-up throws, 60 ft (off the mound)
    ▪ 20 pitches, 60 ft (off the mound)
    ▪ Rest 10 minutes
    ▪ 10 warm-up throws, 60 ft (off the mound)
    ▪ 20 pitches, 60 ft (off the mound)

- Day 24
  - Off
- Day 25
  - 10 warm-up throws, 120–150 ft (lobbing)
  - 10 warm-up throws, 60 ft (off the mound)
  - 30 pitches, 60 ft (off the mound)
  - Rest 8 minutes
  - 20 pitches, 60 ft (off the mound)
  - Rest 8 minutes
  - 20 pitches, 60 ft (off the mound)
  - Rest 8 minutes
  - 20 pitches, 60 ft (off the mound)

At this point the pitcher is ready to begin a normal routine, from throwing batting practice to pitching in the bullpen. This program can and should be adjusted as needed by the physical therapist. Each phase may take longer or shorter time than listed, and the program should be monitored by your athletic trainer, physical therapist, and physician. Keep in mind that you must work hard but not overdo it.

WALKING PROGRAM—WALKING FOR THE HEALTH OF IT

ICD-9
There will be a wide variety of ICD-9 codes for which a walking program to enhance fitness may be appropriate.

This guideline is for returning to active sports participation and is appropriate after the subacute phase of rehabilitation has been completed. Following initial assessment and instruction by the physical therapist, the program outlined will be primarily performed independently (at home or in a health club). Periodic assessment by the physical therapist, with the incorporation of physician recommendations, will allow progression toward goals. The guideline has been formatted so that it can be copied and distributed to the patient as a home program.

CONDITIONS

Individuals not meeting the following criteria should be directed to the appropriate guideline for further assessment or treatment.
- Lower extremity functional ROM:
  - Hip: 0–100°
  - Knee: 5–100°
  - Ankle: 8° dorsiflexion, 40° plantarflexion
- Absence of cardiovascular or other medical conditions that may be contraindications to exercise for fitness
- Any structural biomechanical aspects that may contribute to overuse injuries have been addressed, including the use of orthotics or special footwear as appropriate
- Pain-free gait pattern without assistive devices

EVALUATION

It is assumed that the patient was thoroughly evaluated in the earlier stages of his or her rehabilitation process. However, if this is the patient's initial presentation, conduct a full evaluation in addition to gathering the sport-specific information below.
- Previous walking history
  - Mileage
  - Pace
  - Shoe style
  - Terrain
  - Recent racing history
- Cross-training preferences
- Previous lower quarter injuries/surgeries

PROGRESSION

On the basis of the home program model, 1–3 visits are suggested. However, the guideline can be adapted to the clinical setting and the visits adjusted according to the physician/physical therapist recommendations.

PATIENT INSTRUCTION

- Instruct patient in self-monitoring of heart rate
- Instruct patient in self-monitoring of perceived exertion
- Instruct patient in proper training protocol per the patient's individual fitness level
- Instruct patient in monitoring the signs of overtraining:
  - Elevated resting morning heart rate
  - General sense of listlessness or fatigue
  - Soreness/aching/effusion
- Instruct patient regarding the importance of each segment of training, including aerobic conditioning, flexibility, strengthening, and neuromuscular/balance/proprioceptive reeducation in the overall scheme of returning to full fitness

GOALS/OUTCOMES

- Patient will be able to monitor his or her own heart rate
- Patient will be able to pursue the walking program without exacerbation of symptoms
- Patient displays a good understanding of the walking program progression and the risks of either overtraining or returning to a sedentary lifestyle

RETURN TO SPORT | WALKING PROGRAM—WALKING FOR THE HEALTH OF IT   635

REFERENCES

1. American College of Sports Medicine. *Guidelines for Exercise Testing and Prescription.* 3rd ed. Lea & Febiger; 1986.

2. Gray G. *Lower Extremity Functional Profile.* Adrian, MI: Wynn Marketing; 1995.

3. Lee IM, Paffenbarger RS Jr. Physical activity and its relation to cancer risk: a prospective study of college alumni. *Med Sci Sports Exerc.* 1994;26:831-837.

4. Morris JN. Exercise in the prevention of coronary heart disease: today's best buy in public health. *Med Sci Sports Exerc.* 1994;26:807-814.

5. Paffenbarger RS Jr, Kampert JB, Lee IM, Hyde RT, Leung RW, Wing AL. Changes in physical activity and other lifeway patterns influencing longevity. *Med Sci Sports Exerc.* 1994;26:857-865.

6. Powell KE, Blair SN. The public health burdens of sedentary living habits: theoretical but realistic estimates. *Med Sci Sports Exerc.* 1994;26:844-850.

7. Wood PD. Physical activity, diet and health: independent and interactive effects. *Med Sci Sports Exerc.* 1994;26:838-843.

WALKING FOR THE HEALTH OF IT

PATIENT INFORMATION SHEET

For most of us, walking is perhaps one of the most natural forms of exercise we can do. It requires a minimum of equipment and no special facility. There are no membership dues to pay. In spite of this great simplicity, it remains one of the most popular and effective forms of exercise. Walking for fitness can easily become one part of your journey toward better health. In addition to the exercises your therapist has taught you, a regular program of walking can enhance the body's natural ability to recover from injury by promoting circulation and strengthening the muscles. Walking has also been shown to help control high blood pressure and high blood cholesterol, strengthen the heart muscle, improve lung capacity, promote better posture, and stimulate factors within the immune system. With all these benefits in mind, let's get started!

In order to minimize the risk of injury, it is a good idea to start slowly. At first, you will do less than you think you can, to ensure that you don't overdo it. Your therapist will help you determine how much walking is appropriate for you, but a general rule of thumb, when you're recovering from an injury is to start with 7–10 minutes of slow walking on level ground and to increase that duration by no more than 20–30% per week. To monitor your level of effort, you will use one of two methods: heart rate monitoring or the "talk test." Your therapist will help you determine which method is appropriate for you.

The "talk test" is the easiest method for determining your level of effort. When you first start out on your walk, you should be able to carry on a continuous conversation and even be able to sing without difficulty in breathing (this is considered warming up). After a few minutes you will speed up a little, to a level where you can still talk comfortably but would find singing a real challenge. If at any point during your walk you find talking difficult, or you feel "out of breath," you are walking too fast for your current fitness level and you should slow down.

Monitoring your heart rate may seem awkward at first, but it is a reliable method for determining your level of effort. To take your pulse, place the first and second fingers of one hand on the wrist of the other hand (palm side up) at the base of the thumb where it joins the wrist. While pressing lightly, count the number of pulses you feel with your fingertips in a 15-second period. Multiply this number by four and you have your heart rate in beats per minute. There are two formulas you can use to determine what your working heart rate should be. The first one is for beginners and those recovering from injuries. The second is for individuals who have recently been on a regular exercise program or who are ready for a bit more of a challenge.

- Method 1:
  - 220 - Age = Maximum Heart Rate
  - Maximum Heart Rate x .60 = Training Heart Rate (60% of maximum)
  - For example, a 30-year old individual would train at a heart rate of 114 beats per minute, to work at 60% of maximum capacity.
        220 - 30 = 190   190 x .60 = 114

- Method 2:
  - 220 - Age = Maximum Heart Rate
  - (Maximum Heart Rate - Resting Heart Rate) x .60 + Resting Heart Rate = Training Heart Rate
  - For example, using this method, a 30–year old individual with a resting heart rate of 72 would train at a heart rate of 143 beats per minute to work at 60% of maximum capacity.
        220 - 30 = 190   190 - 72= 118
        118 x .60 = 71   71 + 72 = 143
  (Although the second method is somewhat harder to calculate, it has been shown to be a more accurate

RETURN TO SPORT | PATIENT INFORMATION SHEET—WALKING FOR THE HEALTH OF IT   637 estimate of the proper training heart rate; the first method tends to underestimate the effort level slightly.)

Building your endurance takes time. If you started with a 7–10 minute walk and increased your duration 25% per week, your training profile would look something like this:

- Week 1: Walk an average of 7–10 minutes (1–3 times per day)
- Week 2: Walk an average of 9–12 minutes (1–3 times per day)
- Week 3: Walk an average of 12–15 minutes (1–3 times per day)
- Week 4: Walk an average of 15–19 minutes per day
- Week 5: Walk an average of 19–24 minutes per day

Your therapist may determine that you are ready to start with more than a 7–10 minute walk, but don't jump the gun without discussing it with your therapist first. Many a walking program has been short-lived because of injuries that occurred from doing too much too soon. *Remember, increase your duration by no more than 25–30% per week.*

Training smart will help you avoid injuries over the long haul. Don't walk the same distance or duration every day. Take a "hard/easy" approach for best results. By giving your body "rest" days, you promote tissue healing and growth. Rest days are not necessarily days of inactivity. They can be days when the duration of your walk is somewhat less than usual or your pace is somewhat slower. These rest days are alternated with days when you walk your normal duration. For example, a typical week might look like this:

Sun	**Mon**	**Tues**	**Wed**	**Thurs**	**Fri**	**Sat**
40 min	20 min	30 min	off	40 min	20 min	off

The only equipment you'll need is a good pair of walking or running shoes. Your therapist may make specific recommendations for shoes, but some general guidelines may be helpful. Look for a lace-up shoe with a firm heel counter (the part that wraps around your heel) and plenty of room in the toe box. You should have at least ¼-½" of space between the end of your longest toe and the end of the toe box. You should replace your shoes every 6–9 months to ensure that the cushioning and support of the shoe are not compromised.

Now it's up to you. Remember that every journey starts with a single step. Take that first step now toward better health and you'll be glad you did in the days to come.

ACTIVITY QUESTIONNAIRE FOR RUNNERS/WALKERS

PATIENT INFORMATION SHEET

This questionnaire is designed to help your therapist determine training patterns and other things that may have been significant in the onset of your symptoms. Please take the time to answer the questions fully, and feel free to discuss these items with your therapist during your evaluation.

NAME:_____

Activities

- ❏ Running_____miles/week ❏ Cycling_____miles/week
- ❏ Golf_____holes/week ❏ Hiking_____miles/week
- ❏ Walking_____miles/week ❏ Swimming_____hours/week
- ❏ Other_____

- Please indicate the number of days per week you train on the following types of terrain:

  Treadmill_____ Indoor track_____

  Asphalt_____ Concrete_____ Running track_____ Trails_____

- What kind of running/walking shoes are you using?_____
  - How old are your running/walking shoes?____months or _____miles
- Please describe a typical training week, including miles per day, pace per mile (if known), terrain, as well as other types of exercise used as cross-training.
  - Sunday_____
  - Monday_____
  - Tuesday_____
  - Wednesday_____
  - Thursday_____
  - Friday_____
  - Saturday_____
- Are you currently training for a specific event? ❏ Yes ❏ No
  - Please specify (5K, 10K, marathon, triathlon, etc.)_____
- Have you experienced injuries in the past which caused you to cease training for a period of more than one week? ❏ Yes ❏ No
  - Please explain_____
- Do you currently participate in a consistent stretching program? ❏ Yes ❏ No
- Do you currently wear custom-molded orthotics? ❏ Yes ❏ No
  - How old are they?_____
  - Who prescribed/fitted them for you?_____
  - Do you wear them for all activities?_____
  - Were they prescribed for this injury?_____

RETURN TO SPORT | PATIENT INFORMATION SHEET—ACTIVITY QUESTIONNAIRE FOR RUNNERS/WALKERS **639**

General Medicine

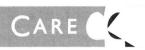

GENERAL MEDICINE

Amputations	643
Time of Fitting the Prosthesis	649
Arthritis	653
Geriatric Rehabilitation	659
Muscle Weakness—General	663
Vestibular Rehabilitation	667
Wound Management	673

642   GENERAL MEDICINE

AMPUTATIONS
SUMMARY OVERVIEW

ICD-9

250	353.6	755.2	755.3	885	886	887	895	896
897	997.6							

APTA Preferred Practice Pattern: **4K, 7A, 7E**

EXAMINATION

- History and Systems Review
- Tests and Measures
  Systems review per APTA's *Guide to Physical Therapy Practice*
  - Anthropometric characteristics
  - Gait, locomotion, and balance
  - Integumentary integrity
  - Muscle performance
  - Pain
  - Posture
  - Prosthetic requirements
  - ROM
  - Self care and home management
  - Sensory integrity
- Establish Plan of Care

GOALS/OUTCOMES

- ROM: Within normal limits for residual limb
- Strength: 4/5 for residual limb
- Independence in bed mobility and transfers, with wheelchair if necessary
- Independence in proper wound/limb care
- Independence in functional activity, with or without assistive device
- Independence with application of prosthetic device
- Wound closed, without complications
- Pain: Less than 5/10

INTERVENTION
NUMBER OF VISITS: 20–48

- Patient Instruction
  - Basic Anatomy and Biomechanics
  - Handouts
  - Functional Considerations
  - Description of Surgical Procedure

- Direct Interventions
  - Lower-Extremity Amputations, Acute Phase: 5–15 Visits, 1–2 Weeks Post-Amputation
  - Lower-Extremity Amputations, Subacute Phase: 5–18 Visits, 2 Weeks Post-Amputation. If Prosthetic Candidate, 10–15 Additional Visits.
  - Upper-Extremity Amputations, Acute Phase: 5–15 Visits, 1–2 Weeks Post-Amputation
  - Upper-Extremity Amputations, Subacute Phase: 5–18 Visits, 2 Weeks Post-Amputation. If Prosthetic Candidate, 10–15 Visits.

DISCHARGE PLANNING AND PATIENT RESPONSIBILITY

- Criteria for Discharge
  - Patient demonstrates proper application of compression device and understanding of times of application
  - Patient demonstrates ability to don and doff prosthesis and understands precautions
  - Patient has achieved independence with prosthetic device
  - Patient is independent with ADLs
  - Patient is independent with home exercise program
- Circumstances Requiring Additional Visits
  - Comorbidity
  - Obesity
  - Cognitive dysfunction
  - Circulatory condition
  - Condition of contralateral extremity
  - Wound healing
- Home Program
  - Stretching exercises for maintenance of ROM
  - Conditioning program
  - Daily limb hygiene for skin integrity
- Monitoring

SUMMARY OVERVIEW | GENERAL MEDICINE | AMPUTATIONS **643**

AMPUTATIONS

ICD-9

250	Diabetes mellitus
353.6	Phantom limb (syndrome)
755.2	Congenital reduction deformities of upper limb
755.3	Congenital reduction deformities of lower limb
885	Traumatic amputation of thumb (complete) (partial)
886	Traumatic amputation of other finger(s) (complete) (partial)
887	Traumatic amputation of arm and hand (complete) (partial)
895	Traumatic amputation of toe(s) (complete) (partial)
896	Traumatic amputation of foot (complete) (partial)
897	Traumatic amputation of leg(s) (complete) (partial)
997.6	Amputation stump complication

APTA Preferred Practice Pattern: 4K, 7A, 7E

EXAMINATION

History and Systems Review

- History of current condition
  - Date of amputation
  - Type of amputation
  - Reason for amputation
- Past medical/surgical history
- Medications
- Functional status and activity level (current/prior)
- Living environment
  - Stairs/barriers
  - Support system
- Occupation/employment
- Psychosocial
  - Support system
  - Caregiver resources
- Health status
  - Cognitive status
  - Physical function
  - Prosthetic candidate
  - Signs and symptoms of depression
- Patient's functional goals

Tests and Measures

Systems review per APTA's *Guide to Physical Therapy Practice*
- Anthropometric characteristics
  - Residual limb
    - Length
      a. Below-the-knee amputation: Medial tibial plateau to end of tibia

b. Above-the-knee amputation: Ischial tuberosity to end of femur
c. Below-the-elbow amputation: Lateral epicondyle to end of residual limb
  - Circumference
    a. Measure by marking limb every two inches
  - Note what activities increase edema in limb
  - Shape of end of residual limb (cylindrical, conical, bulbous)
  - Abnormalities in shape (such as "dog ears")
  - Soft-tissue appearance
- Gait, locomotion, and balance
  - Static and dynamic sitting/standing balance: Eyes open/eyes closed
  - Wheelchair mobility
  - Gait analysis, with or without prosthesis
    - Parallel bars vs. assistive device
    - Weight-bearing ability
    - Stride length and weight shifting
- Integumentary integrity
  - Incision assessment for drainage, odor, size, color
  - Trophic changes (shiny skin, skin texture, nail beds)
  - Assessment of residual limb temperature compared to other extremities
  - Pulses (upper extremity: Brachial, i.e., femoral, popliteal, dorsal pedis)
- Muscle performance
  - Residual limb (be specific with remaining muscle groups without increasing pain)
  - General strength, extremities, trunk
  - Trunk stability

644   AMPUTATIONS | GENERAL MEDICINE

- Pain
  - Measured on visual analog scale
- Posture
  - Standing, focus on extension
- Prosthetic requirements
  - Assess patient's ability to don and doff prosthesis
  - Adherence to wearing schedule
  - Ability to care for residual limb and prosthesis
  - Ability to learn and retain new information
  - Motivation
- ROM
  - Functional ROM
  - ROM with goniometer, especially with affected limb
    - Note contractures
- Self care and home management
  - Bed mobility
  - Transfers
  - Safety awareness
  - Dressing
  - ADLs
- Sensory integrity
  - Tactile sensibility (hyper/hypoesthesia)
  - Position sense
  - Color of residual limb
  - Temperature (hot vs. cold)
  - Phantom pain or sensation
    - Continuous or intermittent
    - Local or diffuse
    - Burning, squeezing, shooting, or cramping
  - Neuromas

Establish Plan of Care
- Based on history, tests, and measures

GOALS/OUTCOMES
- ROM: Within normal limits for residual limb
- Strength: 4/5 for residual limb
- Independence in bed mobility and transfers, with wheelchair if necessary
- Independence in proper wound/limb care
- Independence in functional activity, with or without assistive device
- Independence with application of prosthetic device
- Wound closed, without complications
- Pain: Less than 5/10

INTERVENTION
NUMBER OF VISITS: 20–48

Coordination, Communication, and Documentation
- Provision of services between admission and discharge that facilitate cost-effective and efficient integration or reintegration to home, community, or work
- Documentation of therapeutic intervention is required for each episode of care and serves as the basic foundation for communication
- Coordination and additional communication will depend on the patient's impairment and home/work/community/leisure situation and requirements. Such services may include:
  - Case management
  - Coordination of care and collaboration with those integral to the patient's rehabilitation program
  - Coordination and monitoring of the delivery of available resources
  - Referrals to other health-care professionals
  - Identification of resources, support groups, or advocacy services
  - Provision of educational or training information
  - Technical assistance
- Specific coordination and communication provisions:
  - Dietician
  - Vocational counselor
  - Social worker/case manager
  - Occupational therapy
  - Recreational therapy
  - Prosthetist

Patient Instruction

Basic Anatomy and Biomechanics
- Pertinent Gray's Anatomy of involved musculature and joint
- Education on peripheral vascular disease

Handouts
- Gaily & Gaily, *Prosthetic Gait Training Program for LE Amputees*, PO Box 561533, Miami, FL 33256
- "DO NOT" pictures for lower extremity amputees
- Proper wrapping of residual limb
- Specific home program

Functional Considerations

- Review of proper hygiene and skin care
- Review of proper bandaging, wrapping
- Re-instruct in desensitization techniques
- Check-out home environment for safety, adaptations
- Review of proper shoe fit

Description of Surgical Procedure

- Review of operative procedure and relation to joint biomechanics, rehabilitation, and function

Direct Interventions

Lower-Extremity Amputations, Acute Phase: 5–15 Visits, 1–2 Weeks Post-Amputation

The focus is on wound healing, residual limb care, and general physical conditioning. See *Wound Management* guideline. If a patient is a prosthetic candidate, another 10–15 visits are expected.

- Therapeutic exercise and home program
  - Positioning
    - To avoid contractures
    - Prone position
    - Avoid prolonged sitting
    - Posterior splint in wheelchair for knee extension
    - Avoid elevation of residual limb
  - ROM
    - Residual limb: Active and active/assisted ROM
    - Stretching exercises to all muscle groups that are being strengthened
      a. Contract/relax
      b. Focus on hip flexors, hamstrings
    - Deep breathing and coughing: Instruct patient in proper limb position
  - Strengthening
    - Resistive exercise to uninvolved limbs, such as pull-ups using trapeze, press-ups in wheelchair, and resistive band exercises
    - Isometric knee flexion: Hamstrings for below-the-knee amputation
    - Straight-leg raises
    - Hip flexion with knee flexion
    - Knee flexion and extension
    - Hip abduction
    - Hip extension with knee extension and flexion
    - Quadriceps sets
    - Bridging
    - Gluteal sets

  - Breathing exercise
- Functional training
  - Bed mobility
    - Transfer training
  - Gait training with appropriate devices
    - Wheelchair mobility
- Manual therapy
  - Joint mobilization
  - Passive ROM to decrease contracture
- Electrotherapeutic modalities
  - TENS for phantom pain and neuroma
- Physical agents and mechanical modalities
  - To decrease pain or promote healing
  - Ultrasound
  - Whirlpool
  - Intermittent pressure device
- Goals/outcomes
  - Minimum assistance level with mobility, transfers
  - Proper breathing techniques
  - Decreased limb edema
  - Promote wound healing
  - Prevent contractures/maintain ROM
  - Control pain
  - Maintain/increase strength

Lower-Extremity Amputations, Subacute Phase: 5–18 Visits, 2 Weeks Post-Amputation. If Prosthetic Candidate, 10–15 Additional Visits.

Treatment focus, frequency, and duration will depend on the patient's qualification as a prosthetic candidate. This may not be decided for several months postoperatively. If the patient is not a candidate, the focus is on functional independence.

- Therapeutic exercises
  - Continue exercises as in acute phase
  - Progressive resistive exercises and proprioceptive neuromuscular facilitation
- Functional training
  - Residual limb hygiene
  - Bed mobility
  - Transfer training
  - Gait training
    - Pre-gait training for balance
    - Weight shifts
    - Use of parallel bars
    - Temporary fitting of prosthesis
    - Gait analysis with prosthesis

- Prosthetic training
  - Pre-gait training exercises
- Manual therapy
  - ROM to residual limb to prevent and/or decrease contractures
  - Massage, taping, stroking for limb desensitization once sutures are out and incision is healed
- Therapeutic devices and equipment
  - Appropriate assistive devices
  - Prosthetic fitting
- Electrotherapeutic modalities
  - As needed for pain management
- Physical agents
  - Continue use as needed
- Goals/outcomes
  - Good limb integrity
  - ROM of residual limb at mean within functional limits
  - Maintain shape of limb
  - Independence in ADLs
  - Independence in donning/doffing of prosthesis if appropriate

Upper-Extremity Amputations, Acute Phase: 5–15 Visits, 1–2 Weeks Post-Amputation

The focus is on wound healing, residual limb care, and general physical conditioning. See *Wound Management* guideline.

- Therapeutic exercise
  - Concentrate on muscles that perform above movements
  - Resisted exercise to uninvolved extremities
  - Isometric exercise: Wrist flexors and extensors, biceps and triceps
- Manual therapy
  - Massage therapy
  - Passive ROM focusing on:
    - Scapular abduction, shoulder depression, shoulder extension, shoulder abduction, shoulder flexion, elbow flexion, elbow extension, forearm supination/pronation, chest expansion
- Electrotherapeutic modalities
  - TENS for phantom pain and neuroma
- Physical agents
  - Ultrasound: Prescription for neuroma
  - Chemical blocks (lidocaine or mepivacaine) for treatment of reflex sympathetic dystrophy

- Goals and outcomes
  - Promote wound healing
  - Control incisional and phantom pain
  - Maintain ROM
  - Maximize physical conditioning

Upper-Extremity Amputations, Subacute Phase: 5–18 Visits, 2 Weeks Post-Amputation. If Prosthetic Candidate, 10–15 Visits.

The focus is on wound healing, residual limb care maximizing function, and general physical conditioning. See *Wound Management* guideline.

- Therapeutic exercises and home program
  - Progressive resistive exercises and proprioceptive neuromuscular facilitation
  - Isometric exercise to increase supinators and pronators muscle bulk
- Functional training
  - Proper washing of residual limb
  - Bed mobility
  - Transfer training
  - Gait training
  - Prosthetic training
- Manual therapy
  - Massage, taping, and stroking for limb desensitization (once sutures are out and incision is healed)
  - ROM: As in acute phase
  - Soft-tissue mobilization to reduce adhesions
- Therapeutic devices and equipment
  - Compression types to reduce edema and shape
    - Elastic bandage
    - Intermittent positive pressure
    - Tubular elastic bandage
  - Appropriate assistive devices
  - Prosthetic fitting
- Goals/outcomes
  - Desensitization of residual limb
  - Maintenance of ROM of residual limb
  - Maintain shape of limb
  - Proper hygiene
  - Independence with prosthetic donning and doffing
  - Independence with ADLs

GENERAL MEDICINE | AMPUTATIONS   647

DISCHARGE PLANNING AND PATIENT RESPONSIBILITY

Criteria for Discharge
- Patient demonstrates proper application of compression device and understanding of times of application
- Patient demonstrates ability to don and doff prosthesis and understands precautions
- Patient has achieved independence with prosthetic device
- Patient is independent with ADLs
- Patient is independent with home exercise program

Circumstances Requiring Additional Visits
- Comorbidity
- Obesity
- Cognitive dysfunction
- Circulatory condition
- Condition of contralateral extremity
- Wound healing

Home Program
- Stretching exercises for maintenance of ROM
- Conditioning program
- Daily limb hygiene for skin integrity

Monitoring
- Instruct patient to contact physician if excessive swelling occurs or if drainage from incision is noted
- Contact physical therapist or prosthetist if prosthesis is not fitting properly
- Arrange follow-up visits with physical therapist and prosthetist if prosthesis not fitting or functioning properly

REFERENCES

1. American Physical Therapy Association. *Guide to Physical Therapist Practice.* Alexandria, VA: APTA; 1997.
2. Gray H; Williams PL, ed. *Gray's Anatomy.* 38th ed. New York, NY: Churchill Livingstone; 1995.
3. Hart A, Hopkins C, Ford B. *ICD-9-CM Expert for Physicians, Volume 1&2.* 7th ed. USA: Ingenix. 2005.
4. Ikuma L, Gardella M, Yost L, et al. *Above Knee Amputations.* (Unpublished paper).
5. Kathrins RJ. Lower extremity amputations. In: Logigian MK, ed. *Adult Rehabilitation: A Team Approach for Therapists.* Boston, MA: Little Brown & Co; 1982:82-89.
6. Kulkarni J. Falls in patients with lower limb amputations: prevalence and contributing factors. *Physiotherapy.* 1996;82(2):130-135.
7. Kunrar VN. Stump complications and management. In: Banerjee SN, ed. *Rehabilitation Management of Amputees.* Baltimore, MD: Williams & Wilkins; 1982:372-390.
8. Mensch G, Ellis P. Physical therapeutic management for lower extremity amputees. In: Banerjee SN, ed. *Rehabilitation Management of Amputees.* Baltimore, MD: Williams & Wilkins; 1982:162-236.
9. O'Sullivan B, Schmitz T. *Physical Rehabilitation and Treatment.* Philadelphia, PA: FA Davis; 1994.
10. Shurr DG, Cook TM. *Prosthetics and Orthotics.* Norwalk, CT: Appleton & Lange. 1990:151-171.
11. Brooks D, Hunter JP, Parsons J, et al. Reliability of the two-minute walk test in individuals with transtibial amputation. *Arch Phys Med Rehabil.* November 2002;83(11):1562-1565.
12. Devlin M, Sinclair L, Colman D, et al. Patient preference and gait efficiency in geriatric population with transfemoral amputation using a free-swinging versus a locked prosthetic knee joint. *Arch Phys Med Rehabil.* Feb. 2002;83(2):246-249.
13. Tsai HA, Kirby RL, MacLeod DA, Graham MM. Aided gait of people with lower-limb amputations: comparison of 4-footed and 2-wheeled walkers. *Arch Phys Med Rehabil.* 2003;84(4):584-591.
14. Esquenazi A, DiGiacomo R. Rehabilitation after amputation. *J Am Podiatric Med Assoc.* 2001;91(1):13-22.

TIME OF FITTING THE PROSTHESIS

In general, the earlier a prosthesis is fitted, the better it is for the amputee. One of the most difficult problems facing the amputee and the treatment team is edema, or swelling of the stump, owing to the accumulation of fluids. Edema will be present to some extent in all cases, and it makes fitting of the prosthesis difficult, but certain measures can be taken to reduce the amount of edema.

The use of a rigid dressing seems to control edema. After the rigid dressing has been removed and when a prosthesis is not being worn, elastic bandages are used to keep edema from developing.

The patient is taught the proper technique for bandaging and is generally expected to do this for him or herself as detailed below.

For the average adult, one or two elastic bandages 6" wide are used. During application, the bandages should be stretched almost to the limit of the elastic, and the greatest tension should be around the end of the stump.
The stump should be bandaged constantly, but the bandage should be changed every 4 or 6 hours. It must never be kept in place for more than 12 hours without rebandaging. *If throbbing should occur, remove the bandage and rewrap.* Special elastic "shrinker" socks are available for use instead of elastic bandages, and while not considered by some to be as effective as a properly applied elastic bandage, a "shrinker" sock is better than a poorly applied elastic bandage. Whether elastic bandage or shrinker sock is used, *it should be removed at least 3 times daily and the stump should be massaged vigorously for 10–15 minutes. The bandage or sock must be reapplied immediately after the massage.*

WRAPPING TECHNIQUE FOR BELOW-THE-KNEE AMPUTATION

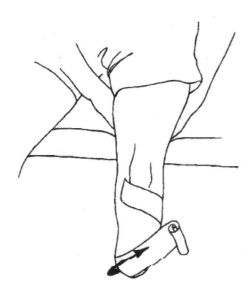

All turns should be on the diagonal. Never use horizontal turns, as they tend to constrict circulation.

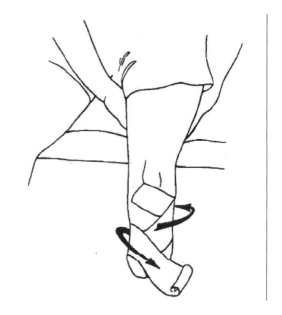

Do not encircle the end of the residual limb with one turn, as this tends to cause skin creases in the scar. Alternatively cover the inside and outside of the end in successive turns.

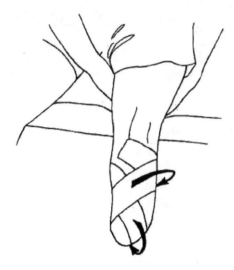

Continue making diagonal turns, exerting firm pressure over the distal end of the residual limb.

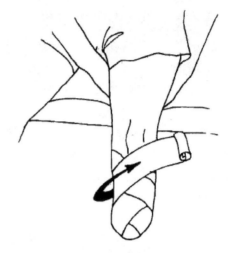

Bandage pressure should become lighter as you continue to wrap proximally.

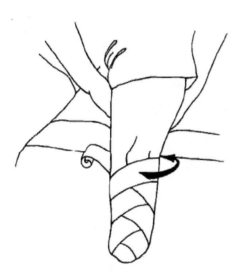

Extend the wrap above the knee. There should be at least one turn above the kneecap.

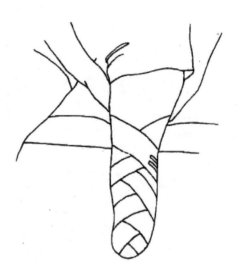

Return to below the knee. If there is bandage remaining, finish the bandage with diagonal turns over the end of the residual limb. Anchor the bandage with tape. Do not use safety pins. Rewrap the residual limb every 3–4 hours or more often if necessary.

Source: Reprinted from L.A. Karacoloff, C.S. Hammersley, and F.J. Schneider, *Lower Extremity Amputation: A Guide to Functional Outcomes in Physical Therapy Management*, pp. 16–18, © 1992, Aspen Publishers, Inc.

WRAPPING TECHNIQUES FOR ABOVE THE KNEE AMPUTATION

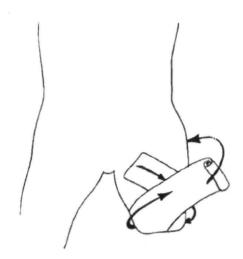

Start with the bandage in the groin area. Roll toward the outside, then behind and around the residual limb, covering the medial thigh. Be certain to keep the bandage smooth. Avoid wrinkles, as they may cause skin irritation.

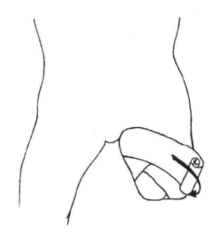

Roll around the posterior residual limb. Continue down and around the lateral half of the distal end.

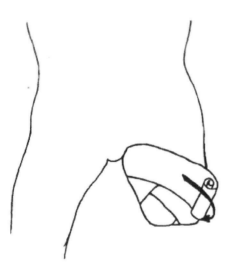

Continue making diagonal turns around the residual limb until all skin is covered with at least two layers of bandage and firm pressure is obtained over the end. Avoid encircling the end with one turn, as this tends to cause skin creases in the scar. Never use circular turns, as this constricts circulation. Pressure should be greatest at the end, becoming lighter as you wrap toward the hip. Include all soft tissue on the medial thigh at the groin

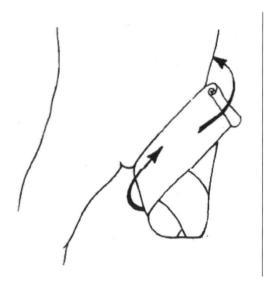

Begin the hip spica as shown here. The bandage should be placed as high as possible on the medial thigh and then crossed over the hip joint.

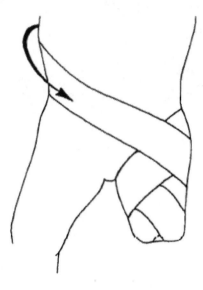 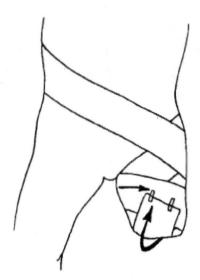

Carry the bandage behind and around the pelvis, crossing just below the waist on the sound side. Returning to the amputated side, cross over the hip joint again.

Finish the bandage by making diagonal turns around the end of the residual limb. Anchor the bandage with tape. Do not use safety pins. The bandage should not cause pain. If so, remove the bandage and rewrap. Rewrap the residual limb every 3–4 hours or more often if necessary.

Source: Reprinted from L.A. Karacoloff, C.S. Hammersley, and F.J. Schneider, *Lower Extremity Amputation: A Guide to Functional Outcomes in Physical Therapy Management*, pp. 16–18, © 1992, Aspen Publishers, Inc.

ARTHRITIS
SUMMARY OVERVIEW

ICD-9

714   715

APTA Preferred Practice Pattern: **4A, 4B, 4C, 4D, 4F, 4G, 4H, 4I, 4J, 6B**

EXAMINATION

- History and Systems Review
- Tests and Measures
  Systems review per APTA's *Guide to Physical Therapy Practice*
  - Aerobic capacity and endurance
  - Anthropometric characteristics
  - Arousal, attention, and cognition
  - Assistive and adaptive devices
  - Environmental, home, and work barriers
  - Ergonomics and body mechanics
  - Gait, locomotion, and balance
  - Integumentary integrity
  - Joint integrity and mobility
  - Motor function
  - Muscle performance
  - Orthotic, protective, and support devices
  - Postural assessment
  - ROM
  - Reflex integrity
  - Self care and home management
  - Sensory integrity
- Establish Plan of Care

GOALS/OUTCOMES

- Increase ROM to a minimum of 70% of AMA guidelines for L6, L5, shoulder, hip, knee, elbow, wrist, and foot
- Pain: 3/10 with ROM of affected joint
- Strength: Grade 4/5 of major muscles of affected joint
- Improve gait with or without assistive devices, and maximize use of appropriate muscles and energy conservation
- Optimize functional independence
- Functional use of affected joint with or without assistive device
- Increase aerobic endurance

INTERVENTION
NUMBER OF VISITS: 6–14

- Patient Instruction
  - Basic Anatomy and Biomechanics
  - Handouts
  - Functional Considerations
- Direct Interventions
  - Acute Phase: 3–6 Visits
  - Subacute/Chronic Phase: 3–8 Visits

DISCHARGE PLANNING AND PATIENT RESPONSIBILITY

- Criteria for Discharge
  - Patient demonstrates ability to perform exercises correctly and in compliance with program
  - Functional use of joint with or without assistive supportive device
  - Independence of care and use of assistive device
- Circumstances Requiring Additional Visits
  - More than one arthritic joint
  - Contracture of joint
  - Deconditioned patient
  - Other cardiac, vascular, pulmonary conditions
- Home Program
  - AROM exercise
  - Isotonics with or without resistance if not in a flare-up
  - Isometrics in flare-up state
  - Stretching exercises
  - Cardiovascular conditioning
- Monitoring

SUMMARY OVERVIEW | GENERAL MEDICINE | ARTHRITIS   653

ARTHRITIS

ICD-9

714	Rheumatoid arthritis and other inflammatory polyarthropathies
715	Osteoarthrosis and allied disorders

APTA Preferred Practice Pattern: 4A, 4B, 4C, 4D, 4F, 4G, 4H, 4I, 4J, 6B

EXAMINATION

History and Systems Review

- History of current condition
  - Current therapeutic intervention
  - Current self-care intervention
  - Date of onset, progression of symptoms, and current pattern of symptoms
  - Patient's emotional response to current condition
- Past history of current condition
  - Prior therapeutic interventions
  - Prior medications
- Other tests and measures
  - Blood tests
  - X-rays, MRIs, bone scans
  - Review of diet and nutrition
- Medication
  - Medication for current condition
  - Side effects of current medication
  - Medications for other conditions
- Past medical/surgical history
  - Endocrine/metabolic
  - Cardiopulmonary
  - Musculoskeletal
  - Neuromuscular
  - Prior hospitalizations, surgeries
  - History of trauma
- Functional status and activity level (current/prior)
  - Current functional status in self-care and ADLs
- Health status
  - General health perception
  - Physical function (mobility, sleep patterns, fatigue)
  - Psychological function (depression, memory)
  - Social function (social support and interaction)
- Family history
  - Family members with history of similar condition
  - Familial health risks
- Living environment

- Growth and development
  - Developmental history
    - Congenital hip malposition
- General demographics
  - Age
  - Ethnicity
  - Sex
- Patient's functional goals

Tests and Measures

Systems review per APTA's *Guide to Physical Therapy Practice*

- Aerobic capacity and endurance
  - Perceived exertion during exercise
  - Assess pulse with treadmill or exercise protocol
- Anthropometric characteristics
  - Assessment of edema with girth measurements
  - Assessment of muscle atrophy with girth measurements
  - Observation of contractures and/or deformities
- Arousal, attention, and cognition
  - Assess attention and motivation
- Assistive and adaptive devices
  - Analyze benefits and practicality (energy conservation)
  - Analysis of patient's ability to use device and adherence to use of device
  - Assess alignment and fit
  - Safety assessment
- Environmental, home, and work barriers
  - Analysis of physical space
  - Assessment of barriers
- Ergonomics and body mechanics
  - Preferred postures
  - Dexterity and coordination of selected tasks and activities
  - Determine limitations during specific work/play activities
- Gait, locomotion, and balance
  - Gait analysis with and without assistive device

654 ARTHRITIS | GENERAL MEDICINE

- Static and dynamic balance assessment
- Assessment up/down stairs with and without assistive device
- Integumentary integrity
  - Palpation of skin temperature
  - Palpation of edema
  - Observation of skin color
- Joint integrity and mobility
  - Assess joint hypermobility and hypomobility through joint glides and accessory movements
  - Stress affected joint ligaments for sprains
  - Combined motion tests for spine
  - Special manual provocation tests specific to affected joints
    - Cervical spine (compression tests, traction, craniovertebral scan)
    - Lumbar spine (torsional stress test, posterior anterior pressures, compression)
    - Hip (Scouering, FABRE)
    - Elbow (Figure 8, Scouering)
- Motor function
  - Assessment of trunk mobility
- Muscle performance
  - Assessment of muscle strength and endurance of affected joints
  - Assessment of muscle tone of affected joints
  - Pain and soreness of muscles
  - EMG of weak muscles
  - Key muscle testing for spinal involvement
- Orthotic, protective, and support devices
  - Analyze benefits and practicality (energy conservation)
  - Analysis of patient's ability to use device and adherence to use of device
  - Assess alignment and fit
  - Safety assessment
- Postural assessment
  - Static and dynamic postures
- ROM
  - Active, overpressure, resistance to affected joints, assessment of end-feel of affected joints
- Reflex integrity
  - Assessment of normal reflexes
  - Assessment of pathological reflexes (Clonus, Babinski, Hoffman's)
- Self care and home management
  - Assessment: Sit/stand, sit/supine

- Adaptive skills assessment
- Safety assessment
- Sensory integrity
  - Assessment of sharp/dull, light to touch, and vibration for spinal involvement
  - Dural tests for spinal involvement

Establish Plan of Care

- Based on history, tests, and measures

GOALS/OUTCOMES

- Increase ROM to a minimum of 70% of AMA guidelines for L6, L5, shoulder, hip, knee, elbow, wrist, and foot
- Pain: 3/10 with ROM of affected joint
- Strength: Grade 4/5 of major muscles of affected joint
- Improve gait with or without assistive devices and maximize use of appropriate muscles and energy conservation
- Optimize functional independence
- Functional use of affected joint with or without assistive device
- Increase aerobic endurance

INTERVENTION

NUMBER OF VISITS: 6–14

Patient Instruction

Basic Anatomy and Biomechanics

- Anatomy of affected joint
- Biomechanics of joint and relationship of symptoms
  - Movement of joint
  - Muscle imbalance or weakness
  - Excessive strain to joint
  - Adjacent joints mobility
- Education of pathogenesis of arthritis
- Joint protection techniques

Handouts

- Proper posture and body mechanics
- Arthritis magazine
- Specific home program
- Community education programs
- VHI ADLs with adaptive equipment

Functional Considerations

- Review of aggravating positions and activities
- Instruction on position of rest
- Instruction on proper use and care of adaptive device, orthotic, protective device
- Instruction in positive and body mechanics for various activities
  - Sleeping
  - Sitting
  - Walking
  - Lifting/carrying
  - Specific ADLs and vocational tasks

Direct Interventions

Acute Phase: 3–6 Visits

- Therapeutic exercise
  - PROM and AAROM within proper range
  - Gentle stretching to joint and muscles and aggressive stretching to adjacent joints
  - Isometrics
  - Home use of ice/cold
  - Home program of isometrics and pain free ROM
- Functional training
  - Self care and home management
    - ADLs training
    - Gait training
    - Assistive and adaptive device training
    - Orthotic, protective, or supportive device training
  - Community work
    - Work or leisure task adaptation
    - Job simulation
- Manual therapy techniques
  - Soft-tissue techniques
    - Soft-tissue mobilization
    - Myofascial release
    - Trigger-point technique
  - Joint mobilization
    - Grades I-II to reduce pain
    - Grades I-II traction to joint to reduce pain
    - Grades II-IV mobilization to adjacent hypomobile joints
- Therapeutic devices and equipment
  - Application, fabrication, and fitting of device and equipment in conjunction with OT
- Electrotherapeutic modalities
  - Electric stimulation

- Biofeedback
- Neuromuscular electrical stimulation
- Physical agents and mechanical modalities
  - Cryotherapy/heat
  - Ultrasound
  - Hydrotherapy
  - Phonophoresis
  - Paraffin baths
  - Fluidotherapy®
- Goals/outcomes
  - Pain: 5/10 or less
  - Independence in isometrics and pain-free ROM
  - 50% pain-free ROM

Subacute/Chronic Phase: 3–8 Visits

- Therapeutic exercise
  - Manual resistance to muscles of joint
  - Progress from AAROM to AROM moving into pain range
  - Isotonics to all major muscles of joint with and without resistance
  - Appropriate neuromuscular, balance, and proprioceptive exercises
  - Posture or training
  - Aerobic exercises
    - Treadmill/walking program
    - Aquatic exercise
    - Stationary bike
- Functional training
  - Community and work
    - Ergonomic modifications of work site
    - More job simulation
  - Self-care and home management
    - Gait training
    - ADLs training
    - Assistive or adaptive device training
- Manual therapy techniques
  - Soft-tissue techniques
    - Continue soft-tissue mobilization
  - Joint mobilization
    - Grades II-IV to affected joint and adjacent joints
    - Progress graded traction to Grades II-IV
- Electrotherapeutic modalities
- Physical agents and mechanical modalities

- Goals/outcomes
  - Pain: 2/10 with rest, 3/10 with ADLs
  - Strength: 4/5 on manual muscle test for major muscles of joint
  - 70% pain-free ROM of joint

DISCHARGE PLANNING AND PATIENT RESPONSIBILITY

Criteria for Discharge
- Patient demonstrates ability to perform exercises correctly and in compliance with program
- Functional use of joint with or without assistive supportive device
- Independence of care and use of assistive device

Circumstances Requiring Additional Visits
- More than one arthritic joint
- Contracture of joint
- Deconditioned patient
- Other cardiac, vascular, or pulmonary conditions

Home Program
- AROM exercise
- Isotonics with or without resistance if not in a flare-up
- Isometrics in flare-up state
- Stretching exercises
- Cardiovascular conditioning

Monitoring
- Patient is to recheck/call at 2 weeks post-discharge to report progression toward previous functional status for recreational and sports activities
- If necessary, schedule a 4-week follow-up at clinic to monitor objective parameters and progress the home exercise program

REFERENCES

1. American Physical Therapy Association. *Guide to Physical Therapist Practice*. Alexandria, VA: APTA; 1997.
2. Cyriax JH. *Orthopaedic Medicine*. Oxford, England: Butterworth-Heinemann; 1993.
3. Ettinger Jr WH, Burs S. A randomized trial comparing aerobic exercise with a health education program in older adults with knee osteoarthritis. *JAMA*. 1997;277:25-31.
4. Gelber LH, Hick JE. Surgical rehabilitation options in the treatment of the rheumatoid arthritis patient resistant to pharmacologic agents. *Rheum Dis Clin North Am*. 1995;21:19-39.
5. Goodman C, Snyder T. *Differential Diagnosis in Physical Therapy*. Philadelphia, PA: WB Saunders; 1990.
6. Gray H; Williams PL, ed. *Gray's Anatomy*. 38th ed. New York, NY: Churchill Livingstone; 1995.
7. Grieve GP. The hip. *Physiotherapy*. 1983;69:196-204.
8. Hart A, Hopkins C, Ford B. *ICD-9-CM Expert for Physicians, Volume 1&2*. 7th ed. USA: Ingenix. 2005.
9. Hoppenfield S. *Physical Examination of the Spine and Extremities*. New York, NY: Appleton-Century-Crofts; 1976.
10. Magee D. *Orthopedic Physical Assessment*. Philadelphia, PA: WB Saunders; 1992.
11. Marks R. Muscles as a pathogenic factor in osteoarthritis. *Physiother Can*. 1993;45(4):251-259.
12. Reid DC. *Sports Injury Assessment and Rehabilitation*. New York, NY: Churchill Livingstone; 1992.
13. Schumacher HR. *Primer on Rheumatic Diseases*. Atlanta, GA: Arthritis Foundation; 1993.
14. Threikeld JA, Currier D. Osteoarthritis: effects on synovial joint tissues. *Phys Ther*. 1998;68:364-370.
15. Walker J. Joint lubrication: a review. *Physiother Can*. 1981;30:237-257.
16. Wyke B. The neurology of joints: a review of general principles. *Clin Rheumatol Dis*. 1983:7:223-239.
17. Munneke M, de Jong Z, Zwinderman AH, et al. Adherence and satisfaction of rheumatoid arthritis patients with a long-term intensive dynamic exercise program (RAPIT program). *Arthritis Rheum*. 2003;49(5):665-672.
18. MacDonald CW, Whitman JM, Cleland JA, Smith M, Hoeksma HL. Clinical outcomes following manual physical therapy and exercise for hip osteoarthritis: a case series. *J Orthop Sports Phys Ther*. 2006;36(8):588-599.
19. Dellhag B, Wollersjö I, Bjelle A. Effect of active hand exercise and wax bath treatment in rheumatoid arthritis patients. *Arthritis Care Res*. 1992;5(2):87-92.

GERIATRIC REHABILITATION

This guideline is intended to supplement all other guidelines when treating the older patient. Unique features for geriatric rehabilitation are detailed and should be considered in coordination with the appropriate diagnostic guide.

EXAMINATION

History and Systems Review

- History of current condition
  - Date of injury/onset
  - Complications and/or surgical procedure
- Past medical/surgical history
- Medications
  - Effects on balance, vision, cardiopulmonary
- Other tests and measures
  - Nutritional status
  - Diagnostic tests
  - Hearing, use of aid
  - Vision
- Functional status and activity level (current/prior)
  - Hobbies and leisure interest may help show activity level (actual vs. reported)
- Living environment
  - Present environment/anticipated discharge environment
    - Situation
      a. Alone
      b. With family
      c. Retirement community
      d. Board and care/assisted living/foster care
    - Accessibility/floor plan
    - Caregiver availability
    - Family support
  - Environment and home barriers
  - Household barriers: Stairs (with or without railings), throw rugs, wheelchair accessibility, safety
  - Assess for safety hazards (throw rugs, slippery floors)
  - Home access problems (stairs, narrow doorways)
  - Glare from windows or lights
- Social history
  - Family and/or caregiver resources
  - Social support systems
  - Occupational history
  - Family dynamics

Tests and Measures

Systems review per APTA's *Guide to Physical Therapy Practice*

- Arousal, attention, and cognition
  - Cognitive ability may decline with age
  - Orientation to person, place, time, and event
  - Recall assessment (for short- and long-term memory)
  - Ability to follow directions and stay focused on task
  - Ability to verbally communicate
  - Safety awareness
- Assistive and adaptive devices
  - Ability to use device properly
  - Proper adjustment of device
- Gait, locomotion, and balance
  - Sitting and standing balance
  - Gait with and without assistive device
  - Gait and balance on varied terrain
  - Stairs
  - Safety awareness
  - Wheelchair mobility if applicable
- Muscle performance
  - Manual muscle testing of all extremities unless limited by acute pain shunt, some type of surgical procedure, or inability of patient to follow directions
    - Muscle tone
    - Pain with muscle contraction
    - Trunk stability/strength
  - Testing muscle performance in the older adult
    - Manual muscle testing may be difficult since some strength loss is normal with increased aging
    - Speed of movement (is the patient able to raise the arms in time to prevent a fall)
    - Functional testing (ability to get up and down from a seated position)
    - Isokinetic testing is important for looking at torque generating capacity throughout the available ROM
- Orthotics, protective and supportive devices
  - Assess patient's ability to use and/or apply device (brace, splint, corset, sling) properly
  - Is device effective/utilized
  - Fit and condition of the device

GENERAL MEDICINE | GERIATRIC REHABILITATION   659

- Pain
  - Measured on visual analog scale
  - Assess factors that cause pain
  - Patient's reaction to pain
- ROM
  - With age tendons/ligaments become more rigid/less pliable/elastic
  - Access functional ROM (such as ability to get up from floor)
  - Use goniometer if ROM is significantly impaired and limits function
  - Assess muscle, joint, or soft tissue during ROM
- Self-care and home management
  - Bed mobility and transfer assessment
- Sensory integrity
  - Light touch, sharp/dull, temperature
  - Proprioception
  - Gross assessment of vision and hearing
  - Age related changes include decreased sensation, vision, hearing, and vestibular response/balance
- Ventilation, respiration, and circulation
  - Postural changes resulting from increased kyphosis, decreased thoracic flexibility and strength contribute to less-efficient respiratory function
  - Cough and sputum
  - Pulse oximetry
  - Lung auscultation

Establish Plan of Care
- Based on history, tests, and measures

GOALS/OUTCOMES
- Goals and outcomes will be specific to the patient's diagnosis and are detailed on individualized guidelines
- Goals and outcomes may have to be modified for the older population with consideration of:
  - Pre-incident physical status
  - Comorbidity
  - Endurance
  - Cognitive involvement
  - Pulmonary function
  - Environmental situation
  - Family/caregiver issues

INTERVENTION

Coordination, Communication, and Documentation
- Services should be provided between admission and discharge that facilitate cost-effective and efficient integration or reintegration to home, community, or work
- Documentation of therapeutic intervention is required for each episode of care and serves as the basic foundation for communication
  - Medicare requirements
  - Recertification every 30 days
  - Physician certificate of plan of care
- Coordination and additional communication will depend on the patient's impairment and home/work/community/leisure situation and requirements. Such services may include:
  - Case management
  - Coordination of care and collaboration with those integral to the patient's rehabilitation program
  - Coordination and monitoring of the delivery of available resources
  - Referrals to other health-care professionals
  - Identification of resources, support groups, or advocacy services
  - Provision of educational or training information
  - Technical assistance
- Specific coordination and communication provisions:
  - Social services/case manager

Patient Instruction

Handouts
- *Home Exercise Programs* (Therapy Skill Builder, 3820 E. Bellevue, PO Box 42050, Tucson, AZ 85733)
- Transfer techniques—dos and don'ts

Functional Considerations
- Assistive equipment, use and care of
- Caregiver instructions

Direct Interventions

Special consideration should be taken when treating older patients with the potential for increased bleeding, hemorrhage, disruption of fragile tissues, fracture, spread of infection, cardiovascular or neurologic compromise, or enhanced growth or metastasis of cancer (Guccione. 1993).

Acute Phase

- Therapeutic exercise and home program
  - Age-related strength loss can be reduced or reversed with appropriate exercise interventions
  - Participation in a regular exercise program is an effective intervention to reduce and prevent a number of physical declines associated with aging
  - When using exercise with the elderly, appropriate precautions should be taken. Severe osteoporosis may limit ROM exercise. Strengthening exercises may place a hypertensive patient at risk for a dangerous elevation in blood pressure if the patient performs a valsalva maneuver.
- Functional training
  - Bed mobility, transfer, and gait training
  - Walking with flexed posture requires greater energy expenditure
  - Training with orthotic, supportive, or protective device
- Manual therapy techniques
  - Joint mobilization and passive ROM with patients with rheumatoid arthritis or osteoporosis may be used with caution
- Therapeutic devices and equipment
  - Assess for appropriate devices (walker, crutches, canes, braces, corsets, oxygen, raised toilet seats, and chairs). With ambulatory devices, care must be taken not to overload the joints of the upper extremity.
  - There is an increase in energy expenditure when using a walker
- Airway clearance techniques
- Electrotherapeutic modalities
  - The patient must have sensation to light touch wherever electrodes are placed
- Physical agents
  - Physical agents may be selected with appropriate diagnoses. If patient has pain and temperature sensation, the use of hot packs, cold packs (ice), or ultrasound may be contraindicated. Traction is contraindicated with a diagnosis of osteoporosis.

Whirlpool may be contraindicated if the patient has impaired circulation.
  - Thermal injury may be prevented by:
    - Avoiding deep heating technique in joints involved with arthritis
    - Lowering temperatures of heating agents and increasing those of cooling agents
    - Decreasing the rate of temperature change
    - Decreasing treatment times

Functional Carryover

- Maximum independent bed mobility, transfers, and gait
- Correct use and maintenance of assistive devices
- Caregiver/family training

DISCHARGE PLANNING AND PATIENT RESPONSIBILITY

Criteria for Discharge

- Patient may be discharged prior to meeting all rehab goals for specific condition
- Caregiver/family training for assisting in functional activities and with home exercise program
- Patient unable to tolerate therapy at the present time

Circumstances Requiring Additional Visits

- Comorbidity
- Cognitive
- Decreased physical condition
- Pulmonary complication
- With age, there is a slower rate of tissue healing

Home Program

- As stated in individual guideline
- Modification for enhancing learning/compromised memory
- Involvement of family/caregiver

REFERENCES

1. American Physical Therapy Association. *Guide to Physical Therapist Practice.* Alexandria, VA: APTA; 1997.
2. Gray H; Williams PL, ed. *Gray's Anatomy.* 38th ed. New York, NY: Churchill Livingstone; 1995.
3. Guccione AA ed. *Geriatric Physical Therapy.* St Louis, MO: CV Mosby; 1993.
4. Hart A, Hopkins C, Ford B. *ICD-9-CM Expert for Physicians, Volume 1&2.* 7th ed. USA: Ingenix. 2005.

662   GERIATRIC REHABILITATION | GENERAL MEDICINE

MUSCLE WEAKNESS—GENERAL
SUMMARY OVERVIEW

ICD-9

    728.87   728.89   780.79

APTA Preferred Practice Pattern: **4D, 4F, 4B, 4C**

EXAMINATION

- History and Systems Review
- Tests and Measures
  Systems review per APTA's *Guide to Physical Therapy Practice*
  - Aerobic capacity/endurance
  - Anthropometric characteristics
  - Arousal, attention, and cognition
  - Assistive and adaptive devices
  - Circulation
  - Cranial and peripheral nerve integrity
  - Environmental, home, and work (job/school/play) barriers
  - Ergonomics and body mechanics
  - Gait, locomotion, and balance
  - Integumentary integrity
  - Joint integrity and mobility
  - Motor function
  - Muscle performance
  - Neuromotor development and sensory integration
  - Orthotics, protective and supportive devices
  - Pain
  - Posture
  - Prosthetic requirements
  - ROM
  - Reflex integrity
  - Self-care and home management
  - Sensory integrity
  - Ventilation and respiration/gas exchange
  - Work (job/school/play), community, and leisure integration or reintegration
- Establish Plan of Care

GOALS/OUTCOMES

- Strength: 4/5 on manual muscle test of all trunk and extremity muscles
- Good postural control in sitting, standing, and walking
- Return to pre-morbid gait and balance
- Return to functional status and activity level (current/prior) for ADLs and vocational, recreational, and sports activities as identified by the patient
- Independence in a progressive home exercise program

INTERVENTION
NUMBER OF VISITS 5–10

- Patient Instruction
  - Basic Anatomy and Biomechanics
  - Handouts
  - Functional Considerations
- Direct Interventions
  - Acute Phase: 2–5 Visits
  - Subacute Phase: 3–5 Visits
- Functional Carryover

DISCHARGE PLANNING AND PATIENT RESPONSIBILITY

- Criteria for Discharge
  - Independence in home exercise program
  - Goals/outcomes achieved
  - Patient has initiated progress toward previous level of strength and functional status
  - Patient understands and is aware of functional deficits and demonstrates safety with all activities
- Circumstances Requiring Additional Visits
  - Severe degenerative changes
  - History of other pathology
  - Presence of other medical conditions
  - Contractures
  - Cognitive limitations
  - Postoperative complications
  - Excessive environmental barriers to discharge
  - Persistent functional strength less than or equal to 3/5 on manual muscle test
  - Persistent balance or safety deficits requiring further training and education
- Home Program
  - Strengthening exercises that address deficits to improve tolerance to activity
  - Stretching exercises to improve and maintain muscle elasticity
  - Functional exercises to improve ADLs and task accomplishment
- Monitoring

SUMMARY OVERVIEW | GENERAL MEDICINE | MUSCLE WEAKNESS—GENERAL   **663**

MUSCLE WEAKNESS—GENERAL

ICD-9

728.87	Muscle weakness (generalized)
728.89	Other disorders of muscle, ligament, and fascia
780.79	Other malaise and fatigue

APTA Preferred Practice Pattern: 4D, 4F, 4B, 4C

EXAMINATION

History and Systems Review

- History of current condition
  - Age
  - Medication
  - Mechanism of injury/onset of weakness
  - Location, nature, and behavior of symptoms
  - General fatigue/malaise, weight loss, depression
  - Presence of cauda equina symptoms
  - Generalized disease symptoms
    - Loss of weight
    - Anemia
    - Pyrexia
- Past history of current condition
  - Hospitalization
  - Surgical intervention
  - Extremity or spine problems
  - Bracing, injections, etc
  - Systemic pathology
    - Appendix
    - Abdominal
    - Pancreas
    - Large intestine
    - Kidney
    - Genital/urinary
      a. Bladder
      b. Ureter
      c. Prostate gland
      d. Cervix
      e. Uterus
    - Iritis
    - Cardiac
    - Respiratory
    - Central nervous system disorders
    - Psoriasis
    - Irritable bowel symptoms
- Other tests and measures
- Functional status and activity level (current/prior)
  - Gait

- Upper extremity function
- Tolerance for sitting, standing, and walking
- Patient's functional goals

Tests and Measures

Systems review per APTA's *Guide to Physical Therapy Practice*

- Aerobic capacity/endurance
- Anthropometric characteristics
- Arousal, attention, and cognition
  - Spell same word backwards and forwards (w-o-r-l-d/d-l-r-o-w is most common)
  - Repeating integers forward and backward (normal: >6 forward, >4 backward)
  - Months forward and backward (normal: Up to twice as long backward as forward)
- Assistive and adaptive devices
- Circulation (arterial, venous, lymphatic)
- Cranial and peripheral nerve integrity
  - Basic cranial nerve screen testing sensory and motor function
  - Responses to light touch and pin prick in all dermatomes
- Environmental, home, and work (job/school/play) barriers
- Ergonomics and body mechanics
  - Determination of dynamic capabilities and limitations during specific activities
- Gait, locomotion, and balance
- Integumentary integrity
- Joint integrity and mobility
  - End feel, arthrokinematic/osteokinematic motion and assessment of patient reaction
- Motor function (motor control and motor learning)
- Muscle performance (including strength, power, and endurance)
- Neuromotor development and sensory integration
  - Rapid alternating movements

664 MUSCLE WEAKNESS—GENERAL | GENERAL MEDICINE

- Orthotics, protective and supportive devices
- Pain
- Posture
- Prosthetic requirements
- ROM (including muscle length)
  - Assessment of muscle, joint, or soft-tissue characteristics
  - Assessment of scapulohumeral rhythm
- Reflex integrity
- Self-care and home management (including ADLs and instrumental ADLs)
- Sensory integrity
- Ventilation and respiration/gas exchange
- Work (job/school/play), community, and leisure integration or reintegration (including instrumental ADLs)

Establish Plan of Care
- Based on history, tests, and measures

GOALS/OUTCOMES
- Strength: 4/5 on manual muscle test of all trunk and extremity muscles
- Good postural control in sitting, standing, and walking
- Return to pre-morbid gait and balance
- Return to functional status and activity level (current/prior) for ADLs and vocational, recreational, and sports activities as identified by the patient
- Independence in a progressive home exercise program

INTERVENTION
NUMBER OF VISITS 5–10

Coordination, Communication, and Documentation
- Provision of services between admission and discharge that facilitate cost-effective and efficient integration or reintegration to home, community, or work
- Documentation of therapeutic intervention is required for each episode of care and serves as the basic foundation for communication
- Coordination and additional communication will depend on the patient's impairment and home/work/community/leisure situation and requirements. Such services may include:
  - Case management

  - Coordination of care and collaboration with those integral to the patient's rehabilitation program
  - Coordination and monitoring of the delivery of available resources
  - Referrals to other health-care professionals
  - Identification of resources, support groups, or advocacy services
  - Provision of educational or training information
  - Technical assistance
- Specific coordination and communication provisions

Patient Instruction

Basic Anatomy and Biomechanics
- Physiology of muscle function information
- Health benefits of an active lifestyle

Handouts
- Education material relative to the cause of weakness
- Home program
  - Computer generated individualized home exercise programs (such as VHI)
  - Specific home program for muscle strengthening, endurance, and functional mobility
  - Specific home program for flexibility and balance training

Functional Considerations
- Strengthen postural muscles to increase activity tolerance (sitting, standing, sleeping, and driving)
- Consider assistive devices (crutches, canes, walkers, collars, tape, etc.) to compensate for weakness
- Be aware of precautions related to exercise safety, pacing, and energy conservation
- Recommend alteration of ADLs—use adaptive equipment if needed to compensate for weakness
- Avoid prolonged postures to prevent muscle shortening, contractures, and over-fatigue of postural muscles
- Body mechanic instruction for lifting, pushing, pulling, etc.
- Training recommendations (cross training, periodization, etc.)
- Avoid a sedentary lifestyle

GENERAL MEDICINE | MUSCLE WEAKNESS—GENERAL   665

Direct Interventions

Acute Phase: 2–5 Visits
- Therapeutic strengthening exercises: active assistive, progressing to active, progressing to resistive
- Stretching relative to length deficits
- Balance, proprioception, and coordination exercises through the upper and/or lower extremities
- Instruct in home program
- Instructions in patient log for self-tracking and compliance

Subacute Phase: 3–5 Visits
- Progression and periodization of therapeutic exercises
  - Initiation of functional, closed-kinetic chain exercises (squats, lunges, step ups, upper-extremity weight bearing exercise, etc.)
- Progress and review home program
  - Reassessment of posture, strength, balance, and AROM

Functional Carryover
- Integration of home exercise program into vocational environment
- Completion of ergonomic adjustments to home, automobile, and vocational areas
- Incorporation of proper posture and body mechanics to avoid exacerbation of symptoms
- Recognition/avoidance of activities that increase or exacerbate radiating symptoms
- Social reintegration related to increased functional ability

DISCHARGE PLANNING AND PATIENT RESPONSIBILITY

Criteria for Discharge
- Home exercise program independence
- Goals/outcomes achieved
- Patient has initiated progress toward previous level of strength and functional status
- Patient understands and is aware of functional deficits and demonstrates safety with all activities

Circumstances Requiring Additional Visits
- Severe degenerative changes
- History of other pathology
- Presence of other medical conditions
- Contractures
- Cognitive limitations
- Postoperative complications
- Excessive environmental barriers to discharge
- Persistent functional strength less than or equal to 3/5 on manual muscle test
- Persistent balance or safety deficits requiring further training and education

Home Program
- Strengthening exercises that address deficits to improve tolerance to activity
- Stretching exercises to improve and maintain muscle elasticity
- Functional exercises to improve ADLs and task accomplishment

Monitoring
- Instruct patient to call for advice should progression halt or negative trends occur
- May consider a follow-up call 60 days post-discharge to monitor patient compliance with lifestyle change and exercise integration

REFERENCES
1. American Physical Therapy Association. *Guide to Physical Therapist Practice.* Alexandria, VA: APTA; revised 2003.
2. Blumenfeld H. *Neuroanatomy through Clinical Cases.* Sinauer Associates Inc; 2002.
3. Cahalin LP, DeTurk WE. *Cardiovascular and Pulmonary Physical Therapy: An Evidence-based Approach.* McGraw Hill Medical Publishing Division; 2004.
4. Hart A, Hopkins C, Ford B. *ICD-9-CM Expert for Physicians, Volume 1&2.* 7th ed. USA: Ingenix. 2005.
5. Magee DJ. *Orthopedic Physical Assessment: 4th Edition.* Saunders: An Imprint of Elsevier Science; 2002.

VESTIBULAR REHABILITATION
SUMMARY OVERVIEW

ICD-9

386.50   386.51   386.56   780.4   781.2   781.3

APTA Preferred Practice Pattern: **4B, 4C, 4H, 4K, 5B**

EXAMINATION

- History and Systems Review
- Tests and Measures
  Systems review per APTA's *Guide to Physical Therapy Practice*
  - Arousal, attention, and cognition
  - Gait, locomotion, and balance
  - Laboratory tests results/dates
  - Motor performance
  - Pain
  - Postural assessment
  - ROM
  - Reflex integrity
  - Sensory integrity
  - Special tests
  - Ventilation, respiration, and circulation
- Establish plan of care

GOALS/OUTCOMES

- No falls, minimize fear of falling
- Decreased feelings of jumpy vision with head movement
- Decreased intensity and frequency of identified symptoms
- Adaptive techniques for varied environments
- Knowledge of adaptation process and basic physiology and need for movement
- General improvement and confidence in physical activity level
- Return to previous functional status for ADLs and vocational, recreational, and sports activities as identified by patient
- Improvement in performance tests
- Decrease visual dependence

INTERVENTION
NUMBER OF VISITS: 4–12

- Patient Instruction
  - Basic Anatomy and Biomechanics
  - Handouts

- Direct Interventions
  - Treatment for Benign Positional Paroxsysmal Vertigo: 2–4 Visits
  - Asymmetric, Bilateral, or Non-Specific Dizziness: 4–12 Visits
  - Progression of Eye/Head Exercises, Balance Exercises

DISCHARGE PLANNING AND PATIENT RESPONSIBILITY

- Criteria for Discharge
  - Client demonstrates knowledge and ability to progress exercises on his or her own
  - All goals/outcomes have been achieved
  - Intensity, frequency of dizziness improved and not interfering with function
  - Home exercise independence
- Circumstances Requiring Additional Visits
  - Head injury
  - Stroke
  - Post-concussive syndrome
  - Severe neurological condition impairing adaptation process
  - Recurrence of existing impairments
  - Multiple system involvement
- Home Program
  - Benign positional paroxsysmal vertigo
  - For eye/head impairments use progressive movements in safe surroundings, such as in a corner, back to counter, chair in front
  - Balance exercises using progressions, environments, and principals above
  - General fitness exercises with emphasis on stationary bike, walking
  - Functional application of principals to ADLs, work
  - Education of the fall risks that accompany busy visual environments, use of night lights, and caregiver training on appropriate assistance levels
- Monitoring

SUMMARY OVERVIEW | GENERAL MEDICINE | VESTIBULAR REHABILITATION   667

VESTIBULAR REHABILITATION

ICD-9

386.50	Labyrinthine dysfunction, unspecified
386.51	Hyperactive labyrinth, unilateral
386.56	Loss of labyrinthine reactivity, bilateral
780.4	Dizziness and giddiness
781.2	Abnormality of gait
781.3	Lack of coordination

APTA Preferred Practice Pattern: 4B, 4C, 4H, 4K, 5B

EXAMINATION

History and Systems Review

- History of current condition
  - Functional activities associated with symptoms
  - Change in condition
  - Prior level of function (including assistive devices)
  - Description of symptoms, chronology
  - Falls, fear
- Past history of current condition
  - Past episodes of dizziness
- Other tests and measures
  - Dizziness Handicap Index
  - Diagnostic tests (vestibular and others, including electronstagmography, caloric testing, posturography, MRI, CT scan, audiological)
  - Date of last comprehensive visual examination
- Medications
- Past medical/surgical history
  - Surgeries
  - Other medical problems (osteoarthritis, diabetes mellitus, hypertension, cervical vascular accident)
- Functional status and activity level (current/prior)
- Living environment
- Occupation/employment
- Patient's functional goals

Tests and Measures

Systems review per APTA's *Guide to Physical Therapy Practice*

- Arousal, attention, and cognition
  - Cognitive status: Mini mental, orientation, interview of function, job performance, neuropsych testing results
  - Change in status

- Gait, locomotion, and balance
  - Ambulation status
    - Gait speed with and without devices
    - Gait deviations
  - Functional balance performance tests
    - Dynamic Gait Index
    - Functional reach
    - Single-leg stance
    - Romberg/Sharpened Romberg
    - Berg Functional Balance test
    - Timed "Get Up and Go" test
    - Clinical test for sensory interaction for balance
    - Tinetti assessment tool
  - Static balance
    - Active weight shifts (detection of asymmetry, ankle vs. hip strategy use, fear, percent of normal of shift)
    - Reactive balance
    - Perturbed balance (detection of ability to recover from imbalance, strategy used, fear)
  - Dynamic balance
    - Walk: Gait deviations, speed, devices
    - Walk with head turns with and without eye movement
    - Pivot turns
    - Endurance, distance of walking, etc.
- Laboratory tests results/dates: Optometric, MRI, CT, audiologic, ENG, posturography, calorics, rotation, VAT, eCog etc.
- Motor performance
  - Upper- and lower-extremity strength
  - Motor behaviors: past pointing, tremors, ataxia, disregard of limbs, etc.
  - Motor control: Synergetic behaviors, Fugal-Meyer tests
- Pain
  - Measured on visual analog scale

668   VESTIBULAR REHABILITATION | GENERAL MEDICINE

- Postural assessment
- ROM
  - Upper- and lower-extremity flexibility
  - Cervical scan
- Reflex integrity
- Sensory integrity
  - Vision screening: Gaze, occulomotor control, smooth pursuits, saccades (normal and abnormal)
  - Proprioception: Integrity of ability to detect movement or pressure with weight shifts. Vibration sense can be good indicator. Emphasis to ankles, feet.
  - Vestibular: Vision-vestibular ocular testing (head movement focusing on a stationary target). Eyes and head movement.
    - Ability to do in progressively balance-challenging position (sitting, standing and walking). Note dyscoordination, abnormal saccadic eye movements, nausea, aversion, imbalance.
    - Fukada stepping test to identify a labyrinth deficit
    - Vertiginous Positioning
      a. Dix-Hallpike test for posterior canal benign positional paroxsysmal vertigo (BPPV)
      b. Horizontal Canal BPPV tests
      c. Cumulative aversion or dizziness to head movement
- Special tests
  The clinician should choose the appropriate tests based on age, ability, cognitive status, and symptoms.
  - Oculomotor exam with and without Frenzel lenses
    - Spontaneous nystagmus
    - Gaze-holding nystagmus (engaze nystagmus)
    - Smooth pursuit
    - Saccadic eye movements
    - Visual vestibular occular reflex (VVOR) cancellation
    - VVOR clinical, head moving focusing on stationary object (sit, stand, walk)
    - VVOR to slow and rapid head movements
    - Static and dynamic visual acuity
  - Performance tests: Dizziness Handicap Index, Berg Balance test, timed "Get Up and Go," Dynamic Gait Index (see Shumway-Cook. 2000)
  - Vertiginous positional testing, vertiginous positioning (description see Herdman. 2000)
    - Dix-Hallpike for BPPV, right and left
    - Roll test
    - Complete cervical scan (vertebral artery test is critical) head right, left, up, and down

- Ventilation, respiration, and circulation
  - Pulses
    - Resting
    - After exercise

Establish Plan of Care
- Based on history, tests, and measures

GOALS/OUTCOMES
- No falls, minimize fear of falling
- Decreased feelings of jumpy vision with head movement
- Decreased intensity and frequency of identified symptoms
- Adaptive techniques for varied environments
- Knowledge of adaptation process and basic physiology and need for movement
- General improvement and confidence in physical activity level
- Return to previous functional status for ADLs and vocational, recreational, and sports activities as identified by patient
- Improvement in performance tests
- Decreased visual dependence

INTERVENTION
NUMBER OF VISITS: 4–12

Patient Instruction

Basic Anatomy and Biomechanics
- Use of written, oral, and Internet instruction on vestibular anatomy, vestibular adaptation process, symptom education, sensory organization, and dysfunction (see references)
- Definitions may include but are not limited to: Adaptation, compensation, vestibular responses (unilateral, bilateral, asymmetrical), BPPV, and asymmetric or bilateral vestibular dysfunction
- Information should be provided on the purpose of vestibular therapy as well as goal and prognosis
- Vestibular Disorders Association (VEDA) (vestibular.org. Last accessed 10/5/2007)

Handouts
- Krames Communication

Direct Interventions

Treatment for Benign Positional Paroxsysmal Vertigo: 2–4 Visits
- Canalithic repositioning procedure(s)
- Epley vs. Semont procedures for posterior canal
- Horizontal roll for horizontal canal (Brandt, Epley, Herdman)

Asymmetric, Bilateral or Non-Specific Dizziness: 4–12 Visits
- Eye/head exercise for asymmetric and bilateral dysfunction: VVOR x1 and VVOR x2 progressions, eye and head exercises. All with increased balance challenge of sitting to standing to walking to increase in environmental visual information. Adaptation exercise to promote gaze stabilization coupled with increased visual information and balance challenge.
- Attention to feet exercise: Increase in ability for person to disregard visual information and increase ability to use available proprioception. Decrease visual overload and dependence.
- Exercise for use of sensory substitution if senses are unavailable. Opportunity and promotion for increase use of cervical ocular—vestibular responses and use.
- Exercise for decreasing abnormal saccadic movements and then use of corrective saccades with eye/head exercises

Progression of Eye/head Exercises, Balance Exercises
- Excursion of head movement, speed of head movement, vary distance from target, increase balance challenge with increase change in position of exercise (sitting to standing to slight offset tandem, to walk stop, then head movement to simultaneous walk with head movement to various balance challenge of BABST, 2x4 etc, uneven ground. Progress to VVOR x2.
- Habituation other than eye/head exercises selected carefully and monitored for effectiveness
- VVOR eye/head exercises vs. eye and head exercises
- Increase environmental busyness: Blank wall for target, to static busyness, then moving busyness, mall etc.
- Balance exercises: Promotion of ankle strategies, such as weight shifts, start-stop, high reaching, awareness/

attention to feet vs. vision for balance progressions, BABST, 2x4 etc.
- Twisting exercises, rotation reaching high etc.
- Various assistive device training environmentally dependent

Functional Carryover
- Independence changing positions, gait, and changing directions while ambulating

DISCHARGE PLANNING AND PATIENT RESPONSIBILITY

Criteria for Discharge
- Client demonstrates knowledge and ability to progress exercises on own
- All goals/outcomes have been achieved
- Intensity, frequency of dizziness improved and not interfering with function
- Home exercise independence

Circumstances Requiring Additional Visits
- Head injury
- Stroke
- Post-concussive syndrome
- Severe neurological condition impairing adaptation process
- Recurrence of existing impairments
- Multiple system involvement

Home Program
- BPPV: Generally thought to restrict pitch plane head movement for up to 48 hours after CRP. Then encourage movement to see effectiveness of procedure within 1 week.
- For eye/head impairments use progressive movements in safe surroundings, such as in a corner, back to counter, chair in front
- Balance exercises using progressions, environments, and principles above
- General fitness exercises with emphasis on stationary bike (because of lack of head movement for conditioning) or walking
- Functional application of principles to ADLs, work. There is fine line between doing ADLs, work without

impairing dizziness vs. doing supplemental eye/head exercises for adaptation. Much support and monitoring.

- Education of the fall risks that accompany busy visual environments, use of night lights, and caregiver training on appropriate assistance levels

Monitoring

- Instruct patient to call for advice should progression halt or negative trends occur
- Communicate with physician regarding need of follow-up

REFERENCES

1. Allison L, Fuller K. Balance and vestibular disorders. In Umphred DA (ed): *Neurological Rehabilitation.* 4th ed. St Louis, MO; Mosby; 2001:616-660.

2. Epley JM. The Canalithic repositioning procedure; for treatment of benign paroxysmal positional vertigo. *Otolaryngol Head Neck Surg.* 1992;107:399-404.

3. Hart A, Hopkins C, Ford B. *ICD-9-CM Expert for Physicians, Volume 1&2.* 7th ed. USA: Ingenix; 2005.

4. Herdman SJ, ed. *Vestibular Rehabilitation. 2nd.* Philadelphia, Pennsylvania: FA Davis; 2000.

5. LaJoie Y, Teasdale N, Bard C, et al. Attentional demands for static and dynamic equilibrium. *Exp Brain Res.* 1993;97:139-144.

6. Shumway-Cook A, Woollacott M. Attentional demands and postural control: the effect of sensory context. *J Gerontol A Biol Sci Med Sci.* 2000;55:10-16.

7. Shumway-Cook A, Woollacott M. *Motor Control: Theory and Practical Application.* 2nd ed. Philadelphia, Pennsylvania: Lippinocott Williams and Wilkins; 2001.

WOUND MANAGEMENT
SUMMARY OVERVIEW

ICD-9

879	880	881	882	883	884	885	886	887
890	891	892	893	894	895	896	897	911
912	913	914	915	916	917			

APTA Preferred Practice Pattern: **4D, 4K, 7A, 7C, 7E**

EXAMINATION

- History and Systems Review
- Tests and Measures
  Systems review per APTA's *Guide to Physical Therapy Practice*
  - Arousal, attention, and cognition
  - Integumentary integrity
  - Pain
  - Ventilation, respiration, and circulation
  - General physical therapy evaluation as appropriate
- Establish Plan of Care

GOALS/OUTCOMES

- Patient displays understanding of phases of wound healing, signs and symptoms of infection, home management
- Pain: 2/10 or less
- Absence of necrotic tissue
- Eliminate infection
- Heal wound to 100% epithelialization
- Return to previous functional status for ADLs and vocational, recreational, and sports activities as identified by patient

INTERVENTION
NUMBER OF VISITS: 5-10

- Patient Instruction
  - Handouts
  - Functional Considerations
- Direct Interventions
  - Inflammation Phase
  - Proliferation Phase
  - Remodeling Phase
- Functional Carryover

DISCHARGE PLANNING AND PATIENT RESPONSIBILITY

- Criteria for Discharge
  - Patient may move from inpatient to outpatient or home health setting once wound is stable and can be managed
  - Marked deteriorations/no progression
  - Understanding of home program/wound prevention
  - Medical instability
- Circumstances Requiring Additional Visits
  - Diabetes
  - Peripheral vascular disease
  - Decreased sensation
  - Smoker
  - Recurrent infection
  - Poor patient compliance
- Home Program
  - Home management program
  - Nursing management program
- Monitoring

SUMMARY OVERVIEW | GENERAL MEDICINE | WOUND MANAGEMENT   673

WOUND MANAGEMENT

ICD-9

879	Open wound of other and unspecified sites, except limbs
880	Open wound of shoulder and upper arm
881	Open wound of elbow, forearm, and wrist
882	Open wound of hand except finger(s) alone
883	Open wound of finger(s)
884	Multiple and unspecified open wound of upper limb
885	Traumatic amputation of thumb (complete) (partial)
886	Traumatic amputation of other finger(s) (complete) (partial)
887	Traumatic amputation of arm and hand (complete) (partial)
890	Open wound of hip and thigh
891	Open wound of knee, leg [except thigh], and ankle
892	Open wound of foot except toe(s) alone
893	Open wound of toe(s)
894	Multiple and unspecified open wound of lower limb
895	Traumatic amputation of toe(s) (complete) (partial)
896	Traumatic amputation of foot (complete) (partial)
897	Traumatic amputation of leg(s) (complete) (partial)
911	Superficial injury of trunk
912	Superficial injury of shoulder and upper arm
913	Superficial injury of elbow, forearm, and wrist
914	Superficial injury of hand(s) except finger(s) alone
915	Superficial injury of finger(s)
916	Superficial injury of hip, thigh, leg, and ankle
917	Superficial injury of foot and toe(s)

APTA Preferred Practice Pattern: 4D, 4K, 7A, 7C, 7E

EXAMINATION

History and Systems Review
- History of current conditions
  - Mechanics of injury/onset of wound
  - Date of injury/onset of wound
  - Location, nature, and behavior of symptoms
    - Radiating symptoms
    - Aggravating/relieving factors
  - Allergies
- Past history of current condition
  - Contributing diagnosis
  - Diabetes, peripheral neuropathy, spinal cord injury, etc.
  - Hospitalization
  - Surgical intervention
  - Lower-extremity problems
  - Bracing interventions
- Other tests and measures
  - Nutritional status
- Medications
- Functional status and activity level (current/prior)
- Patient's functional goals/prior functional level

Tests and Measures
Systems review per APTA's *Guide to Physical Therapy Practice*
- Arousal, attention, and cognition
  - Cognitive status
- Integumentary integrity
  - For lower-extremity ulcers: Determine if venous or arterial
    - Characteristics of venous ulcers
      a. Most commonly on medial malleolus
      b. Vary in size and shape
      c. May occur anywhere between ankle and knee

674   WOUND MANAGEMENT | GENERAL MEDICINE

d. Tend to be superficial (not exposing tendon or bone)

e. Usually have moderate to severe exudate

f. Usually painful when desiccated

g. Pain frequently relieved by elevation

h. May have edematous lower leg and ankle

- Characteristics of arterial ulcers

a. Tend to be very painful

b. Pain may be decreased with dependency

c. Tend to be dry (very little exudate)

d. May occur anywhere on the lower extremity/foot

e. Associated with discoloration of tissue

f. Associated with decreased tissue temperature

○ Measurement

- Width horizontally

- Length head to toe

- Depth of wound from surface to bottom of wound bed

- Tunneling using the clock method

- Surrounding area dark red, necrotic

○ Wound categorization

- Stage I: Non-blanchable erythema of intact skin

- Stage II: Partial thickness skin loss

- Stage III: Full thickness skin loss which may extend to fascia

- Stage IV: Full thickness skin loss with extensive damage to muscle, bone, or supporting structure

○ Description of wound

- Percentage of necrotic tissue

- Undermining

- Surrounding skin integrity

- Granulation tissue

- Color, smell, and amount of exudate

a. Minimal: Discharge within periphery of bandage

b. Moderate: Larger than lesion, soaked through immediate dressing

c. Severe: Drainage beyond immediate dressing

○ Photograph of wound

- Stamp with patient's name plate

- Label anatomical position and date, preferably top of photo toward head of patient

- Attach to wound care evaluation sheet

- Reevaluate and photograph wound every 7 days

- Pain

○ Measured on visual analog scale

- Ventilation, respiration, and circulation
  ○ Ankle/brachial index
- General physical therapy evaluation as appropriate. Depending on wound etiology and patient's medical status, a general physical therapy evaluation should be conducted to examine the impact of the wound on the patient's functional mobility. The general physical therapy evaluation should include, but is not limited to:
  ○ Aerobic capacity
  ○ Gait, locomotion, and balance
  ○ Muscle performance
  ○ ROM
  ○ Reflex integrity
  ○ Self-care and home management
  ○ Sensory integrity

Establish Plan of Care
- Based on history, tests, and measures

GOALS/OUTCOMES
- Patient displays understanding of phases of wound healing, signs and symptoms of infection, home management
- Pain: 2/10 or less
- Absence of necrotic tissue
- Eliminate infection
- Heal wound to 100% epithelialization
- Return to previous functional status for ADLs and vocational, recreational, and sports activities as identified by patient

INTERVENTION
NUMBER OF VISITS: 5–10

Coordination, Communication, and Documentation
- Provision of services between admission and discharge that facilitate cost-effective and efficient integration or reintegration to home, community, or work
- Documentation of therapeutic intervention is required for each episode of care and serves as the basic foundation for communication

- Coordination and additional communication will depend on the patient's impairment and home/work/community/leisure situation and requirements. Such services may include:
  - Case management
  - Coordination of care and collaboration with those integral to the patient's rehabilitation and wound management program
  - Coordination and monitoring of the delivery of available resources
  - Referrals to other health-care professionals
  - Identification of resources, support groups, or advocacy services
  - Provision of educational or training information
  - Technical assistance
- Specific coordination and communication provisions; referral to:
  - Dermatologist
  - Registered dietician
  - Plastic surgeon
  - Internal medicine physician
  - Podiatrist
  - Social worker/case manager
  - Occupational therapist

Patient Instruction

Handouts
- Appropriate positioning for pressure relief
- Positioning schedule to change weight-bearing surfaces
- Appropriate assistive device for pressure relief
  - Ambulatory aide
  - Cushion
- Signs of infection, when to call physical therapy or physician
- Wound care
  - Keep dressing dry
  - Soak foot
  - Home dressing instructions
- Importance of diet/fluid intake
- Smoking cessation to promote wound healing
- Nutrition and supplements
- Footwear recommendations

Functional Considerations
- Use of orthotics, protective device
- Weight-bearing considerations
- Avoidance of movements causing an aggravation of symptoms, including the need for off loading to facilitate wound healing
- Total contact casting

Direct Interventions

Special considerations for treatment
- Venous ulcers
  - Apply compression if ankle brachial index is greater than 0.8
  - Encourage elevation
- Arterial ulcers
  - Refer to vascular specialist: If underlying pathophysiology is not addressed, wound will not heal

Inflammation Phase
- Description
  - Characterized by erythema, heat, and edema
  - Usually lasts from 48–72 hours but can be up to 2 weeks
  - Treatment should be daily to twice a day, dependent on size of wound, patient tolerance, and patient's disposition (i.e., in hospital vs. outpatient)
- Wound management
  - Dressing
    - Xeroform/adaptic
    - Hydrocolloids: Duoderm®
    - Hydrogels: Carrasyn®
    - Transparent film (i.e., Tegaderm™)
    - Silvadene/antibiotic ointment as recommended by physician
      a. Burn wound topical cerium nitrate with silver sulfadiazine
    - Wrap
    - Kerlex®
    - Kling®
    - Bandnet™
    - Montgomery strapping
      Note: Dressing to be done by physical therapist staff after wound care treatments. If greater frequency than twice a day, nursing to do subsequent dressings.

○ Debridement

- Sharp debridement of nonviable tissue with physician's order
  a. Utilizing scalpel or scissors
  b. To be performed only by specially trained physical therapist or physical therapist assistant under close supervision
- Mechanical debridement with physician's order
  a. Utilize 4 x 4s or soft material to debride slough

• Electrotherapeutic modalities
  ○ HVPC
  - Polarity: Negative
  - Pulses per second: 30–50
  - Intensity: 100–200 volts
  - Conduction: Normal saline or water
  - Regularity: Daily or twice a day
  - Duration: 45–60 minutes

• Physical agents and mechanical modalities
  ○ Precautions, antiseptic procedures
  - Gown and gloves for all wound care (mask and goggles for Surgivac®)
  - Lab cultures of whirlpool/Hubbard tanks
    a. Clean tank
    b. Take culture and send to lab if requested by physical therapist or infection control department or at minimum quarterly
    c. Wound culture only on wounds with signs and symptoms of localized infection by nursing services or by physical therapist
  ○ Ultrasound
  - Nonthermal: Superficial wounds
    a. Conduction: Diagnostic US hydrogel sheet or water
    b. Frequency: 1 or 3 MHz
    c. Pulse: 20%
    d. Intensity: .5W/cm^2
    e. Regularity: 5–7 times per week
    f. Duration: 5 minutes
  - Thermal: Deep wounds, periwound tissue
    a. Conduction: Water or conductive gel
    b. Frequency: 1 MHz
    c. Pulse
       - Continuous if noncompromised circulation
       - 20% pulsed if compromised circulation
    d. Intensity: 0.5–1.0W/cm^2
    e. Regularity: 5–7 times per week for 1 week
    f. Duration: 8–10 minutes

○ Whirlpool will be used on heavily exuding wounds only due to potential maceration and delay in wound healing. Once clean, change treatment to ultrasound or HVPC.
  - Temperature: 92–96°F (33.5–35.5°C)
  - Agitation: Moderate
  - Duration: 5–20 minutes
  - Regularity: Depends on necrotic tissue and exudate
○ Surgivac®/Orthovac/Pulsavac®, etc.
  - 1 L. saline solution—warmed for 1 minute in microwave
  - Antibiotic solution—room temperature
  - Regularity: Depends on necrotic tissue and exudates
○ Vacuum-assisted wound closure (VAC therapy)
○ Negative pressure wound dressing

Proliferation Phase

• Description
  ○ Characterized by granulation tissue forming and a beefy red appearance
  ○ Usually lasts 4–8 weeks
  ○ Treatment should be between daily to 2–7 times per week depending on progress of wound and disposition of patient (i.e., acute vs. outpatient)

• Wound management
  ○ Debridement (see "Inflammation Phase")
  ○ Dressing (see "Inflammation Phase")

• Electrotherapeutic modalities
  ○ HVPC
  - Polarity: Alternate every 3 days
  - Pulses per second: Negative 30–50; positive 100–128
  - Intensity: 100–200 volts
  - Conduction: Normal saline or water
  - Regularity: Daily
  - Duration: 45–60 minutes

• Physical agents and mechanical modalities
  ○ Ultrasound
  - Nonthermal: Superficial wounds
    a. Conduction: Diagnostic US hydrogel sheet
    b. Frequency: 1 or 3 MHz
    c. Pulse: 20%
    d. Intensity: 0.5W/cm^2
    e. Regularity: 5–7 times per week for 2–3 weeks
    f. Duration: 5 minutes

Remodeling Phase

- Description
  - Characterized by scar formation. Wound at this point is being covered by epithelial tissue and at end will be closed
  - Can last from several weeks to months
  - Treatment can be from daily to 2–3 times per week depending on progress of wound
- Wound management
  - Dressing (See "Inflammation Phase")
- Electrotherapeutic modalities
  - HVPC
    - Polarity: Alternate every 3 days
    - Pulses per second: 64
    - Intensity: 100–200 volts
    - Conduction: Normal saline or water
    - Regularity: Every day
    - Duration: 45–60 minutes

Functional Carryover

- Avoidance of pressure or compromising positions
- Nutritional program
- Wound care hygiene

DISCHARGE PLANNING AND PATIENT RESPONSIBILITY

Criteria for Discharge

- Patient may move from inpatient to outpatient or to home health setting once wound is stable and can be managed
- Marked deterioration/no progression
- Understanding of home program/wound prevention
- Medical instability

Circumstances Requiring Additional Visits

- Diabetes
- Peripheral vascular disease
- Decreased sensation
- Smoker
- Recurrent infection
- Poor patient compliance

Home Program

- Home management program
  - Written instructions by physical therapist on what to do for wound (moisturizing skin, etc.)
  - Inspect skin daily for reddened areas, broken skin, bruised areas, blisters, and swelling
  - Active/passive ROM activities
  - Pressure relief/off-loading
- Nursing management program
  - Written instructions on appropriate treatment for stage of wound and on when to call physical therapist or physician

Monitoring

- Patient to call if detecting increased skin breakdown or decreased wound healing

REFERENCES

1. Alon G. *High Voltage Stimulation: A Monograph.* Chattanooga, TN: Chattanooga Corp; 1984.
2. American Physical Therapy Association. *Guide to Physical Therapist Practice.* Alexandria, VA: APTA; 1997.
3. Burks, RI. Providone-iodine solution in wound treatment. *Phys Ther.* 1998;78:212-218.
4. Busch K, Chantelau E. Effectiveness of a new brand of stock "diabetic" shoes to protect against diabetic ulcer relapse: a prospective cohort study. *Diabetic Med.* 2003;20(8):665-669.
5. Consensus Development Conference on Diabetic Foot Wound Care. 7-8 April 1999, Boston, MA. *Adv Wound Care.* 1999;12(7):353-361.
6. Cukjati D, Robnik-Sikonja M, Rebersek S, Kononenko I, Miklavcic D. Prognostic factors, prediction of chronic wound healing by electrical stimulation. *Med Biol Eng Comput.* 2001;39(5):542-550.
7. De Gracia CG. An open study comparing topical silver sulfadiazine and topical silver sulfa cerium nitrate in the treatment of moderate and severe burns. *Burns.* 2001;27(1):67-74.
8. Eginton MT, Brown KR, Seabrook GR, Towne JB, Cambria RA. A prospective randomized evaluation of negative pressure wound dressing for diabetic foot wounds. *Ann Vasc Surg.* 2003;17(6):645-649.
9. Gray H; Williams PL, ed. *Gray's Anatomy.* 38th ed. New York, NY: Churchill Livingstone; 1995.
10. Herscovici Jr D, Sanders RW, Scaduto JM, Infante A, DiPasquale T. Vacuum-assisted wound closure

(VAC therapy) for the management of patients with high-energy soft tissue injuries. *J Orthop Trauma.* 2003;17(10):683-688.

11. Houghton PE, Kincaid CB, Lovel M, et al. Effect of electrical stimulation on chronic leg ulcer size and appearance. *Phys Ther.* 2003;83(1):17-28.

12. Klein L, Boarini J, Burton CS, et al. *Pressure Ulcers: A Practical Nursing Reference for the Chronic Wound Environment.* Dow B Hickman Inc; 1991.

13. Hart A, Hopkins C, Ford B. *ICD-9-CM Expert for Physicians, Volume 1&2.* 7th ed. USA: Ingenix; 2005.

14. Morgan D, Hoelscher J. Pulsed lavage: promoting comfort and healing in home care. *Ostomy Wound Manage.* 2000;46(4):44-49.

15. Mosher BA, Cuddigan J, Thomas DR, Boudreau DM. Outcomes of 4 methods of debridement using a decision analysis methodology. *Adv Wound Care.* 1999;12(2):81-88.

16. Mulder G. Treatment of open skin wounds with electrical stimulation. *Arch Phys Med Rehab.* 1991;72:375-377.

17. Rodheaver G, Baharestani MM, Barabec ME. Wound healing and wound management: focus on debridement: an interdisciplinary round table. September 18, 1992. Jackson Hole, WY. *Adv Wound Care.* 1994(7)1:22-24, 26-29, 32-36, 37-39.

18. Sussman C et al. *Woundcare Management in a Managed Care Environment.* Fifth Annual Physical Therapy Management Conference. Oct 25-27, 1993. Torrance, CA: Woundcare Management Services.

19. Sussman C. *Ultrasound for Wound Healing: A Monograph.* Chattanooga, TN: Chattanooga Corp; 1994.

20. Thomas DR. Pressure ulcers. In: Cassel CK, et al, eds. *Geriatric Medicine.* 3rd ed. New York, NY: Springer-Verlag; 1997.

21. Vetra H, Whittaker D. Hydrotherapy and topical collagenase for decubitus ulcers. *Geriatrics.* August 1975;30:53-58.

22. Wethe J, Fowler E, Sussman C, et al. *Interactive Debridement Course.* October 1994. Torrance, CA: Woundcare Management Services.

Neurological

CARE CONNECTIONS *Clinical Practice Guidelines*

NEUROLOGICAL CONDITIONS

Cerebral Vascular Accident 683

Guillain-Barré Syndrome 693

Multiple Sclerosis 699

Parkinson's Disease 705

682 NEUROLOGICAL CONDITIONS

CEREBRAL VASCULAR ACCIDENT
SUMMARY OVERVIEW

ICD-9

342   431   433   434   435   436   442   728.85   781.2   781.9

APTA Preferred Practice Pattern: 4B, 4G, 5B, 5C

EXAMINATION

- History and Systems Review
- Tests and Measures
  Systems review per APTA's *Guide to Physical Therapy Practice*
  - Arousal, attention, and cognition
  - Assistive and adaptive devices
  - Cranial nerve integrity
  - Gait, locomotion, and balance
  - Motor function
  - Muscle performance
  - Orthotics, protective and supportive devices
  - Pain
  - ROM
  - Self-care and home management
  - Sensory integrity
- Establish Plan of Care

GOALS/OUTCOMES

- Prevent contractures, deformity, and skin breakdown
- Minimize pain through maintenance of normal joint alignment and positioning
- Maintain/increase ROM in all joints
- Normalize muscle tone and movement patterns to allow for patient's maximizing independence with endurance, mobility, ambulation/wheelchair, transfers, sitting, standing and dynamic balance, and functional ability in completion of ADLs
- Independence in progressive home exercise program emphasizing function and pacing

INTERVENTIONS
NUMBER OF VISITS: 10–30

- Patient Instruction
  - Handouts
  - Functional Considerations
- Direct Interventions
  - Acute Inpatient Phase: 5–12 Visits per Week, 2–5 Weeks
  - Subacute Outpatient Phase: 5–18 Visits
- Functional Carryover

DISCHARGE PLANNING AND PATIENT/FAMILY RESPONSIBILITY

- Criteria for Discharge
  - All patient/family rehabilitation goals achieved
  - Patient demonstrates compliance with home program
  - Patient noncompliant with rehabilitation program
  - Monitoring: Follow-up visits may be needed to address difficulties with return to previous activities
- Circumstances Requiring Additional Visits
  - Cognitive dysfunction
  - Comorbidity
  - Arthritis
  - Previous incidents
- Home Program
  - Self ROM
  - Strengthening
  - Maintain aerobic conditioning
  - Balance exercise
- Monitoring

SUMMARY OVERVIEW | NEUROLOGICAL CONDITIONS | CEREBRAL VASCULAR ACCIDENT   683

CEREBRAL VASCULAR ACCIDENT

ICD-9

342	Hemiplegia and hemiparesis
431	Intracerebral hemorrhage
433	Occlusion and stenosis of precerebral arteries
434	Occlusion of cerebral arteries
435	Transient cerebral ischemia
436	Acute, but ill-defined, cerebrovascular disease
442	Other aneurysm
728.85	Spasm of muscle
781.2	Abnormality of gait
781.9	Other symptoms involving nervous and musculoskeletal systems

APTA Preferred Practice Pattern: **4B, 4G, 5B, 5C**

INTRODUCTION

No standard program can be established for the cerebral vascular accident (CVA) patient, as the location and the extent of the neurological damage present unique symptoms. Treatment is a dynamic, ever-changing process. Therefore, the approach must be individualized, but the purpose is the same: To provide patients with a treatment program that will help them achieve their maximal functional recovery. This guideline was developed to provide basic content for treatment of the CVA patient. With the changes in health care and reimbursement, the patient's typical hospital course and rehabilitation program have been reduced and require a more concentrated, aggressive, and focused therapy program and plan of care to achieve optimal results.

Treatment goals stated in the guideline are general examples. The therapist must tailor goals toward each patient's level and living environment. Other factors affecting goals are motivation and cooperative behavior. In today's decreased length of stay in acute and inpatient rehab facilities, home health and outpatient physical therapists are seeing more involved cases. Therapists must try to extend the patient's rehab program over the longest period of time to ensure maximal functional outcome. Functional recovery from a stroke can continue for months to years. The degree of motor recovery depends on factors such as the size and location of the lesion. Patients need an intensive multidisciplinary team to help them reach all goals.

Treatment programs should emphasize functional, meaningful activities, not just straight, linear exercise. The activity chosen should coincide with level of deficit and should directly or indirectly be focused on helping the achievement of functional goals. The therapist must vary activities and not expect perfection before moving on to a higher level activity. The patient should be challenged but not pushed so hard as to create associated reactions or to be passively "carried through" the activity by the therapist. For example, if a patient has poor trunk control in sitting, work on trunk control in standing (a higher level activity), and it may improve trunk control in sitting.

EXAMINATION

History and Systems Review

- History of current conditions
  - Type of stroke
  - Date of injury/onset
  - Clinical course
    - Duration of stay and therapy interventions
    - Complications
    - Surgical procedures

- Other tests and measures
  - Diagnostic procedures (MRI, CT, etc.) and results
- Past medical history/surgical history
  - Previous cerebral vascular accidents
  - Surgical procedures (unrelated/related to CVA)
  - Other medical problems/diagnoses (diabetes mellitus, rheumatoid arthritis, osteoarthritis, chronic obstructive pulmonary disease, etc.)

684   CEREBRAL VASCULAR ACCIDENT | NEUROLOGICAL CONDITIONS

- Functional status and activity level (current/prior)
  - Living situation
    - Environment
    - Family/caregiver support
    - Accessibility, ease of mobility
  - Occupation/employment
- Social history
  - Family caregiver resources
  - Support systems
- Patient/family functional goals

Tests and Measures

Systems review per APTA's *Guide to Physical Therapy Practice*

The order of the following assessment depends on the therapist's approach. The specific, objective information can be obtained/observed during a functional mobility assessment. Keep in mind normal movement—if abnormal movement is observed, more specific testing may be done (see beginning of "Addendum").

- Arousal, attention, and cognition
  - Consultation with the speech language pathologist
  - Consciousness
    - Alert
    - Lethargic
    - Unresponsive
    - Eye contact/visual tracking
  - Orientation
    - Person
    - Place
    - Time
    - Purpose
    - Utilization of standardized tests (MMPI)
  - Confusion/cognition
  - Ability to follow directions
  - Memory (long- and short-term)
  - Attention span
  - Safety judgement
  - Affect
    - Agitated
    - Labile
    - Depressed
    - Appropriate
- Assistive and adaptive devices
  - Selection
  - Utilization/outcome
  - Ability to use safely

- Cranial nerve integrity
  - Swallowing
  - Auditory
  - Gustatory
  - Olfactory
  - Visual
  - Vestibular
- Gait, locomotion, balance
  Balance is a multisystem phenomenon that requires an adequate combination of proprioception, somatosensation, vision, vestibular function, strength, postural alignment, and flexibility. Patients must have adequate control of the trunk and bilateral extremities to maintain an upright position. Many tests are available to objectively assess balance. These include the Tinetti assessment tool, the "Get Up and Go" test, and the Berg Functional Balance Test. Balance can also be assessed functionally by looking at static/dynamic sitting, standing, and walking activities. In addition, a standard grading scale may be used (see "Addendum"). When assessing balance, it is also important to note potential reasons for balance loss (e.g., in sitting, an excessive posterior pelvic tilt may contribute to a loss of balance in the posterior direction).
  - Gait
    - Pattern (stance phase, swing phase of uninvolved vs. involved)
    - Distance
    - Velocity
    - Type of surface
    - Use of assistive devices
    - Orthotics
  - Wheelchair mobility and operation (brakes, footrests)
- Motor function
  - Analysis of head, trunk management
  - Posture in supine, sitting, standing, trunk control
  - Postural, equilibrium, and righting reactions
- Muscle performance
  A state of readiness of muscle to move
  - Traditional synergistic patterns of upper and lower extremities:
    - Flexion in upper extremity (scapular retraction, depression; shoulder adduction, internal rotation; forearm pronation; elbow, wrist, finger flexion)
    - Extension in lower extremity (pelvic retraction; hip extension, adduction, internal rotation; knee extension; ankle plantarflexion)

- Tone (see "Addendum")
  - Normal
  - Abnormal
  - Hypotonic/flaccid
  - Hypertonic: Expressed in two forms; rigidity and spasticity
  - Mixed
  - Changing with functional movement
- Orthotics, protective and supportive devices
  - Effects and benefits
  - Alignment and fit
  - Safety
  - Donning/doffing
  - Functional retraining
- Pain (see "Addendum")
  - Pain behavior and reaction with specific movement (alleviation with motions/positions)
  - Muscle soreness
  - Pain with joint movement
  - Pain perception or qualifiers (ache, throb, sharp, dull, etc.)
  - Measured on visual analog scales
  - Observation (if unable to report numerical score, observe facial expressions/behavior)
- ROM
  - Passive /active
    - Faulty postural/limb alignment may be the cause of decreased ROM, synergistic patterns, and/or decreased balance
  - Observation
    - Pattern and quality of movement
    - Movement of associated joints or substitutions
- Self-care and home management
  - Bed mobility: Rolling, bridging, scooting, supine-sit
  - Transfers: Sit/stand, bed/chair, wheelchair/mat, car, commode
  - Level of assistance to complete the task and what components need assistance (see "Addendum")
  - Verbal cues
    - Level, degree, specifics
    - Orientation, safety initiation, sequencing
- Sensory integrity (gross receptive abilities) (see "Addendum")
  - Light touch/deep pressure
  - Sharp/dull
  - Proprioception
  - Temperature

- Neglect: One-sided neglect should be noted during functional mobility as well as sensorimotor testing

Establish Plan of Care
- Based on history, tests, and measures

GOALS/OUTCOMES
Specific goals may vary depending on the setting
- Prevent contractures, deformity, skin breakdown
- Minimize pain through maintenance of normal joint alignment and positioning
- Maintain/increase ROM in all joints
- Normalize muscle tone and movement patterns to allow for patient's maximizing independence with:
  - Endurance
  - Mobility, ambulation/wheelchair
  - Transfers
  - Sitting, standing, and dynamic balance
  - Functional ability in completion of ADLs
- Independence in progressive home exercise program emphasizing function and pacing

INTERVENTIONS
NUMBER OF VISITS: 10–30

Coordination, Communication, and Documentation
- Provision of services between admission and discharge that facilitate cost-effective and efficient integration or reintegration to home, community, or work
- Documentation of therapeutic intervention is required for each episode of care and serves as the basic foundation for communication
- Coordination and additional communication will depend on the patient's impairment and home/work/community/leisure situation and requirements. Such services may include:
  - Case management
  - Coordination of care and collaboration with those integral to the patient's rehabilitation program
  - Coordination and monitoring of the delivery of available resources
  - Referrals to other health-care professionals
  - Identification of resources, support groups, or advocacy services
  - Provision of educational or training information
  - Technical assistance

- Specific coordination and communication provisions:
  - Multidisciplinary approach addressing all patient needs
    - Occupational therapy
    - Speech therapy
    - Social worker/case manager
    - Recreational therapy
  - Recommend further physical therapy as patient progresses in continuum of care from inpatient to home health to outpatient

Patient Instruction

Handouts
- Written exercises/activities
  - Self ROM
  - Strengthening
- Written handouts may include:
  - Specific home program/safety for each patient
  - US Department of Health Services, *Recovering After a Stroke—Patient and Family Guide* (available from Krames Communications, 1100 Grundy Lane, San Bruno, CA 94066)
  - Prevention handouts (e.g., from American Stroke Association, 7272 Greenville Avenue, Dallas, TX 20037)
  - Support groups: A list of stroke support groups in the area may be given to patient/caregiver
  - Community resources (senior centers, transportation, Meals on Wheels, etc.)

Functional Considerations
- Patient/caregiver training
  - Safety, technique, body mechanics, and independence in all ADLs/functional activities
  - Proper/safe use of equipment (orthotics, assistive devices, wheelchairs)
  - Positioning to avoid pain, skin breakdown, contractures
  - Bed mobility, transfers, gait
  - Understanding of home exercise program

Direct Interventions

Acute Inpatient Phase: 5–12 Visits per Week, 2–5 Weeks
[see Subacute Outpatient Phase below]

Subacute Outpatient Phase: 5–18 Visits
Most therapists recognize that there are a variety of treatment approaches when managing the neurological patient. The therapist treating neurological patients must know normal movement and biomechanical alignment in order to best facilitate functional recovery in their clients. Activities will depend on the patient's level and the discharge environment. Functional changes, no matter how big or small, are the goal of all treatment approaches. Each patient's participation in activities will vary. All interventions can be performed in any setting.
- Positioning program to provide support, normal sensory input, inhibit abnormal tone, promote symmetry, relieve pain, and provide comfort
  - Coordinated schedule with nursing, staff, and family
  - Frequent change in position every hour
  - Check for skin breakdown
  - Supine and bilateral sidelying it is generally recommended
    - Upper extremity in a position of slight scapular protraction, shoulder abduction with humeral, not forearm external rotation, elbow extension abduction
    - Lower extremity in a position of pelvic protraction, hip extension to neutral with hip abduction, slight knee flexion, and with no pressure on the ball of the foot
  - Wheelchair
    - Upper extremity is adequately supported
    - Seat cushion needs to provide support as to allow for a normal lordotic curve with weight bearing directly over the ischial tuberosities
    - Knees and feet in line with the hips
- Head/trunk control activities/balance activities, motor function training/retraining
  - Normal alignment in sitting with facilitation of an active trunk (co-contraction)
  - Weight-bearing and forced use/facilitation of the involved side in sitting
  - Weight-bearing symmetrical and asymmetrical scooting
  - Early transition sit to stand from a high surface
  - Normal alignment in standing with upper and lower extremity weight-bearing
  - Incorporate functional activities in early sitting and standing activities

NEUROLOGICAL CONDITIONS | CEREBRAL VASCULAR ACCIDENT   687

- ROM/stretching
  - Mobilization as needed
    - Special attention to thoracic and lumbar spine, scapulae, and pelvis
- Neuromuscular education/re-education
  - Facilitation: Promote desired response (see "Addendum")
    - Progress facilitation from isometric to eccentric to concentric muscle activity
  - Inhibition: Decrease/discourage undesired response example: Movements, postures, behaviors, etc.
  - Facilitation/inhibition should be combined with functional activity for carry over
- Functional training
  - ADLs training (see "Addendum")
    - Bed mobility activities (emphasis is on head and neck control as well as midline orientation)
      a. Bridging
      b. Bridging with weight shift
      c. Scooting upper body/head lift
      d. Placing and maintaining affected limbs
      e. Half bridging
      f. Rolling
      g. Moving up in bed
      h. Supine to sit
      i. Sit to supine
    - Transfer training (including affected upper extremity as able) (See "Addendum")
      a. Early sit to stand
      b. Level surface sit to sit pivot transfer in small increments
      c. Bed to/from wheelchair, commode, mat, chair, sofa, etc.
         Examples of progression:
         - Even surfaces
         - Uneven surfaces (high to low, low to high, varied surfaces)
         - With or without arms
      d. Transfer followed by immediate functional activity (sit to/from stand followed by activity such as stepping and turning to reach)
         - Organized functional training programs in real/simulated environment
    - Assist with community and/or vocational reintegration
    - Gait activities: Emphasize quality/safety, not quantity (with/without assistive devices)

a. Even surfaces
b. Uneven surfaces (ramp, gravel, grass, carpet, etc.)
c. Stairs (reciprocal pattern emphasized to increase control of involved extremity)
d. Functional activities during gait (change in direction and velocity, open/close doors, closets, carrying items, stooping, with distractions, obstacles/object negotiation, etc.)

- Therapeutic devices and equipment
  - Determine/reassess equipment needs (wheelchair, orthotics, assistive devices) ambulatory aids

Functional Carryover
- Home evaluation with recommendations for safety and maximal functional independence
- Appropriate medical supplier names/numbers/addresses will be given to patient/caregiver for future equipment maintenance and replacement needs

DISCHARGE PLANNING AND PATIENT/FAMILY RESPONSIBILITY

Criteria for Discharge
- All patient/family rehabilitation goals achieved
- Patient demonstrates compliance with home program
- Patient noncompliant with rehabilitation program
- Monitoring: Follow-up visits may be needed to address difficulties with return to previous activities

Circumstances Requiring Additional Visits
- Cognitive dysfunction
- Comorbidity
- Arthritis
- Previous incidents

Home Program
- Self ROM
- Strengthening
- Maintain aerobic conditioning
- Balance exercise

Monitoring
- Ongoing contact with therapist to maintain functional status and equipment viability

ADDENDUM

The following information is provided as an explanation of issues common to assessment and treatment of an individual with a CVA.

- Normal movement. The 5 basic components of normal movement for functional activities are:
  - Trunk mobility and control
  - Midline orientation (perceptual line that divides the body into right and left and center of mass and gravity)
  - Weight shift over base of support
  - Head control
  - Limb function
- Balance
  - Normal: The patient maintains the position safely and can withstand maximal challenges to the position in all planes
  - Good: The patient maintains the position safely, however can withstand only moderate challenges to the position in all planes
  - Fair: The patient maintains the position, however can withstand no challenges to the position
  - Poor: The patient maintains the position only with assistance from the therapist
  - Zero: The patient is totally dependent and unable to maintain the position
- Tone
  - Normal: Tone that is high enough to sustain or move against gravity, yet low enough to allow for movement
  - Abnormal:
    - Hypotonic/flaccid: Reduced resistance to passive stretch displayed as inability to hold resting posture; limp, floppy extremity during passive movement; depressed deep tendon stretch reflexes
    - Hypertonic: Expressed in two forms; rigidity and spasticity
      a. Rigidity: Increased tone uniformly in both agonists and antagonists, although the motor performance and reflexes are not affected. It may be uniform throughout the range of movement (plastic/lead pipe) or it may be interrupted by a series of jerks (cogwheel—Parkinson's). Brainstem lesions can produce either decerebrate rigidity or decorticate rigidity.

b. Spasticity: A velocity-dependent increase in tonic stretch reflex with exaggerated tendon jerks. It is a result of the release of the gamma system, and very rarely the alpha, from higher inhibitory control. Passive stretch of a spastic muscle may produce an initial high resistance, followed by a sudden inhibition, or letting go of resistance, termed the "clasp-knife" reflex. Clonus, characterized by the cyclical, spasmodic hyperactivity of antagonistic muscles occurring at a regular frequency, may occur with sustained stretch of a spastic muscle.

- Pain:
Pain may occur at any phase of the hemiplegic patient's rehab phase and can be due to a variety of causes. Some typical causes of pain are muscle imbalance, improper movement patterns, joint dysfunction, improper weight-bearing patterns, muscle shortening, or central nervous system in origin. Assessment of the type, anatomical location, presence of soft tissue dysfunction, and description of body position during the active movement that causes pain or the exact passive movement that causes pain will assist in planning treatment. Any pain scale may be used to quantify the amount of pain before, during, and after treatment. A standard numerical (0–10) scale is best. The therapist needs to be extremely gentle when handling the hemiplegic patient's upper extremity. Properly positioning the upper extremity before all activities is imperative. In order to prevent and control pain, mobilizations, and tone management, modalities may need to precede facilitation of the extremity for functional activities or passive/active ROM exercise.
- Level of assistance:
  - Max: The patient is able to perform less than 25% of the work
  - Mod: The patient is able to perform 50% of the work
  - Min: The patient is able to perform more than 75% of the work
  - Stand by assist/contact guard assist: The patient performs the task inconsistently, requiring occasional minimal assistance and supervision for safety

- Supervision: The patient performs the task completely, requiring hands-on supervision for safety, but no physical assistance
- Independent: The patient performs the task completely in different settings with good safety judgment, with no assistance from the therapist

• Sensory

While some patients may experience a total loss of tactile and/or proprioceptive sensation, the majority experience partial impairment, which usually affects the higher discriminatory sensations. For example, patients may feel touch, but be unable to localize it, may interpret pressure as light touch, or may be unable to distinguish variations in temperature. With impaired sensation and sensory feedback, the patient loses control and coordination of movement. The loss of movement control may also affect the good side of the body. Finally, even if the patient has suffered no sensory loss, abnormal sensations from spastic muscles and abnormal feedback provided from joints could result in abnormal sensory feedback from the periphery to the central nervous system.

• Facilitation:

When a therapist desires a movement, a recommended sequence for problem solving:

- Step 1: Ask the patient to perform the movement (indirectly or directly). If able, go directly to Step 5.
- Step 2: If unable, facilitate the movement (hands-on demonstration)

  When trying to gain muscle activity, keep in mind that isometric control precedes eccentric control precedes concentric control. In other words, a concentric contraction may be most difficult to perform. In addition, movement should begin in slow and small ranges of motion and then advance to normal ranges and speed.
- Step 3: Take the patient through the motion passively. Then go back to facilitation, or if a restriction is present, go to Step 4.
- Step 4: Mobilize, stretch, and/or inhibit. Then go back to Steps 1, 2, or 3.
- Step 5: Challenge, repeat, vary, increase the complexity, change the environment, and make it functional

• Upper extremity:

- Limb use: Therapists need to look at all aspects of limb use in rehab to have true functional gains. All

of the following normal characteristics of upper and lower extremities should be included in treatment:

- Support (part or all of the limb)
- Manipulation: Besides the hand and arm, lower extremities can manipulate as well (the foot manipulates into a shoe, etc.)
- Balance
- Expression (body language, gestures, hugging, waving, shrugging shoulders, etc.)
- Tools (writing, touching, scratching, opening bottles, etc.)

- Upper extremity control sequence: The following is a general weight-bearing sequence to develop upper extremity control in coordination with the body:

- Body movement on arm
- Arm movements on the body
- Arm and body moving together
- Variety and repetition
- Develop upper extremity control for support during transitional movement
- Develop upper extremity control for support for functional activities

- Shoulder dysfunction: Primary shoulder problems of the hemiplegic patient are subluxation, pain, and lack of functional movement patterns. Subluxation may occur in both the flaccid and spastic stage secondary to the interruption of glenohumeral joint stability. Prevention of subluxation requires (1) proper assessment of low tone vs. high tone, (2) appropriate treatment in accordance with assessment, and (3) prevention of shoulder capsule stretch.

• Motor function (motor control learning)

- Postural stability: Situations in which the center of mass falls within the base of support
- Postural response: Alterations in posture that occur in order to keep the center of mass over the base of support
- Righting and equilibrium reactions: Specific balance responses designed to keep the body and head in a vertical position

REFERENCES

1. American Physical Therapy Association. *Guide to Physical Therapist Practice.* Alexandria, VA: APTA; 1997.

2. Bobath B. *Adult Hemiplegia: Evaluation and Treatment.* 3rd ed. Oxford, England: Butterworth-Heinemann; 1990.

3. Bogataj U, Gros N, Kijajic M, Acimonc R, Malezic M. The rehabilitation of gait in patients with hemiplegia: a comparison between conventional therapy and multi-channel functional electrical stimulation therapy. *Phys Ther.* 1995;75:490-502.

4. Brown Jr RD, Ransom J, Haoss S, et al. Use of nursing home after stroke and dependency on stroke severity: a population based study. *Stroke.* 1999;30(5):924-929.

5. Course syllabus, NDT (Bobath) 3-Week Course in the Treatment of Adult Hemiplegia. Daniel Freeman Memorial Hospital, Inglewood, CA, August/November 1996. Primary instructor: Waleed Al-Oboudi OTR.

6. Dancer S. Redesigning care for the nonhemorrhagic stroke patient. *J Neurosci Nurs.* 1996;28(3):183-189.

7. Davis PM. *Steps to Follow: A Guide to Treatment of Adult Hemiplegia.* New York, NY: Springer-Verlag; 1985.

8. Fisher B, Yakura J. Movement analysis: a different perspective. *Orthop Phys Ther Clin North Am.* 1993:1-14.

9. Flick C. Stroke rehabilitation 4: stroke outcome and psychosocial consequences. *Arch Phys Med Rehabil.* May 1999;80:521-526.

10. Gill-Body KM, Papat RA, Parker SW, Krebs DE. Rehabilitation of balance in two patients with cerebellar dysfunction. *Phys Ther.* 1997;77(5):534-552.

11. Gray H; Williams PL, ed. *Gray's Anatomy.* 38th ed. New York, NY: Churchill Livingstone; 1995.

12. Hart A, Hopkins C, Ford B. *ICD-9-CM Expert for Physicians, Volume 1&2.* 7th ed. USA: Ingenix. 2005.

13. Indredavik MD, Bakke F, Slordahl SA, Rokseth R, Haheim LL. Treatment in a combined acute and rehabilitation stroke unit: which aspects are most important? *Stroke.* 1999;30(5):917-923.

14. Kristeins AE, Black-Schaffer RM, Richard RL. Stroke rehabilitation 3: rehabilitation management. *Arch Phys Med Rehabil.* May 1999;80:517-520.

15. Landel R, Fisher B. Musculoskeletal considerations in the neurologically impaired patient. *Orthop Phys Ther Clin North Am.* March 1993:15-24.

16. Maki BE, McIlroy WE. The role of limb movements in maintaining upright stance: the "change in support" strategy. *Phys Ther.* 1997;77(5):488-507.

17. Noback CR, Strominger NL, Demarest RJ. *The Human Nervous System: Introduction and Review.* Philadelphia, PA: Lea & Febiger; 1991.

18. O'Sullivan SB, Schmitz TJ. *Physical Rehabilitation: Assessment and Treatment.* 3rd ed. Philadelphia, PA: FA Davis; 1994.

19. Peat M. Functional anatomy of the shoulder complex. *Phys Ther.* 1986;66(12):1855-1865.

20. Rancho Los Amigos Medical Center: The Pathokinesiology Department And The Physical Therapy Department. *Observational Gait Analysis Handbook.* Downey, CA: Los Amigos Research and Educational Institute; 1996.

21. Umphred DA. *Neurological Rehabilitation.* 2nd ed. St. Louis, MO: CV Mosby; 1990.

22. US Dept of Health and Human Services. *Recovering After a Stroke: Patient and Family Guide.* Washington, DC: USDHHS; 1995. AHCPR publication 95-0664.

23. Velozo CA, Magalhaes LC, Pan A-W, Leiter P. Functional scale discrimination to admission and discharge: Rasch analysis of the level of rehabilitation scale III. *Arch Phys Med Rehabil.* August 1995;76:705-712.

GUILLAIN-BARRÉ SYNDROME
SUMMARY OVERVIEW

ICD-9

357.0

APTA Preferred Practice Pattern: **5E, 6B, 6F, 6G**

EXAMINATION

- History and Systems Review
- Tests and Measures
  Systems review per APTA's *Guide to Physical Therapy Practice*
  - Aerobic capacity and endurance
  - Arousal, attention, cognition
  - Assistive devices/orthotics
  - Cranial nerve integrity
  - Gait, locomotion, and balance
  - Motor function
  - Muscle performance
  - Pain
  - ROM
  - Self-care and home management
  - Sensory integrity
- Establish Plan of Care

GOALS/OUTCOMES

- Prevent contractures, deformities
- Functional ROM
- Pain 3/10 or lower
- Normalize muscle tone
- Independence in all functional activity with assistive device or caregiver as needed
- Independence in home exercise program emphasizing function
- Avoid permanent muscle damage from overfatigue and overwork

INTERVENTION
NUMBER OF VISITS: 12–50

- Patient Instruction
  - Education
  - Handouts
  - Functional Considerations
- Direct Interventions
  - Initial-Onset Phase: 2–10 Visits
  - Mid Phase: 5–20 Visits
  - End Phase: 5–20 Visits
- Functional Carryover

DISCHARGE PLANNING AND PATIENT RESPONSIBILITY

- Criteria for Discharge
  - All rehabilitation goals achieved
  - All patient/family goals achieved
  - Patient demonstrates compliance with home program
- Circumstances Requiring Additional Visits
  - Comorbidities
  - Age
  - Ventilator dependence
  - Complications
  - Severity of disease
  - Use of plasmophoresis/intravenous immunoglobulin therapy
  - Cranial nerve involvement
  - Contractures
  - Cognitive dysfunction
  - Excessive muscle belly tenderness
- Home Program
  - ROM
  - Strengthening
  - Cardiovascular activities

SUMMARY OVERVIEW | NEUROLOGICAL CONDITIONS | GUILLAIN-BARRÉ SYNDROME 693

GUILLAIN-BARRÉ SYNDROME

ICD-9
357.0   Acute infective polyneuritis
APTA Preferred Practice Pattern: **5E, 6B, 6F, 6G**

INTRODUCTION
This guideline is organized into three phases:
- Initial onset phase: symptoms (approx. 3–7 days)
- Mid Phase: Peak involvement to include plateau (1–6 weeks)
- End Phase: Recovery (6–9 months)

You may see the patient at any phase. Guillain-Barré Syndrome (GBS) is a demyelinating disease that affects the mixed peripheral nerves. There is damage to the myelin sheath, which causes slowed conduction, impaired conduction, or complete conduction block. GBS is characterized by relatively symmetrical ascending weakness that rapidly evolves from distal to proximal. Motor weakness can range from mild in distal lower extremities to total paralysis. Most patients will return to their prior functional status with the occasional long-term deficits. Weak anterior tibial musculature is the most common, followed by weak foot and hand intrinsics, quadriceps, and gluteals. Progression of recovery is from proximal to distal.

The point of maximal weakness, the rate of recovery, and residual weakness will vary for each patient. Therapists may see patients at varying levels of weakness/functional ability in different settings. A multidisciplinary approach addressing all patient needs enhances maximum recovery.

EXAMINATION

History and Systems Review
- History of current condition
  - Date of original diagnosis
  - Past and current therapeutic interventions
  - Description of symptoms
  - Patient and family therapeutic/functional goals
- Medications
  - For current condition
- Past medical/surgical history
  - Prior hospitalization
  - Previous surgeries
  - Pre-existing conditions
- Functional status and activity level (current/prior)
- Social history
  - Family/caregiver resources
  - Social activity/support systems
- Living environment
  - Home vs. board and care vs. extended care facility
    - Stairs/railings/carpet/wheelchair access, etc.
  - Alone vs. family support/caregiver
  - Desired discharge destination
- Occupation/employment
  - Current and prior work/school
- Patient's functional goals

Tests and Measures
Systems review per APTA's *Guide to Physical Therapy Practice*
- Aerobic capacity and endurance
  - Perceived exertion
  - Chest expansion with inspiration
  - Breathing pattern
- Arousal, attention, cognition
  - Orientation
    - Person
    - Place
    - Time
    - Purpose
  - Motivation level
  - Ability to follow directions
  - Memory (long and short term)
- Assistive devices/orthotics
  - Needs assessment
  - Effects and benefits
- Cranial nerve integrity
- Gait, locomotion, and balance
  - Static and dynamic balance
    - Tinetti, Berg, "Get Up and Go" (If applicable)

694   GUILLAIN-BARRÉ SYNDROME | NEUROLOGICAL CONDITIONS

○ Gait analysis/characteristics
   ▪ Phases of gait
      a. Swing and stance
      b. Single vs. double limb support
      c. Analysis of head, trunk, upper extremities, and lower extremities
      d. Note deviations
   ▪ Cadence, velocity, and stride length
   ▪ Varied terrains
      a. Smooth, uneven, incline/decline
○ Wheelchair mobility/management
   ▪ Manual vs. electric
○ Safety
   ▪ Level of assistance required
• Motor function
   ○ Dexterity and coordination
      ▪ Grasp and release object
      ▪ Finger to nose and heel to shin
   ○ Head, trunk, and limb movement
      ▪ Postural, equilibrium, and righting reactions
   ○ Trunk mobility/control
      ▪ Lying, sitting, standing, locomotion
      ▪ Transition from supine, sitting, standing to wheelchair
   ○ Initiation of movement
   ○ Quality of movement
   ○ Voluntary vs. involuntary movement
   ○ Ability to transfer
   ○ Bed mobility
• Muscle performance
   ○ Manual muscle test (if applicable)
   ○ Functional muscle strength
   ○ Daily assessment of muscle belly tenderness and muscle strength to avoid over stretch or overwork
   ○ Tone
      ▪ Hypertonicity/weakness/flaccid paralysis most common
• Pain
   ○ Visual analog scale
   ○ Observation of facial expression/behavior
   ○ Body chart
• ROM
   ○ Passive/active
   ○ Functional ROM
   ○ Substitutions
   ○ Cause of limitation

• Self-care and home management
   ○ ADLs scale
      ▪ Barthel index
• Sensory integrity
   ○ Light touch and temperature
   ○ Proprioception

Establish Plan of Care
• Based on history, tests, and measures

GOALS/OUTCOMES
• Prevent contractures, deformities
• Functional ROM
• Pain 3/10 or lower
• Normalize muscle tone
• Independence in all functional activity with assistive device or caregiver as needed
• Independence in home exercise program emphasizing function
• Avoid permanent muscle damage from over fatigue and overwork

INTERVENTION
NUMBER OF VISITS: 12–50

Coordination, Communication, and Documentation
• Provision of services between admission and discharge that facilitate cost-effective and efficient integration or reintegration to home, community, or work
• Documentation of therapeutic intervention is required for each episode of care and serves as the basic foundation for communication
• Coordination and additional communication will depend on the patient's impairment and home/work/community/leisure situation and requirements. Such services may include:
   ○ Case management
   ○ Coordination of care and collaboration with those integral to the patient's rehabilitation program
   ○ Coordination and monitoring of the delivery of available resources
   ○ Referrals to other health-care professionals
   ○ Identification of resources, support groups, or advocacy services
   ○ Provision of educational or training information
   ○ Technical assistance

- Specific coordination and communication provisions:
  - A multidisciplinary approach addressing all patient needs
    - Occupational therapy
    - Speech therapy
    - Respiratory therapy
    - Recreation therapy
    - Social worker/case manager

Patient Instruction

Education
- Information on rehabilitation program in relation to symptom progression

Handouts
- Home program
  - ROM to all extremities
  - Positioning for pressure relief
  - Energy conservation

Functional Considerations
- Proper and safe use of all equipment
- Caregiver training
- Avoidance of overfatigue of involved muscle

Direct Interventions

Initial-Onset Phase: 2–10 Visits
- Therapeutic exercise
  - Positioning program
    - Hand and foot splinting, physiologic position
      a. Towel roll for hands
    - Pressure relief program
      a. Padding for bony prominences
  - ROM
    - Passive ROM
      a. Physiologic joint movement
      b. Longer duration of stretching is beneficial
      c. Joint mobilization
      d. PROM at least 2 times daily
- Manual therapy techniques
  - Chest stretching
    - Manual thoracic mobilization
    - Myofascial release
  - Massage
    - Adjunct to ROM if no hyperesthesia

- Airway clearance techniques
  - Postural drainage
- Functional training
  - Upright tolerance
    - Head of bed elevation in increments/tilt table
    - Progress to sitting position if tolerable
    - Monitor autonomic response
    - Stabilize muscle groups less than 3/5 strength
    - Proceed only as per patient tolerance
- Therapeutic devices and equipment
  - Use of foot cradle in bed
    - Pain management and positioning
- Physical agents and mechanical modalities
  - Compression garments
    - Pain management
- Goals/outcomes
  - Prevent contractures
  - Prevent decubitus ulcers/pressure sores
  - Maintain joint integrity and ROM
  - Minimize pain/sensitivity
  - Prevent deep vein thrombosis
  - Increase tolerance and endurance to upright posture
  - Avoid pulmonary complications
  - Avoid muscle overwork and overstretch

Mid Phase: 5–20 Visits
- Therapeutic exercise
  - Progression from PROM to active assisted to active exercise
    - Muscle facilitation/reeducation
      a. Facilitory techniques
  - Gentle strengthening
    - Isometric, isotonic, isokinetic, manual resistive, progressive resistive, proprioceptive neuromuscular facilitation (PNF)
    - Tailored to strength of each muscle group
    - Avoid overfatigue, may impede recovery
    - Frequent rest periods
    - Use low repetition with higher frequency of exercise
    - Progression of recovery is proximal distal
  - Progress exercise to functional activity
  - Pre-gait activities
    - Tilt table, monitor autonomic response
    - Weight shifting
    - Standing table

696 GUILLAIN-BARRÉ SYNDROME | NEUROLOGICAL CONDITIONS

- Parallel bars to initiate pre-gait/standing, erect posture of trunk
  - Progress to gait training, if able with assistive device
- Electrotherapeutic modalities
  - Electrical stimulation/facilitation of contraction neuromuscular electrical stimulator
- Functional training
  - Bed mobility training/transfer training
    - PNF and neurodevelopmental treatment techniques
    - Trunk initiation and control
  - Wheelchair mobility
    - Initiate training
    - Compensatory strategies (proximal muscles)
    - Increase sitting tolerance—avoid fatigue of axial muscle
- Therapeutic devices and equipment
  - Reevaluate need for current strength status
- Goals/outcomes
  - Facilitate return of strength
  - Prevent injury to weakened muscles
  - Facilitate functional movements/mobility
  - Improve tolerance to sitting in wheelchair
  - Continue re-evaluation of orthotic needs

End Phase: 5–20 Visits
- Therapeutic exercise
  - Progression from active to resistive exercise
    - PNF, manual resistive, weight training
    - Avoid fatigue: Look for decreased strength, tingling, paresthesia's with exercise, if found, then exercise is too strenuous
  - Functionally directed exercise training
  - Progression of sitting tolerance—avoid fatigue of axial muscles
  - Progression of trunk control
    - Dynamic sitting exercise
      a. Trunk movement in all planes
    - Swiss ball sitting exercise
  - Endurance training: Upper-extremity/lower-extremity ergometer, and treadmill
- Electrotherapeutic modalities
  - Electrical stimulation/facilitation of contraction neuromuscular electrical stimulator—continue muscle reduction

- Functional training
  - Progress independence of bed mobility
    - Adaptations if necessary
  - Progress transfer training
    - Adaptations if necessary
  - Progression of gait training
    - Assistive device
    - Orthotics
  - Progression of wheelchair mobility
- Goals/outcomes
  - Facilitate strengthening with functional activity
  - Facilitate good trunk control in upright activities
  - Increase endurance with functional activities
  - Maximize gait with appropriate device/orthotics
  - Continue to avoid over-fatigue and injury to weakened muscles

Functional Carryover
- Instruction in energy conservation techniques
- Decrease utilization of assistive device

DISCHARGE PLANNING AND PATIENT RESPONSIBILITY

Criteria for Discharge
- All rehabilitation goals achieved
- All patient/family goals achieved
- Patient demonstrates compliance with home program

Circumstances Requiring Additional Visits
- Comorbidities
- Age
- Ventilator dependence
- Complications
- Severity of disease
- Use of plasmophoresis/intravenous immunoglobulin therapy
- Cranial nerve involvement
- Contractures
- Cognitive dysfunction
- Excessive muscle belly tenderness

Home Program
- ROM
- Strengthening
- Cardiovascular activities

REFERENCES

1. American Physical Therapy Association. *Guide to Physical Therapist Practice*. Alexandria, VA: APTA; 1997.

2. Beghi E, Bono A, Bogliun G, et al. The prognosis and main prognostic indicators of Guillain-Barré syndrome: a multicenter prospective study of 297 patients. *Brain J Neurol*. 1996:119:2053-2061.

3. Foster E. Functional mobility and length of hospital stay in the acute rehabilitation of individuals with Gillian-Barré Syndrome. *J Neurol Phys Ther*. Dec 2004.

4. Gray H; Williams PL, ed. *Gray's Anatomy*. 38th ed. New York, NY: Churchill Livingstone; 1995.

5. Hart A, Hopkins C, Ford B. *ICD-9-CM Expert for Physicians, Volume 1&2*. 7th ed. USA: Ingenix. 2005.

6. Itahn A. Guillain-Barré syndrome. *Lancet*. 1998;352:635-641.

7. Meythaler JM, DeVivo MJ, Braswell WC. Rehabilitation outcomes of patients who have developed Guillain-Barré syndrome. *Am J Phys Med Rehab*. 1997;76:411-419.

8. Meythaler JM. Rehabilitation of Guillain-Barré syndrome. *Arch Phys Med Rehabil*. 1997;78:872-879.

9. O'Sullivan SB, Schmitz TJ. *Physical Rehabilitation: Assessment and Treatment*. Philadelphia, PA: FA Davis; 1994.

10. Pitetti KH, Barrett PJ, Abbas D. Endurance exercise training in Guillain-Barré syndrome. *Arch Phys Med Rehabil*. 1993;74:761-765.

11. Umphred DA. *Neurological Rehabilitation*. St. Louis, MO: CV Mosby; 1995.

MULTIPLE SCLEROSIS
SUMMARY OVERVIEW

ICD-9

   340

APTA Preferred Practice Pattern: **5C, 6B, 6F, 6G, 7A**

EXAMINATION

- History and Systems Review
- Tests and Measures
  Systems review per APTA's *Guide to Physical Therapy Practice*
  - Aerobic capacity and endurance
  - Arousal, attention, cognition
  - Assistive devices/orthotics
  - Cranial nerve integrity
  - Gait, locomotion, and balance
  - Motor function
  - Muscle performance
  - Pain
  - ROM
  - Self-care and home management
  - Sensory integrity
- Establish Plan of Care

GOALS/OUTCOMES

- Independence in functional status with/without assistive device or caregiver involvement
- Independent/safe use with all adaptive/assistive equipment
- Maximize respiratory capacity
- Pain: 2/10 with activity
- Maintain ROM and endurance for mobility
- Prevent or delay secondary impairments
- Patient and family independence in assisting functional mobility
- Prevent contractures

INTERVENTION
NUMBER OF VISITS: 2–12

- Patient Instruction
  - Education
  - Handouts
  - Functional Considerations
- Direct Interventions
  - Initial Onset of Symptoms: 2–12 Visits
- Functional Carryover

DISCHARGE PLANNING/ PATIENT RESPONSIBILITY

- Criteria for Discharge
  - Rehab patient/family goals achieved
  - Patient demonstrates compliance with home exercise program
- Circumstances Requiring Additional Visits
  - Comorbidities
  - Cognitive dysfunction
  - Arthritis
  - Pulmonary complications
  - Poor physical condition
- Home Program
  - Strengthening exercises
  - Cardiovascular activities
  - ROM exercises

SUMMARY OVERVIEW | NEUROLOGICAL CONDITIONS | MULTIPLE SCLEROSIS   **699**

MULTIPLE SCLEROSIS

ICD-9

340   Multiple sclerosis

APTA Preferred Practice Pattern: 5C, 6B, 6F, 6G, 7A

INTRODUCTION

Multiple Sclerosis is a demyelinating disease of the central nervous system. Age of onset is approximately 15–50 years of age. It is a progressive disease that can be divided into three patterns:

- Classic pattern: Exacerbations and remissions, there may be minimal residual disability or more severe/progressive symptoms resulting in disability
- Progressive pattern: Progression is usually slow without delineated periods of relapse/remission
- Combination of first two patterns, starts with classic relapsing/remitting course but becomes progressive with limited remission

The most common problems associated with multiple sclerosis include:

- Fatigue
- Gait
- Bowel/bladder
- Pain and other sensations
- Visual disturbances
- Cognitive dysfunction
- Tremors

Overall, the course of the disease is unpredictable; therapists may see clients at any stage. A focus on early intervention, modification, and compensation for existing impairments rather than restoration is essential for successful rehabilitation. The therapist's judgment in relation to the specific needs of each patient will determine the implementation of this guideline.

EXAMINATION

History and Systems Review

- History of current condition
  - Date of original diagnosis
  - Past and current therapeutic interventions
  - Description of symptoms
  - Patient and family therapeutic/functional goals
- Medications
  - For current condition
- Past medical/surgical history
  - Prior hospitalization
  - Previous surgeries
  - Pre-existing conditions
- Functional status and activity level (current/prior)
- Social history
  - Family/caregiver resources
  - Social activity/support systems
- Living environment
  - Home vs. board and care vs. extended care facility
    - Stairs/railings/carpet/wheelchair access, etc.
    - Alone vs. family support/caregiver
    - Desired discharge destination
- Occupation/employment
  - Current and prior work/school
- Patient's functional goals

Tests and Measures

Systems review per APTA's *Guide to Physical Therapy Practice*

- Aerobic capacity and endurance
  - Perceived exertion
  - Chest expansion with inspiration
  - Breathing pattern
  - Fatigue assessment
  - Modified fatigue impact scale
- Arousal, attention, cognition
  - Orientation
    - Person
    - Place
    - Time
    - Purpose

700   MULTIPLE SCLEROSIS | NEUROLOGICAL CONDITIONS

- Motivation level
- Ability to follow directions
- Memory (long and short term)
- Assistive devices/orthotics
  - Needs assessment
  - Effects and benefits
- Cranial nerve integrity
  - Visual disturbances
- Gait, locomotion, and balance
  - Assessment of presence of vertigo
  - Static and dynamic balance
    - Tinetti, Berg, "Get Up and Go" (if applicable)
  - Gait analysis/characteristics
    - Phases of gait
      a. Swing and stance
      b. Single- vs. double-limb support
      c. Analysis of head, trunk, upper, and lower extremities
      d. Note deviations
    - Cadence, velocity, and stride length
    - Test gait on varied terrains
      a. Smooth, uneven, incline/decline, etc.
  - Wheelchair mobility/management
    - Manual vs. electric
  - Safety
- Motor function
  - Dexterity and coordination
    - Grasp and release object
    - Finger to nose and heel to shin
  - Head, trunk, and limb movement
    - Postural, equilibrium, and righting reactions
  - Trunk mobility/control
    - Lying, sitting, standing, locomotion
    - Transition from supine, sitting, standing to wheelchair
  - Initiation of movement
  - Quality of movement
  - Voluntary vs. involuntary movement
  - Transfers
  - Bed mobility
- Muscle performance
  - Manual muscle test (if applicable)
  - Functional muscle strength
  - Tone
    - Hypotonic vs. hypertonic
  - Spasticity
    - Ashworth scale

- Involuntary muscle spasms
  - Most common in lower extremities
- Tremors
- Pain
  - Neuralgia vs. musculoskeletal
  - Visual analog scale
  - Observation of facial expression/behavior
  - Body chart
- ROM
  - Passive/active
  - Functional ROM
  - Substitutions
  - Cause of limitation
- Self-care and home management
  - Bowel/bladder dysfunction
  - ADLs scale
    - Barthel Index
- Sensory integrity
  - Light touch and temperature
  - Proprioception

Establish Plan of Care
- Based on history, tests, and measures

GOALS/OUTCOMES
- Independence in functional status with/without assistive device or caregiver involvement
- Independent/safe use with all adaptive/assistive equipment
- Maximize respiratory capacity
- Pain: 2/10 with activity
- Maintain ROM and endurance for mobility
- Prevent or delay secondary impairments
- Patient and family independence in assisting functional mobility
- Prevent contractures

INTERVENTION

NUMBER OF VISITS: 2–12

Coordination, Communication, and Documentation

- Provision of services between admission and discharge that facilitate cost-effective and efficient integration or reintegration to home, community, or work
- Documentation of therapeutic intervention is required for each episode of care and serves as the basic foundation for communication
- Coordination and additional communication will depend on the patient's impairment and home/work/community/leisure situation and requirements. Such services may include:
  - Case management
  - Coordination of care and collaboration with those integral to the patient's rehabilitation program
  - Coordination and monitoring of the delivery of available resources
  - Referrals to other health-care professionals
  - Identification of resources, support groups, or advocacy services
  - Provision of educational or training information
  - Technical assistance
- Specific coordination and communication provisions:
  - Multiple disciplinary approach addressing all patient needs
    - Occupational therapy
    - Recreational therapy
    - Social worker/case manager
    - Respiratory therapy
    - Speech therapy

Patient Instruction

Education

- Information on disease progression and rehabilitation component

Handouts

- Home exercise program to increase general endurance/cardiovascular condition, ROM, and function

Functional Considerations

- Safety education with all mobility and use of equipment
- Energy conservation techniques: Avoid fatigue; plan activities at time of day when energy is highest
- Family/attendant training based on patient/client need
- Cooling techniques with activity instruction
- Environmental modifications/use of adaptive/assistive devices

Direct Interventions

Initial Onset of Symptoms: 2–12 Visits

Ongoing monitoring: 2–12 visits per episode of symptom exacerbation (see summary page). Coordinate care with other services to avoid excessive fatigue

- ROM
  - Daily passive and active stretching
    - Self ROM
- Strengthening
  - Strengthen non-affected muscles to prevent weakness and atrophy
  - Strengthen agonists and relax antagonist (to help regulate/control spasticity)
  - Emphasize proximal strengthening to help energy conservation/stability with functional activities
  - Aerobic exercise
- Positioning program
  - Proper bed and wheelchair positioning to maximize normal tone and alignment/posture and to decrease reflexive activity
  - Reclining vs. upright wheelchair
  - Balance time in and out of wheelchair or bed
  - Increase sitting tolerance
  - Ankle-foot orthosis
- Trunk mobility and control
  - Trunk mobilization exercises with inhibition of spastic muscles
  - Focus on activities that promote trunk flexion with trunk rotation due to extensor tone tending to predominate. Example: Proprioceptive neuromuscular facilitation bilateral upper extremity/diagonal trunk patterns: chopping and lifting
  - Facilitate trunk stabilization to help decrease limb and trunk ataxia. Examples:
    - Rhythmic stabilization
    - Prone on elbows

702   MULTIPLE SCLEROSIS | NEUROLOGICAL CONDITIONS

- Quadriped
- Approximation
- Combine above with functional activities in sitting, standing, and during transitions
- Balance training/upright motor control
  - Utilization of above trunk control training will enhance all balance/upright motor control
  - Static balance training progress to dynamic balance training. Examples:
    - Trunk perturbations in sit/standing
    - Weight shifting in sit/standing on stable surface
    - Sitting activities on Swiss ball/stimulate righting reactions
    - Standing activities on rockerboard
    - Frenkel's exercises: Exercise progress from postures of greatest stability to postures of greatest challenge (less stability)
    - Weighted cuffs or manual resistance to increase proprioceptive feedback during activities for ataxic limbs
    - Vestibular exercise program
  - Give frequent verbal feedback: Knowledge of results and performance improves motor learning
  - Visual feedback may improve performance
  - Sensory stimulation/compensatory strategies
- Gait/locomotion
  - Utilization of above upright motor control training will enhance gait training ability and is essential for progression to gait
  - Pre-gait
    - High stepping to strengthen hip flexors
    - Heel walking to strengthen dorsiflexors
    - Partial squats to strengthen quadriceps and prevent hyperextension of knee
    - Controlled stepping forward and back with weight shift to facilitate quad control and prevent hyperextension
    - Hip abduction in standing
    - Increase sitting/standing tolerance/endurance gradually

  - Gait training
    - Change of direction (forward, backward, sidestepping)
    - Change of surface
    - Monitor fatigue levels
    - Assess need for assistive device
- Breathing strategies
  - Diaphragmatic breathing
  - Resistive breathing
- Manual therapy
  - Soft-tissue mobilization
- Physical agents and mechanical modalities
  - Pain management
- Functional training in home/community
  - Bed mobility training
  - Transfer training based on individual needs/ability of client
    - Sliding board
    - From different heights/surfaces
    - Sit to/from stand
    - Bed to/from wheelchair or commode
- Therapeutic devices and equipment
  - Wheelchair
    - Manual vs. electric
    - Standard vs. reclining
    - Cushions/seating systems
  - Crutches
  - Walker
  - Cane
  - Wheelchair mobility program
  - Ankle-foot orthosis
  - Danish clogs for limited ankle mobility
  - Adaptations to home/work environment
  - Fall recovery training

Functional Carryover
- Caregiver training
- Positioning program
- Energy conservation

DISCHARGE PLANNING/ PATIENT RESPONSIBILITY

Criteria for Discharge
- Rehab patient/family goals achieved
- Patient demonstrates compliance with home exercise program

Circumstances Requiring Additional Visits
- Comorbidities
- Cognitive dysfunction
- Arthritis
- Pulmonary complications
- Poor physical condition

Home Program
- Strengthening exercises
- Cardiovascular activities
- ROM exercises

REFERENCES

1. American Physical Therapy Association. *Guide to Physical Therapist Practice.* Alexandria, VA: APTA; 2003.
2. Brar SP, Smith MB, Nelson LM, Franklin GM, Cobble ND. Evaluation of treatment protocols on minimal to moderate spasticity in multiple sclerosis. *Arch Phys Med Rehab.* 1991;72:186-189.
3. Chiara T, Carlos J Jr, Martin D, Miller R, Nadeau S. Cold effect on oxygen uptake, perceived exertion and spasticity in patients with multiple sclerosis. *Arch Phys Med Rehabil.* 1998;79:503-528.
4. DiFabio RP, Soderberg J, Choi T, Hansen CR, Schapiro RT. Extended outpatient rehabilitation: its influence on symptom frequency, fatigue and functional status for persons with progressive multiple sclerosis. *Arch Phys Med Rehabil.* 1998;9:141-146.
5. DiFabio RP, Choi T, Soderberg J, Hansen CR. Health-related quality of life for patients with progressive multiple sclerosis: influence of rehabilitation. *Phys Ther.* 1997;77:1704-1716.
6. Freeman JA, Langdon DW, Hobart JC, Thompson AJ. The impact of inpatient rehabilitation on progressive multiple sclerosis. *Ann Neurol.* 1997;42:236-244.
7. Gray H; Williams PL, ed. *Gray's Anatomy.* 38th ed. New York, NY: Churchill Livingstone; 1995.
8. Hart A, Hopkins C, Ford B. *ICD-9-CM Expert for Physicians, Volume 1&2.* 7th ed. USA: Ingenix. 2005.
9. Langgartner M, Langgartner I, Drlicek M. The patient's journey: multiple scerosis. *BMJ.* 2005;330:885-888.
10. O'Sullivan SB, Schmitz TJ. *Physical Rehabilitation: Assessment and Treatment.* Philadelphia, PA: FA Davis; 1994.
11. Provance, PG. *Physical Therapy in Multiple Sclerosis Rehabilitation. Clinical Bulletin; Information for Health Professionals.* National MS Society; 2004.
12. Schwid SR, Goodman AD, Mattson DH, et al. The measurement of ambulatory impairment in multiple sclerosis. *Neurology.* 1997;49:1419-1424.
13. Stulfbergen AK. Physical activity and perceived health status in persons with multiple sclerosis. *J Neurosci Nurs.* 1997;29:238-243.
14. Umphred DA. *Neurological Rehabilitation.* St. Louis, MO: CV Mosby; 1995.

PARKINSON'S DISEASE
SUMMARY OVERVIEW

ICD-9

332

APTA Preferred Practice Pattern: **5C, 6B, 6F, 6G, 7A**

EXAMINATION

- History and Systems Review
- Tests and Measures
  Systems review per APTA's *Guide to Physical Therapy Practice*
  - Aerobic capacity and endurance
  - Arousal, attention, cognition
  - Assistive and adaptive devices/orthotics
  - Cranial nerve integrity
  - Gait, locomotion, and balance
  - Motor function
  - Muscle performance
  - Pain
  - ROM
  - Self-care and home management
  - Sensory integrity
- Establish Plan of Care

GOALS/OUTCOMES

- Promote full functional ROM all joints
- Prevent contractures
- Correct posture deficits
- Prevent muscle weakness
- Increase chest expansion
- Promote functional mobility
- Facilitate fluidity of movement
- Maintain or increase trunk and pelvis mobility
- Improve postural and equilibrium reactions
- Improve initiation of movements
- Independence with home exercise program
- Fall recovery
- Maintain or improve oral motor function and fluidity of expression

INTERVENTION
NUMBER OF VISITS: 4–7

- Patient Instruction
  - Education
  - Home Program
  - Functional Considerations
- Direct Interventions
- Functional Carryover

PATIENT RESPONSIBILITY

- Criteria for Discharge
  - Rehab caregiver/patient goals achieved
  - Patient demonstrates compliance with home exercise program
- Circumstances Requiring Additional Visits
  - Comorbidity
  - Cognitive dysfunction
  - Caregiver issues
  - Pulmonary complications
  - Contractures
- Home Program
  - ROM and strengthening
  - Group activity
  - Low-impact aerobics
  - Exercise to music
  - Warm-up exercise large joints prior to exercise/activity
  - Ballroom dancing
  - Stationary bike
  - Swimming

SUMMARY OVERVIEW | NEUROLOGICAL CONDITIONS | PARKINSON'S DISEASE   705

PARKINSON'S DISEASE

ICD-9
> 332   Parkinson's disease

APTA Preferred Practice Pattern: **5C, 6B, 6F, 6G, 7A**

INTRODUCTION

Parkinson's disease is a chronic, progressive disease of the central nervous system. Most commonly it is idiopathic in nature. It is classified by a deficiency of the neurotransmitter dopamine in the basal ganglia. Classic signs and symptoms include: Rigidity, bradykinesia, resting tremor, postural abnormalities, decreased equilibrium reactions, masked face, and "freezing" episodes in which there is great difficulty in initiating movement. There have also been cases of Parkinson's disease with dementia, depression, and autonomic changes. This guideline is designed to help in the management of clients with Parkinson's disease. Therapists may see clients at any stage of the disease from early onset with slight deficits to severe involvement.

EXAMINATION

History and Systems Review

- History of current condition
  - Date of original diagnosis
  - Past and current therapeutic interventions
  - Description of symptoms
  - Patient and family therapeutic/functional goals
- Medications
  - For current condition
- Past medical/surgical history
  - Prior hospitalization
  - Previous surgeries
  - Pre-existing conditions
- Functional status and activity level (current/prior)
- Social history
  - Family/caregiver resources
  - Social activity/support systems
- Living environment
  - Home vs. board and care vs. extended care facility
    - Stairs/railings/carpet/wheelchair access, etc.
  - Alone vs. family support/caregiver
  - Desired discharge destination
- Occupation/employment
  - Current and prior work/school
- Patient's functional goals

Tests and Measures

Systems review per APTA's *Guide to Physical Therapy Practice*

- Aerobic capacity and endurance
  - Perceived exertion
  - Chest expansion with inspiration
  - Breathing pattern
- Arousal, attention, cognition
  - Orientation
    - Person
    - Place
    - Time
    - Purpose
  - Motivation level
  - Ability to follow direction
  - Memory (long and short term)
- Assistive and adaptive devices/orthotics
  - Needs assessment
  - Effects and benefits
- Cranial nerve integrity
- Gait, locomotion, and balance
  - Static and dynamic balance
    - Tinetti, Berg, "Get Up and Go" (if applicable)
  - Gait analysis/characteristics
    - Phases of gait
      a. Swing and stance
      b. Single vs. double limb support
      c. Analysis of head, trunk, upper extremities, and lower extremities
      d. Note deviations
    - Cadence, velocity, and stride length
    - Varied terrains
      a. Smooth, uneven, incline/decline, etc.
  - Wheelchair mobility/management
    - Manual vs. electric
  - Safety

706   PARKINSON'S DISEASE | NEUROLOGICAL CONDITIONS

- Motor function
  - Dexterity and coordination
    - Grasp and release object
    - Finger to nose and heel to shin
  - Head, trunk, and limb movement
    - Postural, equilibrium, and righting reactions
  - Trunk mobility/control
    - Lying, sitting, standing, locomotion
    - Transition from supine, sitting, standing to wheelchair
  - Initiation of movement
  - Quality of movement
  - Voluntary vs. involuntary movement
  - Ability to transfer
  - Bed mobility
  - Ability to change directions
- Muscle performance
  - Manual muscle test (if applicable)
  - Functional muscle strength
  - Tone
    - Hypertonicity is most common
    - Rigidity
- Pain
  - Visual analog scale or Universal Pan Assessment Tool
  - Observation of facial expression/behavior
  - Body chart if motor skills allow
- ROM
  - Passive/active
  - Functional ROM
  - Substitutions
  - Cause of limitation
- Self-care and home management
  - ADLs scale
    - Barthel Index
- Sensory integrity
  - Light touch and temperature
  - Proprioception

Establish Plan of Care
- Based on history, tests, and measures

GOALS/OUTCOMES
- Promote full functional ROM all joints
- Prevent contractures
- Correct posture deficits
- Prevent muscle weakness
- Increase chest expansion
- Promote functional mobility
- Facilitate fluidity of movement
- Maintain or increase trunk and pelvis mobility
- Improve postural and equilibrium reactions
- Improve initiation of movements
- Independence with home exercise program
- Fall recovery
- Maintain or improve oral motor function and fluidity of expression

INTERVENTION
NUMBER OF VISITS: 4–7

Coordination, Communication, and Documentation
- Provision of services between admission and discharge that facilitate cost-effective and efficient integration or reintegration to home, community, or work
- Documentation of therapeutic intervention is required for each episode of care and serves as the basic foundation for communication
- Coordination and additional communication will depend on the patient's impairment and home/work/community/leisure situation and requirements. Such services may include:
  - Case management
  - Coordination of care and collaboration with those integral to the patient's rehabilitation program
  - Coordination and monitoring of the delivery of available resources
  - Referrals to other health-care professionals
  - Identification of resources, support groups, or advocacy services
  - Provision of educational or training information
  - Technical assistance
- Specific coordination and communication provisions:
  - Multidiscipline referrals will depend on stage and progression of disease
    - Social worker
    - Speech/language pathology
    - Occupational therapy

NEUROLOGICAL CONDITIONS | PARKINSON'S DISEASE   707

Patient Instruction

Education
- Information on disease progression and rehabilitation component
  - Krames Communications (1100 Grundy Lane, San Bruno, CA 94066):
    - *Parkinson's Disease*

Home Program
- ROM/stretching instruction
- Relaxation instruction

Functional Considerations
- Safety with all mobility
- Fall recovery instruction

Direct Interventions
- Number of Visits
  - Initial onset of symptoms: 2–3 visits
  - Ongoing monitoring: 2–4 visits per episode
- Therapeutic exercise and home program
  - ROM
    - Relaxation techniques to reduce rigidity
      a. Gentle, slow rocking, rotation of trunk and extremities
      b. Yoga
      c. Sitting position improves relaxation
      d. Proprioceptive neuromuscular facilitation (PNF) rhythmic initiation
      e. Passive to active
      f. Small range to full range
    - Start distal and move proximal
    - Start with bilateral and symmetrical movements
    - Progress to unilateral and reciprocal movements
    - Movement through full range
    - Neurodevelopmental treatment (NDT)/ mobilization of scapulæ and pelvis
    - Progress to functional movement patterns
    - Avoid excessive stretching and pain
    - Increase anterior pelvic tilt
    - Emphasize pelvis mobility, trunk rotation and extension
    - Facial muscle expressions (mimic examples)
  - Equilibrium reactions
    - All planes of motion

- Rhythmic stabilization (monitor resistance, avoid increased trunk rigidity)
- Slow, gradual resistance
- Allow extra time for patient to match resistance
- Start with low-velocity weight shifts: Sitting and standing
  - Swiss ball: Sitting activities for postural reactions and trunk mobility
    a. Lower extremity marching and upper extremity swing
    b. Perturbation
  - Respiratory considerations
    - Breathing exercise
      a. Diaphragmatic breathing
    - Chest stretching
      a. Trunk extension
      b. Prone on elbows, prone extension
      c. Standing with arms raised against wall
      d. Manual thoracic mobilization
      e. Myofascial release
    - In conjunction with upper extremity exercises
      a. Bilateral upper extremity flexion/extension pattern (diagonal 2)
    - Reciprocal arm swing—upright activity and gait training
- Functional training
  - Bed mobility training
    - Firm bed
    - Reduce friction on surface, increase ease
    - Rolling with PNF and NDT patterns
  - Transfer training
    - Initiate with anterior/posterior trunk rocking for relaxation and reduced tone
    - PNF/NDT techniques
    - Initiation of sit to stand, sitting and bouncing on Swiss ball
  - Gait training
    - Practice changing directions
      a. Forward, backward, sideways, braiding
    - Visual cues
      a. Floor markings for increased stride
      b. Stepping over objects
    - Auditory cues
      a. Counting: 1-2, 1-2
      b. Music
      c. Metronome

- Assistive device may/may not be beneficial due to coordination for cane, tendency for increase of festinating gait with walker
- Emphasize heel-toe gait pattern
  a. Duck walking
- Increase arm swing
  a. With wands
- Facilitate trunk rotation
  ○ Pre-gait activity
  - Weight shifting (sagittal plane)
  - Sit to stand
  - PNF/NDT
  ○ Fall recovery
  - Safety techniques getting up off floor

Functional Carryover
- Instruction on use of assistive/adaptive device
- Home modification/safety
- Coordination of activity with medication

DISCHARGE PLANNING AND PATIENT RESPONSIBILITY

Criteria for Discharge
- Rehab caregiver/patient goals achieved
- Patient demonstrates compliance with home exercise program

Circumstances Requiring Additional Visits
- Comorbidity
- Cognitive dysfunction
- Caregiver issues
- Pulmonary complications
- Contractures

Home Program
- ROM and strengthening
- Group activity
- Low-impact aerobics
- Exercise to music
- Warm-up exercise large joints prior to exercise/activity
- Ballroom dancing
- Stationary bike
- Swimming

REFERENCES

1. American Physical Therapy Association. *Guide to Physical Therapist Practice.* Alexandria, VA: APTA; 2003.
2. Bridgewater KJ, Sharpe MH. Trunk performance in early Parkinson's disease. *Phys Ther.* 1998;78:566-575.
3. Caglar AT, Gurses NH, Mutlvay FK, Kiziltan G. Effects of home exercise on motor performance in patients with Parkinsons disease. *Clinical Rehabilitation.* 2005;19, 870-877.
4. Corcos DM. Strategies underlying the control of disordered movement. *Phys Ther.* 1991;7:25-38.
5. Gray H; Williams PL, ed. *Gray's Anatomy.* 38th ed. New York, NY: Churchill Livingstone; 1995.
6. Hart A, Hopkins C, Ford B. *ICD-9-CM Expert for Physicians, Volume 1&2.* 7th ed. USA: Ingenix. 2005.
7. Horak FB, et al. Patients with Parkinson's disease perseverate postural adjustments for compensatory stepping. *Neurol Rep.* 1998;22(5):180-181.
8. O'Sullivan SB, Schmitz TJ. *Physical Rehabilitation: Assessment and Treatment.* Philadelphia, PA: FA Davis; 1994.
9. Smithson F, Morris ME, Lansek R. Performance on clinical tests of balance in Parkinson's disease. *Phys Ther.* 1998;78:577-585.
10. Stelmach GE, Phillips JG. Movement disorders - limbo movement and the basal banglia. *Phys Ther.* 1991;71:60-67.
11. Umphred DA. *Neurological Rehabilitation.* St. Louis, MO: CV Mosby; 1995.

Appendix/Index

APPENDIX

ICD-9	Diagnosis	APTA Preferred Practice Pattern	Rehabilitation Guidelines	Page #
250	Diabetes mellitus	4K, 7A, 7E	Amputations	643
250.8	Diabetes with other specified manifestations	5E, 6B, 7A, 7B, 7C, 7D, 7E	Diabetic Foot	43
307.81	Tension headache	4B, 4C, 4D, 4E, 4F, 4G, 4I, 5D	Headache	367
307.81	Tension headache	4B, 4C, 4D, 4E, 4F, 4G, 4I, 5D, 7A	Stress Management	384
332	Parkinson's disease	5C, 6B, 6F, 6G, 7A	Parkinson's Disease	705
337.20	Reflex sympathetic dystrophy, unspecified	4D	Reflex Sympathetic Dystrophy of the Upper Extremity	593
337.21	Reflex sympathetic dystrophy of the upper limb	4D	Reflex Sympathetic Dystrophy of the Upper Extremity	593
337.29	Reflex sympathetic dystrophy of other specified site	4D	Reflex Sympathetic Dystrophy of the Upper Extremity	593
340	Multiple sclerosis	5C, 6B, 6F, 6G, 7A	Multiple Sclerosis	699
342	Hemiplegia and hemiparesis	4B, 4G, 5B, 5C	Cerebral Vascular Accident	683
346	Migraine	4B, 4C, 4D, 4E, 4F, 4G, 4I, 5D	Headache	367
346	Migraine	4B, 4C, 4D, 4E, 4F, 4G, 4I, 5D, 7A	Stress Management	384
350.2	Atypical face pain	4B, 4C, 4D, 4E, 4F, 4G, 4I, 5D	Headache	367
350.2	Atypical face pain	4B, 4C, 4D, 4E, 4F, 4G, 4I, 5D, 7A	Stress Management	384
353.0	Brachial plexus lesions	4F, 5D	Thoracic Outlet Syndrome	353
353.2	Cervical root lesions, not elsewhere classified	4F, 5D	Thoracic Outlet Syndrome	353
353.3	Thoracic root lesions, not elsewhere classified	4F, 5D	Thoracic Outlet Syndrome	353
353.5	Neuralgic amyotrophy	4F, 5D	Thoracic Outlet Syndrome	353
353.6	Phantom limb (syndrome)	4K, 7A, 7E	Amputations	643
353.8	Other nerve root and plexus disorders	4D, 4E, 4F, 4H, 5D	Rib Dysfunction	341
353.8	Other nerve root and plexus disorders	4F, 5D	Thoracic Outlet Syndrome	353
353.9	Unspecified nerve root and plexus disorder	4F, 5D	Thoracic Outlet Syndrome	353
354.0	Carpal tunnel syndrome	4F	Carpal Tunnel Syndrome	537
354.0	Carpal tunnel syndrome	4F	Postoperative Carpal Tunnel Release	565
354.2	Lesion of ulnar nerve	4E, 5F	Ulnar Nerve Lesion	530

APPENDIX   711

ICD-9	Diagnosis	APTA Preferred Practice Pattern	Rehabilitation Guidelines	Page #
355.5	Tarsal tunnel syndrome	4A, 4B, 4C, 4D, 4E, 4F, 4G, 4H, 4I, 4J, 4K, 5D, 6B	Biomechanical Lower Extremity Dysfunction	33
355.6	Lesion of plantar nerve	4A, 4B, 4C, 4D, 4E, 4F, 4G, 4H, 4I, 4J, 4K, 5D, 6B	Biomechanical Lower Extremity Dysfunction	33
356.1	Peroneal muscular atrophy	4A, 4B, 4F, 4G, 4H, 4J, 5E, 6F	Scoliosis	347
357.0	Acute infective polyneuritis	5E, 6B, 6F, 6G	Guillain-Barré Syndrome	693
386.50	Labyrinthine dysfunction, unspecified	4B, 4C, 4H, 4K, 5B	Vestibular Rehabilitation	667
386.51	Hyperactive labyrinth, unilateral	4B, 4C, 4H, 4K, 5B	Vestibular Rehabilitation	667
386.56	Loss of labyrinthine reactivity, bilateral	4B, 4C, 4H, 4K, 5B	Vestibular Rehabilitation	667
431	Intracerebral hemorrhage	4B, 4G, 5B, 5C	Cerebral Vascular Accident	683
433	Occlusion and stenosis of precerebral arteries	4B, 4G, 5B, 5C	Cerebral Vascular Accident	683
434	Occlusion of cerebral arteries	4B, 4G, 5B, 5C	Cerebral Vascular Accident	683
435	Transient cerebral ischemia	4B, 4G, 5B, 5C	Cerebral Vascular Accident	683
436	Acute, but ill-defined, cerebrovascular disease	4B, 4G, 5B, 5C	Cerebral Vascular Accident	683
442	Other aneurysm	4B, 4G, 5B, 5C	Cerebral Vascular Accident	683
524.6	Temporomandibular joint disorders	4I, 4J	Postoperative Rehabilitation of the Temporomandibular Joint	373
524.6	Temporomandibular joint disorders	4B, 4C, 4D, 4E, 4F, 4G, 4I, 5D, 7A	Stress Management	384
524.6	Temporomandibular joint disorders	4B, 4C, 4D, 4E, 4F, 4G, 4H, 4I	Temporomandibular Dysfunction	389
524.9	Unspecified dentofacial anomalies	4B, 4C, 4D, 4E, 4F, 4G, 4J	Postural Dysfunction	263
524.9	Unspecified dentofacial anomalies	4B, 4C, 4D, 4E, 4F, 4G, 4I, 5D, 7A	Stress Management	384
526.9	Unspecified disease of the jaws	4B, 4C, 4D, 4E, 4F, 4G, 4H, 4I	Temporomandibular Dysfunction	389
564.8	Other specified functional disorders of intestine	4A, 4B, 4C, 4D, 4E, 4F, 4G, 4H, 7A, 7C, 7D	Pelvic Floor Dysfunction	249
569.42	Anal or rectal pain	4A, 4B, 4C, 4D, 4E, 4F, 4G, 4H, 7A, 7C, 7D	Pelvic Floor Dysfunction	249
595.1	Chronic interstitial cystitis	4A, 4B, 4C, 4D, 4E, 4F, 4G, 4H, 7A, 7C, 7D	Pelvic Floor Dysfunction	249
596.59	Other functional disorder of bladder	4A, 4B, 4C, 4D, 4E, 4F, 4G, 4H, 7A, 7C, 7D	Pelvic Floor Dysfunction	249
618.8	Other specified genital prolapse	4A, 4B, 4C, 4D, 4E, 4F, 4G, 4H, 7A, 7C, 7D	Pelvic Floor Dysfunction	249
625.0	Dyspareunia	4A, 4B, 4C, 4D, 4E, 4F, 4G, 4H, 7A, 7C, 7D	Pelvic Floor Dysfunction	249
625.1	Vaginismus	4A, 4B, 4C, 4D, 4E, 4F, 4G, 4H, 7A, 7C, 7D	Pelvic Floor Dysfunction	249
625.6	Stress incontinence, female	4A, 4B, 4C, 4D, 4E, 4F, 4G, 4H, 7A, 7C, 7D	Pelvic Floor Dysfunction	249

ICD-9	Diagnosis	APTA Preferred Practice Pattern	Rehabilitation Guidelines	Page #
625.8	Other specified symptoms associated with female genital organs	4A, 4B, 4C, 4D, 4E, 4F, 4G, 4H, 7A, 7C, 7D	Pelvic Floor Dysfunction	249
625.9	Unspecified symptom associated with female genital organs	4A, 4B, 4C, 4D, 4E, 4F, 4G, 4H, 7A, 7C, 7D	Pelvic Floor Dysfunction	249
696.5	Other and unspecified pityriasis	4A, 4B, 4C, 4D, 4E, 4F, 4G, 4H, 7A, 7C, 7D	Pelvic Floor Dysfunction	249
707.10	Ulcer of lower limb, unspecified	5E, 6B, 7A, 7B, 7C, 7D, 7E	Diabetic Foot	43
707.13	Ulcer of ankle	5E, 6B, 7A, 7B, 7C, 7D, 7E	Diabetic Foot	43
707.14	Ulcer of heel and midfoot	5E, 6B, 7A, 7B, 7C, 7D, 7E	Diabetic Foot	43
707.15	Ulcer of other part of foot	5E, 6B, 7A, 7B, 7C, 7D, 7E	Diabetic Foot	43
707.19	Ulcer of other part of lower limb	5E, 6B, 7A, 7B, 7C, 7D, 7E	Diabetic Foot	43
714	Rheumatoid arthritis and other inflammatory polyarthropathies	4A, 4B, 4C, 4D, 4F, 4G, 4H, 4I, 4J, 6B	Arthritis	653
715	Osteoarthrosis and allied disorders	4A, 4B, 4C, 4D, 4F, 4G, 4H, 4I, 4J, 6B	Arthritis	653
715.00	Osteoarthrosis, generalized, site unspecified	4C, 4D, 4E, 4F, 4G, 4H, 4I, 4J, 6B	Hip Pain in Runners—Return to Sport	623
715.09	Osteoarthrosis, generalized, multiple sites	4C, 4D, 4E, 4F, 4G, 4H, 4I, 4J, 6B	Hip Pain in Runners—Return to Sport	623
715.35	Osteoarthrosis, localized, not specified whether primary or secondary, pelvic region and thigh	4A, 4F, 4H, 6B	Hip Degenerative Joint Disease	171
715.90	Osteoarthrosis, unspecified whether generalized or localized, site unspecified	4B, 4C, 4D, 4E, 4F, 4G, 4H, 4I, 4J, 5F, 6B	Cervical/Thoracic General Pain	295
715.90	Osteoarthrosis, unspecified whether generalized or localized, site unspecified	4B, 4C, 4D, 4E, 4F, 4G, 4H, 4I, 4J, 5F, 6B	Low Back General Pain	209
715.95	Osteoarthrosis, unspecified whether generalized or localized, pelvic region and thigh	4A, 4B, 4C, 4D, 4E, 4F, 4G, 4H, 4I, 4J, 4K, 5D, 6B	Biomechanical Lower Extremity Dysfunction	33
715.95	Osteoarthrosis, unspecified whether generalized or localized, pelvic region and thigh	4B, 4C, 4D, 4E, 4F, 4G, 4H, 4I, 4J, 5F, 6B	Low Back General Pain	209
715.96	Osteoarthrosis, unspecified whether generalized or localized, lower leg	4A, 4B, 4C, 4D, 4E, 4F, 4G, 4H, 4I, 4J, 4K, 5D, 6B	Biomechanical Lower Extremity Dysfunction	33
715.96	Osteoarthrosis, unspecified whether generalized or localized, lower leg	4B, 4C, 4D, 4E, 4F, 4G, 4I, 4J, 6B, 7A	Knee Arthroscopy	95
715.96	Osteoarthrosis, unspecified whether generalized or localized, lower leg	4C, 4D, 4F, 4G, 4H, 4I, 4J, 6B	Knee Degenerative Joint Disease	105
715.97	Osteoarthrosis, unspecified whether generalized or localized, ankle and foot	4A, 4B, 4C, 4D, 4E, 4F, 4G, 4H, 4I, 4J, 4K, 5D, 6B	Biomechanical Lower Extremity Dysfunction	33
715.98	Osteoarthrosis, unspecified whether generalized or localized, other specified sites	4B, 4C, 4D, 4E, 4F, 4G, 4H, 4I, 4J, 5F, 6B	Cervical/Thoracic General Pain	295

ICD-9	Diagnosis	APTA Preferred Practice Pattern	Rehabilitation Guidelines	Page #
715.98	Osteoarthrosis, unspecified whether generalized or localized, other specified sites	4B, 4C, 4D, 4E, 4F, 4G, 4H, 4I, 4J, 5F, 6B	Low Back General Pain	209
716.91	Arthropathy, unspecified, shoulder region	4D, 4E, 4F, 4G, 4J, 7A	Adhesive Capsulitis	399
716.91	Arthropathy, unspecified, shoulder region	4B,4C, 4D, 4E, 4F, 4G, 4I, 5D, 5H	Elbow/Shoulder Injury—Return to Tennis	615
716.91	Arthropathy, unspecified, shoulder region	4D, 4E, 4F, 4G, 4J	Shoulder Bursitis	447
716.91	Arthropathy, unspecified, shoulder region	4F, 4D, 4G, 7A	Shoulder Degenerative Joint Disease	455
716.91	Arthropathy, unspecified, shoulder region	4B, 4D, 4E, 4F, 4G, 4H, 4J, 7A	Shoulder Sprain/Strain	475
716.91	Arthropathy, unspecified, shoulder region	4D, 4E, 4F, 4G, 4J, 7A	Shoulder Tendinitis	483
716.94	Arthropathy, unspecified, hand	4D, 4E, 4F	Hand Arthropathy	557
717.0	Old bucket handle tear of medial meniscus	4E, 4I, 4J	Meniscal Repair	129
717.0	Old bucket handle tear of medial meniscus	4I, 4D, 4H	Meniscus Tear	135
717.1	Derangement of anterior horn of medial meniscus	4E, 4I, 4J	Meniscal Repair	129
717.1	Derangement of anterior horn of medial meniscus	4I, 4D, 4H	Meniscus Tear	135
717.2	Derangement of posterior horn of medial meniscus	4E, 4I, 4J	Meniscal Repair	129
717.2	Derangement of posterior horn of medial meniscus	4I, 4D, 4H	Meniscus Tear	135
717.3	Other and unspecified derangement of medial meniscus	4E, 4I, 4J	Meniscal Repair	129
717.3	Other and unspecified derangement of medial meniscus	4I, 4D, 4H	Meniscus Tear	135
717.4	Derangement of lateral meniscus	4E, 4I, 4J	Meniscal Repair	129
717.4	Derangement of lateral meniscus	4I, 4D, 4H	Meniscus Tear	135
717.5	Derangement of meniscus, not elsewhere classified	4E, 4I, 4J	Meniscal Repair	129
717.5	Derangement of meniscus, not elsewhere classified	4I, 4D, 4H	Meniscus Tear	135
717.7	Chondromalacia of patella	4A, 4D, 4E, 4F, 4G, 4H, 4I, 4J	Patellofemoral Syndrome	147
717.83	Old disruption of anterior cruciate ligament	4B, 4C, 4D, 4E, 4F, 4G, 4I, 4J, 6B, 7A	Knee Arthroscopy	95
717.84	Old disruption of posterior cruciate ligament	4E, 4J	Posterior Cruciate Ligament Reconstruction	153
717.9	Unspecified internal derangement of knee	4B, 4C, 4D, 4E, 4F, 4G, 4I, 4J, 6B, 7A	Knee Arthroscopy	95
717.9	Unspecified internal derangement of knee	4E, 4I, 4J	Meniscal Repair	129
717.9	Unspecified internal derangement of knee	4I, 4D, 4H	Meniscus Tear	135
717.9	Unspecified internal derangement of knee	4A, 4D, 4E, 4F, 4G, 4H, 4I, 4J	Patellofemoral Syndrome	147

ICD-9	Diagnosis	APTA Preferred Practice Pattern	Rehabilitation Guidelines	Page #
718.21	Pathological dislocation, shoulder region	4B,4C, 4D, 4E, 4F, 4G, 4I, 5D, 5H	Elbow/Shoulder Injury—Return to Tennis	615
718.21	Pathological dislocation, shoulder region	4B, 4D, 4E, 4F, 4G, 4J	Postoperative Rehabilitation For Shoulder Instability	423
718.31	Recurrent dislocation of joint, shoulder region	4B,4C, 4D, 4E, 4F, 4G, 4I, 5D, 5H	Elbow/Shoulder Injury—Return to Tennis	615
718.31	Recurrent dislocation of joint, shoulder region	4B, 4D, 4E, 4F, 4G, 4J	Postoperative Rehabilitation For Shoulder Instability	423
718.31	Recurrent dislocation of joint, shoulder region	4B, 4D, 4E, 4F, 4G, 4J	Shoulder Anterior Dislocation	441
718.56	Ankylosis of joint, lower leg	4A, 4B, 4E, 4H, 4I, 4J	Knee Hypomobility/Infrapatellar Contracture Syndrome (IPCS)	117
718.81	Other joint derangement, not elsewhere classified, shoulder region	4B,4C, 4D, 4E, 4F, 4G, 4I, 5D, 5H	Elbow/Shoulder Injury—Return to Tennis	615
718.81	Other joint derangement, not elsewhere classified, shoulder region	4B, 4D, 4E, 4F, 4G, 4J	Postoperative Rehabilitation For Shoulder Instability	423
718.81	Other joint derangement, not elsewhere classified, shoulder region	4B, 4D, 4E, 4F, 4G, 4J	Shoulder Anterior Dislocation	441
718.81	Other joint derangement, not elsewhere classified, shoulder region	4B, 4D, 4E, 4F, 4G, 4H, 4J, 7A	Shoulder Sprain/Strain	475
718.86	Other joint derangement, not elsewhere classified, lower leg	4B, 4C, 4D, 4E, 4F, 4G, 4I, 4J, 6B, 7A	Knee Arthroscopy	95
718.91	Unspecified derangement of joint, shoulder region	4B,4C, 4D, 4E, 4F, 4G, 4I, 5D, 5H	Elbow/Shoulder Injury—Return to Tennis	615
718.91	Unspecified derangement of joint, shoulder region	4F, 4H, 4I	Shoulder Joint Pathology	467
719.41	Pain in joint, shoulder region	4D, 4E, 4F, 4G, 4J, 7A	Adhesive Capsulitis	399
719.41	Pain in joint, shoulder region	4B,4C, 4D, 4E, 4F, 4G, 4I, 5D, 5H	Elbow/Shoulder Injury—Return to Tennis	615
719.41	Pain in joint, shoulder region	4F, 4D, 4G, 7A	Shoulder Degenerative Joint Disease	455
719.41	Pain in joint, shoulder region	4B, 4D, 4E, 4F, 4G, 4H, 4J, 7A	Shoulder Sprain/Strain	475
719.41	Pain in joint, shoulder region	4D, 4E, 4F, 4G, 4J, 7A	Shoulder Tendinitis	483
719.42	Pain in joint, upper arm	4D, 4E, 4J, 7A	Elbow Sprain/Strain	511
719.42	Pain in joint, upper arm	4B,4C, 4D, 4E, 4F, 4G, 4I, 5D, 5H	Elbow/Shoulder Injury—Return to Tennis	615
719.42	Pain in joint, upper arm	4E, 4F, 4J, 4D, 7A	Lateral Epicondylitis	517
719.42	Pain in joint, upper arm	4D, 4E, 4F, 4H, 4J, 7A	Medial Epicondylitis	523
719.43	Pain in joint, forearm	4D, 7A	Elbow Joint Pathology	506
719.43	Pain in joint, forearm	4B,4C, 4D, 4E, 4F, 4G, 4I, 5D, 5H	Elbow/Shoulder Injury—Return to Tennis	615
719.44	Pain in joint, hand	4D, 4E, 4F	Hand Arthropathy	557
719.45	Pain in joint, pelvic region and thigh	4A, 4B, 4C, 4D, 4E, 4F, 4G, 4H, 7A, 7C, 7D	Pelvic Floor Dysfunction	249
719.45	Pain in joint, pelvic region and thigh	4B, 4C, 4E, 4F, 4G, 4J, 7A	Sacroiliac Dysfunction	271

ICD-9	Diagnosis	APTA Preferred Practice Pattern	Rehabilitation Guidelines	Page #
719.46	Pain in joint, lower leg	4B, 4C, 4D, 4E, 4F, 4G, 4I, 4J, 6B, 7A	Knee Arthroscopy	95
719.47	Pain in joint, ankle and foot	4A, 4B, 4C, 4D, 4E, 4F, 4G, 4H, 4I, 4J, 4K, 5D, 6B	Biomechanical Lower Extremity Dysfunction	33
719.47	Pain in joint, ankle and foot	7B	Foot Contusion	51
719.51	Stiffness of joint, not elsewhere classified, shoulder region	4B,4C, 4D, 4E, 4F, 4G, 4I, 5D, 5H	Elbow/Shoulder Injury—Return to Tennis	615
719.51	Stiffness of joint, not elsewhere classified, shoulder region	4F, 4H, 4I	Shoulder Joint Pathology	467
719.52	Stiffness of joint, not elsewhere classified, upper arm	4B,4C, 4D, 4E, 4F, 4G, 4I, 5D, 5H	Elbow/Shoulder Injury—Return to Tennis	615
719.52	Stiffness of joint, not elsewhere classified, upper arm	4F, 4H, 4I	Shoulder Joint Pathology	467
719.55	Stiffness of joint, not elsewhere classified, pelvic region and thigh	4A, 4C, 4D, 4F, 4G, 4H, 4I, 4J, 7A	Hip Fracture/Total Hip Replacement—Inpatient	183
719.55	Stiffness of joint, not elsewhere classified, pelvic region and thigh	4A, 4C, 4D, 4F, 4G, 4H, 4I, 4J, 7A	Hip Fracture/Total Hip Replacement—Outpatient	177
719.56	Stiffness of joint, not elsewhere classified, lower leg	4A, 4B, 4E, 4H, 4I, 4J	Knee Hypomobility/Infrapatellar Contracture Syndrome (IPCS)	117
719.57	Stiffness of joint, not elsewhere classified, ankle and foot	4A, 4B, 4C, 4D, 4E, 4F, 4G, 4H, 4I, 4J, 4K, 5D, 6B	Biomechanical Lower Extremity Dysfunction	33
719.57	Stiffness of joint, not elsewhere classified, ankle and foot	7B	Foot Contusion	51
719.66	Other symptoms referable to joint, lower leg	4A, 4B, 4C, 4D, 4E, 4F, 4G, 4H, 4I, 4J, 4K, 5D, 6B	Biomechanical Lower Extremity Dysfunction	33
719.7	Difficulty in walking	4A, 4B, 4C, 4D, 4E, 4F, 4G, 4H, 4I, 4J, 4K, 5D, 6B	Biomechanical Lower Extremity Dysfunction	33
719.91	Unspecified disorder of joint, shoulder region	4B,4C, 4D, 4E, 4F, 4G, 4I, 5D, 5H	Elbow/Shoulder Injury—Return to Tennis	615
719.91	Unspecified disorder of joint, shoulder region	4F, 4H, 4I	Shoulder Joint Pathology	467
720.0	Ankylosing spondylitis	4F, 4G	Ankylosing Spondylitis	201
720.2	Sacroiliitis, not elsewhere classified	4A, 4B, 4C, 4D, 4E, 4F, 4G, 4H, 4I, 4J, 4K, 5D, 6B	Biomechanical Lower Extremity Dysfunction	33
721.0	Cervical spondylosis without myelopathy	4B, 4C, 4D, 4E, 4F, 4G, 4H, 4I, 4J, 5F, 6B	Cervical/Thoracic General Pain	295
721.1	Cervical spondylosis with myelopathy	4F, 5H, 4I	Cervical Spondylolysis with Myelopathy	308
721.3	Lumbosacral spondylosis without myelopathy	4B, 4C, 4D, 4E, 4F, 4G, 4H, 4I, 4J, 5F, 6B	Low Back General Pain	209

ICD-9	Diagnosis	APTA Preferred Practice Pattern	Rehabilitation Guidelines	Page #
721.4	Thoracic or lumbar spondylosis with myelopathy	4B, 4C, 4D, 4E, 4F, 4G, 4H, 4I, 4J, 5F, 6B	Low Back General Pain	209
721.4	Thoracic or lumbar spondylosis with myelopathy	4F, 4I, 5H	Lumbar Spondylolysis with Myelopathy	235
721.91	Spondylosis of unspecified site, with myelopathy	4F, 5H, 4I	Cervical Spondylolysis with Myelopathy	308
721.91	Spondylosis of unspecified site, with myelopathy	4F, 4I, 5H	Lumbar Spondylolysis with Myelopathy	235
722.0	Displacement of cervical intervertebral disc without myelopathy	4A, 4B, 4F, 4G, 4H, 4J, 5F	Cervical Disc Pathology	301
722.10	Displacement of lumbar intervertebral disc without myelopathy	4A, 4B, 4E, 4F, 4G, 4J	Lumbar Disc Pathology	219
722.2	Displacement of intervertebral disc, site unspecified, without myelopathy	4A, 4B, 4E, 4F, 4G, 4J	Lumbar Disc Pathology	219
722.4	Degeneration of cervical intervertebral disc	4A, 4B, 4F, 4G, 4H, 4J, 5F	Cervical Disc Pathology	301
722.52	Degeneration of lumbar or lumbosacral intervertebral disc	4A, 4B, 4E, 4F, 4G, 4J	Lumbar Disc Pathology	219
722.6	Degeneration of intervertebral disc, site unspecified	4A, 4B, 4E, 4F, 4G, 4J	Lumbar Disc Pathology	219
722.71	Intervertebral disc disorder with myelopathy, cervical region	4A, 4B, 4F, 4G, 4H, 4J, 5F	Cervical Disc Pathology	301
722.73	Intervertebral disc disorder with myelopathy, lumbar region	4F, 4I, 5H	Lumbar Spondylolysis with Myelopathy	235
722.80	Postlaminectomy syndrome, unspecified region	4B, 4G, 4H, 4J	Lumbar Surgery—Inpatient	243
722.80	Postlaminectomy syndrome, unspecified region	4B, 4G, 4H, 4J	Postoperative Rehabilitation of the Lumbar Spine	255
722.81	Postlaminectomy syndrome, cervical region	4D, 4G, 4H, 4J	Postoperative/Postfracture Rehabilitation of the C/T Spine	335
722.82	Postlaminectomy syndrome, thoracic region	4D, 4G, 4H, 4J	Postoperative/Postfracture Rehabilitation of the C/T Spine	335
722.83	Postlaminectomy syndrome, lumbar region	4B, 4G, 4H, 4J	Lumbar Surgery—Inpatient	243
722.83	Postlaminectomy syndrome, lumbar region	4B, 4G, 4H, 4J	Postoperative Rehabilitation of the Lumbar Spine	255
722.93	Other and unspecified disc disorder, lumbar region	4A, 4B, 4E, 4F, 4G, 4J	Lumbar Disc Pathology	219
723.0	Spinal stenosis in cervical region	4G	Cervical Stenosis	313
723.1	Cervicalgia	4B, 4C, 4D, 4E, 4F, 4G, 4H, 4I, 4J, 5F, 6B	Cervical/Thoracic General Pain	295
723.1	Cervicalgia	4B, 4C, 4D, 4E, 4F, 4G, 4J	Postural Dysfunction	263
723.4	Brachial neuritis or radiculitis NOS	4A, 4B, 4F, 4G, 4H, 4J, 5F	Cervical Disc Pathology	301
724.00	Spinal stenosis, unspecified region	4F, 4G, 4J	Spinal Stenosis	279
724.01	Spinal stenosis, thoracic region	4F, 4G, 4J	Spinal Stenosis	279
724.02	Spinal stenosis, lumbar region	4F, 4G, 4J	Spinal Stenosis	279

APPENDIX   717

ICD-9	Diagnosis	APTA Preferred Practice Pattern	Rehabilitation Guidelines	Page #
724.1	Pain in thoracic spine	4B, 4C, 4D, 4E, 4F, 4G, 4H, 4I, 4J, 5F, 6B	Cervical/Thoracic General Pain	295
724.1	Pain in thoracic spine	4B, 4C, 4D, 4E, 4F, 4G, 4J	Postural Dysfunction	263
724.2	Lumbago	4B, 4C, 4D, 4E, 4F, 4G, 4H, 4I, 4J, 5F, 6B	Low Back General Pain	209
724.2	Lumbago	4B, 4C, 4D, 4E, 4F, 4G, 4J	Postural Dysfunction	263
724.3	Sciatica	4E, 4F, 4J	Hip Soft Tissue Pain	187
724.3	Sciatica	4A, 4B, 4E, 4F, 4G, 4J	Lumbar Disc Pathology	219
724.4	Thoracic or lumbosacral neuritis or radiculitis, unspecified	4A, 4B, 4E, 4F, 4G, 4J	Lumbar Disc Pathology	219
724.5	Backache, unspecified	4B, 4C, 4D, 4E, 4F, 4G, 4H, 4I, 4J, 5F, 6B	Low Back General Pain	209
724.6	Disorders of sacrum	4B, 4C, 4E, 4F, 4G, 4J, 7A	Sacroiliac Dysfunction	271
724.79	Other disorders of coccyx	4A, 4B, 4C, 4D, 4E, 4F, 4G, 4H, 7A, 7C, 7D	Pelvic Floor Dysfunction	249
724.8	Other symptoms referable to back	4B, 4C, 4D, 4E, 4F, 4G, 4H, 4I, 4J, 5F, 6B	Low Back General Pain	209
724.9	Other unspecified back disorders	4B, 4C, 4D, 4E, 4F, 4G, 4H, 4I, 4J, 5F, 6B	Low Back General Pain	209
726.0	Adhesive capsulitis of shoulder	4D, 4E, 4F, 4G, 4J, 7A	Adhesive Capsulitis	399
726.0	Adhesive capsulitis of shoulder	4B, 4C, 4D, 4E, 4F, 4G, 4I, 5D, 5H	Elbow/Shoulder Injury—Return to Tennis	615
726.1	Rotator cuff syndrome of shoulder and allied disorders	4B, 4C, 4D, 4E, 4F, 4G, 4I, 5D, 5H	Elbow/Shoulder Injury—Return to Tennis	615
726.1	Rotator cuff syndrome of shoulder and allied disorders	4B, 4C, 4D, 4E, 4F, 4J	Postoperative Rehabilitation of the Rotator Cuff	429
726.1	Rotator cuff syndrome of shoulder and allied disorders	4D, 4E, 4F, 4G, 4J	Shoulder Bursitis	447
726.1	Rotator cuff syndrome of shoulder and allied disorders	4B, 4D, 4E, 4F, 4G, 4H, 4J, 7A	Shoulder Sprain/Strain	475
726.1	Rotator cuff syndrome of shoulder and allied disorders	4D, 4E, 4F, 4G, 4J, 7A	Shoulder Tendinitis	483
726.2	Other affections of shoulder region, not elsewhere classified	4D, 4E, 4F, 4G, 4J, 7A	Adhesive Capsulitis	399
726.2	Other affections of shoulder region, not elsewhere classified	4B, 4C, 4D, 4E, 4F, 4G, 4I, 5D, 5H	Elbow/Shoulder Injury—Return to Tennis	615
726.2	Other affections of shoulder region, not elsewhere classified	4B, 4D, 4E, 4F, 4G, 4H, 4J, 7A	Shoulder Sprain/Strain	475
726.3	Enthesopathy of elbow region	4D, 4E, 4F, 4I	Elbow and Hand Enthesopathy	498
726.3	Enthesopathy of elbow region	4B, 4C, 4D, 4E, 4F, 4G, 4I, 5D, 5H	Elbow/Shoulder Injury—Return to Tennis	615
726.31	Medial epicondylitis	4D, 4E, 4F, 4H, 4J, 7A	Medial Epicondylitis	523
726.32	Lateral epicondylitis	4E, 4F, 4J, 4D, 7A	Lateral Epicondylitis	517
726.4	Enthesopathy of wrist and carpus	4D, 4E, 4F, 4I	Elbow and Hand Enthesopathy	498

ICD-9	Diagnosis	APTA Preferred Practice Pattern	Rehabilitation Guidelines	Page #
726.5	Enthesopathy of hip region	4A, 4B, 4C, 4D, 4E, 4F, 4G, 4H, 4I, 4J, 4K, 5D, 6B	Biomechanical Lower Extremity Dysfunction	33
726.5	Enthesopathy of hip region	4C, 4D, 4E, 4F, 4G, 4H, 4I, 4J, 6B	Hip Pain in Runners—Return to Sport	623
726.5	Enthesopathy of hip region	4E, 4F, 4J	Hip Soft Tissue Pain	187
726.6	Enthesopathy of knee	4E, 4D, 4I	Knee Enthesopathy	111
726.64	Patellar tendinitis	4A, 4B, 4C, 4D, 4E, 4F, 4G, 4H, 4I, 4J, 4K, 5D, 6B	Biomechanical Lower Extremity Dysfunction	33
726.64	Patellar tendinitis	4D, 4E, 4F, 4J	Patellar Tendinitis	141
726.64	Patellar tendinitis	4A, 4D, 4E, 4F, 4G, 4H, 4I, 4J	Patellofemoral Syndrome	147
726.7	Enthesopathy of ankle and tarsus	4A, 4B, 4C, 4D, 4E, 4F, 4G, 4H, 4I, 4J, 4K, 5D, 6B	Biomechanical Lower Extremity Dysfunction	33
726.7	Enthesopathy of ankle and tarsus	4B, 4C, 4D, 4E, 4F, 4H, 4I, 4J, 6B	Foot Reconstruction	57
726.70	Enthesopathy of ankle and tarsus, unspecified	4E, 4D, 4I	Ankle Enthesopathy	15
726.71	Achilles bursitis or tendinitis	4D, 4E, 4F, 4J	Achilles Tendinitis	3
726.72	Tibialis tendinitis	4D, 4E, 4F, 4J	Posterior Tibialis Tendinitis (Shin Splints)	75
726.73	Calcaneal spur	4D, 4E, 4F, 4J	Plantar Fasciitis	69
726.91	Exostosis of unspecified site	4B, 4C, 4D, 4E, 4F, 4G, 4I, 5D, 5H	Elbow/Shoulder Injury—Return to Tennis	615
726.91	Exostosis of unspecified site	4D, 4E, 4F, 4G, 4J, 7A	Shoulder Tendinitis	483
727	Synovitis and tenosynovitis	4D, 4E, 4F, 4I	Elbow and Hand Enthesopathy	498
727.00	Synovitis and tenosynovitis, unspecified	4D, 4E, 4F, 4J	Achilles Tendinitis	3
727.01	Synovitis and tenosynovitis in diseases classified elsewhere	4D, 4E, 4F, 4J	Achilles Tendinitis	3
727.04	Radial styloid tenosynovitis	4F	DeQuervain's Tendinitis	543
727.04	Radial styloid tenosynovitis	4F	Postoperative DeQuervain's Syndrome	571
727.06	Tenosynovitis of foot and ankle	4D, 4E, 4F, 4J	Achilles Tendinitis	3
727.1	Bunion	4I	Bunion	39
727.3	Other bursitis	4B, 4C, 4D, 4E, 4F, 4G, 4I, 5D, 5H	Elbow/Shoulder Injury—Return to Tennis	615
727.3	Other bursitis	4D, 4E, 4F, 4G, 4J	Shoulder Bursitis	447
727.61	Complete rupture of rotator cuff	4B, 4C, 4D, 4E, 4F, 4G, 4I, 5D, 5H	Elbow/Shoulder Injury—Return to Tennis	615
727.61	Complete rupture of rotator cuff	4B, 4C, 4D, 4E, 4F, 4J	Postoperative Rehabilitation of the Rotator Cuff	429
727.62	Nontraumatic rupture of tendons of biceps (long head)	4E, 4I	Biceps Tendon Rupture	405

APPENDIX   719

ICD-9	Diagnosis	APTA Preferred Practice Pattern	Rehabilitation Guidelines	Page #
727.62	Nontraumatic rupture of tendons of biceps (long head)	4B, 4C, 4D, 4E, 4F, 4G, 4I, 5D, 5H	Elbow/Shoulder Injury—Return to Tennis	615
727.67	Nontraumatic rupture of Achilles tendon	4D, 4E, 4F, 4J	Achilles Tendon Repair	9
728.5	Hypermobility syndrome	4B, 4C, 4D, 4E, 4F, 4H, 4I, 4J, 6B	Foot Reconstruction	57
728.6	Contracture of palmar fascia	4D, 4J	Postoperative Dupuytren's Fasciectomy	577
728.71	Plantar fascial fibromatosis	4A, 4B, 4C, 4D, 4E, 4F, 4G, 4H, 4I, 4J, 4K, 5D, 6B	Biomechanical Lower Extremity Dysfunction	33
728.71	Plantar fascial fibromatosis	4D, 4E, 4F, 4J	Plantar Fasciitis	69
728.85	Spasm of muscle	4B, 4G, 5B, 5C	Cerebral Vascular Accident	683
728.87	Muscle weakness (generalized)	4D, 4F, 4B, 4C	Muscle Weakness—General	663
728.89	Other disorders of muscle, ligament, and fascia	4D, 4F, 4B, 4C	Muscle Weakness—General	663
728.9	Unspecified disorder of muscle, ligament, and fascia	4A, 4C, 4D, 4F, 4G, 4H, 4I, 4J, 7A	Hip Fracture/Total Hip Replacement—Inpatient	183
728.9	Unspecified disorder of muscle, ligament, and fascia	4A, 4C, 4D, 4F, 4G, 4H, 4I, 4J, 7A	Hip Fracture/Total Hip Replacement—Outpatient	177
728.9	Unspecified disorder of muscle, ligament, and fascia	4B, 4C, 4D, 4E, 4F, 4G, 4I, 5D, 7A	Stress Management	384
728.9	Unspecified disorder of muscle, ligament, and fascia	4B, 4C, 4D, 4E, 4F, 4G, 4H, 4I	Temporomandibular Dysfunction	389
729.1	Myalgia and myositis, unspecified	4B, 4C, 4D, 4E, 4F, 4G, 4H, 4I, 4J, 5F, 6B	Cervical/Thoracic General Pain	295
729.1	Myalgia and myositis, unspecified	4B, 4C, 4D, 4E, 4F, 4G, 4H, 4I, 4J, 5F, 6B	Low Back General Pain	209
729.1	Myalgia and myositis, unspecified	4B, 4C, 4D, 4E, 4F, 4G, 4J	Postural Dysfunction	263
729.1	Myalgia and myositis, unspecified	4B, 4C, 4D, 4E, 4F, 4G, 4I, 5D, 7A	Stress Management	384
729.1	Myalgia and myositis, unspecified	4B, 4C, 4D, 4E, 4F, 4G, 4H, 4I	Temporomandibular Dysfunction	389
729.5	Pain in limb	7B	Foot Contusion	51
732.0	Juvenile osteochondrosis of spine	4A, 4B, 4F, 4G, 4H, 4J, 5E, 6F	Scoliosis	347
732.1	Juvenile osteochondrosis of hip and pelvis	4A, 4B, 4F, 4G, 4H, 4J, 5E, 6F	Scoliosis	347
732.8	Other specified forms of osteochondropathy	4A, 4B, 4F, 4G, 4H, 4J, 5E, 6F	Scoliosis	347
732.9	Unspecified osteochondropathy	4A, 4B, 4F, 4G, 4H, 4J, 5E, 6F	Scoliosis	347
733.0	Osteoporosis	4A, 4B, 4C, 4G, 4H	Osteoporosis	329
733.10	Pathologic fracture, unspecified site	4A, 4B, 4C, 4D, 4E, 4F, 4G, 4H, 4I, 4J, 4K, 5D, 6B	Biomechanical Lower Extremity Dysfunction	33

ICD-9	Diagnosis	APTA Preferred Practice Pattern	Rehabilitation Guidelines	Page #
733.10	Pathologic fracture, unspecified site	4A, 4B, 4C, 4G, 4H	Osteoporosis	329
733.13	Pathologic fracture of vertebræ	4D, 4H, 4J	Compression Fracture	319
733.13	Pathologic fracture of vertebræ	4D, 4H, 4J	Lumbar Fracture	227
733.13	Pathologic fracture of vertebræ	4A, 4B, 4C, 4G, 4H	Osteoporosis	329
733.14	Pathologic fracture of neck of femur	4A, 4B, 4C, 4D, 4E, 4F, 4G, 4H, 4I, 4J, 4K, 5D, 6B	Biomechanical Lower Extremity Dysfunction	33
733.14	Pathologic fracture of neck of femur	4C, 4D, 4E, 4F, 4G, 4H, 4I, 4J, 6B	Hip Pain in Runners—Return to Sport	623
733.15	Pathologic fracture of other specified part of femur	4A, 4B, 4C, 4D, 4E, 4F, 4G, 4H, 4I, 4J, 4K, 5D, 6B	Biomechanical Lower Extremity Dysfunction	33
733.15	Pathologic fracture of other specified part of femur	4C, 4D, 4E, 4F, 4G, 4H, 4I, 4J, 6B	Hip Pain in Runners—Return to Sport	623
733.16	Pathologic fracture of tibia or fibula	4A, 4B, 4C, 4D, 4E, 4F, 4G, 4H, 4I, 4J, 4K, 5D, 6B	Biomechanical Lower Extremity Dysfunction	33
733.19	Pathologic fracture of other specified site	4A, 4B, 4C, 4D, 4E, 4F, 4G, 4H, 4I, 4J, 4K, 5D, 6B	Biomechanical Lower Extremity Dysfunction	33
733.19	Pathologic fracture of other specified site	4A, 4B, 4C, 4G, 4H	Osteoporosis	329
733.2	Cyst of bone	4A, 4B, 4C, 4G, 4H	Osteoporosis	329
733.40	Aseptic necrosis of bone, site unspecified	4A, 4B, 4C, 4G, 4H	Osteoporosis	329
733.49	Aseptic necrosis of bone, other	4A, 4B, 4C, 4G, 4H	Osteoporosis	329
733.7	Algoneurodystrophy	4A, 4B, 4C, 4G, 4H	Osteoporosis	329
733.90	Disorder of bone and cartilage, unspecified	4A, 4B, 4C, 4G, 4H	Osteoporosis	329
733.91	Arrest of bone development or growth	4A, 4B, 4C, 4G, 4H	Osteoporosis	329
733.92	Chondromalacia	4A, 4D, 4E, 4F, 4G, 4H, 4I, 4J	Patellofemoral Syndrome	147
733.95	Stress fracture of other bone	4A, 4B, 4C, 4G, 4H	Osteoporosis	329
733.99	Other disorder of bone and cartilage	4A, 4B, 4C, 4G, 4H	Osteoporosis	329
735.0	Hallux valgus (acquired)	4A, 4B, 4C, 4D, 4E, 4F, 4G, 4H, 4I, 4J, 4K, 5D, 6B	Biomechanical Lower Extremity Dysfunction	33
735.0	Hallux valgus (acquired)	4B, 4C, 4D, 4E, 4F, 4H, 4I, 4J, 6B	Foot Reconstruction	57
735.2	Hallux rigidus	4A, 4B, 4C, 4D, 4E, 4F, 4G, 4H, 4I, 4J, 4K, 5D, 6B	Biomechanical Lower Extremity Dysfunction	33
735.2	Hallux rigidus	4B, 4C, 4D, 4E, 4F, 4H, 4I, 4J, 6B	Foot Reconstruction	57
735.4	Other hammer toe (acquired)	4B, 4C, 4D, 4E, 4F, 4H, 4I, 4J, 6B	Foot Reconstruction	57
735.5	Claw toe (acquired)	4B, 4C, 4D, 4E, 4F, 4H, 4I, 4J, 6B	Foot Reconstruction	57

ICD-9	Diagnosis	APTA Preferred Practice Pattern	Rehabilitation Guidelines	Page #
735.8	Other acquired deformities of toe	4B, 4C, 4D, 4E, 4F, 4H, 4I, 4J, 6B	Foot Reconstruction	57
736.73	Cavus deformity of foot, acquired	4B, 4C, 4D, 4E, 4F, 4H, 4I, 4J, 6B	Foot Reconstruction	57
737.12	Kyphosis, postlaminectomy	4B, 4G, 4H, 4J	Lumbar Surgery—Inpatient	243
737.12	Kyphosis, postlaminectomy	4B, 4G, 4H, 4J	Postoperative Rehabilitation of the Lumbar Spine	255
737.22	Other postsurgical lordosis	4B, 4G, 4H, 4J	Lumbar Surgery—Inpatient	243
737.22	Other postsurgical lordosis	4B, 4G, 4H, 4J	Postoperative Rehabilitation of the Lumbar Spine	255
737.3	Kyphoscoliosis and scoliosis	4A, 4B, 4F, 4G, 4H, 4J, 5E, 6F	Scoliosis	347
737.4	Curvature of spine associated with other conditions	4A, 4B, 4F, 4G, 4H, 4J, 5E, 6F	Scoliosis	347
738.4	Acquired spondylolisthesis	4B, 4G, 4J	Spondylolisthesis	285
739.1	Nonallopathic lesions, not elsewhere classified, cervical region	4B, 4C, 4D, 4E, 4F, 4G, 4H, 4I, 4J, 5F, 6B	Cervical/Thoracic General Pain	295
739.2	Nonallopathic lesions, not elsewhere classified, thoracic region	4B, 4C, 4D, 4E, 4F, 4G, 4H, 4I, 4J, 5F, 6B	Cervical/Thoracic General Pain	295
739.3	Nonallopathic lesions, not elsewhere classified, lumbar region	4B, 4C, 4D, 4E, 4F, 4G, 4H, 4I, 4J, 5F, 6B	Low Back General Pain	209
739.4	Nonallopathic lesions, not elsewhere classified, sacral region	4B, 4C, 4E, 4F, 4G, 4J, 7A	Sacroiliac Dysfunction	271
754.2	Certain congenital musculoskeletal deformities of spine	4A, 4B, 4F, 4G, 4H, 4J, 5E, 6F	Scoliosis	347
754.62	Talipes calcaneovalgus	4B, 4C, 4D, 4E, 4F, 4H, 4I, 4J, 6B	Foot Reconstruction	57
754.69	Other valgus deformities of feet	4A, 4B, 4C, 4D, 4E, 4F, 4G, 4H, 4I, 4J, 4K, 5D, 6B	Biomechanical Lower Extremity Dysfunction	33
754.71	Talipes cavus	4A, 4B, 4C, 4D, 4E, 4F, 4G, 4H, 4I, 4J, 4K, 5D, 6B	Biomechanical Lower Extremity Dysfunction	33
755.2	Congenital reduction deformities of upper limb	4K, 7A, 7E	Amputations	643
755.3	Congenital reduction deformities of lower limb	4K, 7A, 7E	Amputations	643
755.64	Congenital deformity of knee (joint)	4A, 4D, 4E, 4F, 4G, 4H, 4I, 4J	Patellofemoral Syndrome	147
756.12	Congenital spondylolisthesis	4B, 4G, 4J	Spondylolisthesis	285
780.4	Dizziness and giddiness	4B, 4C, 4H, 4K, 5B	Vestibular Rehabilitation	667
780.79	Other malaise and fatigue	4D, 4F, 4B, 4C	Muscle Weakness—General	663
781.2	Abnormality of gait	4B, 4G, 5B, 5C	Cerebral Vascular Accident	683
781.2	Abnormality of gait	4B, 4C, 4H, 4K, 5B	Vestibular Rehabilitation	667
781.3	Lack of coordination	4B, 4C, 4H, 4K, 5B	Vestibular Rehabilitation	667

ICD-9	Diagnosis	APTA Preferred Practice Pattern	Rehabilitation Guidelines	Page #
781.9	Other symptoms involving nervous and musculoskeletal systems	4B, 4G, 5B, 5C	Cerebral Vascular Accident	683
784.0	Headache	4B, 4C, 4D, 4E, 4F, 4G, 4I, 5D	Headache	367
784.0	Headache	4B, 4C, 4D, 4E, 4F, 4G, 4H, 4I	Temporomandibular Dysfunction	389
784	Symptoms involving head and neck	4B, 4C, 4D, 4E, 4F, 4G, 4I, 5D, 7A	Stress Management	384
787.6	Incontinence of feces	4A, 4B, 4C, 4D, 4E, 4F, 4G, 4H, 7A, 7C, 7D	Pelvic Floor Dysfunction	249
788.3	Urinary incontinence	4A, 4B, 4C, 4D, 4E, 4F, 4G, 4H, 7A, 7C, 7D	Pelvic Floor Dysfunction	249
788.4	Frequency of urination and polyuria	4A, 4B, 4C, 4D, 4E, 4F, 4G, 4H, 7A, 7C, 7D	Pelvic Floor Dysfunction	249
788.6	Other abnormality of urination	4A, 4B, 4C, 4D, 4E, 4F, 4G, 4H, 7A, 7C, 7D	Pelvic Floor Dysfunction	249
802.2	Fracture of mandible, closed	4I, 4J	Postoperative Rehabilitation of the Temporomandibular Joint	373
805.0	Closed fracture of cervical vertebra without mention of spinal cord injury	4D, 4H, 4J	Compression Fracture	319
805.0	Closed fracture of cervical vertebra without mention of spinal cord injury	4D, 4G, 4H, 4J	Postoperative/Postfracture Rehabilitation of the C/T Spine	335
805.1	Open fracture of cervical vertebra without mention of spinal cord injury	4D, 4G, 4H, 4J	Postoperative/Postfracture Rehabilitation of the C/T Spine	335
805.2	Closed fracture of dorsal [thoracic] vertebra without mention of spinal cord injury	4D, 4H, 4J	Compression Fracture	319
805.2	Closed fracture of dorsal [thoracic] vertebra without mention of spinal cord injury	4D, 4G, 4H, 4J	Postoperative/Postfracture Rehabilitation of the C/T Spine	335
805.3	Open fracture of dorsal [thoracic] vertebra without mention of spinal cord injury	4D, 4G, 4H, 4J	Postoperative/Postfracture Rehabilitation of the C/T Spine	335
805.4	Closed fracture of lumbar vertebra without mention of spinal cord injury	4D, 4H, 4J	Lumbar Fracture	227
805.8	Closed fracture of unspecified part of vertebral column without mention of spinal cord injury	4D, 4H, 4J	Lumbar Fracture	227
807	Fracture of rib(s), sternum, larynx, and trachea	4D, 4G, 4H, 4J	Postoperative/Postfracture Rehabilitation of the C/T Spine	335
807	Fracture of rib(s), sternum, larynx, and trachea	4D, 4E, 4F, 4H, 5D	Rib Dysfunction	341
808.0	Closed fracture of acetabulum	4A, 4C, 4D, 4F, 4G, 4H, 4I, 4J, 7A	Hip Fracture/Total Hip Replacement—Inpatient	183
808.0	Closed fracture of acetabulum	4A, 4C, 4D, 4F, 4G, 4H, 4I, 4J, 7A	Hip Fracture/Total Hip Replacement—Outpatient	177
810	Fracture of clavicle	4B, 4C, 4D, 4E, 4F, 4G, 4I, 5D, 5H	Elbow/Shoulder Injury—Return to Tennis	615
810	Fracture of clavicle	4D, 4H, 4I, 4J	Shoulder Fracture	461

APPENDIX   723

ICD-9	Diagnosis	APTA Preferred Practice Pattern	Rehabilitation Guidelines	Page #
812.00	Closed fracture of unspecified part of upper end of humerus	4D, 4H, 4I, 4J	Postoperative Total Shoulder Arthroplasty	435
812.0	Closed fracture of upper end of humerus	4G, 4H, 4I	Humerus Fracture	411
812	Fracture of humerus	4B,4C, 4D, 4E, 4F, 4G, 4I, 5D, 5H	Elbow/Shoulder Injury—Return to Tennis	615
812	Fracture of humerus	4D, 4H, 4I, 4J	Shoulder Fracture	461
812.19	Other open fracture of upper end of humerus	4G, 4H, 4I	Humerus Fracture	411
812.20	Closed fracture of unspecified part of humerus	4D, 4H, 4I, 4J	Postoperative Total Shoulder Arthroplasty	435
812.21	Closed fracture of shaft of humerus	4G, 4H, 4I	Humerus Fracture	411
812.30	Open fracture of unspecified part of humerus	4G, 4H, 4I	Humerus Fracture	411
813.00	Closed fracture of upper end of forearm, unspecified	4D, 4E, 4F, 4H, 4J, 7A	Medial Epicondylitis	523
813.0	Closed fracture of upper end of radius and ulna	4G, 4I	Elbow Fracture	493
813.0	Closed fracture of upper end of radius and ulna	4B,4C, 4D, 4E, 4F, 4G, 4I, 5D, 5H	Elbow/Shoulder Injury—Return to Tennis	615
813.4	Closed fracture of lower end of radius and ulna	4D, 4H, 4J	Wrist Fracture	599
813.8	Closed fracture of unspecified part of radius and ulna	4D, 4H, 4J	Wrist Fracture	599
814.00	Closed fracture of carpal bone, unspecified	4D, 4H, 4J	Wrist Fracture	599
815.00	Closed fracture of metacarpal bone(s), site unspecified	4G, 4H, 4I	Hand Fracture	561
816.00	Closed fracture of phalanx or phalanges of hand, unspecified	4G, 4H, 4I	Hand Fracture	561
816.01	Closed fracture of middle or proximal phalanx or phalanges of hand	4G, 4H, 4I	Hand Fracture	561
820.00	Closed fracture of unspecified intracapsular section of neck of femur	4A, 4C, 4D, 4F, 4G, 4H, 4I, 4J, 7A	Hip Fracture/Total Hip Replacement—Inpatient	183
820.00	Closed fracture of unspecified intracapsular section of neck of femur	4A, 4C, 4D, 4F, 4G, 4H, 4I, 4J, 7A	Hip Fracture/Total Hip Replacement—Outpatient	177
820.01	Closed fracture of epiphysis (separation) (upper) of neck of femur	4A, 4C, 4D, 4F, 4G, 4H, 4I, 4J, 7A	Hip Fracture/Total Hip Replacement—Inpatient	183
820.01	Closed fracture of epiphysis (separation) (upper) of neck of femur	4A, 4C, 4D, 4F, 4G, 4H, 4I, 4J, 7A	Hip Fracture/Total Hip Replacement—Outpatient	177
820.2	Closed pertrochanteric fracture of neck of femur	4A, 4C, 4D, 4F, 4G, 4H, 4I, 4J, 7A	Hip Fracture/Total Hip Replacement—Inpatient	183
820.2	Closed pertrochanteric fracture of neck of femur	4A, 4C, 4D, 4F, 4G, 4H, 4I, 4J, 7A	Hip Fracture/Total Hip Replacement—Outpatient	177
820.8	Closed fracture of unspecified part of neck of femur	4A, 4C, 4D, 4F, 4G, 4H, 4I, 4J, 7A	Hip Fracture/Total Hip Replacement—Inpatient	183
820.8	Closed fracture of unspecified part of neck of femur	4A, 4C, 4D, 4F, 4G, 4H, 4I, 4J, 7A	Hip Fracture/Total Hip Replacement—Outpatient	177

ICD-9	Diagnosis	APTA Preferred Practice Pattern	Rehabilitation Guidelines	Page #
821.00	Closed fracture of unspecified part of femur	4A, 4C, 4D, 4F, 4G, 4H, 4I, 4J, 7A	Hip Fracture/Total Hip Replacement—Inpatient	183
821.00	Closed fracture of unspecified part of femur	4A, 4C, 4D, 4F, 4G, 4H, 4I, 4J, 7A	Hip Fracture/Total Hip Replacement—Outpatient	177
822.0	Closed fracture of patella	4A, 4D, 4E, 4F, 4G, 4H, 4I, 4J	Patellofemoral Syndrome	147
822.1	Open fracture of patella	4A, 4D, 4E, 4F, 4G, 4H, 4I, 4J	Patellofemoral Syndrome	147
824	Fracture of ankle	4D, 4H, 4J	Ankle Fracture	21
824.8	Closed fracture of ankle, unspecified	4B, 4C, 4D, 4E, 4F, 4H, 4I, 4J, 6B	Foot Reconstruction	57
825	Fracture of one or more tarsal and metatarsal bones	4D, 4H, 4J	Ankle Fracture	21
827	Other, multiple, and ill-defined fractures of lower limb	4D, 4H, 4J	Ankle Fracture	21
830.0	Closed dislocation of jaw	4I, 4J	Postoperative Rehabilitation of the Temporomandibular Joint	373
831.0	Closed dislocation of shoulder	4B, 4C, 4D, 4E, 4F, 4G, 4I, 5D, 5H	Elbow/Shoulder Injury—Return to Tennis	615
831.0	Closed dislocation of shoulder	4B, 4D, 4E, 4F, 4G, 4J	Postoperative Rehabilitation For Shoulder Instability	423
831.00	Closed dislocation of shoulder, unspecified	4B, 4D, 4E, 4F, 4G, 4J	Shoulder Anterior Dislocation	441
831.01	Anterior dislocation of humerus, closed	4B, 4D, 4E, 4F, 4G, 4J	Shoulder Anterior Dislocation	441
831.1	Open dislocation of shoulder	4B, 4C, 4D, 4E, 4F, 4G, 4I, 5D, 5H	Elbow/Shoulder Injury—Return to Tennis	615
831.1	Open dislocation of shoulder	4B, 4D, 4E, 4F, 4G, 4J	Postoperative Rehabilitation For Shoulder Instability	423
834.0	Closed dislocation of finger	4J	Proximal Interphalangeal Joint Injuries Dorsal Dislocation	589
836.0	Tear of medial cartilage or meniscus of knee, current	4E, 4I, 4J	Meniscal Repair	129
836.0	Tear of medial cartilage or meniscus of knee, current	4I, 4D, 4H	Meniscus Tear	135
836.1	Tear of lateral cartilage or meniscus of knee, current	4E, 4I, 4J	Meniscal Repair	129
836.1	Tear of lateral cartilage or meniscus of knee, current	4I, 4D, 4H	Meniscus Tear	135
836.2	Other tear of cartilage or meniscus of knee, current	4E, 4I, 4J	Meniscal Repair	129
836.2	Other tear of cartilage or meniscus of knee, current	4I, 4D, 4H	Meniscus Tear	135
836.3	Dislocation of patella, closed	4B, 4C, 4D, 4E, 4F, 4G, 4I, 4J, 6B, 7A	Knee Arthroscopy	95
836.3	Dislocation of patella, closed	4A, 4D, 4E, 4F, 4G, 4H, 4I, 4J	Patellofemoral Syndrome	147

APPENDIX   725

ICD-9	Diagnosis	APTA Preferred Practice Pattern	Rehabilitation Guidelines	Page #
836.4	Dislocation of patella, open	4A, 4D, 4E, 4F, 4G, 4H, 4I, 4J	Patellofemoral Syndrome	147
836.59	Other dislocation of knee, closed	4A, 4D, 4E, 4F, 4G, 4H, 4I, 4J	Patellofemoral Syndrome	147
836.6	Other dislocation of knee, open	4B, 4C, 4D, 4E, 4F, 4G, 4I, 4J, 6B, 7A	Knee Arthroscopy	95
837	Dislocation of ankle	4D, 4E, 4F, 4I, 4J	Ankle Sprain/Instability	27
837	Dislocation of ankle	4E, 4J	Ankle Sprain/Instability—Return to Sport	611
838.0	Closed dislocation of foot	4B, 4C, 4D, 4E, 4F, 4H, 4I, 4J, 6B	Foot Reconstruction	57
840	Sprains and strains of shoulder and upper arm	4B,4C, 4D, 4E, 4F, 4G, 4I, 5D, 5H	Elbow/Shoulder Injury—Return to Tennis	615
840	Sprains and strains of shoulder and upper arm	4B, 4D, 4E, 4F, 4G, 4H, 4J, 7A	Shoulder Sprain/Strain	475
840.3	Infraspinatus (muscle) (tendon) sprain	4D, 4E, 4F, 4G, 4J, 7A	Shoulder Tendinitis	483
840.7	Superior glenoid labrum lesion	4D, 4E, 4I	Labrum Tear	417
840.8	Sprain of other specified sites of shoulder and upper arm	4B, 4C, 4D, 4E, 4F, 4G, 4H, 4I, 4J, 5F, 6B	Cervical/Thoracic General Pain	295
840.8	Sprain of other specified sites of shoulder and upper arm	4B, 4C, 4D, 4E, 4F, 4G, 4J	Postural Dysfunction	263
841	Sprains and strains of elbow and forearm	4B,4C, 4D, 4E, 4F, 4G, 4I, 5D, 5H	Elbow/Shoulder Injury—Return to Tennis	615
841.2	Radiohumeral (joint) sprain	4D, 4E, 4J, 7A	Elbow Sprain/Strain	511
841.3	Ulnohumeral (joint) sprain	4D, 4E, 4J, 7A	Elbow Sprain/Strain	511
841.8	Sprain of other specified sites of elbow and forearm	4D, 4E, 4J, 7A	Elbow Sprain/Strain	511
841.9	Sprain of unspecified site of elbow and forearm	4D, 4E, 4J, 7A	Elbow Sprain/Strain	511
841.9	Sprain of unspecified site of elbow and forearm	4E, 4F, 4J, 4D, 7A	Lateral Epicondylitis	517
841.9	Sprain of unspecified site of elbow and forearm	4D, 4E, 4F, 4H, 4J, 7A	Medial Epicondylitis	523
842.0	Wrist sprain	4D, 4I	Wrist Sprain/Strain	605
842.1	Hand sprain	4E, 4J	Proximal Interphalangeal Joint Injuries Collateral Ligament Sprain	583
842.1	Hand sprain	4D, 4I	Wrist Sprain/Strain	605
843.0	Iliofemoral (ligament) sprain	4E, 4F, 4J	Hip Sprain/Strain	193
843.8	Sprain of other specified sites of hip and thigh	4E, 4F, 4J	Hip Sprain/Strain	193
843.9	Sprain of unspecified site of hip and thigh	4D, 4E, 4J, 7B, 7E	Hamstring Injury—Return to Sport	621
843.9	Sprain of unspecified site of hip and thigh	4C, 4D, 4E, 4F, 4G, 4H, 4I,4J, 6B	Hip Pain in Runners—Return to Sport	623
843.9	Sprain of unspecified site of hip and thigh	4E, 4F, 4J	Hip Soft Tissue Pain	187

ICD-9	Diagnosis	APTA Preferred Practice Pattern	Rehabilitation Guidelines	Page #
843.9	Sprain of unspecified site of hip and thigh	4E, 4F, 4J	Hip Sprain/Strain	193
844.0	Sprain of lateral collateral ligament of knee	4A, 4B, 4E, 4H, 4I, 4J	Knee Hypomobility/Infrapatellar Contracture Syndrome (IPCS)	117
844.0	Sprain of lateral collateral ligament of knee	4D, 4E, 4J	Knee Sprain/Strain	123
844.1	Sprain of medial collateral ligament of knee	4D, 4E, 4J	Knee Sprain/Strain	123
844.2	Sprain of cruciate ligament of knee	4E, 4J	Accelerated Anterior Cruciate Ligament Reconstruction	83
844.2	Sprain of cruciate ligament of knee	4E, 4J	Anterior Cruciate Ligament Reconstruction—Return to Sport	613
844.8	Sprain of other specified sites of knee and leg	4D, 4E, 4J	Knee Sprain/Strain	123
844.9	Sprain of unspecified site of knee and leg	4D, 4E, 4J, 7B, 7E	Hamstring Injury—Return to Sport	621
844.9	Sprain of unspecified site of knee and leg	4E, 4F, 4J	Hip Sprain/Strain	193
844.9	Sprain of unspecified site of knee and leg	4D, 4E, 4J	Iliotibial Band Syndrome	89
844.9	Sprain of unspecified site of knee and leg	4D, 4E, 4J	Knee Sprain/Strain	123
845	Sprains and strains of ankle and foot	4D, 4E, 4F, 4I, 4J	Ankle Sprain/Instability	27
845	Sprains and strains of ankle and foot	4E, 4J	Ankle Sprain/Instability—Return to Sport	611
846.0	Lumbosacral (joint) (ligament) sprain	4B, 4C, 4D, 4E, 4F, 4G, 4H, 4I, 4J, 5F, 6B	Low Back General Pain	209
846.1	Sacroiliac ligament sprain	4B, 4C, 4E, 4F, 4G, 4J, 7A	Sacroiliac Dysfunction	271
846.8	Sprain of other specified sites of sacroiliac region	4B, 4C, 4E, 4F, 4G, 4J, 7A	Sacroiliac Dysfunction	271
846.9	Sprain of unspecified site of sacroiliac region	4B, 4C, 4E, 4F, 4G, 4J, 7A	Sacroiliac Dysfunction	271
847.0	Neck sprain	4B, 4C, 4D, 4E, 4F, 4G, 4H, 4I, 4J, 5F, 6B	Cervical/Thoracic General Pain	295
847.0	Neck sprain	4G	Whiplash Syndrome	359
847	Sprains and strains of other and unspecified parts of back	4B, 4C, 4D, 4E, 4F, 4G, 4I, 5D, 7A	Stress Management	384
847.1	Thoracic sprain	4B, 4C, 4D, 4E, 4F, 4G, 4H, 4I, 4J, 5F, 6B	Cervical/Thoracic General Pain	295
847.2	Lumbar sprain	4B, 4C, 4D, 4E, 4F, 4G, 4H, 4I, 4J, 5F, 6B	Low Back General Pain	209
847.3	Sprain of sacrum	4B, 4C, 4E, 4F, 4G, 4J, 7A	Sacroiliac Dysfunction	271
847.9	Sprain of unspecified site of back	4B, 4C, 4E, 4F, 4G, 4J, 7A	Sacroiliac Dysfunction	271
848.1	Jaw sprain	4B, 4C, 4D, 4E, 4F, 4G, 4H, 4I	Temporomandibular Dysfunction	389
848.3	Sprain of ribs	4D, 4E, 4F, 4H, 5D	Rib Dysfunction	341
879	Open wound of other and unspecified sites, except limbs	4D, 4K, 7A, 7C, 7E	Wound Management	673
880	Open wound of shoulder and upper arm	4D, 4K, 7A, 7C, 7E	Wound Management	673
881	Open wound of elbow, forearm, and wrist	4D, 4K, 7A, 7C, 7E	Wound Management	673
882	Open wound of hand except finger(s) alone	4D, 4K, 7A, 7C, 7E	Wound Management	673
882.2	Open wound of hand except finger(s) alone, with tendon involvement	4J, 7E	Flexor Tendon Repair	549

APPENDIX   727

ICD-9	Diagnosis	APTA Preferred Practice Pattern	Rehabilitation Guidelines	Page #
883	Open wound of finger(s)	4D, 4K, 7A, 7C, 7E	Wound Management	673
883.2	Open wound of finger(s) with tendon involvement	4J, 7E	Flexor Tendon Repair	549
884	Multiple and unspecified open wound of upper limb	4D, 4K, 7A, 7C, 7E	Wound Management	673
885	Traumatic amputation of thumb (complete) (partial)	4K, 7A, 7E	Amputations	643
885	Traumatic amputation of thumb (complete) (partial)	4D, 4K, 7A, 7C, 7E	Wound Management	673
886	Traumatic amputation of other finger(s) (complete) (partial)	4K, 7A, 7E	Amputations	643
886	Traumatic amputation of other finger(s) (complete) (partial)	4D, 4K, 7A, 7C, 7E	Wound Management	673
887	Traumatic amputation of arm and hand (complete) (partial)	4K, 7A, 7E	Amputations	643
887	Traumatic amputation of arm and hand (complete) (partial)	4D, 4K, 7A, 7C, 7E	Wound Management	673
890	Open wound of hip and thigh	4D, 4K, 7A, 7C, 7E	Wound Management	673
891	Open wound of knee, leg [except thigh], and ankle	4D, 4K, 7A, 7C, 7E	Wound Management	673
892	Open wound of foot except toe(s) alone	4D, 4K, 7A, 7C, 7E	Wound Management	673
893	Open wound of toe(s)	4D, 4K, 7A, 7C, 7E	Wound Management	673
894	Multiple and unspecified open wound of lower limb	4D, 4K, 7A, 7C, 7E	Wound Management	673
895	Traumatic amputation of toe(s) (complete) (partial)	4K, 7A, 7E	Amputations	643
895	Traumatic amputation of toe(s) (complete) (partial)	4D, 4K, 7A, 7C, 7E	Wound Management	673
896	Traumatic amputation of foot (complete) (partial)	4K, 7A, 7E	Amputations	643
896	Traumatic amputation of foot (complete) (partial)	4D, 4K, 7A, 7C, 7E	Wound Management	673
897	Traumatic amputation of leg(s) (complete) (partial)	4K, 7A, 7E	Amputations	643
897	Traumatic amputation of leg(s) (complete) (partial)	4D, 4K, 7A, 7C, 7E	Wound Management	673
911	Superficial injury of trunk	4D, 4K, 7A, 7C, 7E	Wound Management	673
912	Superficial injury of shoulder and upper arm	4D, 4K, 7A, 7C, 7E	Wound Management	673
913	Superficial injury of elbow, forearm, and wrist	4D, 4K, 7A, 7C, 7E	Wound Management	673
914	Superficial injury of hand(s) except finger(s) alone	4D, 4K, 7A, 7C, 7E	Wound Management	673
915	Superficial injury of finger(s)	4D, 4K, 7A, 7C, 7E	Wound Management	673
916	Superficial injury of hip, thigh, leg, and ankle	4D, 4K, 7A, 7C, 7E	Wound Management	673
917	Superficial injury of foot and toe(s)	4D, 4K, 7A, 7C, 7E	Wound Management	673

ICD-9	Diagnosis	APTA Preferred Practice Pattern	Rehabilitation Guidelines	Page #
924.0	Contusion of hip and thigh	4D, 4E, 4J, 7B, 7E	Hamstring Injury—Return to Sport	621
924.10	Contusion of lower leg	7B	Knee Contusion	101
924.11	Contusion of knee	7B	Knee Contusion	101
924.20	Contusion of foot	7B	Foot Contusion	51
924.3	Contusion of toe	7B	Foot Contusion	51
928.0	Crushing injury of hip and thigh	4D, 4E, 4J, 7B, 7E	Hamstring Injury—Return to Sport	621
953.2	Injury to lumbar nerve root	4A, 4B, 4E, 4F, 4G, 4J	Lumbar Disc Pathology	219
959.09	Other and unspecified injury of face and neck	4B, 4C, 4D, 4E, 4F, 4G, 4H, 4I	Temporomandibular Dysfunction	389
959.2	Other and unspecified injury to shoulder and upper arm	4B, 4C, 4D, 4E, 4F, 4G, 4I, 5D, 5H	Elbow/Shoulder Injury—Return to Tennis	615
959.2	Other and unspecified injury to shoulder and upper arm	4B, 4D, 4E, 4F, 4G, 4H, 4J, 7A	Shoulder Sprain/Strain	475
959.2	Other and unspecified injury to shoulder and upper arm	4D, 4E, 4F, 4G, 4J, 7A	Shoulder Tendinitis	483
959.7	Other and unspecified injury to knee, leg, ankle, and foot	4D, 4E, 4F, 4J	Achilles Tendon Repair	9
997.6	Amputation stump complication	4K, 7A, 7E	Amputations	643
V43.60	Unspecified joint replacement	4A, 4C, 4D, 4F, 4G, 4H, 4I, 4J, 7A	Hip Fracture/Total Hip Replacement—Inpatient	183
V43.60	Unspecified joint replacement	4A, 4C, 4D, 4F, 4G, 4H, 4I, 4J, 7A	Hip Fracture/Total Hip Replacement—Outpatient	177
V43.61	Shoulder joint replacement	4D, 4H, 4I, 4J	Postoperative Total Shoulder Arthroplasty	435
V43.64	Hip joint replacement	4A, 4C, 4D, 4F, 4G, 4H, 4I, 4J, 7A	Hip Fracture/Total Hip Replacement—Inpatient	183
V43.64	Hip joint replacement	4A, 4C, 4D, 4F, 4G, 4H, 4I, 4J, 7A	Hip Fracture/Total Hip Replacement—Outpatient	177
V43.65	Knee joint replacement	4I	Total Knee Replacement—Inpatient	159
V43.65	Knee joint replacement	4I	Total Knee Replacement—Outpatient	163
V43.69	Other joint replacement	4A, 4C, 4D, 4F, 4G, 4H, 4I, 4J, 7A	Hip Fracture/Total Hip Replacement—Inpatient	183
V43.69	Other joint replacement	4A, 4C, 4D, 4F, 4G, 4H, 4I, 4J, 7A	Hip Fracture/Total Hip Replacement—Outpatient	177
V45.4	Postprocedural arthrodesis status	4B, 4G, 4H, 4J	Lumbar Surgery—Inpatient	243
V45.4	Postprocedural arthrodesis status	4B, 4G, 4H, 4J	Postoperative Rehabilitation of the Lumbar Spine	255
V45.4	Postprocedural arthrodesis status	4D, 4G, 4H, 4J	Postoperative/Postfracture Rehabilitation of the C/T Spine	335

730   APPENDIX

INDEX

A

Accelerated Anterior Cruciate Ligament
  Reconstruction 83–88, 613
  Return to Sport 83, 87, 613–614
Achilles Tendinitis 3–8
Achilles Tendon Repair 9–14
Activity Questionnaire for Runners/
  Walkers 623
Adhesive Capsulitis 399–404
Amputations 643–648
Ankle
  Enthesopathy 15–20
  Fracture 21–26
  Sprain/Instability 27–32, 611
  Sprain/Instability, Return to Sport
    611–612
Ankylosing Spondylitis 201–208
Anterior Cruciate Ligament
  Reconstruction 83–88
  Return to Sport 613–614,
Arthritis 653–658
Arthroscopy, Knee 95–100

B

Biceps Tendon Rupture 405–410
Biomechanical Lower Extremity
  Dysfunction 4, 33–38, 70, 76,
    172, 188, 194
Bunion 39–42
Bursitis, Shoulder 447–454

C

Carpal Tunnel Syndrome 537–542
Cerebral Vascular Accident 683–692
Cervical/Thoracic Spine
  Cervical Disc Pathology 301–306
  Cervical Spondylolysis with
    Myelopathy 307–312
  Cervical Stenosis 313–318
  Compression Fracture 319–324

General Pain 295–300, 330, 375, 391
Objective Measurement of Forward
  Head Posture 327–328
Osteoporosis 329–334
Rib Dysfunction 341–346

Scoliosis 347–352
Thoracic Outlet Syndrome 353–358,
  392
Whiplash Syndrome 359–364
Cervical/Thoracic General Pain 295–
  300, 330
Cervical/Thoracic Spine, Postoperative/
  Postfracture Rehabilitation of the
  335–340
Cervical Disc Pathology 301–306
Cervical Spondylolysis with Myelopathy
  307–312
Cervical Stenosis 313–318
Compression Fracture 319–324
Contusion
  Foot 51–56
Cranioverteberal Stability Tests 302,
  325–326
Cruciate Ligament
  Anterior Cruciate Ligament
    Reconstruction 83–88, 613
    Return to Sport 83, 87, 613–614
  Posterior Cruciate Ligament
    Reconstruction 153–158

D

Diabetic
  Diabetic Foot 43–48
  Foot Care Guidelines For the Diabetic
    Patient 49–50
Degenerative Joint Disease
  Hip 171–176
  Knee 105–110
  Shoulder 455–460
DeQuervain's Tendinitis 543–548

Postoperative 572–576
Dislocation
  Proximal Interphalangeal Joint Injuries
    Dorsal Dislocation 589–592
  Shoulder Anterior 441–446
Dupuytren's Fasciectomy, Postoperative
  577–582
Dysfunction
  Biomechanical Lower Extremity 4,
    33–38, 70, 76, 172, 188, 194

  Pelvic Floor 249–254
  Sacroiliac 271–278

E

Elbow
  Enthesopathy 497–504
  Fracture 493–496
  Injury, Return to Tennis 421,
    615–616
  Joint Pathology 505–510
  Lateral Epicondylitis 517–522
  Medial Epicondylitis 523–528
  Sprain/Strain 511–516
  Ulnar Nerve Lesion 529–534
Epicondylitis
  Lateral 517–522
  Medial 523–528

F

Flexor Tendon Repair 549–556
Foot
  Contusion 51–56
  Diabetic Foot 43–48
  Reconstruction 57–62
Fracture
  Ankle 21–26
  Compression 319–324
  Elbow 493–496
  Hand 561–564
  Hip, Inpatient 183–186

INDEX   731

Hip, Outpatient 177–182
Humerus 411–416
Lumbar 227–234
Shoulder 461–466
Wrist 599–604

G

General Pain
Cervical/Thoracic 295–300, 330, 375, 391
Knee 621
Low Back 194, 209–218, 265
Geriatric Rehabilitation 282, 659–662
Guillain-Barré Syndrome 693–698

H

Hamstring Injury, Return to Sport 621–622
Hand
Arthropathy 557–560
Enthesopathy 497–504
Fracture 561–564
Headache 367–372
Hip
Degenerative Joint Disease 171–176
Fracture
Inpatient 183–186
Outpatient 177–182
Pain in Runners, Return to Sport 623–624
Replacement
Inpatient 183–186
Outpatient 177–182
Soft Tissue Pain 187–192, 623
Sprain/Strain 193–198
Humerus Fracture 411–416
Hypomobility
Knee/Infrapatellar Contracture Syndrome 117–122

I

Iliotibial Band Syndrome 89–94
Infrapatellar Contracture Syndrome
See Knee Hypomobility

K

Knee
Accelerated Anterior Cruciate
Ligament Reconstruction 83–88, 613
Return to Sport 83, 87, 613–614
Arthroscopy 95–100
Degenerative Joint Disease 105–110
Enthesopathy 111–116
Hypomobility/Infrapatellar
Contracture Syndrome 117–122
Iliotibial Band Syndrome 89–94
Meniscal Repair 129–134
Meniscus Tear 135–140
Patellar Tendinitis 141–146
Patellofemoral Syndrome 147–152
Replacement
Inpatient 159–162
Outpatient 163–168
Sprain/Strain 123–128

L

Labrum Tear 417–422
Lateral Epicondylitis 517–522
Low Back General Pain 189, 194, 209–218, 221, 229, 237, 265
Lower Extremity, Biomechanical
Dysfunction 4, 33–38, 70, 76, 172, 188, 194
Lumbar
Disc Pathology 219–226
Fracture 227–234
Spondylolysis with Myelopathy 235–242
Surgery—Inpatient 243–248
Lumbar Spine
Ankylosing Spondylitis 201–208
Craniovertebral Stability Tests 302, 325–326
Low Back General Pain 237, 265
Pelvic Floor Dysfunction 249–254
Postoperative Rehabilitation 255–262
Postural Dysfunction 263–270
Sacroiliac Dysfunction 271–278
Spinal Stenosis 279–284

Spondylolisthesis 285–292
Spondylolysis with Myelopathy 235–242
Surgery, Inpatient 243–248

M

Medial Epicondylitis 523–528
Meniscal Repair 129–134
Meniscus Tear 135–140
Multiple Sclerosis 699–704
Muscle Weakness, General 663–666

O

Objective Measurement of Forward
Head Posture 327–328, 391
Orthotics
Commonly Asked Questions 36, 63–64
Choosing the Right Shoe 36, 65–66, 91
Your New Orthotics 36, 67–68
Osteoporosis 320, 329–334

P

Pain
Cervical/Thoracic 295–300, 330, 375, 391
Hip, in Runners 623–624
Hip Soft Tissue 187–192, 623
Parkinson's Disease 705–710
Patellar Tendinitis 141–146
Patellofemoral Syndrome 147–152
Pelvic Floor Dysfunction 249–254
Plantar Fasciitis 69–74
Posterior Cruciate Ligament
Reconstruction 153–158
Posterior Tibialis Tendinitis (Shin Splints) 75–80
Postoperative Carpal Tunnel Release 565–570
Postoperative DeQuervain's Syndrome 572–576
Postoperative Dupuytren's Fasciectomy 577–582

Postoperative Rehabilitation For
Shoulder Instability 423–428
Postoperative Rehabilitation of the
Lumbar Spine 255–262
Postoperative Rehabilitation of the
Rotator Cuff 429–434
Postoperative Rehabilitation of the
Temporomandibular Joint
373–380
Postoperative Total Shoulder
Arthroplasty 435–440
Postoperative/Postfracture
Rehabilitation of the Cervical/
thoracic Spine 335–340
Postural Dysfunction 263–270
Prosthesis, Fitting the 649–652
Proximal Interphalangeal Joint Injuries
Collateral Ligament Sprain 583–588
Dorsal Dislocation 589–592

R

Reconstruction
Accelerated Anterior Cruciate
Ligament 83–88
Anterior Cruciate Ligament, Return to
Sport 83, 87, 613–614
Foot 57–62
Posterior Cruciate Ligament 153–158
Reflex Sympathetic Dystrophy of the
Upper Extremity 593–598
Replacement
Hip, Inpatient 183–186
Hip, Outpatient 177–182
Knee, Inpatient 159–162
Knee, Outpatient 163–168
Return to Sport
Ankle Sprain/Instability 30, 611–612
Anterior Cruciate Ligament
Reconstruction 83, 87, 613–614
Elbow/Shoulder Injury 421, 615–616
Exercise Sequence 617–620
Hamstring Injury 621–622
Hip Pain In Runners 623–624
Exercise Sequence 625–626

Questionnaire for Runners/Walkers
623
Upper Extremity Injury 421, 627–628
Exercise Sequence 629–634
Walking Program 635–636, 637–638
Rib Dysfunction 341–346
Rotator Cuff, Postoperative
Rehabilitation of the 429–434

S

Sacroiliac Dysfunction 271–278
Scoliosis 347–352
Shin Splints. *See* Posterior Tibialis
Tendinitis
Shoe, Choosing the Right 36, 65–66,
91
Shoulder
Adhesive Capsulitis 399–404
Anterior Dislocation 441–446
Arthroplasty, Postoperative 435–440
Biceps Tendon Rupture 405–410
Bursitis 447–454
Degenerative Joint Disease 455–460
Fracture 461–466
Humerus Fracture 411–416
Injury, Return to Tennis 421,
615–616
Instability, Postoperative
Rehabilitation 423–428
Joint Pathology 467–474
Labrum Tear 417–422
Medial Epicondylitis 523–528
Rotator Cuff, Postoperative
Rehabilitation 429–434
Sprain/Strain 430, 475–482
Tendinitis 483–490
Spinal Stenosis 279–284
Spondylolisthesis 285–292
Sprain/Strain
Ankle 27–32
Elbow 511–516
Hip 193–198
Knee 123–128
Proximal Interphalangeal Joint Injuries
Collateral Ligament 583–588

Shoulder 430, 475–482
Wrist 605–608
Stress Management 267, 383–388
Relaxation and 378, 381–382, 386,
394

T

Temporomandibular Dysfunction
389–396
Temporomandibular Joint
Postoperative Rehabilitation 373–380
Tendinitis
Achilles 3–8
DeQuervain's 543–548
Postoperative 572–576
Patellar Tendinitis 141–146
Posterior Tibialis (Shin Splints) 75–80
Shoulder 483–490
Thoracic Outlet Syndrome 353–358,
392
Total Hip Replacement
Inpatient 183–186
Outpatient 177–182
Total Knee Replacement
Inpatient 159–162
Outpatient 163–168
Total Shoulder Arthroplasty,
Postoperative 435–440

U

Ulnar Nerve Lesion 529–534
Upper Extremity
Injury, Return to Throwing 421,
627–628
Exercise Sequence 629–634
Reflex Sympathetic Dystrophy of the
593–598

V

Vestibular Rehabilitation 667–672

W

Walking Program 635–636, 637–638

Whiplash Syndrome 359–364

Wound Management 646, 647,
  673–680

Wrist
  Fracture 599–604
  Sprain/Strain 605–608

Wrist/Hand
  Carpal Tunnel Release, Postoperative
    565–570
  Carpal Tunnel Syndrome 537–542
  DeQuervain's Tendinitis 543–548
  Flexor Tendon Repair 549–556
  Hand Arthropathy 557–560
  Hand Fracture 561–564
  Postoperative Carpal Tunnel Release
    565–570
  Postoperative DeQuervain's Syndrome
    572–576
  Postoperative Dupuytren's Fasciectomy
    577–582
  Proximal Interphalangeal Joint
    Injuries Collateral Ligament
    Sprain 583–588
  Proximal Interphalangeal Joint Injuries
    Dorsal Dislocation 589–592
  Reflex Sympathetic Dystrophy of the
    Upper Extremity 593–598